Differential Diagnosis in Magnetic Resonance Imaging

Francis A. Burgener, M.D.
Professor of Radiology
University of Rochester Medical Center
Rochester, NY, USA

Raymond K. Tan, M.D.
Assistant Professor of Radiology
University of Rochester Medical Center
Rochester, NY, USA

Steven P. Meyers, M.D., Ph.D.
Associate Professor of Radiology
University of Rochester Medical Center
Rochester, NY, USA

Wolfgang Zaunbauer, M.D.
Institute of Radiology
Kantonsspital St. Gallen
St. Gallen, Switzerland

1964 illustrations

Thieme
Stuttgart · New York

Library of Congress Cataloging-in-Publication Data is available from the publisher.

Contributors of illustrations

Kevin G.J. Ibach, M.D., F.R.C.P.C.
Lecturer
University of Toronto
University Health Network
Toronto General Hospital
Toronto, Ontario, Canada

Uresh Patel, M.D.
Radiologist
Ide Group, PC
Rochester, NY, USA

Brian K. Tan, M.D.
Chief Resident
Department of Radiology
University of Rochester Medical Center
Rochester, NY, USA

© 2002 Georg Thieme Verlag,
Rüdigerstraße 14, D-70469 Stuttgart, Germany
Thieme New York, 333 Seventh Avenue,
New York, N.Y. 10001 USA

Cover design by Renate Stockinger, Stuttgart
Drawings by Christiane and Dr. Michael von Solodkoff, Neckargmünd

Typesetting by primustype Robert Hurler GmbH
D-73274 Notzingen, Germany

Printed in Germany by Druckhaus Götz, Ludwigsburg

ISBN 3-13-108121-X (GTV)
ISBN 1-58890-085-1 (TNY)   2 3 4 5

Important Note: Medicine is an ever-changing science undergoing continual development. Research and clinical experience are continually expanding our knowledge, in particular our knowledge of proper treatment and drug therapy. Insofar as this book mentions any dosage or application, readers may rest assured that the authors, editors, and publishers have made every effort to ensure that such references are in accordance with the state of knowledge at the time of production of the book.

Nevertheless this does not involve, imply, or express any guarantee or responsibility on the part of the publishers in respect of any dosage instructions and forms of application stated in the book. Every user is requested to examine carefully the manufacturer's leaflets accompanying each drug and to check, if necessary in consultation with a physician or specialist, whether the dosage schedules mentioned therein or the contraindications stated by the manufacturers differ from the statements made in the present book. Such examination is particularly important with drugs that are either rarely used or have been newly released on the market. Every dosage schedule or every form of application used is entirely at the user's own risk and responsibility. The authors and publishers request every user to report to the publishers any discrepancies or inaccuracies noticed.

Foreword

Since 1985, when I had the pleasure and honor of publishing the first edition of the textbook "Differential Diagnosis in Conventional Radiology" with Dr. Francis A. Burgener, it has become customary to use a similar approach in writing radiological textbooks, i.e. to structure the books on the basis of radiographic findings instead of disease entities. When the book first appeared, the approach was well received by radiology residents preparing for their specialist examinations. Even non-radiologist physicians, occasionally called upon to interpret radiographic findings, used the text as it does not require extensive reading to find the essential diagnostic criteria.

In 1996 we published another textbook using a similar approach, namely "Differential Diagnosis in Computed Tomography," which also proved successful. Even then, we had plans to continue the series by writing another volume on differential diagnosis in magnetic resonance imaging. To my sincere dismay, I was unable to invest enough time and energy to finish my part of the planned MRI textbook in time. So it was a great relief both to myself and Dr. Burgener that he found three talented and proficient younger radiologists, Dr. Stephen P. Meyers, M.D. Ph.D and Raymond K. Tan, M.D. of the University of Rochester Medical Center, Rochester, N.Y., and Wolfgang Zaunbauer, M.D. of Kantonsspital, St. Gallen, Switzerland to complete the book on differential diagnosis in MRI without undue delay.

MRI is still developing rapidly and new imaging sequences are published almost daily. New diagnostic signs continue to be discovered in great numbers. With this overflow of new information, selecting the essential information for a single-volume textbook has become a very demanding task. It goes without saying that a differential diagnostic textbook about MRI will be substantially larger than one on CT. The authors are to be congratulated for their success in fitting a significant amount of essential radiological information, hundreds of differential diagnostic tables, and approximately 2000 state-of-the-art drawings, charts, and MR images into a textbook of almost 700 pages.

The structure and layout of Differential Diagnosis in Magnetic Resonance Imaging is essentially similar to the previous two differential diagnostic textbooks, published by Thieme, of which Dr. Burgener is the first author. It is divided into anatomical sections, including the brain, head and neck, spine, musculoskeletal system, chest, abdomen, and pelvis. The book covers the most common diseases and a multitude of rare and unusual conditions, providing quick access to differential diagnostic information.

I am convinced that this guide to differential diagnosis in MRI will receive the same enthusiastic acceptance as the previous books in this series. It will be helpful to radiologists and other physicians involved in interpreting MR images. Residents and fellows will find it an invaluable board preparation tool.

Martti Kormano, M.D.
Professor and Chairman
Department of Diagnostic Radiology
University of Turku
Turku, Finland

Preface

All good things must come to an end. After having co-authored with Dr. Martti Kormano the textbooks "Differential Diagnosis in Conventional Radiology" and "Differential Diagnosis in Computed Tomography," which were translated into five languages and produced several spin-off books, Dr. Kormano had to back out at the last minute from this project because of too many other professional commitments as chairman of a radiology department and many national and international societies, as clinician, researcher, and teacher, and last but not least as berry farmer. It was impossible to replace Dr. Kormano with his extensive knowledge in the entire field of diagnostic radiology by a single person. I was, however, fortunate enough to find three colleagues and friends of mine to write the part originally assigned to Dr. Kormano and I believe they performed an outstanding job.

MRI has gained worldwide acceptance and, in addition to many new indications, has replaced other diagnostic imaging techniques. MRI is no longer the exclusive domain of the radiologist, but is also practiced and/or interpreted by a large number of clinicians and surgeons. With each examination, one is confronted with a number of MRI findings that require interpretation in order to arrive at a general diagnostic impression and a reasonable differential diagnosis. To assist the physician in attaining this goal, our book is based upon MRI findings. This offers a contrast to most other radiology textbooks, which are disease oriented. Since many diseases present with MRI in a variety of manifestations, some overlap in the text is unavoidable. To minimize repetition, the differential diagnosis is presented in tabular form wherever feasible. The tables list not only the various diseases that may present with MRI in a specific way, but also include the characteristically associated MRI findings and pertinent clinical data in a succinct form. Illustrations and drawings are enclosed to visually demonstrate the MRI findings under discussion.

This book is intended for radiologists and physicians with some expertise in diagnostic imaging who wish to strengthen their diagnostic acumen in MRI. It is a comprehensive outline of MRI findings and we expect it to be particularly useful to radiology residents who are preparing for their specialist examinations. Any physician involved in the interpretation of MRI studies should find this book helpful in direct proportion to his or her curiosity. It is my hope that this new textbook will be as well received by medical students, interns, residents, radiologists, and physicians—all being involved in the interpretation of MRI examinations—as my previous texts "Differential Diagnosis in Conventional Radiology" and "Differential Diagnosis in Computed Tomography," written with Dr. Kormano, which were based on the same concept.

Francis A. Burgener, M.D.

Acknowledgements

It is impossible to thank individually all those who helped to prepare this textbook. We wish to acknowledge the Thieme staff, in particular Dr. Clifford Bergman and Mr. Gert A. Krüger.

We wish also to express our gratitude to many radiologists whose cooperation helped make this illustrative collection of MRI cases available. We are indebted to Drs. Barry R. Armandi Jr., Ja-Kwei Chang, Gary M. Hollenberg, Deborah J. Klein, Valeh Levy, Amit L. Mehta, Bradley R. Peters, Rodolfo Queiroz, Stuart J. Rubin, Gwy Suk Seo, John G. Strang, Eric P. Weinberg, Per-Lennart Westesson, and Ian J. Wilson, all current or former members of the University of Rochester Radiology Department, and to Drs. Masoom Haider and Naeem Merchant of the University of Toronto, who all supplied cases from their personal files. Valuable assistance in preparation and execution of the manuscript was given by Drs. Mark J. Adams, Patrick J. Fultz, and Johnny U. V. Monu, all of the University of Rochester Radiology Department, and by Dr. Claude Jean-Pierre of the Radiology Department of the University of Oslo, Norway.

We wish to express our thanks to Therese Burgener for preparing a large number of drawings and to Catherine Tan, M.D. for typing and proofreading a portion of the manuscript. Iona Mackey's work in preparing the references is also greatly appreciated. Last, but not least, we are most grateful to Alyce Norder who orchestrated the execution of this project. Not only did she do a superb job in typing, editing, and proofreading the manuscript, but she was also in charge of the transatlantic coordination of this undertaking. Without Alyce there would be no manuscript yet.

Finally, we appreciate the support of our families. They have generously given of their precious family time for the preparation of this book.

Table of Contents

Abbreviations

ABC	aneurysmal bone cyst
ACTH	adrenocorticotropic hormone
ADEM	acute disseminated encephalomyelitis
AFP	alpha-fetoprotein
AIDS	acquired immune deficiency syndrome
ALL	acute lymphoblastic leukemia
AML	acute myeloblastic leukemia
ANCA	antineutrophil cytoplasmotic autoantibodies
ANT	anterior
AP	anteroposterior
APUD	amine precursor uptake and decarboxylation
APVR	anomalous pulmonary venous return
ARDS	acute respiratory distress syndrome
ATN	acute tubular necrosis
AV	arteriovenous
AVF	arteriovenous fistula
AVM	arteriovenous malformation
AVN	avascular necrosis
Bx	biopsy
+C	after gadolinium contrast enhancement
Ca	calcium
CAD	coronary artery disease
CAM	cystic adenomatoid malformation
CBD	common bile duct
CHD	common hepatic duct
CHF	congestive heart failure
CLL	chronic lymphatic leukemia
CMV	cytomegalovirus
CNS	central nervous system
COPD	chronic obstructive pulmonary disease
CPA	cerebellopontine angle
CPPD	calcium pyrophosphate dihydrate deposition disease
CRMD	chronic recurrent multifocal osteomyelitis
CSF	cerebrospinal fluid
CSI	chemical shift imaging
CT	computed tomography
2D	two-dimensional
3D	three-dimensional
DD	differential diagnosis
DDH	developmental dysplasia of the hip
DES	diethylstilbestrol
3DFT	three-dimensional Fourier transform
DIC	disseminated intravascular coagulation
DISH	diffuse idiopathic skeletal hyperostosis
DISI	dorsal intercalated segmental instability
EAC	external auditory canal
ECA	external carotid artery
EG	eosinophilic granuloma
ERCP	endoscopic retrograde cholangiopancreatography
F	female
FAST	Fourier-acquired steady state
FISP	fast imaging with steady-state precession
FLAIR	fluid attenuated inversion recovery
FLASH	fast low-angle shot
FNH	follicular nodular hyperplasia
FS	fat-suppressed (saturation)
FSE	fast spin echo
FSPGR	fast spoiled gradient-recalled echo
GB	gallbladder
Gd	gadolinium chelates
GD-contrast	gadolinium chelate contrast
Gd-DTPA	gadolinium diethylene-triamine-pentaacetic acid
GE	gastroesophageal
GI	gastrointestinal
GRASS	gradient-refocused acquisition in the steady state
GRE	gradient-refocused echo pulse sequence
GTD	gestational trophoblastic disease
GU	genitourinary
Hb	hemoglobin
HD	Hodgkin disease
HIV	human immunodeficiency virus
HRCT	high-resolution CT
Hx	history
IAC	internal auditory canal
ICA	internal carotid artery
IM	intramuscular
IMA	inferior mesenteric artery
IMV	inferior mesenteric vein
IR	inversion recovery
IS	ileosacral, internal standard
IV	intravenous
IVC	inferior vena cava
IVP	intravenous pyelogram
L	left
LA	left atrium
LCH	Langerhans cell histiocytosis
LDH	lactate dehydrogenase
LE	lupus erythematosus
LL	lower lobes
LLL	left lower lobe
LLQ	left lower quadrant
LUL	left upper lobe
LUQ	left upper quadrant
LV	left ventricle
M	male
MAI	Mycobacterium avium intracellulare
MCK	multicystic kidney
MCP	metacarpophalangeal
MEA	multiple endocrine adenomas
MEN	multiple endocrine neoplasia
MFH	malignant fibrous histiocytoma
MIP	maximum intensity projection
ML	middle lobe
MPGR	multiplanar gradient recall
MPS	mucopolysaccharidosis
MR	magnetic resonance
MRA	magnetic resonance angiography
MRC	magnetic resonance cholangiography
MRCP	magnetic resonance cholangiopancreatography
MRI	magnetic resonance imaging
MRS	magnetic resonance spectroscopy
MTP	metatarsophalangeal
NHL	non-Hodgkin lymphoma

NUC	nuclear medicine		SI	sacroiliac
PA	posteroanterior		SLAC	scapholunate advanced collapse
PAPVR	partial anomalous pulmonary venous return		SLE	systemic lupus erythematosus
PATH	pathology		SMA	superior mesenteric artery
PAVM	pulmonary arteriovenous malformation		SMV	superior mesenteric vein
PCKD	polycystic kidney disease		SR	surface-rendering
PCP	Pneumocystis carinii pneumonia		SR	saturation recovery
PD	proton density weighted imaging (long TR/ short TE sequences)		STIR	short tau (T1) inversion recovery
			SVC	superior vena cava
PDA	patent ductus arteriosus		T1	spin-lattice or longitudinal relaxation time
PDWI	proton density weighted imaging		T2	spin-spin or transverse relaxation time
PE	pulmonary embolism		T2*	effective spin-spin relaxation time
PET	positron emission tomography		T1W1	T1-weighted imaging
PHPV	persistent hyperplastic primary vitreous		T2WI	T2-weighted imaging
PIP	proximal interphalangeal		TAPVR	total anomalous pulmonary venous return
PNET	primitive neuroectodermal tumor		TB	tuberculosis
PO	per oral		TE	echo time
PSA	prostate specific antigen		TFC	triangular fibrocartilage
PTHC	percutaneous transhepatic cholangiography		TFCC	triangular fibrocartilage complex
PVNS	pigmented villonodular synovitis		TI	inversion time
RA	rheumatoid arthritis		TNM	tumor-node-metastasis
RA	right atrium		TOF	time-of-flight
RBC	red blood cell		TR	repetition time
RDS	respiratory distress syndrome		TURP	transurethral resection of prostate
RES	reticuloendothelial system		UGI	upper gastrointestinal series
RF	radio frequency		UPJ	ureteropelvic junction
RLL	right lower lobe		US	ultrasound
RLQ	right lower quadrant		VIP	vasoactive intestinal peptides
RML	right middle lobe		VISI	volar intercalated segmental instability
RSD	reflex sympathetic dystrophy		WBC	white blood cells
RUL	right upper lobe		WDHA	watery diarrhea, hypokalemia, achlorhydria
RV	right ventricle		WDHH	watery diarrhea, hypokalemia, hypochlorhydria
SE	spin echo			

Introduction

Magnetic Resonance Imaging (MRI) is a method which can provide in vivo anatomic images of portions of the human body with high soft-tissue contrast resolution. The magnetic resonance (MR) images can be obtained in multiple planes, i.e. sagittal, axial, coronal, or various oblique combinations. The "signal" used to generate an MR image comes from hydrogen nuclei (protons) within a human body. In essence, MRI is basically a hydrogen scan.

The hydrogen nucleus has a net charge of +1 and spins at a frequency that is dependent on the ambient magnetic field and its particular physical characteristic known as its gyromagnetic ratio. The spinning charge of each hydrogen nucleus gives off a tiny magnetic field perpendicular to the axis of spin, thus acting like a tiny bar magnet. Outside of the bore of a magnet, the net magnetic properties (magnetic moment) of a person will be zero because the spinning hydrogen nuclei will be oriented randomly resulting in an overall cancellation of the sum total of tiny magnetic fields. Once placed into a high field strength magnet, spinning hydrogen nuclei within the human body become aligned or magnetized along the magnetic field of the magnet. This net magnetization of hydrogen nuclei is oriented in a low energy alignment (ground state) that is parallel to the magnetic field of the magnet. The hydrogen nuclei spin (precess) at a frequency proportional to their specific gyromagnetic ratio and the magnetic field, in a relationship known as the Larmor equation. The precessional frequency of hydrogen nuclei at 1.5 T (tesla) is 64 MHz.

To generate an MR signal, energy is transferred to the hydrogen nuclei within the magnet by using a radio frequency (RF) pulse at the Larmor frequency. The Larmor frequency is dependent on the field strength of the magnetic device and the gyromagnetic ratio–which is specific for the element or molecule of interest. For MRI, that element is the hydrogen nucleus. The hydrogen nuclei absorb this energy and move out of their ground-state alignment. When the RF pulse is turned off, the energy absorbed by the hydrogen nuclei is emitted at the same frequency. This emitted energy, or MR signal, can be detected by the receiver coils (which act like antennae) in the magnet, and used to produce an MR image. Soft-tissue contrast results from: 1) the densities of protons (hydrogen nuclei) within different tissues; 2) the different rates at which the protons in various tissues realign themselves with the magnetic field of the magnet (also referred to as T1 relaxation, longitudinal or spin-lattice relaxation); 3) rates of signal decay or dephasing (also referred to as T2 relaxation, transverse or spin-spin relaxation). Using these biophysical properties of different normal and abnormal tissues allows MRI to have greater soft-tissue contrast than computed tomography (CT).

The main components of a typical MRI scanner include: 1) a large-bore magnet with high field strength (0.3 to 1.5 T); 2) RF coils within the magnet which can transmit and receive properly tuned RF pulses, as well as set spatially-dependent magnetic fields (gradients) that allow localization of specific regions of anatomic interest; 3) a computer that operates the device and processes the RF signal data received from the patient to form an anatomic image. To generate an MR image, a person is placed onto a table that can be specifically located within the bore of the magnet. Once in the magnet, the operator selects programs that include the RF pulse sequences necessary to generate images with the desired contrast parameters based on the proton densities, T1 and T2 values of the various tissues. The data received from the subject or patient is processed by the computer using computer algorithms (2D or 3D Fourier transformation). The images are displayed on the monitor console and transferred to film or other computers. Many systems store the image data on digital tape or optical discs for easy retrieval.

Not all patients can have MRI examinations. Intracranial aneursym clips, cardiac pacemakers, and metallic foreign bodies in the eyes are absolute contraindications for MRI. In addition, the presence of surgical clips, metallic rods, wires, and other orthopedic hardware can produce artifacts obscuring visualization of the anatomic structures in the region of interest.

Section I

Brain

Introduction

Major advantages of MRI include excellent soft-tissue contrast resolution, multiplanar imaging capabilities, dynamic rapid data acqustion, and various available contrast agents. MRI has proven to be a powerful imaging modality in the evaluation of: 1) congenital anomalies of the brain; 2) disorders of histogenesis; 3) neoplasms of the central nervous system; cranial nerves, pituitary gland, meninges, and skull base; 4) traumatic lesions; 5) intracranial hemorrhage; 6) ischemia and infarction; 7) infectious and noninfectious diseases; 8) metabolic disorders; and 9) dysmyelinating and demyelinating diseases. MR data can also be used to generate images of arteries and veins (MR angiography [MRA]) in displays similar to conventional angiography. Another option with clinical MRI scanners is the acquisition of spectral data to characterize the biochemical properties of selected regions of interest in the brain (MR spectroscopy [MRS]).

The appearance of brain tissue depends on the MRI pulse sequence used as well as the age of the patient imaged. Myelination of the brain begins in the fifth fetal month and progresses rapidly during the first 2 years of life. The degree of myelination affects the appearance of the brain parenchyma on MRI. In adults, the cerebral cortex has intermediate signal on T1WI, which is lower or hypointense relative to normal white matter. On T2WI, gray matter has intermediate signal, which is higher in signal (hyperintense) relative to white matter. For infants less than 6 months of age, this pattern is reversed due to the immature myelination of brain tissue. Maturation or myelination of the brain tissue as seen on T1WI versus T2WI occurs at different rates. The myelination proceeds in a predictable and characteristic pattern with regard to locations and timing. These changes on T1WI become most evident during the first 6 months, whereas the changes are most apparent on T2WI from 6 to 18 months. At around 6 months of age, the adult MRI signal pattern of the gray and white matter begins to progressively emerge. After 18 months, the brain has a mature MRI appearance with regard to the gray and white matter signal patterns.

In addition to the commonly used standard spin-echo (SE) or fast spin-echo (FSE) sequences for evaluation of brain parenchyma, other MRI pulse sequences or imaging options are sometimes used. These include: inversion recovery (STIR, FLAIR, etc), gradient-recall-echo (GRE) imaging, magnetic transfer, diffusion/perfusion MRI, frequency selective chemical saturation, etc. Detailed discussions of these sequences and options can be found elsewhere.

Various pathologic processes can affect the T1 or T2 properties of the involved tissue or organ. For example, intraparenchymal hemorrhage can have variable appearances in the brain depending on the age of the hematoma, oxidation states of the iron in hemoglobin, hematocrit, protein concentration, clot formation and retraction, location, and size. Oxyhemoglobin in a hyperacute blood clot has ferrous iron and is diamagnetic. Oxyhemoglobin does not significantly alter the T1 and T2 values of the tissue environment other than causing possible localized edema. After a few hours during the acute phase of the hematoma,

the oxyhemoglobin loses its oxygen to form deoxyhemoglobin.

Deoxyhemoglobin also has ferrous iron, although it has unpaired electrons and becomes paramagnetic. As a result, deoxyhemoglobin shortens the T2 value of the acute clot but does not significantly change the T1 value. On MRI, deoxyhemoglobin in the clot will have intermediate T1 signal and low signal on SE, FSE or GRE T2WI. Later in the early subacute phase of the hematoma, deoyxhemoglobin becomes oxidized to the ferric state, methemoglobin, which is strongly paramagnetic. Methemoglobin shortens the T1 value of hydrogen nuclei, resulting in high signal on T1WI. While the red blood cells in the clot are intact with intracellular methemoglobin, the T2 values will also be decreased resulting in low signal on T2WI. In the late subacute phase, breakdown of the membranes of the red blood cells results in extracellular methemoglobin, which now results in high signal on both T1WI and T2WI. In the chronic phase, methemoglobin becomes further oxidized and broken down by macrophages into hemosiderin, which has prominent low signal on T2WI and low to intermediate signal on T1WI.

The MRI features of subdural hematomas are variable, although the appearances can progress in patterns similar to intraparenchymal hematomas. Chronic subdural hematomas often have low to intermediate signal on T1WI and high signal on T2WI. Subarachnoid hemorrhage is often difficult to see on T1WI and T2WI, although it can sometimes be identified on long repetition time (TR)/short echo time (TE) (proton density weighted images) or FLAIR images.

Other processes that can result in zones of high signal on T1WI are fat, dermoids (intact or ruptured), teratomas, lipomas, cystic structures with high protein concentration or cholesterol, and pantopaque.

Most other pathologic processes increase the T1 and T2 relaxation coefficients of the involved tissues, resulting in decreased signal on T1WI and increased signal on T2WI relative to adjacent normal tissue. Such processes include ischemia, infarction, inflammation, infection, demyelination, dysmyelination, metabolic or toxic encephalopathy, trauma, neoplasms, gliosis, radiation injury, and encephalomalacic changes. Areas where there is breakdown of the blood-brain barrier from these disorders can also be evaluated with gadolinium(Gd-)based intravenous contrast agents. Leakage of these agents through the blood-brain barrier reduces the T1 values of the hydrogen nuclei localized to the involved regions, resulting in high signal (enhancement) on T1WI. Contrast-enhanced MR images are an important portion of most imaging examinations of the head. In addition to pathologically altered intracranial tissues, Gd-contrast enhancement can be normally seen in dura mater, veins, choroid plexus, anterior pituitary gland, pituitary infundibulum, pineal gland, and area postrema. For this book, MRI signal of the various entities will be described as low, intermediate, high, or mixed on T1WI and T2WI; presence or nonpresence of Gd-contrast-enhancement will also be noted.

Lesions or structures with low signal on T1WI and T2WI can result from calcifications, very high protein or Gd-contrast-chelate concentrations, magnetic susceptibility effects, especially from metal fragments or surgical clips, and artifacts.

Intracranial lesions are typically classified as being extra-axial or intra-axial. Extra-axial lesions arise from the skull, meninges, or tissues other than the brain parenchyma. Extra-axial lesions are characterized as being within epidural, subdural, or subarachnoid spaces or compartments. Lesions involving the meninges can further be categorized as involving the dura mater (such as with benign postoperative dural fibrosis, etc.) or involving the leptomeninges (pia and arachnoid). Abnormalities of the meninges are often best seen after intravenous administration of Gd-contrast material. Dural enhancement usually has a linear configuration, whereas pathology involving the leptomeninges appears as enhancement within the sulci and basilar cisterns. Enhancement of the leptomeninges is usually related to significant pathology such as neoplastic or inflammatory diseases.

Intra-axial lesions are located in the brain parenchyma or brainstem. Differential diagnosis of extra-axial and intra-axial mass-like lesions are presented in Tables 1A.2, 1A.3, 1A.4 and 1A.5. Intra-axial mass-like lesions are presented according to location, supratentorial versus infratentorial. Infratentorial neoplasms are more common in children and adolescents than adults. During childhood, the most common neoplasms are intra-axial tumors such as astrocytomas, medulloblastomas, ependymomas, and brainstem gliomas. In adults, metastatic lesions and hemangioblastomas are the most common intra-axial infratentorial tumors, and acoustic schwannomas and meningiomas are common extra-axial infratentorial neoplasms. Infratentorial lesions are discussed in Table 1A.4, 1A.5.

MRI is an excellent imaging modality for evaluation of the posterior cranial fossa, skull base, orbits, nasopharynx and oropharynx, and floor of mouth because of its multiplanar imaging capabilities, high soft-tissue contrast resolution, and lack of scatter artifacts from bone that are seen with CT. The intracranial portions of the fifth, seventh, and eighth cranial nerves can be routinely seen with MRI. Occasionally, the third cranial nerve can be seen. MRI is the optimal method for imaging the location and extent of lesions at the skull base such as pituitary tumors, acoustic and trigeminal schwannomas, chordomas and chondrosarcomas at the clivus, metastatic tumors, perineural tumor spread through skull foramina, cholestrol granulomas, petrous apicitis, and inflammatory lesions of the cranial nerves.

MRI is the optimal method for evaluation of normal and abnormal brain parenchyma. Congenital and or developmental anomalies of the brain (such as semilobar holoprosencephaly, septo-optic dysplasia, schizencephaly, gray matter heterotopia, cortical dysplasias, unilateral megalencephaly, Dandy-Walker complex) can be characterized in detail by MRI.

Diseases of white matter are classified into two major groups: dysmyelinating and demyelinating diseases. Dysmyelinating diseases, also known as leukodystrophies, are a group of disorders resulting from enzyme deficiencies that cause abnormal formation and metabolism of myelin. Demyelinating diseases are a group of disorders in which myelin is degraded or destroyed after it has formed in a normal fashion.

Abnormalities involving the lateral third and fourth ventricles as well as the cerebral aqueduct are well seen with MRI because of the difference of MRI signal characteristics between the brain parenchyma and cerebrospinal fluid (CSF). CSF has prolonged T1 and T2 relaxation values, with resultant low signal on T1WI and high signal on T2WI. CSF production occurs in the choroid plexus within the ventricles. CSF circulates from the lateral ventricles through the foramen of Monro into the third ventricle. The third ventricle communicates with the fourth ventricle via the cerebral aqueduct. CSF from the fourth ventricle enters the subarachnoid space through the foramina of Luschka and Magendie. Mass lesions along the CSF pathway can result in obstructive hydrocephalus with dilatation of the ventricles proximal to the blockage.

Some asymmetry of the lateral ventricles can be seen normally. Altered morphology of the ventricles can result from various congenital anomalies (e.g., holoprosencephaly, septo-optic dysplasia, unilateral hemimegalencephaly, gray matter heterotopia, Dandy-Walker malformation), as well as from distortion from intra-axial or extra-axial mass lesions.

The sizes of sulci can vary depending on multiple variables such as age, congential malformations, vascular abnormalities (e.g., cerebral infarcts, Sturge-Weber, arteriovenous malformation [AVM]), intra-axial or extra-axial mass lesions, hydrocephalus, or inflammatory diseases. Sulci should have CSF signal within them. The presence of Gd-contrast enhancement within the sulci and basilar cisterns is usually associated with pathology such as inflammatory or neoplastic disease. Subarachnoid hemorrhage can sometimes have increased signal on proton density weighted, or FLAIR images.

MRI is a powerful imaging modality for evaluating normal and abnormal blood vessels. The appearance of blood vessels on MRI depends on various factors such as the type of MRI pulse sequence, pulsatility and range of velocities in the vessels of interest, and size, shape, and orientation of the vessels relative to the image plane. Useful anatomic information of blood vessels can be gained by using SE pulse sequences that can display patent vessels as zones of signal void (black-blood images), or GRE pulse sequences that display the moving hydrogen atomic nuclei (protons) in blood as zones of high signal (bright-blood images). The GRE pulse sequences can also be adapted to produce MR angiograms. MRA has proven to be clinically useful in the evaluation of intracranial arteries, veins, and dural venous sinuses. Pathologic processes involving intracranial blood vessels–such as aneurysms, AVM, arterial occlusions, and dural venous sinus thrombosis–can be seen with MRA.

1A Brain

Table 1A.1 Congenital malformations of brain

Disease	MRI Findings	Comments
Holoprosencephaly	*Alobar:* Large monoventricle with posterior midline cyst, lack of hemisphere formation with absence of falx, corpus callosum, and septum pellucidum. Fused thalami. *Semilobar* (Fig. 1A.**1**): Monoventricle with partial formation of interhemispheric fissure, occipital and temporal horns, partially fused thalami. Absent corpus callosum and septum pellucidum. Associated with mild craniofacial anomalies. *Lobar:* Near complete formation of interhemispheric fissure and ventricles. Fused inferior portions of frontal lobes, dysgenesis of corpus callosum, absence of septum pellucidum, separate thalami, neuronal migration disorders. *Septo-optic dysplasia (de Morsier syndrome)* (Fig. 1A.**2**): Mild form of lobar holoprosencephaly. Dysgenesis or agenesis of septum pellucidum, optic hypoplasia, squared frontal horns. Association with schizencephaly in 50%.	*Holoprosencephaly:* Disorders of diverticulation (4–6 weeks of gestation) characterized by absent or partial cleavage and differentiation of the embryonic cerebrum (prosenecephalon) into hemispheres and lobes.
Neuronal migration disorders:		
Lissencephaly (Fig. 1A.**3**)	Absent or incomplete formation of gyri and sulci with shallow sylvian fissures and "figure 8" appearance of brain on axial images. Abnormally thick cortex, gray matter heterotopia with smooth gray-white matter interface.	Severe disorder of neuronal migration (7–16 weeks of gestation) with absent or incomplete formation of gyri, sulci, and sylvian fissures. Associated with severe mental retardation and seizures, early death. Other associated CNS anomalies include dysgenesis of corpus callosum, microcephaly, hypoplastic thalami, cephaloceles.
Pachygyria (nonlissencephalic cortical dysplasia) (Fig. 1A.4)	Thick gyri with shallow sulci involving all or portions of the brain. Thickened cortex with relatively smooth gray-white interface. May have areas of high T2 signal in the white matter (gliosis).	Severe disorder of neuronal migration. Clinical findings related to degree of extent of this malformation.
Gray matter heterotopia (Figs. 1A.5–1A.7)	*Laminar heterotopia:* appears as band(s) of isointense gray matter within the cerebral white matter (Fig. 1A.**5**). *Nodular heterotopia:* appears as nodule(s) of isointense gray matter along the ventricles (Fig. 1A.**6**) or within the cerebral white matter (Fig. 1A.**7**).	Disorder of neuronal migration (7–22 weeks of gestation) where a collection or layer of neurons is located beween the ventricles and cerebral cortex. Can have a band-like (laminar) or nodular appearance isointense to gray matter, may be unilateral or bilateral. Associated with seizures, schizencephaly.

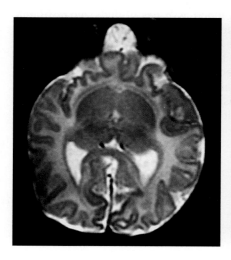
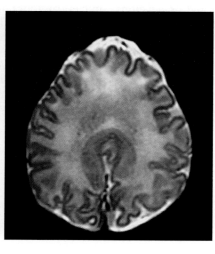

Fig. 1A.**1** **Semilobar holoprosencephaly. a, b** Axial T2WI of an 8-day old male shows fused frontal lobes and partial formation of interhemispheric fissure posteriorly.

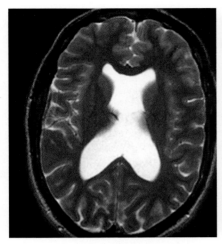

Fig. 1A.**2** **Septo-optic dysplasia (de Morsier syndrome).** **a** Axial T2WI shows absence of septum pellucidum and squared frontal horns of lateral ventricles.

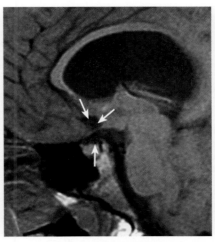

Fig. 1A.**2 b** Sagittal T1WI shows optic nerve hypoplasia (arrows).

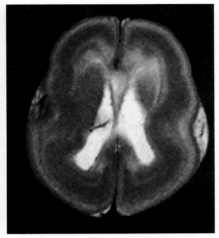

Fig. 1A.**3** **Lissencephaly.** Axial T2WI of a 2-day old male shows absent formation of gyri and sulci with shallow sylvian fissures and "figure 8" appearance of brain. Abnormally thick cortex, gray matter heterotopia with smooth gray-white matter interface.

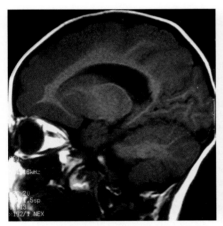

Fig. 1A.**4** **Pachygyria (nonlissencephalic cortical dysplasia).** **a** Sagittal T1WI shows thick gyri with shallow sulci involving portions of the brain.

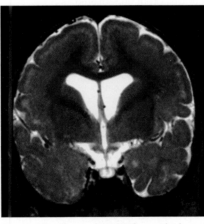

Fig. 1A.**4 b** Coronal T2WI shows thickened cortex with relatively smooth gray-white interface.

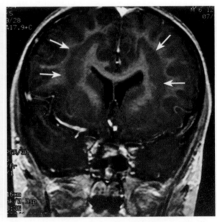

Fig. 1A.**5 a** **Gray matter heterotopia.** Laminar heterotopia. Coronal T1WI (arrows).

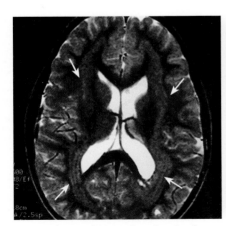

Fig. 1A.**5 b** Axial T2WI show bands of isointense heterotopic gray matter within the cerebral white matter (arrows).

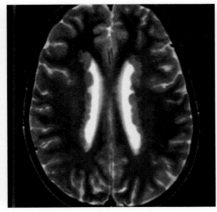

Fig. 1A.**6** **Gray matter heterotopia.** Nodular heterotopia. Axial T2WI shows nodules of isointense heterotopic gray matter along the lateral ventricles.

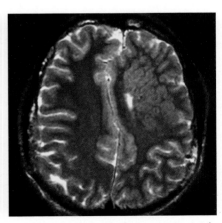

Fig. 1A.**7** **Gray matter heterotopia.** Axial T2WI shows isointense heterotopic gray matter within the cerebral white matter of the left frontal lobe.

Table 1A.**1** (Cont.) Congenital malformations of brain

Disease	MRI Findings	Comments
Schizencephaly (split brain) (Figs. 1A.8, 1A.9)	Cleft in brain extending from ventricle to cortical surface, lined by heterotopic gray matter. Cleft may be narrow (closed lip, Fig. 1A.**8**) or wide (open lip, Fig. 1A.**9**).	Association with seizures, blindness, retardation, and other CNS anomalies (e.g., septo-optic dysplasia). Clinical manifestations related to severity of malformation. Ischemia or insult to portion or germinal matrix before hemisphere formation.
Unilateral hemimegalencephaly (Fig. 1A.10)	Nodular or multinodular region of gray matter heterotopia involving all or part of a cerebral hemisphere with associated enlargement of the ipsilateral lateral ventricle and hemisphere.	Neuronal migration disorder associated with hamartomatous overgrowth of the involved hemisphere.
Neural tube closure disorders		
Chiari I malformation (Fig. 1A.11)	Cerebellar tonsils extend more than 5 mm below the foramen magnum in adults, 6 mm in children below 10 years of age. Syringohydromyelia in 20 to 40 %. Hydrocephalus in 25 %. Basilar impression in 25 %. Less common association: Klippel-Feil, atlanto-occipital assimilation.	Cerebellar tonsilar ectopia. Most common anomaly of CNS. Not associated with myelomeningocele.
Chiari II malformation (Arnold-Chiari) (Fig. 1A.12)	Small posterior cranial fossa with gaping foramen magnum through which there is an inferiorly positioned vermis associated with a cervicomedullary kink. Beaked dorsal margin of the tectal plate. Myelomeningoceles in nearly all patients. Hydrocephalus and syringomyelia common. Dilated lateral ventricles posteriorly (colpocephaly).	Complex anomaly involving the cerebrum, cerebellum, brainstem, spinal cord, ventricles, skull, and dura. Failure of fetal neural folds to develop properly results in altered development affecting multiple sites of the CNS.
Chiari III malformation	Features of Chiari II plus lower occipital or high cervical encephalocele.	Rare anomaly associated with high mortality.
Cephaloceles (meningoceles or meningoencephaloceles) (Fig. 1A.13)	Defect in skull through which there is either herniation of meninges and CSF (meningocele) or meninges, CSF, and brain tissue (meningoencephaloceles).	Congenital malformation involving lack of separation of neuroectoderm from surface ectoderm with resultant localized failure of bone formation. Occipital location most common in western hemisphere, frontoethmoidal location most common site in Southeast Asians. Other sites include parietal and sphenoid bones. Cephaloceles can also result from trauma or surgery.
Dysgenesis of the corpus callosum (Fig. 1A.14) (Fig. 1A.16)	Spectrum of abnormalities ranging from complete to partial absence of the corpus callosum. Widely separated and parallel orientations of frontal horns and bodies of lateral ventricles, high position of third ventricle in relation to interhemispheric fissure, colpocephaly. Associated with interhemispheric cysts, lipomas, and anomalies such as Chiari II, gray matter heterotopia, Dandy-Walker malformations, holoprosencephaly, azygous anterior cerebral artery, and cephaloceles.	Failure or incomplete formation of corpus callosum (7–18 weeks of gestation). Axons that normally cross from one hemisphere to the other are aligned parallel along the medial walls of lateral ventricles (bundles of Probst).
Dandy-Walker malformation (Fig. 1A.15)	Vermian aplasia or severe hypoplasia, communication of fourth ventricle with retrocerebellar cyst, enlarged posterior fossa, high position of tentorium and transverse venous sinuses. Hydrocephalus common. Associated with other anomalies such as dysgenesis of the corpus callosum, gray matter heterotopia, schizencephaly, holoprosencephaly, and cephaloceles.	Abnormal formation of roof of fourth ventricle with absent or near incomplete formation of cerebellar vermis.

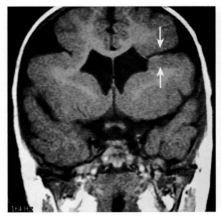

Fig. 1A.**8   Schizencephaly (split brain).** Coronal T1WI shows a narrow cleft (arrows) in brain (closed lip type) extending from ventricle to cortical surface lined by heterotopic gray matter.

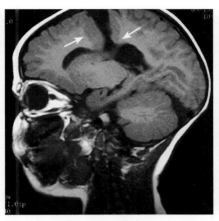

Fig. 1A.**9   Schizencephaly (split brain).** Sagittal T1WI shows a wide cleft in brain (open lip type) extending from ventricle to cortical surface lined by heterotopic gray matter (arrows).

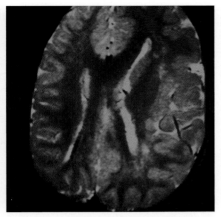

Fig. 1A.**10   Unilateral hemimegalencephaly.** Axial T2WI shows multinodular region of gray matter heterotopia involving an enlarged left cerebral hemisphere with associated enlargement of the left lateral ventricle.

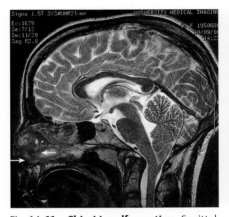

Fig. 1A.**11   Chiari I malformation.** Sagittal T2WI shows the cerebellar tonsils extending 12 mm below the foramen magnum in adults, representing a Chiari 1 malformation (arrows).

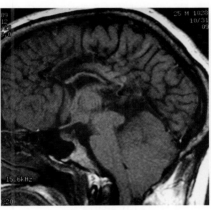

Fig. 1A.**12   Chiari II Malformation (Arnold-Chiari).** Sagittal T1WI shows a small posterior cranial fossa with gaping foramen magnum through which there is an inferiorly positioned vermis associated with an elongated fourth ventricle. Note also dysplasia of the corpus callosum and "beaked" tectum.

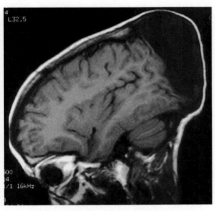

Fig. 1A.**13   Cephaloceles.** Sagittal T1WI shows a defect in the parieto-occipital portion of the skull through which there is herniation of meninges, CSF, and brain tissue (meningoencephalocele).

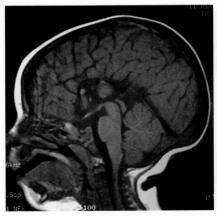

Fig. 1A.**14   Dysgenesis of the corpus callosum.   a** Sagittal T1WI shows absence of the corpus callosum.

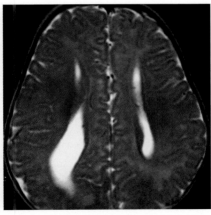

Fig. 1A.**14b**   Axial T2WI shows widely separated and parallel orientations of frontal horns and bodies of lateral ventricles.

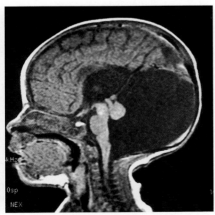

Fig. 1A.**15   Dandy-Walker malformation.** Sagittal T1WI shows severe vermian hypoplasia, communication of fourth ventricle with retrocerebellar cyst, enlarged posterior fossa, high position of tentorium and transverse venous sinuses.

Table 1A.**1** (Cont.) Congenital malformations of brain

Disease	MRI Findings	Comments
Dandy-Walker variant (Fig. 1A.**16**)	Mild vermian hypoplasia with communication of posteroinferior portion of the fourth ventricle with cisterna magna. No associated enlargement of the posterior cranial fossa.	Occasionally associated with hydrocephalus, dysgenesis of corpus callosum, gray matter heterotopia, other anomalies.
Lhermitte-Duclos disease (Fig. 1A.**17**)	Poorly defined zone of low T1 signal, high T2 signal with laminated appearance and localized mass effect in the cerebellum. No enhancement.	Uncommon cerebellar dysplasia with gross thickening of cerebellar folia and disorganized cellular structure.

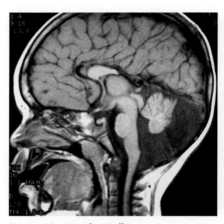

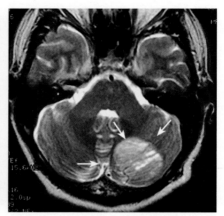

Fig. 1A.**16** **Dandy-Walker variant.** Sagittal T1WI shows mild to moderate vermian hypoplasia with communication of posteroinferior portion of the fourth ventricle with cisterna magna. No associated enlargement of the posterior cranial fossa. Dysgenesis (partial formation) of corpus callosum is also observed.

Fig. 1A.**17** **Lhermitte-Duclos Disease.** Axial T2WI shows a spheroid zone with heterogenous high T2 signal with laminated appearance and localized mass effect located in the left cerebellar hemisphere (arrows).

Table 1A.**2** Supratentorial intra-axial mass lesions

Disease	MRI Findings	Comments
Congenital		
Gray matter heterotopia (see p. 6, Figs. 1A.5–1A.7)		
Unilateral hemimegalencephaly (see p. 8, Fig. 1A.10)		
Neoplastic		
Astrocytoma (Figs.1A.**18**–1A.**21**)	*Low-grade astrocytoma:* Focal or diffuse mass lesion usually located in white matter with low to intermediate signal on T1WI and high signal on T2WI; with or without mild Gd-contrast enhancement. Minimal associated mass effect. *Juvenile pilocytic astrocytoma:* Subtype: solid/cystic focal lesion with low to intermediate signal on T1WI and high signal on T2WI; usually with prominent Gd-contrast enhancement. Lesions located in cerebellum, hypothalamus, adjacent to third or fourth ventricles, brainstem. *Gliomatosis cerebri:* Infiltrative lesion with poorly defined margins with mass effect located in the white matter. Low to intermediate signal on T1WI and high signal on T2WI; usually no Gd-contrast enhancement until late in disease. *Anaplastic astrocytoma:* Often irregularly marginated lesion located in white matter with low to intermediate signal on T1WI and high signal on T2WI, with or without Gd-contrast enhancement.	*Low-grade astrocytoma:* Often occur in children and adults (age 20–40 years). Tumors comprised of well-differentiated astrocytes. Association with neurofibromatosis type 1. Ten-year survival. May become malignant. *Juvenile pilocytic astrocytoma:* Subtype: common in children, usually favorable prognosis if totally resected. *Gliomatosis cerebri:* Diffusely infiltrating astrocytoma with relative preservation of underlying brain architecture. Imaging appearance may be more prognostic than histologic grade. Approximate 2-year survival. *Anaplastic astrocytoma:* Intermediate between low-grade astrocytoma and glioblastoma multiforme. Approximate 2-year survival.

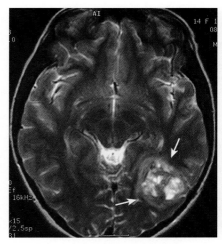

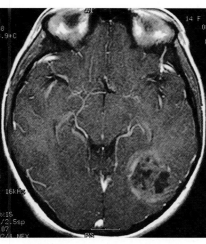

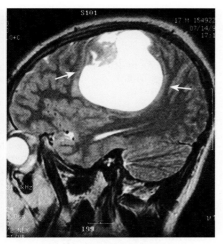

Fig. 1A.18   Low-grade astrocytoma.
a Axial T2WI shows a focal mass lesion in left temporo-occipital region with heterogeneous intermediate to high signal (arrows).

Fig. 1A.18 b   Postcontrast axial T1WI shows a small zone of mild Gd-contrast enhancement in only a small portion of the lesion.

Fig. 1A.19   Juvenile pilocytic astrocytoma, subtype.   a Sagittal T2WI shows a mixed solid and cystic focal lesion in the right frontoparietal region (arrows). The solid component of the lesion has intermediate signal, and the cystic component has high signal.

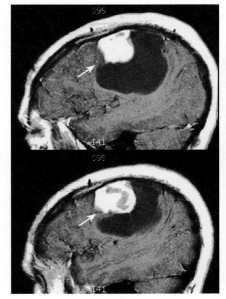

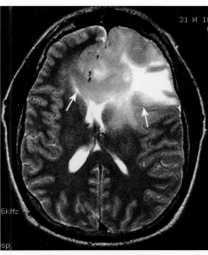

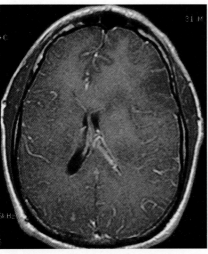

Fig. 1A.19 b   Sagittal postcontrast T1WI shows prominent Gd-contrast enhancement at the solid component of the lesion (arrows).

Fig. 1A.20   Gliomatosis cerebri.   a Axial T2WI shows an infiltrative lesion with heterogenous high signal, poorly defined margins with mass effect located in the left frontal lobe extending through the corpus callosum into the right frontal lobe (arrows).

Fig. 1A.20 b   Postcontrast axial T1WI shows no Gd-contrast enhancement at neoplasm.

Fig. 1A.21   Anaplastic astrocytoma.   a Axial T2WI shows an infiltrative lesion with heterogenous high signal, poorly defined margins with mass effect located in the right frontoparietal region.   **b** Postcontrast axial T1WI shows irregular Gd-contrast enhancement in a portion of the neoplasm.

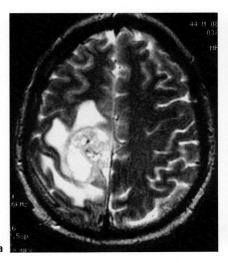

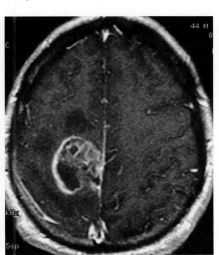

a

b

Table 1A.2 (Cont.) Supratentorial intra-axial mass lesions

Disease	MRI Findings	Comments
Glioblastoma multiforme (Fig. 1A.22)	Irregularly marginated mass lesion with necrosis or cyst. Mixed signal on T1WI and heterogeneous high signal on T2WI. Hemorrhage may be associated. Prominent heterogeneous Gd-contrast enhancement. Peripheral edema. Can cross corpus callosum.	Most common primary CNS tumor. Highly malignant neoplasms with necrosis and vascular proliferation, usually in patients above 50 years. Extent of lesion underestimated by MRI. Survival less than 1 year.
Giant cell astrocytoma–Tuberous sclerosis (Fig. 1A.23)	Circumscribed lesion located near the foramen of Monro with mixed low to intermediate or high signal on T1WI and on T2WI. Cysts and/or calcifications may be associated. Heterogenous or homogenous Gd-contrast enhancement.	Subependymal hamartoma near foramen of Monro, occurs in 15% of patients with tuberous sclerosis below 20 years of age. Slow-growing lesions that can progressively cause obstruction of CSF flow through the foramen of Monro. Long-term survival usual if resected.
Pleomorphic xanthoastrocytoma (Fig. 1A.24)	Circumscribed supratentorial lesion involving cerebral cortex and white matter. Low to intermediate signal on T1WI, intermediate to high signal on T2WI. Cyst(s) may be present. Heterogeneous Gd-contrast enhancement, with or without enhancing mural nodule associated with cyst.	Rare type of astrocytoma occurring in young adults and children, associated with seizure history.
Oligodendroglioma (Fig. 1A.25)	Circumscribed lesion with mixed low to intermediate signal on T1WI and mixed intermediate to high signal on T2WI; areas of signal void at sites of clump-like calcification; heterogenous Gd-contrast enhancement. Involves white matter and cerebral cortex. Can cause chronic erosion of inner table of calvaria.	Uncommon slow-growing gliomas with usually mixed histologic patterns (e.g., astrocytoma). Usually in adults older than 35 years of age, 85% supratentorial. If low-grade 75% 5-year survival; higher grade lesions have a worse prognosis.

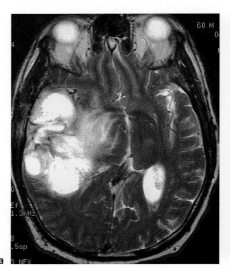
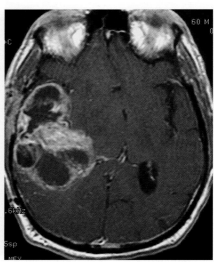

Fig. 1A.**22**   **Glioblastoma multiforme.   a** Axial T2WI shows a large mass lesion with heterogenous high signal containing areas of necrosis, poorly defined margins, and marked mass effect located in the right temporal, frontal, and parietal lobes.   **b** Postcontrast axial T1WI shows prominent irregular Gd-contrast enhancement at the neoplasm.

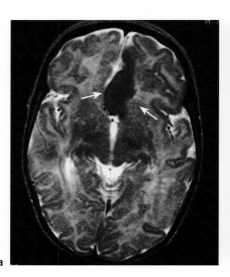
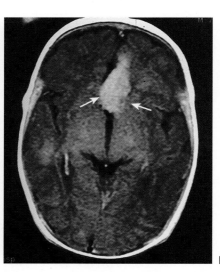

Fig. 1A.**23**   **Giant cell astrocytoma–tuberous sclerosis.   a** Axial T2WI shows a circumscribed lesion located near the foramen of Monro with low to intermediate signal (arrows).   **b** Postcontrast axial T1WI shows Gd-contrast enhancement at lesion (arrows).

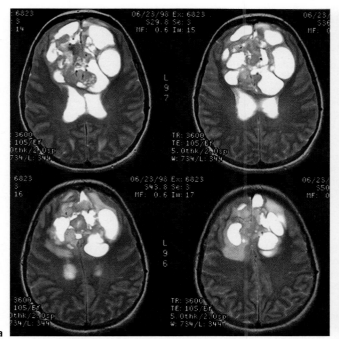

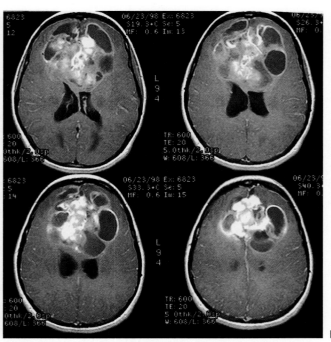

Fig. 1A.**24 Pleomorphic xanthoastrocytoma. a** Axial T2WI shows a large mutilobulated lesion containing solid and cystic zones involving the cerebral cortex and white matter of both frontal lobes, with hetergeneous intermediate to high signal and mass effect.

Fig. 1A.**24 b** Postcontrast axial T1WI shows prominent heterogeneous Gd-contrast enhancement at the lesion

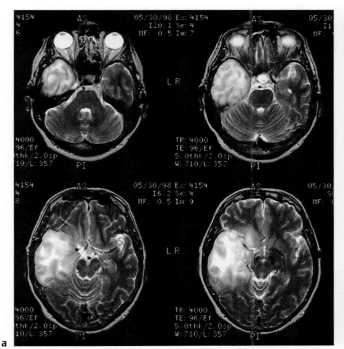

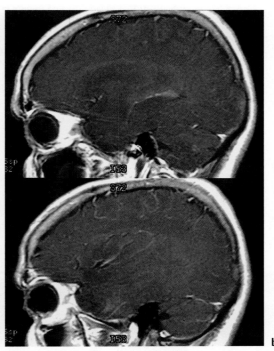

Fig. 1A.**25 Oligodendroglioma. a** Axial T2WI shows a lesion with heterogenous high signal, poorly defined margins with mass effect located in the right temporal lobe.

Fig. 1A.**25 b** Postcontrast sagittal T1WI shows equivocal minimal Gd-contrast enhancement at neoplasm

Table 1A.2 (Cont.) Supratentorial intra-axial mass lesions

Disease	MRI Findings	Comments
Central neurocytoma (Fig. 1A.26)	Circumscribed lesion located at margin of lateral ventricle or septum pellucidum with intraventricular protrusion. Heterogeneous intermediate signal on T1WI; heterogeneous intermediate to high signal on T2WI. Calcifications and/or small cysts may be associated. Heterogeneous Gd-contrast enhancement.	Rare tumors that have neuronal differentiation. Imaging appearance similar to intraventricular oligodendrogliomas. Occur in young adults. Benign slow-growing lesions.
Ganglioglioma, ganglioneuroma, gangliocytoma (Fig. 1A.27)	Circumscribed tumor; usually supratentorial, often temporal or frontal lobes. Low to intermediate signal on T1WI, intermediate to high signal on T2WI. Cysts may be present. With or without Gd-contrast enhancement.	Ganglioglioma (contains glial and neuronal elements), ganglioneuroma (contains only ganglion cells). Uncommon tumors, below 30 years, seizure presentation, slow-growing neoplasms. Gangliocytoma (contains only neuronal elements, dysplastic brain tissue). Favorable prognosis if completely resected.
Ependymoma (Fig. 1A.28)	Circumscribed lobulated supratentorial lesion, often extraventricular. Cysts and/or calcifications may be associated. Low to intermediate signal on T1WI; intermediate to high signal on T2WI. Variable Gd-contrast enhancement.	Occurs more commonly in children than adults. One-third supratentorial, two-thirds infratentorial. 45 % 5-year survival.
Hamartoma–Tuberous sclerosis (Fig. 1A.29)	*Cortical:* Subcortical lesion with high signal on T1WI and low signal on T2WI in neonates and infants; changes to low to intermediate signal on T1WI and high signal on T2WI in older children and adults. Calcifications in 50 % in older children. Gd-contrast enhancement uncommon. *Subependymal hamartomas:* Small nodules located along and projecting into the lateral ventricles. Signal on T1WI and T2WI similar to cortical tubers. Calcification and Gd-contrast enhancement common.	Cortical and subependymal hamartomas are nonmalignant lesions associated with tuberous sclerosis. Tuberous sclerosis is an autosomal dominant disorder associated with hamartomas in multiple organs.
Hypothalamic hamartoma (Fig. 1A.30)	Sessile or pedunculated lesions at the tuber cinereum of the hypothalamus. Often intermediate signal on T1WI and T2WI similar to gray matter, occasionally slightly high signal on T2WI; usually no enhancement. Rarely contain cystic and/or fatty portions.	Usually occur in children with isosexual precocious puberty (age 0–8 years) or seizures (gelastic or partial complex) in second decade. Congenital/developmental heterotopia/hamartoma (non-neoplastic lesions).

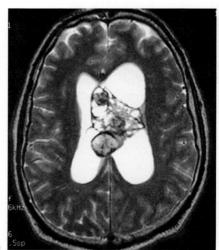

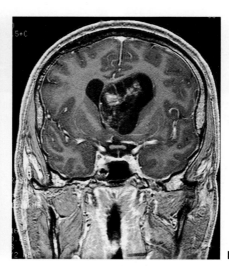

Fig. 1A.26 **Central neurocytoma. a** Axial T2WI shows a circumscribed lesion with heterogenous high signal containing cystic zones, involving the septum pellucidum with extension into both lateral ventricles. **b** Postcontrast coronal (GRE) T1WI shows irregular pattern of Gd-contrast enhancement at neoplasm

a

b

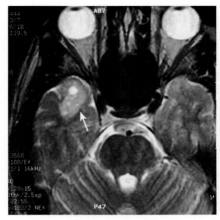

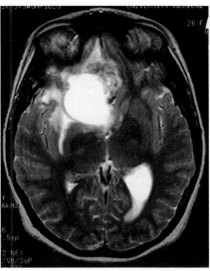

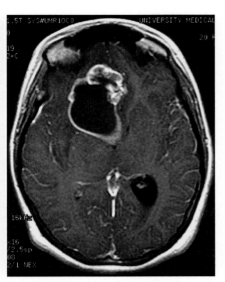

Fig. 1A.**27** **Ganglioglioma, gan-glioneuroma, gangliocytoma.** Axial T2WI shows a lesion with heterogenous high signal containing small cystic zones in the anterior right temporal lobe (arrows). No Gd-contrast enhancement was seen associated with this lesion (images not shown).

Fig. 1A.**28** **Ependymoma.** **a** Axial T2WI shows a lesion with heterogenous high signal containing a cystic zone in the inferior right frontal lobe.

Fig. 1A.**28 b** Postcontrast axial T1WI shows irregular peripheral enhancement at lesion.

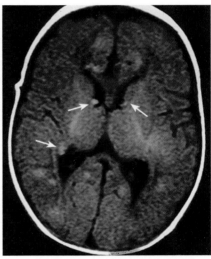

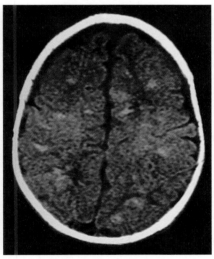

Fig. 1A.**29** **Hamartoma–tuberous sclerosis.** **a** Axial T1WI in a 7-week-old male shows three small nodules with high signal along ventricular margins representing subependymal hamartomas (arrows).

Fig. 1A.**29 b** Axial T1WI shows cortical/subcortical lesions with high signal representing cortical tubers and white matter abnormalities associated with tuberous sclerosis.

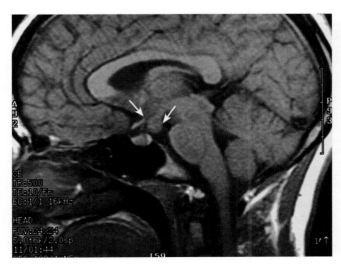

Fig. 1A.**30** **Hypothalamic hamartoma.** Sagittal T1WI shows a pedunculated lesion at the tuber cinereum of the hypothalamus with intermediate signal similar to gray matter (arrow).

Table 1A.**2** (Cont.) Supratentorial intra-axial mass lesions

Disease	MRI Findings	Comments
Primitive neuroectodermal tumor (Fig. 1A.31)	Circumscribed or invasive lesions. Low to intermediate signal on T1WI; intermediate to high signal on T2WI. Variable Gd-contrast enhancement. Frequent dissemination into the leptomeninges.	Highly malignant tumors located in the cerebrum, pineal gland, and cerebellum that frequently disseminate along CSF pathways.
Dysembryoplastic neuroepithelial tumor (Fig. 1A.32)	Circumscribed lesions involving the cerebral cortex and subcortical white matter. Low signal on T1WI; high signal on T2WI. Small cysts may be associated. Usually no Gd-contrast enhancement.	Benign superficial lesions commonly located in the temporal or frontal lobes.
Lymphoma (Fig. 1A.33)	Primary CNS lymphoma: focal or infiltrating lesion located in the basal ganglia, periventricular regions, posterior fossa/brainstem. Low to intermediate signal on T1WI; intermediate to slightly high signal on T2WI. Hemorrhage/necrosis may be associated in immunocompromised patients. Usually Gd-contrast enhancement. Diffuse leptomeningeal enhancement is another pattern of intracranial lymphoma.	Primary CNS lymphoma more common than secondary, usually occurs in adults older than 40 years of age. B cell lymphoma more common than T cell lymphoma. Increasing incidence related to number of immunocompromised patients in population. MRI features of primary and secondary lymphoma of brain overlap. Intracranial lymphoma can involve the leptomeninges in secondary lymphoma more commonly than primary lymphoma.
Hemangioblastoma (Fig. 1A.94)	Circumscribed tumors usually located in the cerebellum and/or brainstem. Small Gd-contrast-enhancing nodule with or without cyst, or larger lesion with prominent heterogeneous enhancement with or without flow voids within lesion or at the periphery. Intermediate signal on T1WI; intermediate to high signal on T2WI. Occasionally lesions have evidence of recent or remote hemorrhage.	Rarely occur in cerebral hemispheres; occur in adolescents, young and middle-aged adults. Lesions are typically multiple in patients with von Hippel-Lindau disease.
Metastases (Fig. 1A.34)	Circumscribed spheroid lesions in brain that can have various intra-axial locations, often at gray-white matter junctions. Usually low to intermediate signal on T1WI; intermediate to high signal on T2WI. Hemorrhage, calcifications, cysts may be associated. Variable Gd-contrast enhancement. Often high signal on T2WI peripheral to nodular enhancing lesion representing axonal edema.	Represent approximately 33% of intracranial tumors, usually from extracranial primary neoplasm in adults older than 40 years of age. Primary tumor source in order of decreaseing frequency: lung, breast, GI, GU, melanoma.
Neurocutaneous melanosis	Extra-axial or intra-axial lesions usually less than 3 cm in diameter with irregular margins in the leptomeninges or brain parenchyma/brainstem (anterior temporal lobes, cerebellum, thalami, inferior frontal lobes) with intermediate to slightly high signal on T1WI secondary to increased melanin. Gd-contrast enhancement. Vermian hypoplasia, arachnoid cysts, Dandy-Walker malformation may be associated.	Neuroectodermal dysplasia with proliferation of melanocytes in leptomeninges associated with large and/or numerous cutaneous nevi. May change into CNS melanoma.

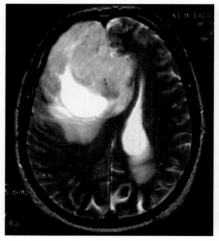
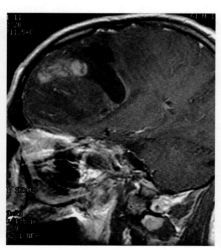

a   b

Fig. 1A.31 Primitive neuroectodermal tumor. a Axial T2WI shows a large lesion with heterogeneous high signal in the right frontal lobe extending across the corpus callosum to the left frontal lobe. **b** Postcontrast sagittal T1WI shows irregular enhancement in a portion of the lesion.

Fig. 1A.34 Metastases. a Axial T2WI ▷ shows multiple intra-axial lesions of varying sizes with high signal in the brain (many at gray-white matter junctions). The larger of the lesions have associated peripheral edema. **b** Postcontrast sagittal T1WI shows nodular and ring-like patterns of enhancement at the intra-axial lesions.

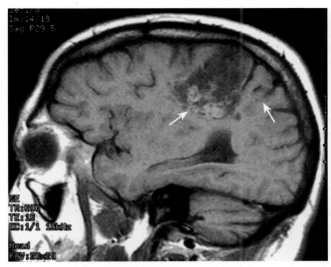
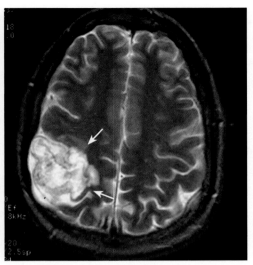

Fig. 1A.**32** **Dysembryoplastic neuroepithelial tumor.** **a** Sagittal T1WI shows a lesion with heterogeneous, predominantly low signal involving the cerebral cortex and subcortical white matter in the right cerebral hemisphere (arrows).

Fig. 1A.**32b** Axial T2WI shows the lesion to have heterogeneous high signal with small cysts. Note also the chronic erosive changes at the adjacent inner table of the skull (arrows).

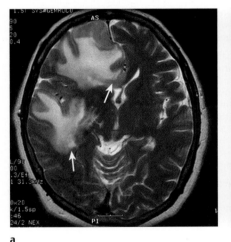
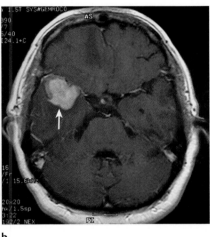
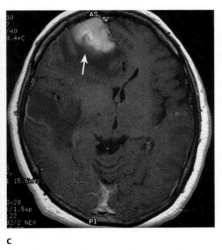

a   **b**   **c**

Fig. 1A.**33** **Lymphoma.** **a** Axial T2WI shows infiltrating lesions with high signal and mass effect located in the right frontal and temporal lobes with involvement of the corpus callosum (arrows). **b, c** Postcontrast axial T1WI shows Gd-contrast enhancement at two sites of intra-axial lymphoma (arrows).

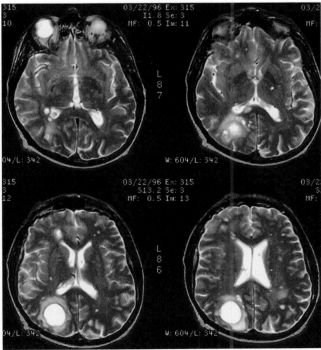
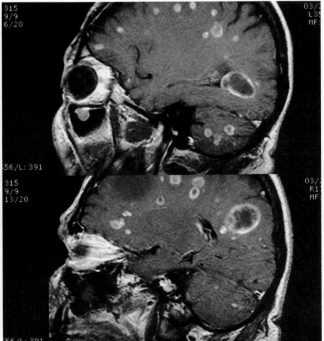
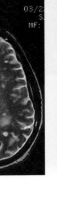

Fig. 1A.**34a**   Fig. 1A.**34b**

Table 1A.2 (Cont.) Supratentorial intra-axial mass lesions

Disease	MRI Findings	Comments
Inflammatory		
Cerebritis (Fig. 1A.35)	Poorly defined zone or focal area of low to intermediate signal on T1WI and intermediate to high signal on T2WI; minimal or no Gd-contrast enhancement. Involves cerebral cortex and white matter for bacterial and fungal infections.	Focal infection/inflammation of brain tissue from bacteria or fungi, secondary to sinusitis, meningitis, surgery, hematogenous source (cardiac and other vascular shunts), and/or immunocompromised status. Can progress to abscess formation.
Pyogenic brain abscess (Fig. 1A.36)	Circumscribed lesion with low signal on T1WI; central zone of high signal on T2WI (air-fluid level may be present) surrounded by a thin rim of low T2 signal; peripheral poorly defined zone of high signal on T2WI representing edema. Ring-like Gd-contrast enhancement that is sometimes thicker laterally than medially.	Formation of brain abscess occurs 2 weeks after cerebritis with liquefaction and necrosis centrally surrounded by a capsule and peripheral edema. Can be multiple. Complication from meningitis and/or sinusitis, septicemia, trauma, surgery, cardiac shunt.
Fungal brain abscess (Fig. 1A.37)	Vary depending on organism. Lesions occur in meninges and brain parenchyma; solid or cystic lesions with low to intermediate signal on T2WI and high signal on T2WI. Nodular or ring enhancement. Peripheral high signal in brain lesions on T2WI (edema).	Occur in immunocompromised or diabetic patients with resultant granulomas in meninges and brain parenchyma; *Cryptococcus* involves the basal meninges and extends along perivascular spaces into the basal ganglia. *Aspergillus* and *Mucor* spread via direct extension through paranasal sinuses or hematogenously invade blood vessels resulting in hemorrhagic lesions and/or cerebral infarcts. Coccidiomycosis usually involves the basal meninges.
Encephalitis , (Fig. 1A.38) (Fig. 1A.95)	Poorly defined zone(s) of low to intermediate signal on T1WI and intermediate to high signal on T2WI; minimal or no Gd-contrast enhancement. Involves cerebral cortex and/or white matter, minimal localized mass effect. Herpes simplex typically involves the temporal lobes/limbic system; hemorrhage may be associated. Cytomegalovirus (CMV) usually in periventricular/subependymal locations. HIV often involves periatrial white matter.	Encephalitis: infection/inflammation of brain tissue from viruses, often in immuncompromised patients (herpes simplex, CMV, HIV, progressive multifocal leukoencephalopathy) or immunocompetent (St Louis encephalitis, Eastern or Western equine encephalitis, Epstein-Barr virus).
Tuberculoma (Fig. 1A.39)	Intra-axial lesions in cerebral hemispheres and basal ganglia (adults), cerebellum (children). Low to intermediate signal on T1WI, central zone of high signal on T2WI with a thin peripheral rim of low signal, occasionally low signal on T2WI. Solid or rim Gd-contrast enhancement. Calcification may be present. Meningeal lesions: nodular or cystic zones of basilar meningeal enhancement.	Occurs in immunocompromised patients and in developing countries. Caseating intracranial granulomas via hematogenous dissemination. Lesions more common in meninges than brain.

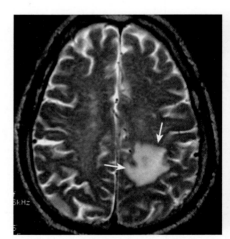

Fig. 1A.35 Cerebritis. a Axial T2WI shows a poorly defined zone of high signal involving the upper left cerebral hemisphere from bacterial infection (arrows).

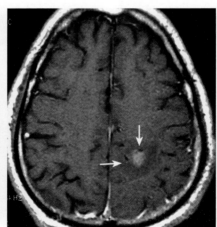

Fig. 1A.35 b Axial T1WI shows Gd-contrast enhancement at site of cerebritis (arrows).

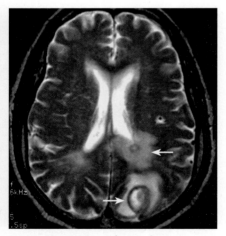

Fig. 1A.36 Pyogenic brain abscess. a Axial T2WI shows two circumscribed lesions with central zones of high signal surrounded by a thin rim of low signal, as well as a more peripheral poorly defined zone of high signal representing edema (arrows).

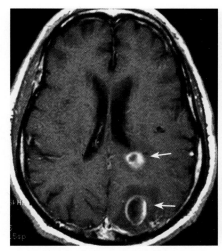

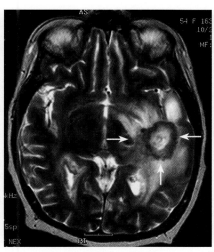

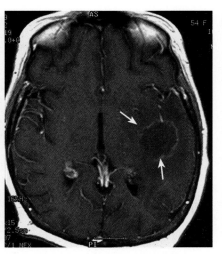

Fig. 1A.**36 b** Postcontrast axial T1WI shows ring-like Gd-contrast enhancement (thicker laterally than medially) at the abscesses (arrows).

Fig. 1A.37 **Fungal brain abscess. a** Axial T2WI shows a fungal abscess (aspergillosis) with a central zone of heterogeneous high signal surrounded by a thick rim of low T2 signal, as well as a more peripheral poorly defined zone of high signal representing edema (arrows).

Fig. 1A.37 b Postcontrast axial T1WI shows ring-like Gd-contrast enhancement at site of fungal abscess (arrows).

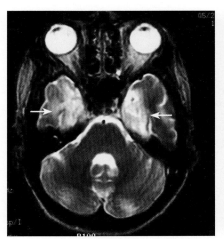

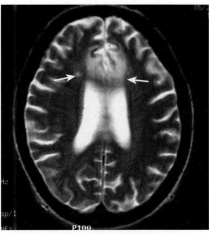

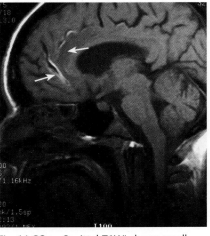

Fig. 1A.**38 Encephalitis. a, b** Axial T2WI shows poorly defined zones of high signal involving the cortex and subcortical white matter of both medial temporal lobes and cingulate gyri representing herpes limbic encephalitis (arrows).

Fig. 1A.**38 c** Sagittal T1WI shows small zones of hemorrhage (methemoglobin) in the cingulate gyri resulting from the herpes infection (arrows).

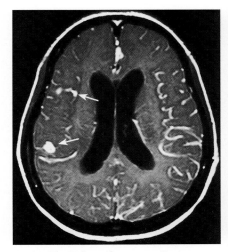

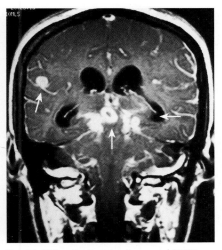

Fig. 1A.**39 Tuberculoma. a** Postcontrast axial T1WI shows two ehancing intraaxial lesions in the right cerebral hemisphere (arrows) as well as abnormal enhancement in the leptomeninges along the sulci.

Fig. 1A.**39 b** Postcontrast coronal T1WI shows a solid enhancing lesion in the right cerebral hemisphere as well as curvilinear zones and ring enhancing lesions in the basal and supratentorial leptomeninges (arrows).

Table 1A.2 (Cont.) Supratentorial intra-axial mass lesions

Disease	MRI Findings	Comments
Parasitic brain lesions		
Toxoplasmosis (Fig. 1A.40)	Single or multiple solid and/or cystic lesions located in basal ganglia and/or corticomedullary junctions in cerebral hemispheres. Low to intermediate signal on T1WI; high signal on T2WI. Nodular or rim pattern of Gd-contrast enhancement, with or without peripheral high T2 signal (edema).	Most common opportunistic CNS infection in AIDS patients, caused by ingestion of food contaminated with parasites (_Toxoplasma gondii_).
Cysticercosis (Fig. 1A.41)	Single or multiple cystic lesions in brain or meninges. _Acute/subacute phase:_ Low to intermediate signal on T1WI and high signal on T2WI. Rim and possible nodular pattern of Gd-contrast enhancement, with or without peripheral high T2 signal (edema). _Chronic phase:_ calcified granulomas.	Caused by ingestion of ova (_Taenia solium_) in contaminated food (undercooked pork). Involves in order of decreasing frequency: meninges, brain parenchyma, ventricles.
Hydatid cyst	_Echinococcus granulosus:_ Single or rarely multiple cystic lesions with low signal on T1WI and high signal on T2WI with a thin wall with low signal on T2WI; typically no Gd-contrast enhancement or peripheral edema unless superinfected. Often located in vascular territory of the middle cerebral artery. _Echinococcus multilocularis:_ Cystic (possibly multilocular) and/or solid lesions. Central zone of low to intermediate signal on T1WI or T2WI, surrounded by a slightly thickened rim of low signal on T2WI; Gd-contrast enhancement. Peripheral zone of high signal on T2WI (edema) and calcifications are common.	Caused by parasites: _Echinococcus granulosus_ (South America, Middle East Australia, New Zealand) or _Echinococcus multilocularis_ (North America, Europe, Turkey, China).CNS involvement in 2% of cases of hydatid infestation.
Radiation necrosis (Fig. 1A.42)	Focal lesion with or without associated mass effect, or poorly defined zone of low to intermediate signal on T1WI and intermediate to high signal on T2WI, with or without Gd-contrast enhancement involving tissue (gray matter and/or white matter) in field of treatment.	Usually occurs from 4–6 months to 10 years after radiation treatment. May be difficult to distinguish from neoplasm. Positron emission tomography (PET) and MR spectroscopy (MRS) might be helpful for evaluation.

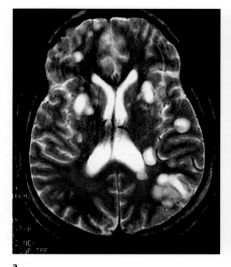

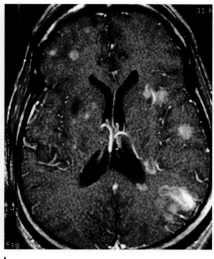

a   b

Fig. 1A.**40 Toxoplasmosis. a** Axial T2WI shows multiple complex cystic-like lesions located in the basal ganglia and corticomedullary junctions in both cerebral hemispheres.   **b** Postcontrast axial T1WI shows rim patterns of Gd-contrast enhancement at lesions.

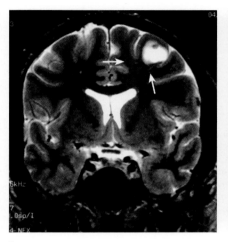

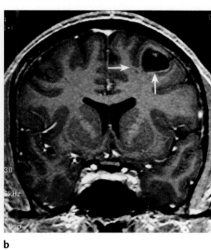

a   b

Fig. 1A.**41 Cysticercosis. a** Coronal T2WI shows a single cystic lesion with high signal containing a small nodule in the upper left cerebral hemisphere (arrows).   **b** Postcontrast coronal (spoiled GRE) T1WI shows minimal rim pattern of Gd-contrast enhancement at cystic lesion as well as at the small nodule (arrows).

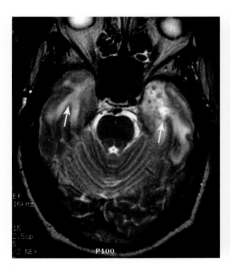

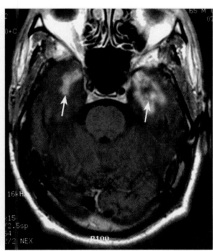

a   b

Fig. 1A.**42 Radiation injury/necrosis. a** Axial T2WI shows poorly defined zones of heterogeneous high signal involving the cerebral cortex and white matter at the anterior portions of both temporal lobes (arrows). Mild localized mass effect is also seen.   **b** Postcontrast axial T1WI shows Gd-contrast enhancement involving tissue (gray and/or white matter) in the field of treatment (arrows).

Table 1A.2 (Cont.) Supratentorial intra-axial mass lesions

Disease	MRI Findings	Comments
Hemorrhage		
Intracerebral hemorrhage (Figs. 1A.43, 1A.44)	The signal of the hematoma depends on its age, size, location, hematocrit, hemoglobin oxidation state, clot retraction, and extent of edema. *Hyperacute phase (4–6 hours):* Hemoglobin primarily as diamagnetic oxyhemoglobin (iron Fe^{+2} state), intermediate signal on T1WI and slightly high signal on T2WI. *Acute phase (12–48 hours):* Hemoglobin primarily as paramagnetic deoxyhemoglobin (iron, Fe^{+2} state), intermediate signal on T1WI and low signal on T2WI, surrounded by a peripheral zone of high T2 signal (edema). *Subacute phase (>2 days):* Hemoglobin becomes oxidized to the iron Fe^{+3} state, methemoglobin, which is strongly paramagnetic. When methemoglobin is initially intracellular: the hematoma has high signal on T1WI, progressing from peripheral to central, and low signal on T2WI, surrounded by a zone of high T2 signal (edema). When methemoglobin eventually becomes primarily extracellular: the hematoma has high signal on T1WI and T2WI. *Chronic phase:* Hemoglobin as extracellular methemoglobin is progressively degraded to hemosiderin. The hematoma progresses from a lesion with high signal on T1WI and T2WI with a peripheral rim of low signal on T2WI (hemosiderin) to predominant hemosiderin composition and low signal on T2WI.	Can result from trauma, ruptured aneurysms or vascular malformations, coagulopathy, hypertension, adverse drug reaction, amyloid angiopathy, hemorrhagic transformation of cerebral infarct, metastases, abscesses, viral infections (herpes simplex, CMV).
Cerebral contusions (Fig. 1A.45)	The MR appearance of contusions is initially one of focal hemorrhage involving the cerebral cortex and subcortical white matter. The MR signal of the contusion depends on its age and presence of oxyhemoglobin, deoxyhemoglobin, methemoglobin, hemosiderin, etc. Contusions eventually appear as focal superficial encephalomalacic zones with high signal on T2WI, with or without small zones of low signal on T2WI from hemosiderin.	Contusions are superficial brain injuries involving the cerebral cortex and subcortical white matter that result from skull fracture and/or acceleration/deceleration trauma to the inner table of the skull. Often involve the anterior portions of the temporal and frontal lobes and inferior portions of the frontal lobes.

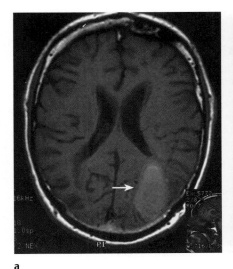

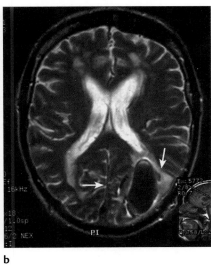

a   b

Fig. 1A.**43** **Subacute intracerebral hemorrhage (intracellular methemoglobin).** **a** Axial T1WI shows a hematoma in the left cerebral hemisphere that has high signal representing methemoglobin (arrows). **b** Axial T2WI shows a large central zone of low signal (intracellular methemoglobin) surrounded by thin irregular zone of high signal (edema) (arrows).

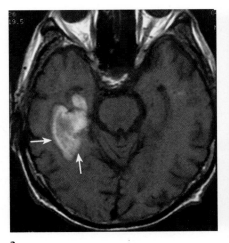

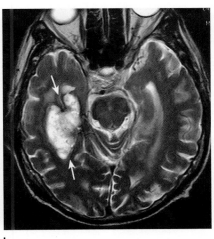

a   b

Fig. 1A.**44** **Subacute intracerebral hemorrhage (extracellular methemoglobin).** **a** Axial T1WI shows a hematoma in the right temporal lobe that has high signal representing methemoglobin (arrows). **b** Axial T2WI shows high signal (extracellular methemoglobin) surrounded by thin irregular zones of low signal (hemosiderin) and high signal (edema) (arrows).

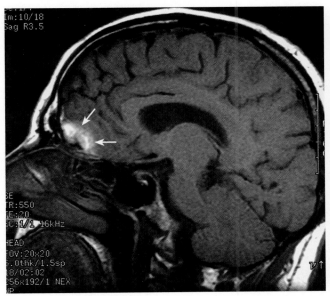

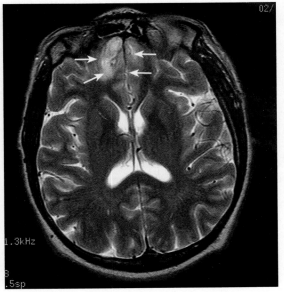

Fig. 1A.**45** **Cerebral contusions.** **a** Sagittal T1WI shows a contusion at the superficial portion of the inferior right frontal lobe where there is high signal representing hemorrhage (methemoglobin) (arrows).

Fig. 1A.**45 b** Axial T2WI shows high signal involving the cerebral cortex and subcortical white matter at the site of contusion (extracellular methemoglobin) (arrows).

Table 1A.**2** (Cont.) Supratentorial intra-axial mass lesions

Disease	MRI Findings	Comments
Metastases (Fig. 1A.46**)**	The MR appearance of a hemorrhagic metastatic lesion is one of an intracerebral hematoma involving a portion or all of the neoplasm. Usually associated with peripheral edema (high signal on T2WI), often multiple.	Metastatic intra-axial tumors associated with hemorrhage include bronchogenic carcinoma, renal cell carcinoma, melanoma, choriocarcinoma, and thyroid carcinoma. May be difficult to distinguish from hemorrhage related to other etiologies, such as vascular malformations and amyloid angiopathy
Vascular		
Arteriovenous malformation (AVM) (Fig. 1A.**47)**	Lesions with irregular margins that can be located in the brain parenchyma–pia, dura, or both locations. AVMs contain multiple tortuous tubular flow voids on T1WI and T2WI secondary to patent arteries with high blood flow; as well as thrombosed vessels with variable signal, areas of hemorrhage in various phases, calcifications, and gliosis. The venous portions often show Gd-contrast enhancement. Gradient-echo (GRE) MRI shows flow-related enhancement (high signal) in patent arteries and veins of the AVM. MRA using TOF or phase contrast techniques can provide additional detailed information about the nidus, feeding arteries, and draining veins, and presence of associated aneurysms. Usually not associated with mass effect except in the case of recent hemorrhage or venous occlusion.	Supratentorial AVMs occur more frequently (80–90%) than infratentorial AVMs (10–20%). Annual risk of hemorrhage. AVMs can be sporadic, congenital, or associated with a history of trauma. Multiple AVMs can be seen in syndromes: Rendu-Osler-Weber, AVMs in brain and lungs, and mucosal capillary telangectasias; Wyburn-Mason, AVMs in brain and retina, cutaneous nevi.

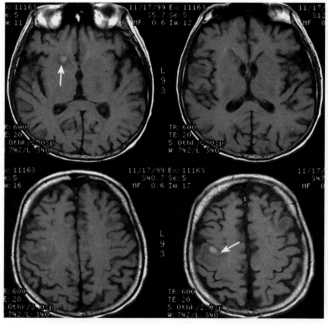

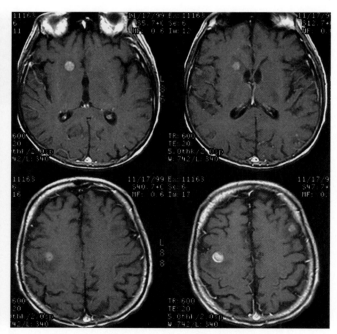

Fig. 1A.**46 Metastases. a** Axial T1WI shows two metastatic lesions from melanoma in the right cerebral hemisphere that have high signal representing methemoglobin (arrows).

Fig. 1A.**46 b** Postcontrast axial T1WI also shows enhancement at both of these metastatic lesions as well as at another lesion in the lateral left frontal lobe.

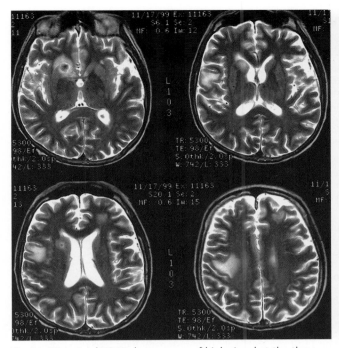

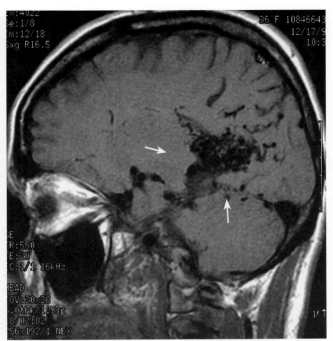

Fig. 1A.**46 c**   Axial T2WI shows zones of high signal at the three metastatic lesions. The anterior of the two lesions in the right cerebral hemisphere also has a central zone of low signal, probably secondary to intracellular methemoglobin versus less likely melanin deposition.

Fig. 1A.**47   AVM.   a** Sagittal T1WI shows a large AVM involving the right cerebral hemisphere containing multiple tortuous tubular flow voids (arrows).

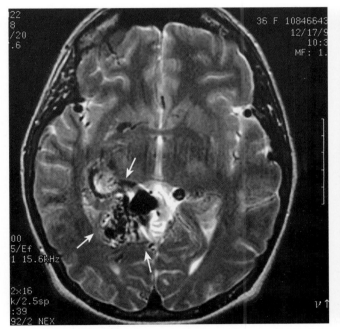

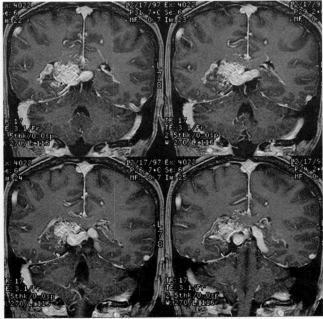

Fig. 1A.**47 b**   Axial T2WI also shows multiple tortuous tubular flow voids at the lesion (arrows).

Fig. 1A.**47 c**   Coronal (spoiled GRE) T1WI show prominent enhancement of arteries and veins at the AVM.

Table 1A.2 (Cont.) Supratentorial intra-axial mass lesions

Disease	MRI Findings	Comments
Cavernous hemangioma (Fig. 1A.48)	Single or multiple multilobulated intra-axial lesions that have a peripheral rim or irregular zone of low signal on T2WI secondary to hemosiderin, surrounding a central zone of variable signal (low, intermediate, high, or mixed) on T1WI and T2WI depending on ages of hemorrhagic portions. GRE techniques useful for detecting multiple lesions.	Supratentorial cavernous angiomas occur more frequently than infratentorial lesions. Can be found in many different locations; multiple lesions >50 %. Association with venous angiomas and risk of hemorrhage.
Venous angioma (Fig. 1A.49)	On postcontrast T1WI, venous angiomas are seen as a Gd-contrast-enhancing transcortical vein draining a collection of small medullary veins (caput Medusa). The draining vein can be seen as a signal void on T2WI.	Considered an anomalous venous formation typically not associated with hemorrhage. Usually an incidental finding except when associated with cavernous hemangioma.
Lipoma (Fig. 1A.50)	Lipomas have MR signal isointense to subcutaneous fat on T1WI (high signal) and on T2WI. Signal suppression occurs with frequency-selective fat suppression (FS) techniques or with a STIR method. Typically no Gd-contrast enhancement or peripheral edema. Lipomas can be nodular or curvilinear. Lipomas can occur in many locations, commonly: corpus callosum, cerebellopontine angle cistern, tectal plate.	Benign fatty lesions resulting from congenital malformation, often located in or near the midline. May contain calcifications and/or traversing blood vessels.
Neuroepithelial cyst (Fig. 1A.51)	Well-circumscribed cysts with low signal on T1WI and high signal on T2WI. Thin walls. No Gd-contrast enhancement or peripheral edema.	Cyst walls have histopathologic features similar to epithelium. Neuroepithelial cysts located in: choroid plexus, choroidal fissure, ventricles, brain parenchyma.

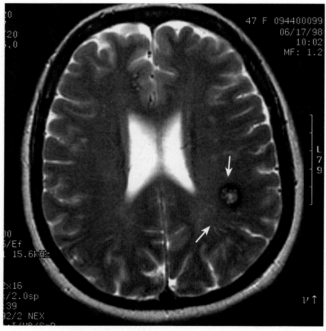

Fig. 1A.**48** **Cavernous hemangioma.** Axial T2WI shows a multilobulated intra-axial lesion in the left cerebral hemiphere that has a thin peripheral irregular zone of low signal secondary to hemosiderin, surrounding a central zone of high signal (arrows).

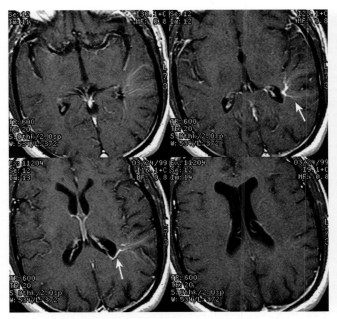

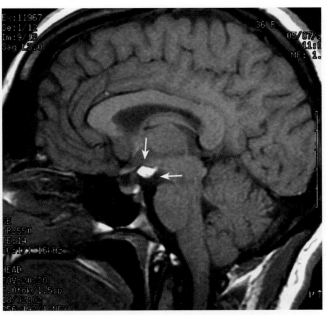

Fig. 1A.**49**   **Venous angioma.** Postcontrast axial T1WI shows enhancing veins draining a collection of small medullary veins (caput Medusa) adjacent to the atrium of the left lateral ventricle (arrows).

Fig. 1A.**50**   **Lipoma.** Sagittal T1WI shows a lipoma at the hypothalamus that has MR signal isointense to subcutaneous fat (arrows).

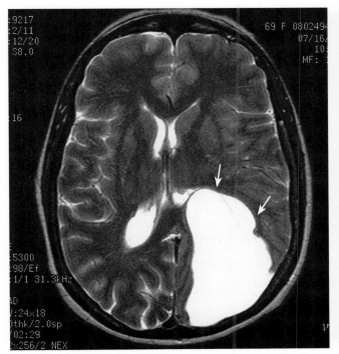

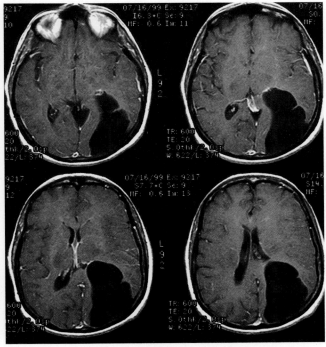

Fig. 1A.**51**   **Neuroepithelial cyst.   a** Axial T2WI shows a well-circumscribed cyst with high signal and thin walls (arrows).

Fig. 1A.**51 b**   Postcontrast axial T1WI shows no Gd-contrast enhancement or peripheral edema associated with the neuroepithelial cyst.

Table 1A.**2** (Cont.) Supratentorial intra-axial mass lesions

Disease	MRI Findings	Comments
Porencephalic cyst (Fig. 1A.52)	Irregular relatively well-circumscribed zone with low signal on T1WI and high signal on T2WI similar to CSF, surrounded by poorly defined thin zone of high T2 signal in adjacent brain tissue. No Gd-contrast enhancement or peripheral edema.	Represent remote sites of brain injury (trauma, infarct, infection, hemorrhage) with evolution into a cystic zone with CSF. MR signal characteristics surrounded by gliosis in adjacent brain parenchyma. Gliosis (high T2 signal) allows differentiation from schizencephaly.
Demyelinating disease– Multiple sclerosis (MS), acute disseminated encephalomyelitis (ADEM) (Figs.1A.53, 1A.54)	Lesions located in cerebral or cerebellar white matter, brainstem. Usually have low to intermediate signal on T1WI and high signal on T2WI. With or without Gd-contrast enhancement. Enhancement can be ring-like or nodular, usually in acute/early subacute phase of demyelination. Lesions rarely can have associated mass effect simulating neoplasms.	MS is the most common acquired demyelinating disease usually affecting women (peak age 20–40 years). Other demyelinating diseases include: ADEM–immune mediated demyelination after viral infection; toxins (exogenous from environmental exposure or ingestion–alcohol, solvents etc.–or endogenous from metabolic disorder–leukodystrophies, mitochondrial encephalopathies, etc.), radiation injury, trauma, vascular disease.

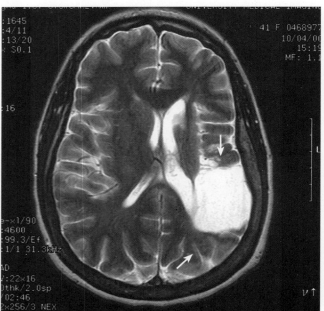

a

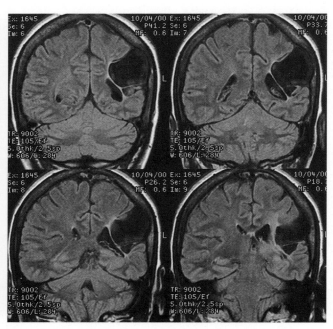

b

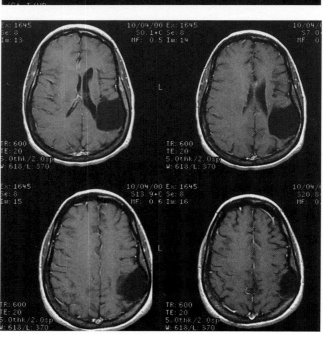

c

Fig. 1A.**52** **Porencephalic cyst.** **a** Axial T2WI shows an irregular, relatively well-circumscribed zone with high signal similar to CSF (arrows). **b** Coronal FLAIR images show the cystic zone to be surrounded by a poorly defined thin zone of high T2 signal in adjacent brain tissue. The cystic lesion is associated with chronic erosive changes of the adjacent skull. **c** Postcontrast axial T1WI shows no enhancement at the cystic lesion.

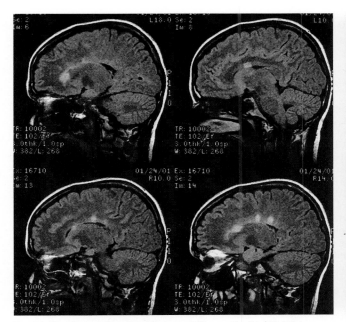

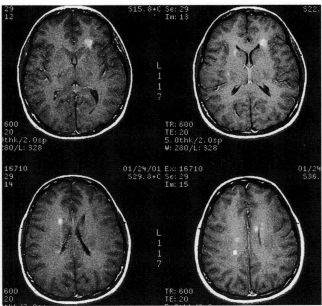

Fig. 1A.**53   Demyelinating disease–MS.   a** Sagittal FLAIR images show multiple foci of high signal in the periventricular white matter and corpus callosum.

Fig. 1A.**53 b**   Postcontrast axial T1WI shows enhancement associated with multiple lesions, indicating areas of active demyelination.

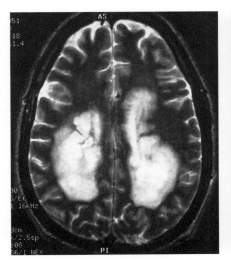

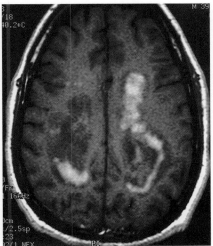

Fig. 1A.**54   Demyelinating disease-ADEM.   a** Axial T2WI shows poorly defined zones with high signal in the periventricular white matter bilaterally with mild mass effect.   **b** Postcontrast axial T1WI shows thick irregular zones of enhancement at sites of active demyelination.

a   **b**

Table 1A.**2** (Cont.) Supratentorial intra-axial mass lesions

Disease	MRI Findings	Comments
Cerebral infarct **(Fig.** 1A.**55)** **(Fig.** 1A.**102)**	MRI features of cerebral and cerebellar infarcts depend on age of infarct relative to time of examination: *<12 hours:* Localized edema, usually isointense signal to normal brain on T1WI and T2WI. Diffusion weighted images can show positive findings related to decreased apparent diffusion coefficients secondary to cytotoxic edema. Absence of arterial flow void or arterial enhancement in the vascular distribution of the infarct. *12–24 hours:* Intermediate signal on T1WI and high signal on T2WI. Localized edema. Signal abnormalities commonly involve the cerebral cortex and subcortical white matter and/or basal ganglia. *24 hours to 3 days:* Low to intermediate signal on T1WI and high signal on T2WI. Localized edema. Hemorrhage may be associated. With or without enhancement. *4 days to 2 weeks:* Low to intermediate signal on T1WI and high signal on T2WI. Edema/mass effect diminishing. Hemorrhage may be associated. With or without enhancement. *2 weeks to 2 months:* Low to intermediate signal on T1WI and high signal on T2WI. Edema resolves. Hemorrhage may be associated. Enhancement may eventually decline. *>2 months:* Low signal on T1WI and high signal on T2WI. Encephalomalacic changes. With or without calcification, hemosiderin.	Cerebral infarcts usually result from occlusive vascular disease involving large, medium, or small arteries. Vascular occlusion may be secondary to atheromatous arterial disease, cardiogenic emboli, neoplastic encasement, hypercoagulable states, dissection, or congenital anomalies. Cerebral infarcts usually result from arterial occlusion involving specific vascular territories; occasionally result from metabolic disorders (e.g., mitochondrial encephalopathies) or intracranial venous occlusion (e.g., thrombophlebitis, hypercoagulable states, dehydration) that do not correspond to arterial distributions.

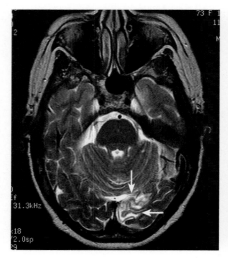

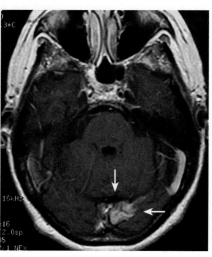

Fig. 1A.**55** **Enhancing cerebral infarct.** **a** Axial T2WI shows abnormal high signal involving the cerebral cortex and subcortical white matter in the medial left occipital lobe (arrows). **b** Postcontrast T1WI shows enhancement at the cerebral infarct (arrows).

a

b

Table 1A.**3** Supratentorial extra-axial mass lesions

Disease	MRI Findings	Comments
Neoplastic		
Meningioma (Fig. 1A.**56**)	Extra-axial, well-circumscribed, dural-based lesions. Locations in order of decreasing frequency: supratentorial, infratentorial, parasagittal, convexity, sphenoid ridge, parasellar, posterior fossa, optic nerve sheath, intraventricular. Intermediate signal on T1WI and intermediate to slightly high signal on T2WI. Usually prominent Gd-contrast enhancement. Calcifications may be associated.	Most common extra-axial tumor. Usually benign neoplasms, typically occurring in adults above 40 years of age, in women more commonly than men. Multiple meningiomas seen with neurofibromatosis type 2. Can result in compression of adjacent brain parenchyma, encasement of arteries, and compression of dural venous sinuses. Rarely invasive/malignant types.
Hemangiopericytoma (Fig. 1A.**57**)	Extra-axial mass lesions, often well-circumscribed. Intermediate signal on T1WI and intermediate to slightly high signal on T2WI; prominent Gd-contrast enhancement (may resemble meningiomas). With or without associated erosive bone changes.	Rare neoplasms in young adults (more common in males than females) sometimes referred to as angioblastic meningioma or meningeal hemangiopericytoma. Arise from vascular cells (pericytes). Frequency of metastases > meningiomas.

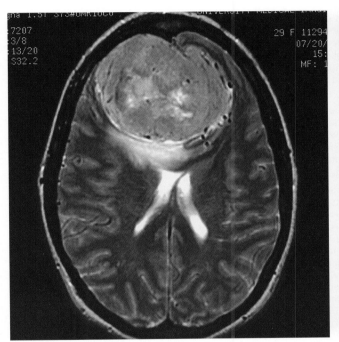
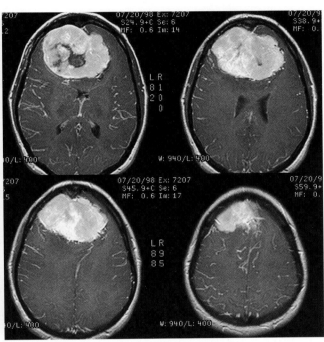

Fig. 1A.**56** **Meningioma.** **a** Axial T2WI shows a large, well-circumscribed, extra-axial dural-based lesion at the anterior falx with heterogeneous intermediate to slightly high signal that results in prominent compression of both frontal lobes.

Fig. 1A.**56 b** Postcontrast axial T1WI shows prominent, slightly heterogenous Gd-contrast enhancement at the meningioma.

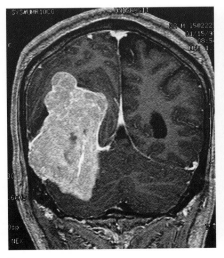
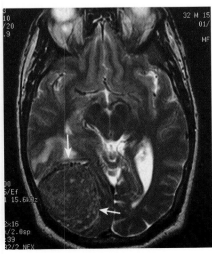

Fig. 1A.**57** **Hemangiopericytoma.** **a** Postcontrast coronal (spoiled GRE) T1WI shows a large, slightly lobulated, prominently enhancing extra-axial dural-based lesion at the tentorium that results in prominent compression of the right cerebral hemisphere superiorly and right cerebellar hemisphere inferiorly. **b** Axial T2WI shows the large extra-axial lesion to have heterogeneous intermediate signal (arrows).

a   b

Table 1A.**3** (Cont.) Supratentorial extra-axial mass lesions

Disease	MRI Findings	Comments
Metastatic tumor (Fig. 1A.**58**)	Single or multiple well-circumscribed or poorly defined lesions involving the skull, dura, leptomeninges, and/or choroid plexus. Low to intermediate signal on T1WI and intermediate to high signal on T2WI; usually Gd-contrast enhancement. Bone destruction and compression of neural tissue or vessels may be present. Leptomeningeal tumor often best seen on postcontrast images.	Metastatic tumor may have variable destructive or infiltrative changes involving single or multiple sites of involvement.
Neurocutaneous melanosis	Extra-axial or intra-axial lesions usually less than 3 cm in diameter with irregular margins in the leptomeninges or brain parenchyma/brainstem (anterior temporal lobes, cerebellum, thalami, inferior frontal lobes) with intermediate to slightly high signal on T1WI secondary to increased melanin. Gd-contrast enhancement. Vermian hypoplasia, arachnoid cysts, Dandy-Walker malformation may be associated.	Neuroectodermal dysplasia with proliferation of melanocytes in leptomeninges associated with large and/or numerous cutaneous nevi. May change into CNS melanoma.
Germinoma (Fig. 1A.**59**)	Circumscribed tumors. With or without disseminated disease. Pineal region, suprasellar region, third ventricle/basal ganglia. Low to intermediate signal on T1WI, occasionally high signal on T1WI; variable low, intermediate, high signal on T2WI. Gd-contrast enhancement of tumor and leptomeninges if disseminated.	Most common type of germ cell tumor; More common in males than females (10–30 years); usually midline neoplasms.
Teratoma (Fig. 1A.**60**)	Circumscribed lesions; pineal region, suprasellar region, third ventricle. Variable low, intermediate, and/or high signal on T1WI and T2WI; with or without Gd-contrast enhancement. May contain calcifications as well as fatty components that can cause a chemical meningitis if ruptured.	Second most common type of germ cell tumors. Occurs in children, males more than females. Benign or malignant types, composed of derivatives of ectoderm, mesoderm, and/or endoderm.
Pituitary adenoma (Fig. 1A.**61**)	*Microadenomas (<10 mm):* Commonly have intermediate signal on T1WI and T2WI. Cysts, hemorrhage, necrosis may be associated. Typically enhance less than normal pituitary tissue–often best seen with dynamic early phase imaging. *Macroadenomas (>10 mm):* Commonly have intermediate signal on T1WI and T2WI similar to gray matter. Necrosis, cyst, hemorrhage may be associated. Usually prominent enhancement. Extension into suprasellar cistern with waist at diaphragma sella, with or without extension into cavernous sinus. Occasionally invades skull base.	Common benign slow-growing tumors representing approximately 50% of sellar/parasellar neoplasms in adults. Can be associated with endocrine abnormalities related to oversecretion of hormones (prolactin, nonsecretory type, growth hormone, ACTH, and others). Prolactinomas: more common in females than males; growth hormone tumors: more common in males than females.

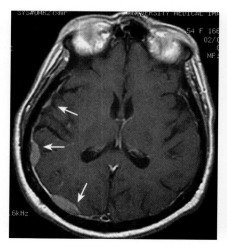

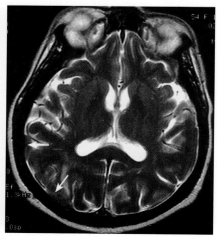

Fig. 1A.**58 Metastatic tumor. a** Postcontrast axial T1WI shows abnormal curvilinear dural enhancement on the right with two zones of nodular thickening representing metastatic breast carcinoma (arrows). **b** Axial T2WI shows the two zones of dural thickening have intermediate signal, which can also be seen with meningiomas (arrows).

a   b

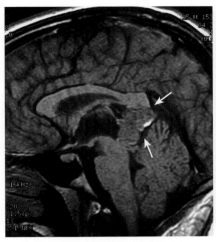

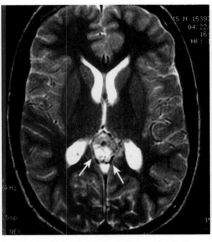

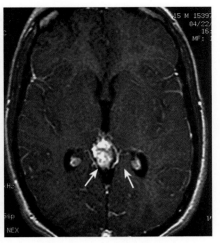

Fig. 1A.**59 Germinoma. a** Sagittal T1WI shows a circumscribed, slightly lobulated tumor with intermediate signal in the pineal recess (arrows).

Fig. 1A.**59 b** Axial T2WI shows the lesion to have heterogeneous, intermediate to high signal with a thin rim of low signal (arrows).

Fig. 1A.**59 c** Postcontrast axial T1WI shows prominent Gd-contrast enhancement of tumor (arrows).

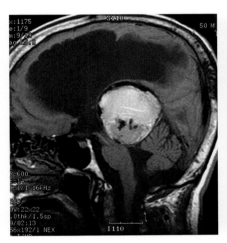

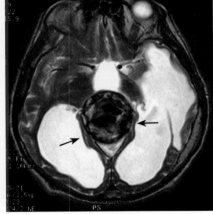

Fig. 1A.**60 Teratoma. a** Sagittal T1WI shows a large spheroid lesion with predominantly high signal as well as smaller zones of low and intermediate signal in the pineal recess and dorsal portion of the third ventricle. The lesion causes obstructive hydrocephalus, involving the third and lateral ventricles. **b** Axial T2WI shows the lesion to have mixed low, intermediate, and high signal (arrows).

a   b

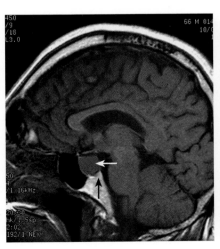

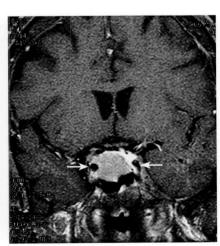

Fig. 1A.**61 Pituitary macroadenoma. a** Sagittal T1WI shows a pituitary macroadenoma with intermediate signal measuring 18 mm in height (arrows). **b** Postcontrast coronal T1WI shows prominent enhancement of the lesion, which extends upward into the suprasellar cistern (arrows).

a   b

Table 1A.3 (Cont.) Supratentorial extra-axial mass lesions

Disease	MRI Findings	Comments
Craniopharyngioma (Fig. 1A.62)	Circumscribed lobulated lesions; both suprasellar and intrasellar location, less commonly suprasellar or intrasellar only. Variable low, intermediate, and/or high signal on T1WI and T2WI. With or without nodular or rim Gd-contrast enhancement. May contain cysts, lipid components, and calcifications.	Usually histologically benign but locally aggressive lesions arising from squamous epithelial rests along Rathke's cleft. Occurs in children (10 years) and adults (above 40 years). Affects males and females equally.
Choroid plexus papilloma or carcinoma (Fig. 1A.63)	Circumscribed and/or lobulated lesions with papillary projections. Intermediate signal on T1WI and mixed intermediate to high signal on T2WI; usually prominent Gd-contrast enhancement. May contain calcifications. Locations: atrium of lateral ventricle (children) more common than fourth ventricle (adults), rarely other locations such as third ventricle. Associated with hydrocephalus.	Rare intracranial neoplasms. MR features of choroid plexus carcinoma and papilloma overlap. Both histologic types can disseminate along CSF pathways and invade brain tissue.
Lymphoma (Fig. 1A.64)	Single or multiple well-circumscribed or poorly defined lesions involving the skull, dura, and/or leptomeninges. Low to intermediate signal on T1WI and intermediate to high signal on T2WI, usually with Gd-contrast enhancement. Bone destruction may be present. Leptomeningeal tumor often best seen on postcontrast images.	Extra-axial lymphoma may have variable destructive or infiltrative changes involving single or multiple sites of involvement.
Myeloma/plasmacytoma (Fig. 1A.65)	Multiple (myeloma) or single (plasmacytoma) well-circumscribed or poorly defined lesions involving the skull and dura. Low to intermediate signal on T1WI and intermediate to high signal on T2WI, usually with Gd-contrast enhancement and with bone destruction.	Myeloma may have variable destructive or infiltrative changes involving the axial and/or appendicular skeleton
Chordoma (Fig. 1A.111)	Well-circumscribed lobulated lesions with low to intermediate signal on T1WI and high signal on T2WI; Gd-contrast enhancement (usually heterogeneous). Locally invasive associated with bone erosion/destruction, encasement of vessels and nerves. Skull base and clivus common location, usually in the midline.	Rare, slow-growing tumors. Detailed anatomic display of extension of chordomas by MRI is important for planning of surgical approaches.
Chondrosarcoma (Fig. 1A.112)	Lobulated lesions with low to intermediate signal on T1WI and high signal on T2WI. With or without matrix mineralization: low signal on T2WI. With Gd-contrast enhancement (usually heterogeneous). Locally invasive associated with bone erosion/destruction, encasement of vessels and nerves. Skull base and petro-occipital synchondrosis common location, usually off midline.	Rare, slow-growing tumors. Detailed anatomic display of extension of chondrosarcomas by MRI is important for planning of surgical approaches.

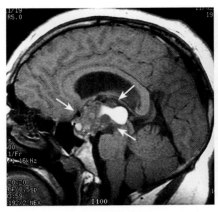 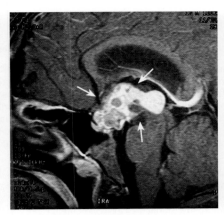 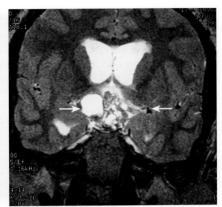

Fig. 1A.**62** **Craniopharyngioma. a** Sagittal T1WI shows a lobulated lesion with mixed low, intermediate, and high signal in the sella and suprasellar cistern with deformation of the third ventricle (arrows).

Fig. 1A.**62 b** Postcontrast sagittal T1WI shows enhancement in portions of the lesion (arrows).

Fig. 1A.**62 c** Coronal T2WI shows the lesion to have mixed low, intermediate, and high signal (arrows).

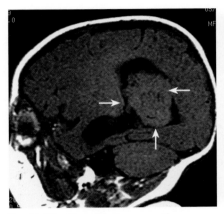 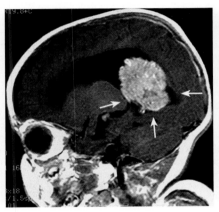 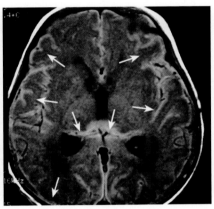

Fig. 1A.**63** **Choroid plexus papilloma. a** Sagittal T1WI shows a circumscribed, slightly lobulated lesion with intermediate signal located in the atrium of the right lateral ventricle (arrows). Hydrocephalus is also present.

Fig. 1A.**63 b** Postcontrast sagittal T1WI shows prominent Gd-contrast enhancement of the lesion (arrows).

Fig. 1A.**64** **Lymphoma.** Postcontrast axial T1WI shows extensive abnormal enhancement within the sulci (leptomeninges), Sylvian fissures, pineal recess, and dorsal third ventricle (arrows).

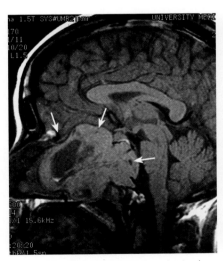 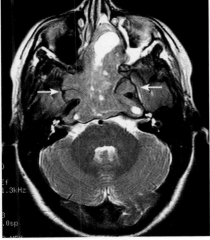 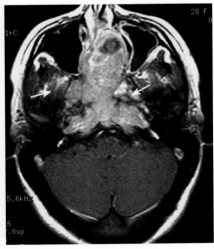

Fig. 1A.**65** **Plasmacytoma. a** Sagittal T1WI shows a large lesion with low and intermediate signal involving the nasal cavity, ethmoidal and sphenoidal sinuses, anterior and mid skull base. The lesion extends into the anterior cranial fossa, displacing the inferior portions of the frontal lobes (arrows).

Fig. 1A.**65 b** Axial T2WI shows the lesion to have mixed intermediate to high signal. The lesion encases portions of the carotid arteries (arrows).

Fig. 1A.**65 c** Postcontrast axial T1WI shows prominent enhancement of the lesion (arrows).

Table 1A.**3** (Cont.) Supratentorial extra-axial mass lesions

Disease	MRI Findings	Comments
Osteogenic sarcoma (Fig. 1A.**66**)	Destructive lesions involving the skull base. Low to intermediate signal on T1WI and mixed low, intermediate, high signal on T2WI. Usually with matrix mineralization/ossification: low signal on T2WI. With Gd-contrast enhancement (usually heterogeneous).	Rare lesions involving the endochondral bone-forming portions of the skull base. More common than chodrosarcomas and Ewing sarcoma. Locally invasive, high metastatic potential. Occurs in children as primary tumors and adults (associated with Paget disease, irradiated bone, chronic osteomyelitis, osteoblastoma, giant cell tumor, fibrous dysplasia).
Ewing sarcoma	Destructive lesions involving the skull base with low to intermediate signal on T1WI and mixed low, intermediate, high signal on T2WI. With or without matrix mineralization: low signal on T2WI, Gd-contrast enhancement (usually heterogeneous).	Usually occurs between the ages of 5 and 30, affects males more than females. Rare lesions involving the skull base. Locally invasive, high metastatic potential.
Sinonasal squamous cell carcinoma	Destructive lesions in the nasal cavity, paranasal sinuses, nasopharynx. With or without intracranial extension via bone destruction or perineural spread. Intermediate signal on T1WI and intermediate to slightly high signal on T2WI; mild Gd-contrast enhancement. Large lesions (necrosis and/or hemorrhage may be associated).	Occurs in adults, more common in males than females, usually above 55 years. Associated with occupational or other exposure to nickel, chromium, mustard gas, radium, manufacture of wood products.
Adenoid cystic carcinoma (Fig. 1A.**67**)	Destructive lesions in the paranasal sinuses, nasal cavity, nasopharynx. With or without intracranial extension via bone destruction or perineural spread. Intermediate signal on T1WI and intermediate to high signal on T2WI; variable mild, moderate, or prominent Gd-contrast enhancement.	Account for 10 % of sinonasal tumors. Arise in any location within sinonasal cavities, usually occurring in adults older than 30 years.
Esthesioneuroblastoma (Fig. 2B.**31**)	Locally destructive lesions with low to intermediate signal on T1WI and intermediate to high signal on T2WI, with prominent Gd-contrast enhancement. Location: superior nasal cavity, ethmoid air cells with occasional extension into the other paranasal sinuses, orbits, anterior cranial fossa, cavernous sinuses.	Tumors also referred to as olfactory neuroblastoma. Arise from olfactory epithelium in the superior nasal cavity. Occurs in adolescents and adults, more common in males than females.
Hemorrhagic		
Epidural hematoma (Fig. 1A.**68**)	Biconvex extra-axial hematoma located between the skull and dura. Displaced dura has low signal on T2WI. The signal of the hematoma itself depends on its age, size, hematocrit, and oxygen tension. With or without associated edema. High signal on T2WI involving the displaced brain parenchyma. Subfalcine, uncal herniation may be associated. *Hyperacute:* intermediate signal on T1WI, intermediate to high signal on T2WI. *Acute:* low to intermediate signal on T1WI, high signal on T2WI. *Subacute:* high signal on T1WI and low or high signal on T2WI.	Epidural hematomas usually result from trauma/tearing of an epidural artery (often the middle meningeal artery) or dural venous sinus. Epidural hematomas do not cross cranial sutures. With or without associated skull fracture.

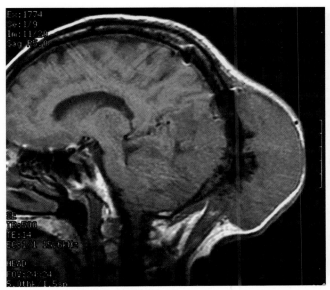 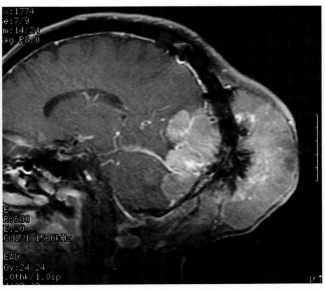

Fig. 1A.**66** **Osteogenic sarcoma.** **a** Sagittal T1WI shows a large destructive lesion involving the skull with intracranial and extracranial soft-tissue components. These have intermediate signal containing irregular zones of low signal, representing matrix mineralization/ossification.

Fig. 1A.**66 b** Postcontrast sagittal T1WI shows prominent enhancement at the soft-tissue portions of the lesion.

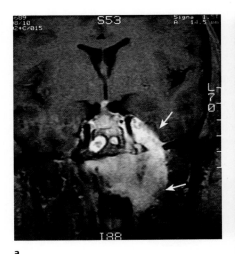 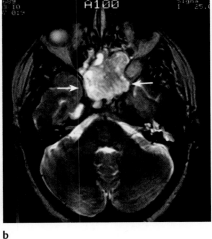

Fig. 1A.**67** **Adenoid cystic carcinoma.** **a** Postcontrast FS coronal T1WI shows an enhancing lesion in the nasopharynx extending superiorly through a widened left foramen ovale (perineural spread) into the left trigeminal cistern and medial left middle cranial fossa (arrows). **b** Axial T2WI shows that the lesion also extends into the sphenoidal and ethmoidal sinuses and has heterogeneous intermediate and high signal (arrows). A left middle ear effusion is also present.

a **b**

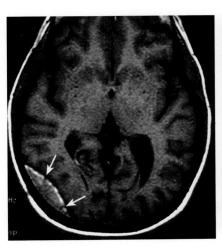 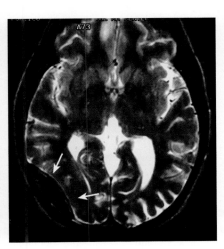

Fig. 1A.**68** **Subacute epidural hematoma.** **a** Axial T1WI biconvex extra-axial hematoma with intermediate to high signal located between the skull and dura in the right occipital region (arrows). **b** Axial T2WI shows the hematoma to have low signal (intracellular methemoglobin) (arrows). The displaced dura has low signal.

a **b**

Table 1A.3 (Cont.) Supratentorial extra-axial mass lesions

Disease	MRI Findings	Comments
Subdural hematoma (Figs. 1A.69–1A.71)	Crescentic extra-axial hematoma located in the potential space between the inner margin of the dura and outer margin of the arachnoid membrane. The signal of the hematoma depends on its age, size, hematocrit,and oxygen tension. With or without associated edema. High signal on T2WI involving the displaced brain parenchyma. Subfalcine, uncal herniation may be associated. *Hyperacute:* intermediate signal on T1WI, intermediate to high signal on T2WI. *Acute:* low to intermediate signal on T1WI, low signal on T2WI. *Subacute:* High signal on T1WI, low signal on T2WI (intracellular methemoglobin) with eventual progression to high signal on T2WI (extracellular methemoglobin). *Chronic:* Variable, often low to intermediate signal on T1WI, high signal on T2WI. With or without enhancement of collection and organizing neomembrane. Mixed MRI signal can result if rebleeding occurs into chronic collection.	Subdural hematomas usually result from trauma/stretching/tearing of cortical veins where they enter the subdural space to drain into dural venous sinuses. Subdural hematomas do cross sites of cranial sutures. Skull fracture may be associated.
Inflammatory		
Subdural/epidural abscess–Empyema (Fig. 1A.72)	Epidural or subdural collections with low signal on T1WI and high signal on T2WI; thin, linear peripheral zones of Gd-contrast enhancement.	Often results from complications related to sinusitis (usually frontal), meningitis, otitis media, ventricular shunts, or surgery. Can be associated with venous sinus thrombosis and venous cerebral or cerebellar infarcts, cerebritis, brain abscess. Mortality 30%.
Leptomeningeal infection/inflammation (Fig. 1A.73)	Single or multiple nodular enhancing lesions and/or focal or diffuse abnormal subarachnoid enhancement. Low to intermediate signal on T1WI, intermediate to high signal on T2WI. Leptomeningeal inflammation often best seen on postcontrast images.	Gd-DTPA enhancement in the intracranial subarachnoid space (leptomeninges) usually is associated with significant pathology (inflammation and/or infection versus neoplasm). Inflammation and/or infection of the leptomeninges can result from pyogenic, fungal, or parasitic diseases as well as tuberculosis. Neurosarcoidosis results in granulomatous disease in the leptomeninges, producing similar patterns of subarachnoid enhancement.

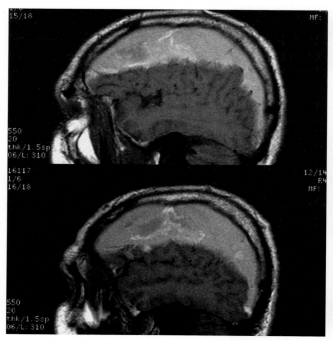

Fig. 1A.69 **Subacute subdural hematoma. a** Sagittal T1WI shows a subacute subdural hematoma with heterogeneous high signal.

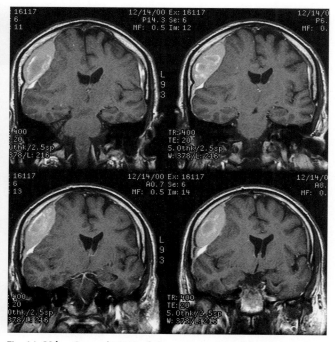

Fig. 1A.69 b Coronal T1WI of the same patient shows bilateral subacute subdural hematomas with prominent compression of the right cerebral hemisphere (midline shift/subfalcine herniation).

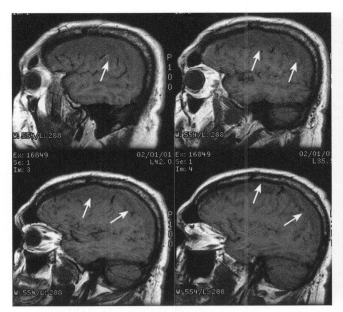

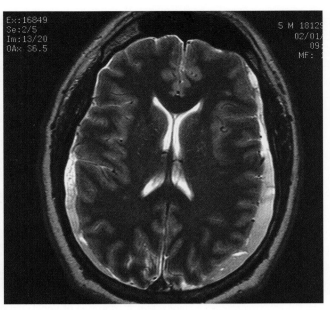

Fig. 1A.**70** **Early chronic subdural hematoma.** **a** Sagittal T1WI shows a subdural hematoma with heterogeneous low to intermediate signal (arrows).

Fig. 1A.**70 b** Axial T2WI shows bilateral subdural hematomas with mixed intermediate to high signal

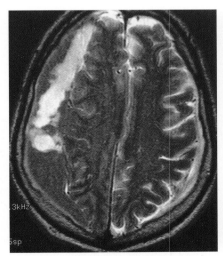

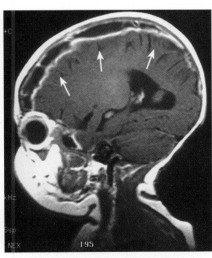

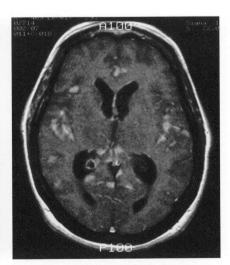

Fig. 1A.**71** **Subdural hematoma (mixed subacute and chronic).** Axial T2WI shows bilateral subdural hematomas with mixed low, intermediate, and high signal, indicating different temporal episodes of bleeding.

Fig. 1A.**72** **Subdural/epidural ebscess–empyema.** Postcontrast sagittal T1WI shows a subdural collection with low signal surrounded by thin irregular linear zones of Gd-contrast enhancement (arrows).

Fig. 1A.**73** **Neurosarcoidosis–lepto-meningeal inflammation.** Postcontrast axial T1WI shows multiple nodular enhancing lesions in the subarachnoid space (leptomeninges).

Table 1A.**3** (Cont.) Supratentorial extra-axial mass lesions

Disease	MRI Findings	Comments
Eosinophilic granuloma (Fig. 1A.74)	Single or mutiple circumscribed soft-tissue lesions in the marrow of the skull associated with focal bony destruction/erosion with extension extracranially, intracranially, or both. Lesions usually have low to intermediate signal on T1WI and mixed intermediate to slightly high signal on T2WI, with Gd-contrast enhancement. With or without enhancement of the adjacent dura.	*Single lesion:* Commonly seen in males more than females (below 20 years). Proliferation of histiocytes in medullary cavity with localized destruction of bone with extension into adjacent soft tissues. *Multiple lesions:* Associated with syndromes such as: Letterer-Siwe disease (lymphadenopathy hepatosplenomegaly), children below 2 years; Hand-Schüller-Christian disease (lymphadenopathy, exophthalmos, diabetes insipidus) children aged 5–10 years.
Other:		
Vascular		
Arterial aneurysm (Figs. 1A.75–1A.77)	*Saccular aneurysm:* Focal well-circumscribed zone of signal void on T1WI and T2WI; variable mixed signal if thrombosed. *Giant aneurysm:* Focal well-circumscribed structure with layers of low, intermediate, and high signal on T2WI secondary to layers of thrombus of different ages, as well as a zone of signal void representing a patent lumen if present. On T1WI, layers of intermediate and high signal can be seen as well as a zone of signal void. *Fusiform aneurysm:* elongated and ectatic arteries, variable intraluminal MR signal related to turbulent or slowed blood flow or partial/complete thrombosis. *Dissecting aneurysms:* The involved arterial wall is thickened and has intermediate to high signal on T1WI and T2WI; the signal void representing the patent lumen is narrowed.	Abnormal fusiform or focal dilatation of artery secondary to: acquired/degenerative etiology, polycystic disease, connective-tissue disease, atherosclerosis, trauma, infection (mycotic), AVM, vasculitis, and drugs. Focal aneurysms are also referred to as saccular aneurysms that typically occur at arterial bifurcations and are multiple in 20%. Saccular aneurysms greater than 2.5 cm in diameter are referred to as giant aneurysms. Fusiform aneurysms are often related to atherosclerosis or collagen vascular disease (e.g., Marfan syndrome, Ehlers-Danlos syndrome). Dissecting aneurysms: hemorrhage occurs in the arterial wall from incidental or significant trauma.
Dural AVMs (Fig. 1A.78)	Dural AVMs contain multiple tortuous tubular flow voids on T1WI and T2WI. The venous portions often show Gd-contrast enhancement. GRE MR images and MR angiography (MRA) using TOF or phase contrast techniques show flow signal in patent portions of the vascular malformation and areas of venous sinus occlusion or recanalization. Usually not associated with mass effect except in cases of recent hemorrhage or venous occlusion.	Dural AVMs are usually acquired lesions resulting from thrombosis or occlusion of an intracranial venous sinus with subsequent recanalization resulting in direct arterial to venous sinus communications. Location in order of decreasing frequency: transverse, sigmoid venous sinuses; cavernous sinus; straight, superior sagittal sinuses.

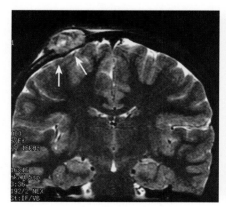

a

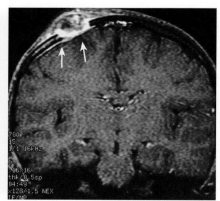

b

Fig. 1A.**74** **Eosinophilic granuloma.** **a** Coronal T2WI shows a soft-tissue lesion with mixed intermediate to high signal in the marrow of the skull, associated with focal bony destruction/erosion (arrows). **b** Postcontrast FS coronal T1WI shows heterogeneous enhancement of the lesion as well as enhancement of the adjacent dura (arrows).

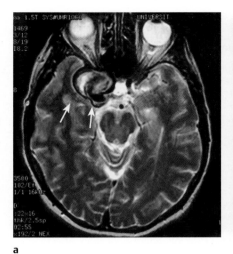

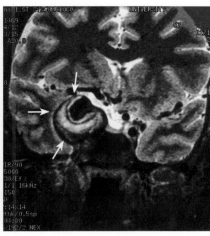

Fig. 1A.**75   Giant arterial aneurysm.   a** Axial T2WI shows a focal well-circumscribed structure involving the cavernous portion of the right internal carotid artery. It contains layers of low, intermediate, and high signal, as well a zone of signal void representing a patent channel (arrows).   **b** Coronal IR (FS) image also shows layers of low, intermediate, and high signal as well as a zone of signal void representing a patent channel (arrows).

a

b

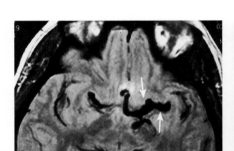

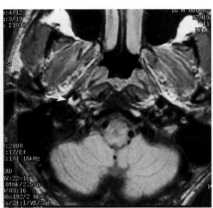

Fig. 1A.**76   Fusiform aneurysm.** Axial proton density weighted (long repetition time[TR]/short echo time[TE]) image shows an elongated and ectatic flow void involving the M1 segment of the left middle cerebral artery (arrows).

Fig. 1A.**77   Dissecting aneurysm.** Axial proton density weighted (long TR/short TE) image shows a crescentic zone of high signal (representing the intramural hematoma) at the petrous portion of the right internal carotid artery (arrow) with narrowing of the signal void of the artery.

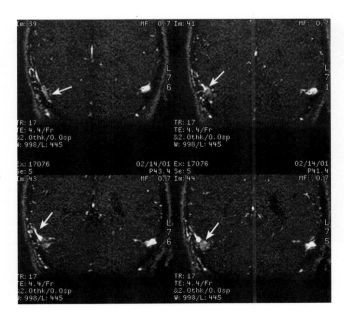

Fig. 1A.**78   Dural AVM.** Coronal GRE MRI shows flow signal in multiple small arteries adjacent to a partially occluded/recanalized right transverse sinus (arrows). Note normal flow signal and configuration of the left transverse venous sinus.

Table 1A.**3** (Cont.) Supratentorial extra-axial mass lesions

Disease	MRI Findings	Comments
Vein of Galen aneurysm (Fig. 1A.**79)**	Multiple tortuous tubular flow voids on T1WI and T2WI involving choroidal and thalamoperforate arteries, internal cerebral veins, vein of Galen (aneurysmal formation), straight and transverse venous sinuses, and other adjacent veins and arteries. The venous portions often show Gd-contrast enhancement. GRE MR images and MRA using TOF or phase contrast techniques show flow signal in patent portions of the vascular malformation.	Heterogeneous group of vascular malformations with arteriovenous shunts and dilated deep venous structures draining into and from an enlarged vein of Galen. Hydrocephalus, hemorrhage, macrocephaly, parenchymal vascular malformation components, and seizures may be associated. High-output congestive heart failure in neonates.
Non-neoplastic lesions		
Arachnoid cyst (Fig. 1A.**80)**	Well-circumscribed extra-axial lesions with low signal on T1WI and high signal on T2WI similar to CSF; no Gd-contrast enhancement. Common locations in order of frequency: anterior middle cranial fossa, suprasellar/quadrigeminal, frontal convexities, posterior cranial fossa.	Non-neoplastic congenital, developmental or acquired extra-axial lesions filled with CSF. Usually mild mass effect on adjacent brain. More often supratentorial than infratentorial location. Affects males more than females. With or without related clinical symptoms.
Rathke's cleft cyst (Fig. 1A.**81)**	Well-circumscribed lesion with variable low, intermediate, or high signal on T1WI and T2WI. On T1WI, two-thirds have high signal and one-third low signal; on T2WI, 50% have high signal, 25% low signal, and 25% intermediate signal. No Gd-contrast centrally, with or without thin peripheral enhancement. Lesion locations: 50% intrasellar, 25% suprasellar, 25% intrasellar and suprasellar.	Uncommon sellar/juxtasellar benign cystic lesion containing fluid with variable amounts of protein, mucopolysaccharide, and/or cholesterol; arise from epithelial rests of the craniopharyngeal duct.
Leptomeningeal cyst (Fig. 1A.**82)**	Well-circumscribed extra-axial lesions with low signal on T1WI and high signal on T2WI similar to CSF; no Gd-contrast enhancement. Associated with erosion of the adjacent skull.	Non-neoplastic extra-axial lesions filled with CSF thought to be secondary to trauma with dural tear/skull fracture. Usually mild mass effect on adjacent brain with progressive erosion of adjacent skull. Occasionally presents as a scalp lesion, more common in children than adults.
Pineal cyst (Fig. 1A.**83)**	Well-circumscribed extra-axial lesions with low signal on T1WI and high signal on T2WI similar to CSF. No central enhancement; thin linear peripheral Gd-contrast enhancement. Rarely atypical appearance with proteinaceous contents: intermediate, slightly high signal on T1WI.	Common, usually incidental non-neoplastic cyst in pineal gland.

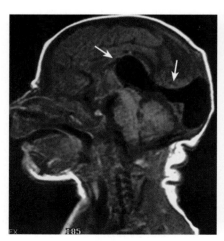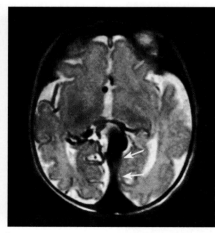

Fig. 1A.79 Vein of Galen aneursym. Sagittal T1WI (**a**) and axial T2WI (**b**) show multiple tortuous tubular flow voids representing arteriovenous shunting, as well as a markedly enlarged vein of Galen (aneurysmal formation) and straight venous sinus (arrows).

a   b

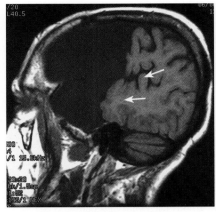

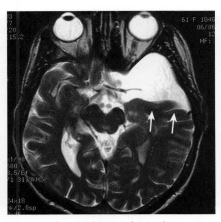

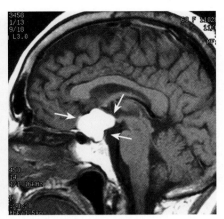

Fig. 1A.**80 Arachnoid cyst. a** Sagittal T1WI shows a well-circumscribed extra-axial lesion with low signal similar to CSF located at the anterior left middle and anterior cranial fossa. It displaces the left temporal and frontal lobes posteriorly (arrows).

Fig. 1A.**80 b** Axial T2WI shows the cyst to have high signal (arrows).

Fig. 1A.**81 Rathke's cleft cyst.** Sagittal T1WI shows a well-circumscribed lesion with high signal located within the sella and suprasellar cistern (arrows).

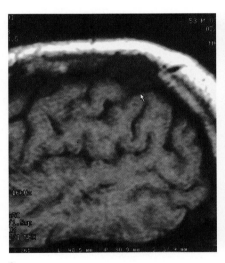

a

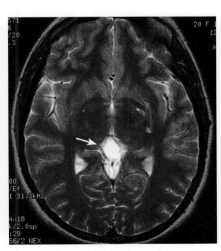

b

Fig. 1A.**82 Leptomeningeal cyst. a** Sagittal T1WI shows a well-circumscribed extra-axial lesion with low signal associated with erosion of the adjacent skull (arrow). **b** Axial T2WI shows the lesion to have high signal similar to CSF.

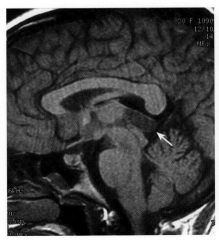

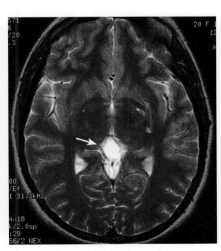

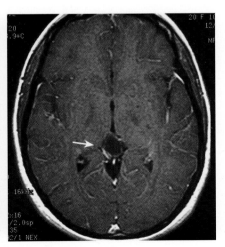

Fig. 1A.**83 Pineal cyst. a** Sagittal T1WI shows a well-circumscribed cyst with low signal in the pineal recess (arrow).

Fig. 1A.**83 b** Axial TWI shows the cyst to have high signal on T1WI similar to CSF (arrow).

Fig. 1A.**83 c** Postcontrast axial T1WI shows thin linear peripheral Gd-contrast enhancement but no central enhancement (arrow).

Table 1A.**3** (Cont.) Supratentorial extra-axial mass lesions

Disease	MRI Findings	Comments
Colloid cyst (Fig. 1A.**84**)	Well-circumscribed spheroid lesions located at the anterior portion of the third ventricle. Variable signal (low, intermediate, or high) on T1WI and T2WI, often high signal on T1WI and low signal on T2WI; no Gd-contrast enhancement.	Common presentation of headaches and intermittent hydrocephalus. Removal leads to cure.
Lipoma (Fig. 1A.**178**)	Lipomas have MR signal isointense to subcutaneous fat on T1WI and T2WI. Signal suppression occurs with frequency-selective FS techniques or with a STIR method. Typically no Gd-contrast enhancement or peripheral edema.	Benign fatty lesions resulting from congenital malformation, often located in or near the midline. May contain calcifications and/or traversing blood vessels.
Epidermoid (Fig. 1A.**85**)	Well-circumscribed, spheroid or multilobulated extra-axial ectodermal-inclusion cystic lesions with low to intermediate signal on T1WI and high signal on T2WI similar to CSF. Mixed low, intermediate, or high signal on FLAIR images; no Gd-contrast enhancement. Often insinuate along CSF pathways, chronic deformation of adjacent neural tissue (brainstem, brain parenchyma). Commonly located in posterior cranial fossa (cerebellopontine angle cistern), parasellar/middle cranial fossa.	Non-neoplastic, congenital or acquired extra-axial off-midline lesions filled with desquamated cells and keratinaceous debris. Usually mild mass effect on adjacent brain. Infratentorial locations more common than supratentorial locations. Affects male and female adults equally. With or without related clinical symptoms.
Dermoid (Fig. 1A.**86**)	Well-circumscribed, spheroid or multilobulated extra-axial lesions, usually with high signal on T1WI and variable low, intermediate, and/or high signal on T2WI. No Gd-contrast enhancement. Fluid-fluid or fluid-debris levels may be present. Can cause chemical meningitis if dermoid cyst ruptures into the subarachnoid space. Commonly located at or near midline; supratentorial more common than infratentorial.	Non-neoplastic, congenital or acquired ectodermal-inclusion cystic lesions filled with lipid material, cholesterol, desquamated cells, and keratinaceous debris. Usually mild mass effect on adjacent brain. Slightly more common in adult males than adult females. With or without related clinical symptoms.

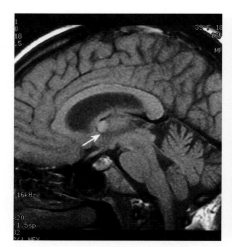

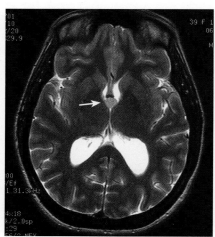

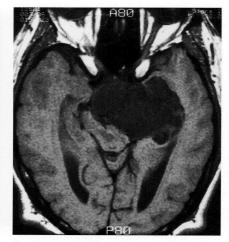

Fig. 1A.**84 Colloid cyst. a** Sagittal T1WI shows a well-circumscribed spheroid lesion (arrow) with slightly high signal located at the anterior portion of the third ventricle.

Fig. 1A.**84 b**   Axial T2WI shows the colloid cyst (arrow) to have intermediate signal.

Fig. 1A.**85 Epidermoid. a** Axial T1WI shows a multilobulated extra-axial lesion with low to intermediate signal. The lesion compresses the left side of the midbrain and medial left temporal lobe.

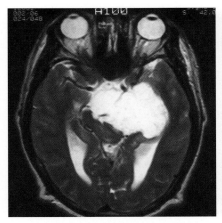

Fig. 1A.**85 b** Axial T2WI shows the lesion to have high signal. Note that there is no abnormal high signal in the compressed midbrain or left temporal lobe.

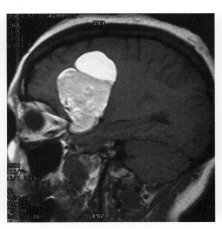

Fig. 1A.**86 Dermoid. a** Sagittal T1WI shows a well-circumscribed multilobulated extra-axial lesion with heterogeneous intermediate to high signal in the anterior left temporal/frontal region.

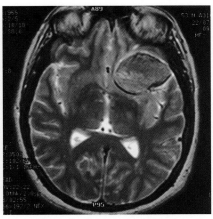

Fig. 1A.**86 b** Axial T2WI shows the lesion to have intermediate signal surrounded by a thin rim of low signal.

Table 1A.**4** Intra-axial lesions in the posterior cranial fossa (infratentorial)

Disease	MRI Findings	Comments
Congenital		
Chiari I malformation (Fig. 1A.11)	Cerebellar tonsils extend more than 5 mm below the foramen magnum in adults, 6 mm in children below 10 years. Syringohydromyelia in 20% to 40%. Hydrocephalus in 25%. Basilar impression in 25%. Less common association: Klippel-Feil, atlanto-occipital assimilation	Cerebellar tonsilar ectopia. Most common anomaly of CNS. Not associated with myelomeningocele.
Chiari II malformation (Arnold-Chiari) (Fig. 1A.12)	Small posterior cranial fossa with gaping foramen magnum through which there is an inferiorly positioned vermis associated with a cervicomedullary kink. Beaked dorsal margin of the tectal plate. Myelomeningoceles in nearly all patients. Hydrocephalus and syringomyelia common. Dilated lateral ventricles posteriorly (colpocephaly).	
Dandy-Walker malformation (Fig. IA.15)	Vermian aplasia or severe hypoplasia, communication of fourth ventricle with retrocerebellar cyst, enlarged posterior fossa, high position of tentorium and transverse venous sinuses. Hydrocephalus common. Associated with other anomalies such as dysgenesis of the corpus callosum, gray matter heterotopia, schizencephaly, holoprosencephaly, cephaloceles.	Abnormal formation of roof of fourth ventricle with absent or near incomplete formation of cerebellar vermis.
Dandy-Walker variant (Fig. 1A.16)	Mild vermian hypoplasia with communication of posteroinferior portion of the fourth ventricle with cisterna magna. No associated enlargement of the posterior cranial fossa.	Occasionally associated with hydrocephalus, dysgenesis of corpus callosum, gray matter heterotopia, other anomalies.
Lhermitte-Duclos disease (Fig. 1A.17)	Poorly defined zone of low T1 signal, high T2 signal with laminated appearance and localized mass effect located in the cerebellum. No enhancement.	Uncommon cerebellar dysplasia with gross thickening of cerebellar folia and disorganized cellular structure. Also known as dysplastic gangliocytoma.

Table 1A.4 (Cont.) Intra-axial lesions in the posterior cranial fossa (infratentorial)

Disease	MRI Findings	Comments
Neoplastic: **Intra-axial lesions** **Astrocytoma** **(Fig. 1A.87, 1A.88)**	*Low-grade astrocytoma:* Focal or diffuse mass lesion usually located in cerebellar white matter or brainstem with low to intermediate signal on T1WI and high signal on T2WI. With or without mild Gd-contrast enhancement. Minimal associated mass effect. *Juvenile pilocytic astrocytoma:* Subtype: Solid/cystic focal lesion with low to intermediate signal on T1WI and high signal on T2WI, usually with prominent Gd-contrast enhancement. Lesions located in cerebellum, brainstem. *Gliomatosis cerebri:* Infiltrative lesion with poorly defined margins with mass effect locate in the white matter, with low to intermediate signal on T1WI. High signal on T2WI; usually no Gd-contrast enhancement until late in disease. *Anaplastic astrocytoma:* Often irregularly marginated lesion located in white matter with low to intermediate signal on T1WI and high signal on T2WI. With or without Gd-contrast enhancement.	*Low-grade astrocytoma:* Often occur in children and adults (20–40 years). Tumors comprised of well-differentiated astrocytes. Association with neurofibromatosis type 1. Ten-year survival. May become malignant. *Juvenile pilocytic astrocytoma:* Subtype: common in children, usually favorable prognosis if totally resected. *Gliomatosis cerebri:* Diffusely infiltrating astrocytoma with relative preservation of underlying brain architecture. Imaging appearance may be more prognostic than histologic grade. Approximate 2-year survival. *Anaplastic astrocytoma:* Intermediate between low-grade astrocytoma and glioblastoma multiforme. Approximate 2-year survival.
Medulloblastoma **(primitive neuroec-** **todermal tumor of the** **cerebellum)** **(Fig. 1A.89)**	Circumscribed or invasive lesions with low to intermediate signal on T1WI and intermediate to high signal on T2WI; variable Gd-contrast enhancement. Frequent dissemination into the leptomeninges.	Highly malignant tumors that frequently disseminate along CSF pathways.

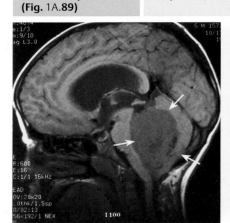

a

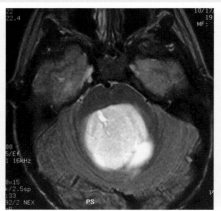

b

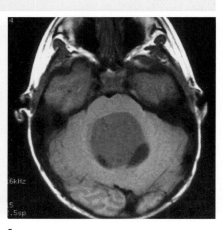

c

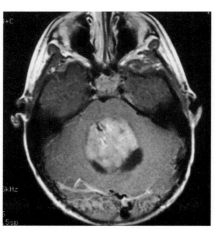

d

Fig. 1A.87 **Low-grade astrocytoma.** **a** Sagittal T1WI shows a mass lesion with low and intermediate signal filling the fourth ventricle (arrows). **b** Axial T2WI shows the lesion to have heterogeneous high signal with peripheral small cystic zones. **c** Axial T1WI shows the lesion to have predominantly intermediate signal with small peripheal zones of low signal fluid. **d** Postcontrast axial T1WI shows prominent heterogeneous enhancement of the solid portion of the lesion.

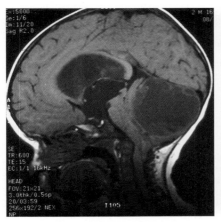

a

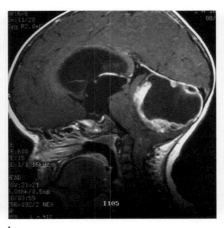

b

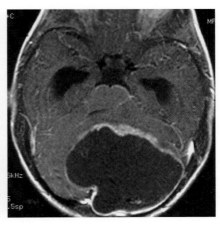

c

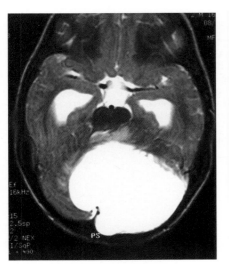

d

Fig. 1A.88 Juvenile pilocytic astrocytoma. a Sagittal T1WI shows a mixed cystic and solid lesion with low and intermediate signal involving the cerebellum, resulting in obstrucive hydrocephalus and downward displacement of the cerebellar tonsils through the foramen magnum. **b** Postcontrast sagittal T1WI shows enhancement at the periphery of the cystic lesion. **c** Postcontrast axial T1WI shows peripheral enhancement of the lesion as well as compression of the fourth ventricle and dilatation of the temporal horns of the lateral ventricles. **d** Axial T2WI shows high signal at the large cystic component of the lesion.

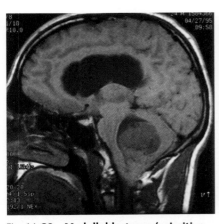

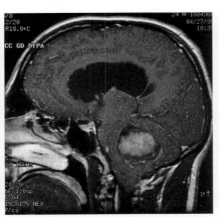

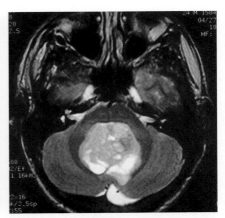

Fig. 1A.89 Medulloblastoma (primitive neuroectodermal tumor of the cerebellum). a Sagittal T1WI shows a lesion with intermediate and low signal involving the cerebellar vermis extending into the fourth ventricle, resulting in obstructive hydrocephalus and downward displacement of the cerebellar tonsils through the foramen magnum.

Fig. 1A.89 b Postcontrast sagittal T1WI shows prominent heterogeneous enhancement of the lesion.

Fig. 1A.89 c Axial T2WI shows the lesion to have heterogeneous high signal.

Table 1A.**4** (Cont.) Intra-axial lesions in the posterior cranial fossa (infratentorial)

Disease	MRI Findings	Comments
Ependymoma (Fig. 1A.90)	Circumscribed spheroid or lobulated infratentorial lesion, usually in the fourth ventricle. Cysts and/or calcifications may be present. Low to intermediate signal on T1WI and intermediate to high signal on T2WI; variable Gd-contrast enhancement. With or without extension through the foramina of Luschka and Magendie.	Occurs more commonly in children than adults; two-thirds infratentorial, one-third supratentorial.
Rhabdoid tumors (Fig. 1A.91)	Circumscribed mass lesions with intermediate signal on T1WI, with or without zones of high signal from hemorrhage on T1WI; variable mixed low, intermediate, and/or high signal on T2WI. Usually prominent Gd-contrast enhancement with or without heterogeneous pattern.	Rare malignant tumors involving the CNS, usually occurring in the first decade. Histologically appear as solid tumors with or without necrotic areas, similar to malignant rhabdoid tumors of the kidney. Associated with a poor prognosis.
Metastases (Fig. 1A.92)	Circumscribed spheroid lesions in brain that can have various intra-axial locations, often at gray-white matter junctions. Usually low to intermediate signal on T1WI and intermediate to high signal on T2WI. Hemorrhage, calcifications, cysts may be associated. Variable Gd-contrast enhancement. Often high signal on T2WI peripheral to nodular enhancing lesion representing axonal edema.	Represent approximately 33% of intracranial tumors, usually from extracranial primary neoplasm in adults above 40 years. Primary tumor source in order of decreasing frequency: lung, breast, GI, GU, melanoma. Metastatic lesions in the cerebellum can present with obstructive hydrocephalus/neurosurgical emergency.
Lymphoma (Fig. 1A.93) (Fig. 1A.64) (Fig. 1A.33)	Primary CNS lymphoma: focal or infiltrating lesion located in the basal ganglia, posterior fossa/brainstem. Low to intermediate signal on T1WI and intermediate to slightly high signal on T2WI. Hemorrhage/necrosis may be associated in immunocompromised patients. Usually Gd-contrast enhancement. Diffuse leptomeningeal enhancement is another pattern of intracranial lymphoma.	Primary CNS lymphoma more common than secondary, usually in adults above 40 years. B cell lymphoma more common than T cell lymphoma. Increasing incidence related to number of immunocompromised patients in population. MR imaging features of primary and secondary lymphoma of brain overlap. Intracranial lymphoma can involve the leptomeninges in secondary lymphoma more commonly than primary lymphoma.

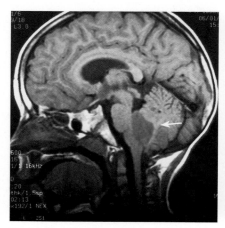

Fig. 1A.**90 Ependymoma. a** Sagittal T1WI shows a circumscribed spheroid lesion with low to intermediate signal in the fourth ventricle (arrow).

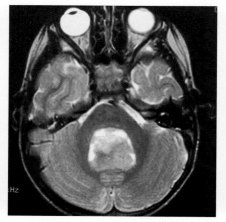

Fig. 1A.**90 b** Axial T2WI shows the lesion to have heterogeneous intermediate and high signal.

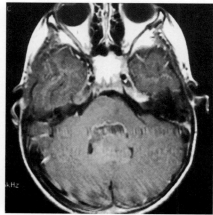

Fig. 1A.**90 c** Postcontrast axial T1WI shows the lesion to have mild heterogeneous enhancement.

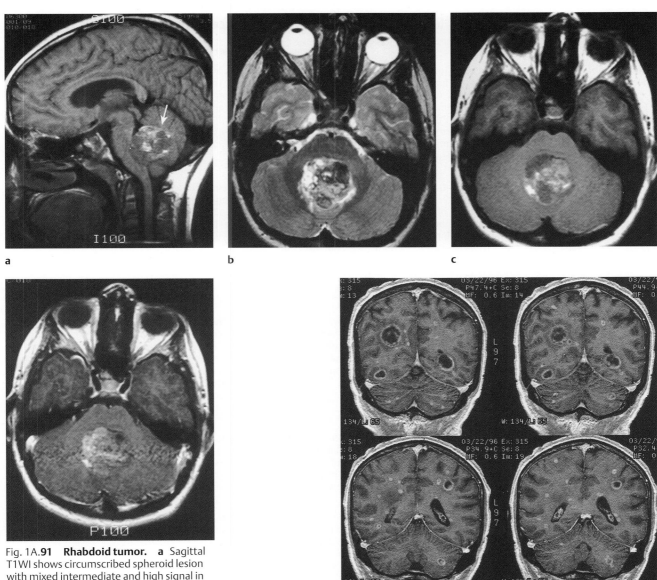

Fig. 1A.**91 Rhabdoid tumor. a** Sagittal T1WI shows circumscribed spheroid lesion with mixed intermediate and high signal in the fourth ventricle (arrow). **b** Axial T2WI shows the lesion to have mixed low, intermediate, and high signal. **c** Axial T1WI shows zones of intermediate and high signal in the lesion filling the fourth ventricle. **d** Post-contrast axial T1WI shows varying degrees of enhancement in portions of the lesion.

Fig. 1A.**92 Metastases.** Postcontrast coronal (spoiled GRE) T1WI show multiple enhancing metastatic lesions in the cerebrum and cerebellum from lung carcinoma.

Fig. 1A.**93 Lymphoma. a** Axial T2WI shows a poorly defined zone of high signal in the inferior left cerebellar hemisphere with mild associated localized mass effect. **b** Postcontrast axial T1WI shows two nodular foci of enhancement in the left cerebellar hemisphere.

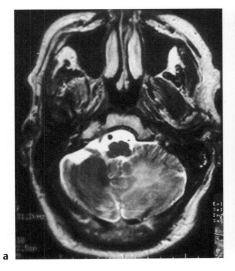

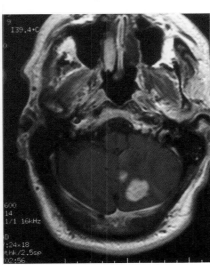

Table 1A.**4** (Cont.) Intra-axial lesions in the posterior cranial fossa (infratentorial)

Disease	MRI Findings	Comments
Hemangioblastoma (Fig. 1A.**94**)	Circumscribed tumors usually located in the cerebellum and/or brainstem. Small Gd-contrast-enhancing nodule with or without cyst, or larger lesion with prominent heterogeneous enhancement with or without flow voids within lesion or at the periphery. Intermediate signal on T1WI and intermediate to high signal on T2WI. Occasionally lesions have evidence of recent or remote hemorrhage.	Occurs in adolescents, young and middle-aged adults. Lesions are typically multiple in patients with von Hippel-Lindau disease.
Neurocutaneous melanosis	Extra-axial or intra-axial lesions usually less than 3 cm in diameter with irregular margins in the leptomeninges or brain parenchyma/brainstem (anterior temporal lobes, cerebellum, thalami, inferior frontal lobes). Intermediate to slightly high signal on T1WI secondary to increased melanin. Gd-contrast enhancement. Vermian hypoplasia, arachnoid cysts, Dandy-Walker malformation may be associated.	Rare neuroectodermal dysplasia with proliferation of melanocytes in leptomeninges associated with large and/or numerous cutaneous nevi. May change into CNS melanoma.
Inflammatory lesions		
Cerebellitis	Poorly defined zone or focal area of low to intermediate signal on T1WI, intermediate to high signal on T2WI; minimal or no Gd-contrast enhancement. Involves cerebellar cortex and white matter. Edema may result in hydrocephalus from compression of fourth ventricle.	Focal infection/inflammation of brain tissue from bacteria or fungi, secondary to sinusitis, meningitis, surgery, hematogenous source (cardiac and other vascular shunts), and/or immunocompromised status. Can progress to abscess formation. Childhood illnesses (Coxsackievirus, rubeola, typhoid fever, polio virus, pertussis, diphtheria, varicella zoster, Epstein-Barr) can cause acute cerebellitis.
Pyogenic brain abscess (Fig. 1A.**36**)	Circumscribed lesion with low signal on T1WI; central zone of high signal on T2WI (air-fluid level may be present) surrounded by a thin rim of low T2 signal; peripheral poorly defined zone of high signal on T2WI representing edema; ring-like Gd-contrast enhancement.	Formation of brain abscess occurs 2 weeks after cerebritis with liquefaction and necrosis centrally surrounded by a capsule and peripheral edema. Can be multiple. Complication from meningitis and/or sinusitis, septicemia, trauma, surgery, caridac shunt.
Fungal brain abscess (Fig. 1A.**37**)	Vary depending on organism. Lesions occur in meninges and brain parenchyma, solid or cystic with low to intermediate signal on T2WI and high signal on T2WI. Nodular or ring-enhancement, peripheral high signal in brain lesions on T2WI (edema).	Occur in immunocompromised or diabetic patients with resultant granulomas in meninges and brain parenchyma.
Encephalitis (Fig. 1A.**95**) (Fig. 1A.**38**)	Poorly defined zone(s) of low to intermediate signal on T1WI and intermediate to high signal on T2WI; minimal or no Gd-contrast enhancement. Involves cerebellar cortex and/or white matter. Minimal localized mass effect.	Encephalitis: infection/inflammation of brain tissue from viruses, often in immuncompromised patients (Herpes simplex, CMV, HIV, progressive multifocal leukoencephalopathy) or immunocompetent (St Louis encephalitis, Eastern or Western equine encephalitis, Epstein-Barr virus).
Tuberculoma (Fig. 1A.**96**)	*Intra-axial lesions in the cerebellum (children):* Low to intermediate signal on T1WI, central zone of high signal on T2WI with a thin peripheral rim of low signal, occasionally low signal on T2WI; solid or rim Gd-contrast enhancement. Calcification may be associated. *Meningeal lesions:* nodular or cystic zones of basilar meningeal enhancement.	Occurs in immunocompromised patients and in developing countries. Caseating intracranial granulomas via hematogenous dissemination. Lesions more common in meninges than brain.

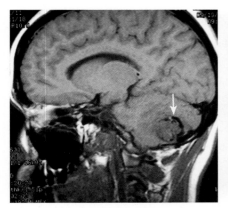

Fig. 1A.**94** **Hemangioblastoma. a** Sagittal T1WI shows a circumscribed lesion in the cerebellum with intermediate signal with peripheral tubular flow voids (arrow).

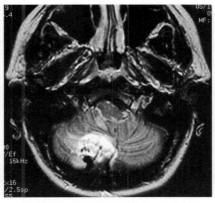

Fig. 1A.**94 b**   Axial T2WI shows a mass lesion in the right cerebellar hemisphere that has heterogeneous, predominantly high signal with peripheral flow voids.

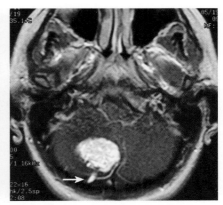

Fig. 1A.**94 c**   Postcontrast axial T1WI shows prominent enhancement of the lesion as well as a prominent vein dorsal to the tumor (arrow).

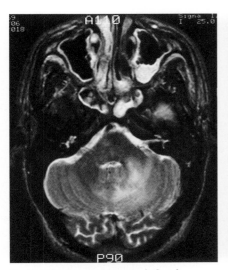

Fig. 1A.**95**   **Progressive multifocal leukoencephalopathy/encephalitis.   a** Axial T2WI shows a poorly defined zone of high signal in the left cerebellar hemisphere and left middle cerebellar peduncle.

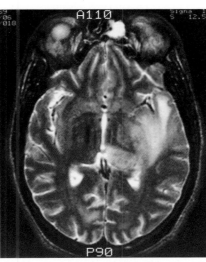

Fig. 1A.**95 b**   Axial T2WI shows a poorly defined zone of high signal in the subcortical white matter of the left temporal lobe.

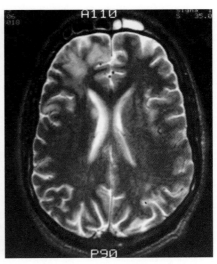

Fig. 1A.**95 c**   Axial T2WI also shows poorly defined zone of high signal in the subcortical white matter of the right frontal lobe.

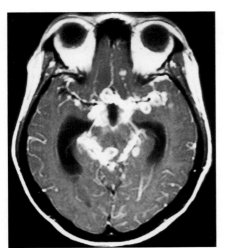

Fig. 1A.**96**   **Tuberculoma.** Postcontrast axial T1WI shows a ring-enhancing lesion in the midbrain as well as multiple ring-enhancing lesions in the basal subarachnoid space/cisterns and sylvian fissures.

Table 1A.**4** (Cont.) Intra-axial lesions in the posterior cranial fossa (infratentorial)

Disease	MRI Findings	Comments
Parasitic brain lesions		
Toxoplasmosis (Fig. 1A.**40**)	Single or multiple solid and/or cystic lesions in cerebellum. Low to intermediate signal on T1WI and high signal on T2WI; nodular or rim pattern of Gd-contrast enhancement, with or without peripheral high T2 signal (edema).	Most common opportunistic CNS infection in AIDS patients, caused by ingestion of food contaminated with parasites (*Toxoplasma gondii*).
Cysticercosis (Fig. 1A.**41**)	Single or multiple cystic lesions in brain or meninges. *Acute/subacute phase:* Low to intermediate signal on T1WI and high signal on T2WI; rim and possible nodular pattern of Gd-contrast enhancement, with or without peripheral high T2 signal (edema). *Chronic phase:* calcified granulomas.	Caused by ingestion of ova (*Taenia solium*) in contaminated food (undercooked pork). Involves in order of decreasing frequency: meninges, brain parenchyma, ventricles.
Hydatid cyst	*Echinococcus granulosus:* Single or rarely multiple cystic lesions with low signal on T1WI and high signal on T2WI with a thin wall with low signal on T2WI. Typically no Gd-contrast enhancement or peripheral edema unless superinfected. Often located in vascular territory of the middle cerebral artery. *Echinococcus multilocularis:* Cystic (possibly multilocular) and/or solid lesions. Central zone of low to intermediate signal on T1WI and T2WI, surrounded by a slightly thickened rim of low signal on T2WI; Gd-contrast enhancement. Peripheral zone of high signal on T2WI (edema) and calcifications are common.	Caused by parasites, *Echinococcus granulosus* (South America, Middle East Australia, New Zealand) or *Echinococcus multilocularis* (North America, Europe, Turkey, China). CNS involvement in 2% of cases of hydatid infestation.
Radiation injury/ necrosis (Fig. 1A.**97**) (Fig. 1A.**42**)	Focal lesion with or without mass effect, or poorly defined zone of low to intermediate signal on T1WI, intermediate to high signal on T2WI. With or without Gd-contrast enhancement involving tissue (gray matter and/or white matter) in field of treatment.	Usually occurs from 4–6 months to 10 years after radiation treatment. May be difficult to distinguish from neoplasm. PET and MRS might be helpful for evaluation.
Hemorrhage		
Cerebellar hemorrhage (Fig. 1A.**98**)	The signal of the hematoma depends on its age, size, location, hematocrit, hemoglobin oxidation state, clot retraction, and extent of edema. *Hyperacute phase (4–6 hours):* intermediate signal on T1WI, slightly high signal on T2WI. *Acute phase (12–48 hours):* Intermediate signal on T1WI, low signal on T2WI; surrounded by a peripheral zone of high T2 signal (edema). *Subacute phase (>2 days):* When methemoglobin is initially intracellular: the hematoma has high signal on T1WI, progressing from peripheral to central, and low signal on T2WI, surrounded by a zone of high T2 signal (edema). When methemoglobin eventually becomes primarily extracellular: the hematoma has high signal on T1WI and T2WI. *Chronic phase:* Hematoma progresses from a lesion with high signal on T1WI and T2WI with a peripheral rim of low signal on T2WI (hemosiderin) to predominant hemosiderin composition and low signal on T2WI.	Can result from trauma, ruptured aneurysms or vascular malformations, coagulopathy, hypertension, adverse drug reaction, amyloid angiopathy, hemorrhagic transformation of cerebral infarct, metastases, abscesses, viral infections (herpes simplex, CMV)
Cerebellar contusions (Fig. 1A.**45**)	The MR appearance of contusions is initially one of focal hemorrhage involving the cerebellar cortex and subcortical white matter. The MR signal of the contusion depends on its age and presence of oxyhemoglobin, deoxyhemoglobin, methemoglobin, hemosiderin, etc. Contusions eventually appear as focal superficial encephalomalacic zones with high signal on T2WI, with or without small zones of low signal on T2WI from hemosiderin.	Contusions are superficial brain injuries involving the cerebellar cortex and subcortical white matter that result from skull fracture and/or acceleration/deceleration trauma to the inner table of the skull.
Metastases (Fig. 1A.**46**)	The MR appearance of a hemorrhagic metastatic lesion is one of an intracerebral hematoma involving a portion or all of the neoplasm. Usually associated with peripheral edema (high signal on T2WI), often multiple.	Metastatic intra-axial tumors associated with hemorrhage include bronchogenic carcinoma, renal cell carcinoma, melanoma, choriocarcinoma, and thyroid carcinoma. May be difficult to distinguish from hemorrhage related to other etiologies.

Table 1A.**4** (Cont.) Intra-axial lesions in the posterior cranial fossa (infratentorial)

Disease	MRI Findings	Comments
Vascular		
Arterial aneurysm (Fig. 1A.99)	*Saccular aneurysm:* Focal well-circumscribed zone of signal void on T1WI and T2WI. Variable mixed signal if thrombosed. *Giant aneurysm:* Focal well-circumscribed structure with layers of low, intermediate, and high signal on T2WI secondary to layers of thrombus of different ages, as well as a zone of signal void representing a patent lumen if present. On T1WI, layers of intermediate and high signal can be seen as well as a zone of signal void. *Fusiform aneurysm:* Elongated and ectatic arteries. Variable intraluminal MR signal related to turbulent or slowed blood flow or partial/complete thrombosis. *Dissecting aneurysms:* The involved arterial wall is thickened and has intermediate to high signal on T1WI and T2WI; the signal void representing the patent lumen is narrowed.	Abnormal fusiform or focal dilatation of artery secondary to: acquired/degenerative etiology, polycystic disease, connective-tissue disease, atherosclerosis, trauma, infection (mycotic), AVM, vasculitis, and drugs.

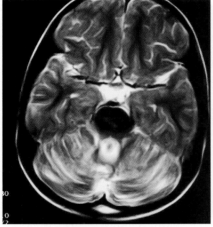 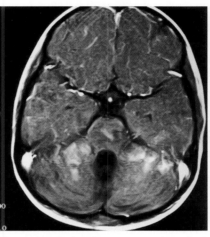 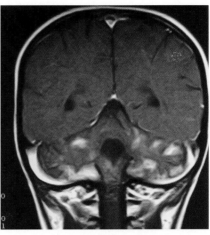

a, b   c

Fig. 1A.**97** **Radiation injury/necrosis. a** Axial T2WI shows poorly defined zones of high signal involving both cerebellar hemispheres and pons with encephalomalacia in the field of radiotherapy.

The patient had undergone resection of a medulloblastoma 7 months earlier. Postcontrast axial (**a**) and coronal (**b**) T1WI show multiple poorly defined zones of enhancement in the cerebellum and pons.

Subsequent MRI showed resolution of the enhancement and progression of encephalomalacia, as well as PET scan findings consistent with radiation necrosis.

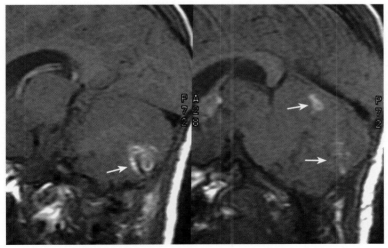 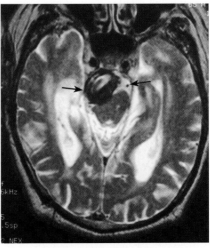

Fig. 1A.**98** **Cerebellar hemorrhage.** Sagittal T1WI shows areas of high signal (arrows) representing methemoglobin from subacute cerebellar hemorrhage, resulting from a vascular malformation.

Fig. 1A.**99** **Giant arterial aneurysm.** Axial T2WI shows a giant aneurysm (arrows) with layers of low, intermediate, and high signal compressing the anterior margin of the right cerebral peduncle.

Table 1A.**4** (Cont.) Intra-axial lesions in the posterior cranial fossa (infratentorial)

Disease	MRI Findings	Comments
AVM (Fig. IA.47)	Lesions with irregular margins that can be located in the brain parenchyma-pia, dura, or both locations. AVMs contain multiple tortuous tubular flow voids on T1WI and T2WI secondary to patent arteries with high blood flow; as well as thrombosed vessels with variable signal, areas of hemorrhage in various phases, calcifications, and gliosis. The venous portions often show Gd-contrast enhancement. GRE MRI shows flow-related enhancement (high signal) in patent arteries and veins of the AVM. MRA using TOF or phase contrast techniques can provide additional detailed information about the nidus, feeding arteries and draining veins, and presence of associated aneurysms. Usually not associated with mass effect except in cases of recent hemorrhage or venous occlusion.	Infratentorial AVMs are much less common than supratentorial AVMs.
Cavernous hemangioma (Fig. 1A.100)	Single or multiple multilobulated intra-axial lesions that have a peripheral rim or irregular zone of low signal on T2WI secondary to hemosiderin, surrounding a central zone of variable signal (low, intermediate, high, or mixed) on T1WI and T2WI depending on ages of hemorrhagic portions. GRE techniques useful for detecting multiple lesions.	Infratentorial lesions are less common than supratentorial. Can be found in many different locations; multiple lesions >50%. Association with venous angiomas and risk of hemorrhage.
Venous angioma (Fig. 1A.101)	On postcontrast T1WI, venous angiomas are seen as a Gd-contrast-enhancing transcortical vein draining a collection of small medullary veins (caput Medusa). The draining vein can be seen as a signal void on T2WI.	Considered an anomalous venous formation typically not associated with hemorrhage. Usually an incidental finding except when associated with cavernous hemangioma.
Lipoma (Fig. 1A.50)	Lipomas have MR signal isointense to subcutaneous fat on T1WI and T2WI. Signal suppression occurs with frequency-selective FS techniques or with a STIR method. Typically no Gd-contrast enhancement or peripheral edema. Lipomas can be nodular or curvilinear. Common locations in the posterior cranial fossa include cerebellopontine angle cisterns and tectal plate.	Benign fatty lesions resulting from congenital malformation, often located in or near the midline, may contain calcifications and/or traversing blood vessels.
Acute demyelinating disease–MS, ADEM (Fig. 1A.53 (Fig. 1A.54)	Lesions located in cerebellar white matter, brainstem. Usually have low to intermediate signal on T1WI and high signal on T2WI, with or without Gd-contrast enhancement. Gd-contrast enhancement can be ring-like or nodular, usually in acute/early subacute phase of demyelination. Lesions rarely can have associated mass effect simulating neoplasms.	Other demyelinating diseases can result from toxins (exogenous from environmental exposure or ingestion–alcohol, solvents etc. or endogenous from metabolic disorder–leukodystrophies, mitochondrial encephalopathies, etc.), radiation injury, trauma, vascular disease.
Cerebellar infarct (Fig. 1A.102)	MRI features of cerebellar infarcts depend on age of infarct relative to time of examination. *<12 hours:* Localized edema, usually isointense signal to normal brain on T1WI and T2WI. Diffusion weighted images can show positive findings related to decreased apparent diffusion coefficients secondary to cytotoxic edema, absence of arterial flow void or arterial enhancement in the vascular distribution of the infarct. *12–24 hours:* Intermediate signal on T1WI and high signal on T2WI. Localized edema. Signal abnormalities commonly involve the cerebral cortex and subcortical white matter and/or basal ganglia. *24 hours to 3 days:* Low to intermediate signal on T1WI, high signal on T2WI. Localized edema. Hemorrhage may be associated. With or without enhancement. *4 days to 2 weeks:* Low to intermediate signal on T1WI and high signal on T2WI. Edema/mass effect diminishing. Hemorrhage may be associated. With or without enhancement. *2 weeks to 2 months:* Low to intermediate signal on T1WI and high signal on T2WI. Edema resolves. Hemorrhage may be associated. Enhancement may eventually decline. *> 2 months:* Low signal on T1WI and high signal on T2WI. Encephalomalacic changes. Calcification, hemosiderin may be present.	Cerebellar infarcts usually result from occlusive vascular disease involving branches from the basilar artery (PICA, AICA). Vascular occlusion may be secondary to atheromatous arterial disease, cardiogenic emboli, neoplastic encasement, hypercoagulable states, dissection, or congenital anomalies. Cerebellar infarcts usually result from arterial occlusion involving specific vascular territories; occasionally result from metabolic disorders (e.g., mitochondrial encephalopathies) or intracranial venous occlusion (e.g., thrombophlebitis, hypercoagulable states, dehydration) that do not correspond to arterial distributions.

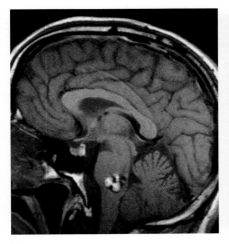
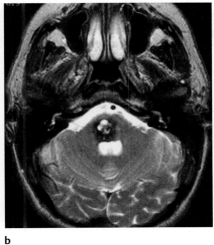

Fig. 1A.**100** **Cavernous hemangioma.** **a** Sagittal T1WI shows a multi-lobulated lesion in the pons with mixed low and high signal. **b** Axial T2WI shows the hemangioma to have a peripheral rim or irregular zone of low signal surrounding an irregular central zone of high signal.

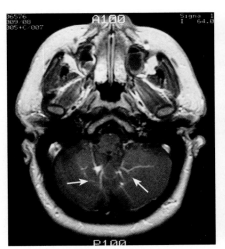
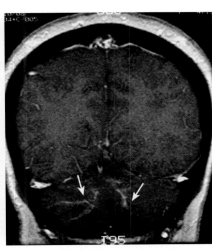

Fig. 1A.**101** **Venous angioma.** Postcontrast axial (**a**) and coronal (**b**) T1WI show venous angiomas in the medial portions of both cerebellar hemispheres where Gd-contrast-enhancing veins drain collections of small medullary veins (caput Medusa) (arrows).

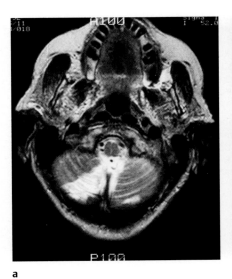
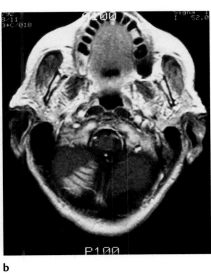

Fig. 1A.**102** **Subacute enhancing cerebellar infarct.** **a** Axial T2WI shows a wedge-shaped zone of high signal at the inferomedial portion of the right cerebellar hemisphere. **b** Postcontrast axial T1WI shows enhancement of the infarct in the vascular distribution of the posterior inferior cerebellar artery.

Table 1A.**4** (Cont.) Intra-axial lesions in the posterior cranial fossa (infratentorial)

Disease	MRI Findings	Comments
Wallerian degeneration	Corticospinal tract involvement from infarct or injury at motor cortex or posterior limb of internal capsule can result in: linear zone of high signal on T2WI in ipsilateral corticospinal tract of brainstem (high signal on T2WI 5–12 weeks after injury results from edema, >12 weeks secondary to gliosis). With or without associated atrophy in brainstem at ipsilateral corticospinal tract. Extensive unilateral cerebral cortical atrophy can result in atrophy of the contralateral middle cerebellar peduncle and cerebellum from interruption of the corticopontocerebellar pathway (which connects the cerebral cortex to the contralateral middle cerbellar peduncle via pontine nuclei).	Refers to pathologic changes (degeneration, myelin degradation, atrophy) in axons secondary to injuries involving the cell bodies of neurons (e.g., hemorrhage, cerebral infarct, contusion, surgery).

Table 1A.**5** (Cont.) Extra-axial lesions in the posterior cranial fossa (infratentorial)

Disease	MRI Findings	Comments
Neoplastic		
Metastatic tumor (Figs. 1A.103, 1A.104)	Single or multiple well-circumscribed or poorly defined lesions involving the skull, dura, leptomeninges, and/or choroid plexus. Low to intermediate signal on T1WI and intermediate to high signal on T2WI; usually Gd-contrast enhancement. Bone destruction, compression of neural tissue or vessels may be associated. Leptomeningeal tumor often best seen on postcontrast images.	Metastatic tumor may have variable destructive or infiltrative changes involving single or multiple sites of involvement.
Schwannoma (neurinoma)–Acoustic, trigeminal, etc. (Figs.1A.105, 1A.106)	Circumscribed or lobulated extra-axial lesions. Low to intermediate signal on T1WI and high signal on T2WI; prominent Gd-contrast enhancement. High signal on T2WI and Gd-contrast enhancement can be heterogeneous in large lesions.	Acoustic (vestibular nerve) schwannoma account for 90% of intracranial schwannomas and represent 75% of lesions in the cerebellopontine angle cisterns. Trigeminal schwannomas are the next most common intracranial schwannomas, followed by facial nerve schwannomas. Multiple schwannomas seen with neurofibromatosis type 2.
Meningioma (Fig. 1A.107)	Extra-axial, well-circumscribed, dural-based lesions. Supratentorial location more common than infratentorial. Intermediate signal on T1WI and intermediate to slightly high signal on T2WI; usually prominent Gd-contrast enhancement. Calcifications may be associated.	Most common extra-axial tumor, usually benign neoplasms. Typically occurs in adults (above 40 years of age), more common in females than males. Multiple meningiomas seen with neurofibromatosis type 2, can result in compression of adjacent brain parenchyma, encasement of arteries, and compression of dural venous sinuses. Rarely invasive/malignant types.
Hemangiopericytoma (Fig. 1A.108)	Extra-axial mass lesions, often well-circumscribed. Intermediate signal on T1WI and intermediate to slightly high signal on T2WI; prominent Gd-contrast enhancement (may resemble meningiomas). With or without associated erosive bone changes.	Rare neoplasms in young adults (more common in males than females), sometimes referred to as angioblastic meningioma or meningeal hemangiopericytoma. Arise from vascular cells (pericytes). Frequency of metastases > meningiomas.

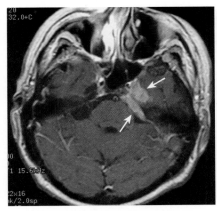

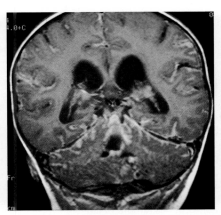

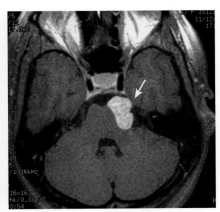

Fig. 1A.**103 Metastatic tumor, dural based.** Postcontrast axial T1WI shows abnormal dural enhancement along the left petrous apex and within the left trigeminal cistern (arrows), representing metastatic disease from breast carcinoma.

Fig. 1A.**104 Disseminated medulloblastoma in the leptomeninges.** Postcontrast coronal T1WI shows diffuse abnormal enhancement within the cerebellar sulci as well as in supratentorial sulci representing disseminated tumor.

Fig. 1A.**105 Trigeminal schwannoma/ neuroma.** Postcontrast axial T1WI shows an enhancing mass lesion involving the left trigeminal nerve as it exits the pons (arrow).

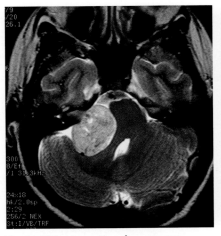

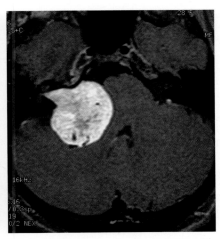

Fig. 1A.**106 Acoustic schwannoma (neurinoma). a** Axial T2WI shows a large mass lesion with heterogenous, slightly high signal in the right cerebellopontine angle cistern extending into the right internal auditory canal.

Fig. 1A.**106 b** Postcontrast axial T1WI with fat suppression shows prominent enhancement of the lesion.

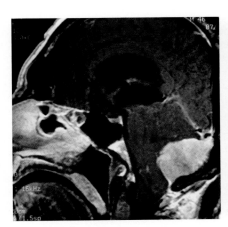

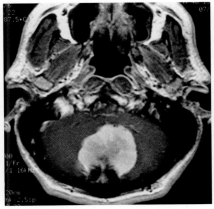

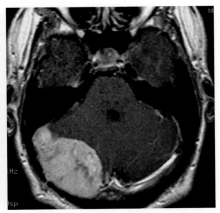

Fig. 1A.**107 Meningioma. a** Postcontrast sagittal T1WI shows a prominantly enhancing extra-axial lesion at the dorsal inferior aspect of the posterior cranial fossa. The lesion results in inferior displacement of the cerebellar tonsils below the foramen magnum. In addition, there is compression of the fourth ventricle.

Fig. 1A.**107 b** Postcontrast axial T1WI shows the enhancing lesion to be centered near the midline.

Fig. 1A.**108 Hemangiopericytoma.** Postcontrast T1WI shows a prominently enhancing extra-axial mass lesion at the dorsal right posterior cranial fossa.

Table 1A.5 (Cont.) Extra-axial lesions in the posterior cranial fossa (infratentorial)

Disease	MRI Findings	Comments
Paraganglioma–Glomus jugulare (Fig. 1A.109)	Extra-axial mass lesions located in jugular foramen, often well-circumscribed. Intermediate signal on T1WI, often heterogeneous intermediate to slightly high signal on T2WI. With or without flow voids. Prominent Gd-contrast enhancement. Often associated erosive bone changes and expansion of jugular foramen.	Lesions, also referred to as chemodectomas, arise from paraganglia in multiple sites in the body and are named accordingly (e.g., glomus jugulare, tympanicum, vagale).
Choroid plexus papilloma or carcinoma (Fig. 1A.63)	Circumscribed and/or lobulated lesions with papillary projections. Intermediate signal on T1WI and mixed intermediate to high signal on T2WI; usually prominent Gd-contrast enhancement. Calcificationsmay be associated. Locations: atrium of lateral ventricle (children) more common than fourth ventricle (adults), rarely other locations such as third ventricle. Associated with hydrocephalus.	Rare intracranial neoplasms. MR features of choroid plexus carcinoma and papilloma overlap. Both histologic types can disseminate along CSF pathways and invade brain tissue.
Lymphoma (Fig. 1A.110)	Single or multiple well-circumscribed or poorly defined lesions involving the skull, dura, and/or leptomeninges. Low to intermediate signal on T1WI and intermediate to high signal on T2WI, usually with Gd-contrast enhancement. Bone destruction may be present. Leptomeningeal tumor often best seen on postcontrast images.	Extra-axial lymphoma may have variable destructive or infiltrative changes involving single or multiple sites of involvement.
Neurocutaneous melanosis	Extra-axial or intra-axial lesions usually less than 3 cm in diameter with irregular margins in the leptomeninges or brain parenchyma/brainstem (anterior temporal lobes, cerebellum, thalami, inferior frontal lobes) with intermediate to slightly high signal on T1WI secondary to increased melanin. Gd-contrast enhancement. Vermian hypoplasia, arachnoid cysts, Dandy-Walker malformation may be associated.	Neuroectodermal dysplasia with proliferation of melanocytes in leptomeninges associated with large and/or numerous cutaneous nevi. May change into CNS melanoma.
Myeloma/plasmacytoma (Fig. 2B.25) (Fig. 1A.65)	Multiple (myeloma) or single (plasmacytoma) well-circumscribed or poorly defined lesions involving the skull and dura. Low to intermediate signal on T1WI and intermediate to high signal on T2WI, usually with Gd-contrast enhancement and with bone destruction.	Myeloma may have variable destructive or infiltrative changes involving the axial and/or appendicular skeleton.
Chordoma (Fig. 1A.111)	Well-circumscribed lobulated lesions with low to intermediate signal on T1WI and high signal on T2WI; Gd-contrast enhancement (usually heterogeneous). Locally invasive associated with bone erosion/destruction, encasement of vessels and nerves. Skull base and clivus common location, usually in the midline.	Rare, slow-growing tumors. Detailed anatomic display of extension of chondrosarcomas by MRI is important for planning of surgical approaches.
Chondrosarcoma (Fig. 1A.112)	Lobulated lesions with low to intermediate signal on T1WI and high signal on T2WI. With or without matrix mineralization: low signal on T2WI. With Gd-contrast enhancement (usually heterogeneous). Locally invasive associated with bone erosion/destruction, encasement of vessels and nerves. Skull base and petro-occipital synchondrosis common location, usually of midline.	Rare, slow-growing tumors. Detailed anatomic display of extension of chondrosarcomas by MRI is important for planning of surgical approaches.
Osteogenic sarcoma (Fig. 2B.29)	Destructive lesions involving the skull base. Low to intermediate signal on T1WI and mixed low, intermediate, high signal on T2WI. Usually with matrix mineralization/ossification: low signal on T2WI. With Gd-contrast enhancement (usually heterogeneous).	Rare lesions involving the endochondral bone-forming portions of the skull base. More common than chodrosarcomas and Ewing sarcoma. Locally invasive, high metastatic potential. Occurs in children as primary tumors and adults (associated with Paget disease, irradiated bone, chronic osteomyelitis, osteoblastoma, giant cell tumor, fibrous dysplasia).
Ewing sarcoma	Destructive lesions involving the skull base with low to intermediate signal on T1WI and mixed low, intermediate, high signal on T2WI. With or without matrix mineralization: low signal on T2WI. With Gd-contrast enhancement (usually heterogeneous).	Usually occurs between the ages of 5 and 30, affects males more than females. Rare lesions involving the skull base. Locally invasive, high metastatic potential.

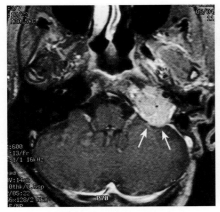

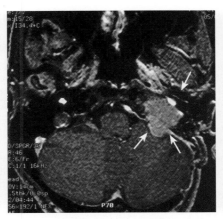

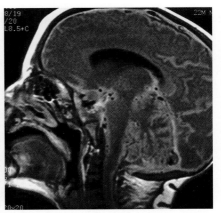

Fig. 1A.**109** **Paraganglioma–glomus jugulare.** **a** Postcontrast axial (FS) T1WI shows an enhancing well-circumscribed lesion located in left jugular foramen (arrows).

Fig. 1A.**109 b** Postcontrast axial (spoiled GRE) T1WI shows the enhancing lesion (straight arrows) located in the left jugular foramen dorsal to the left internal carotid artery (curved arrow).

Fig. 1A.**110** **Lymphoma.** Postcontrast sagittal T1WI shows diffuse abnormal enhancement in the cerebral and cerebellar sulci (intracranial leptomeninges) and basilar cisterns from disseminated lymphoma.

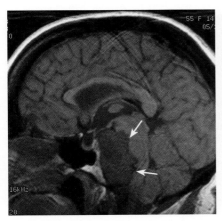

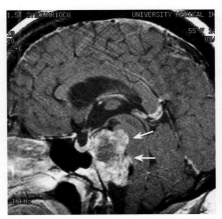

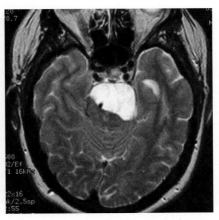

Fig. 1A.**111** **Chordoma.** **a** Sagittal T1WI shows a well-circumscribed lobulated lesion (arrows) with low to intermediate signal located along the endocranial surface of the clivus, resulting in displacement and deformation of the brainstem.

Fig. 1A.**111 b** Postcontrast sagittal T1WI shows heterogeneous Gd-contrast enhancement of the lesion (arrows).

Fig. 1A.**111 c** Axial T2WI shows the lesion to have high signal.

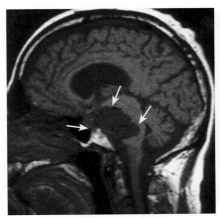

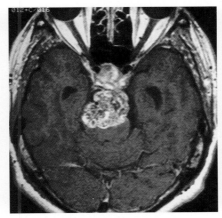

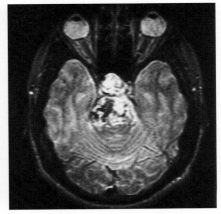

Fig. 1A.**112** **Chondrosarcoma.** **a** Sagittal T1WI shows a well-circumscribed lobulated lesion (arrows) with low to intermediate signal located along the endocranial surface of the clivus, resulting in displacement and deformation of the brainstem. The lesion is associated with bone erosion/destruction of the upper clivus with tumor extension into the sella.

Fig. 1A.**112 b** Postcontrast axial T1WI shows heterogeneous Gd-contrast enhancement of the lesion.

Fig. 1A.**112 c** Axial T2WI shows the lesion to have predominantly high signal, with small zones of low signal representing foci of matrix mineralization.

Table 1A.**5** (Cont.) Extra-axial lesions in the posterior cranial fossa (infratentorial)

Disease	MRI Findings	Comments
Sinonasal squamous cell carcinoma	Destructive lesions in the nasal cavity, paranasal sinuses, nasopharynx. With or without intracranial extension via bone destruction or perineural spread. Intermediate signal on T1WI and intermediate to slightly high signal on T2WI; mild Gd-contrast enhancement. Large lesions (necrosis and/or hemorrhage may be associated).	Occurs in adults, more common in males than females, usually above 55 years. Associated with occupational or other exposure to nickel, chromium, mustard gas, radium, manufacture of wood products.
Adenoid cystic carcinoma (Fig. 1A.**67)**	Destructive lesions in the paranasal sinuses, nasal cavity, nasopharynx. With or without intracranial extension via bone destruction or perineural spread. Intermediate signal on T1WI and intermediate to high signal on T2WI; variable mild, moderate, or prominent Gd-contrast enhancement.	Account for 10 % of sinonasal tumors. Arise in any location within sinonasal cavities, usually occurring in adults older than 30 years.
Non-neoplastic lesions		
Arachnoid cyst (Fig. 1A.**113)**	Well-circumscribed extra-axial lesions with low signal on T1WI and high signal on T2WI similar to CSF; no Gd-contrast enhancement. Common locations in order of frequency: anterior middle cranial fossa, suprasellar/quadrigeminal, frontal convexities, posterior cranial fossa.	Non-neoplastic congenital, developmental or acquired extra-axial lesions filled with CSF. Usually mild mass effect on adjacent brain. More often supratentorial than infratentorial location. More common in males than females. With or without related clinical symptoms.
Lipoma (Fig. 1A.**178)**	Lipomas have MR signal isointense to subcutaneous fat on T1WI and T2WI. Signal suppression occurs with frequency-selective FS techniques or with a STIR method. Typically no Gd-contrast enhancement or peripheral edema.	Benign fatty lesions resulting from congenital malformation, often located in or near the midline. May contain calcifications and/or traversing blood vessels.
Epidermoid (Fig. 1A.**114)**	Well-circumscribed, spheroid or multilobulated extra-axial ectodermal-inclusion cystic lesions with low to intermediate signal on T1WI and high signal on T2WI similar to CSF. Mixed low, intermediate, or high signal on FLAIR images; no Gd-contrast enhancement. Often insinuate along CSF pathways, chronic deformation of adjacent neural tissue (brainstem, brain parenchyma). Commonly located in posterior cranial fossa (cerebellopontine angle cistern), parasellar/middle cranial fossa.	Non-neoplastic, congenital or acquired extra-axial off-midline lesions filled with desquamated cells and keratinaceous debris. Usually mild mass effect on adjacent brain. Infratentorial locations more common than supratentorial locations. Affects male and female adults equally. With or without related clinical symptoms.
Dermoid (Fig. 1A.**86)**	Well-circumscribed, spheroid or multilobulated extra-axial lesions, usually with high signal on T1WI and variable low, intermediate, and/or high signal on T2WI. No Gd-contrast enhancement. Fluid-fluid or fluid-debris levels may be present. Can cause chemical meningitis if dermoid cyst ruptures into the subarachnoid space. Commonly located at or near midline; supratentorial more common than infratentorial.	Non-neoplastic, congenital or acquired ectodermal-inclusion cystic lesions filled with lipid material, cholesterol, desquamated cells and keratinaceous debris. Usually mild mass effect on adjacent brain. Slightly more common in adult males than adult females. With or without related clinical symptoms.

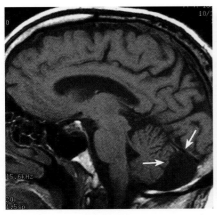

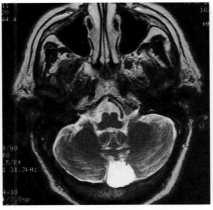

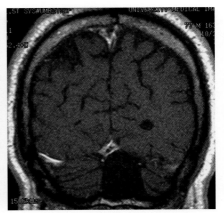

Fig. 1A.**113 Arachnoid cyst. a** Sagittal T1WI shows a well-circumscribed extra-axial structure with low signal located at the dorsal inferior portion of the fourth ventricle (arrows).

Fig. 1A.**113 b** Axial T2WI shows the structure to have high signal comparable to CSF. The lesion mildly deforms the vermis and posteromedial portion of the left cerebellar hemisphere.

Fig. 1A.**113 c** Postcontrast coronal T1WI shows no enhancement of the cyst.

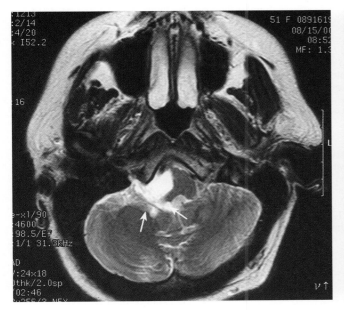

a

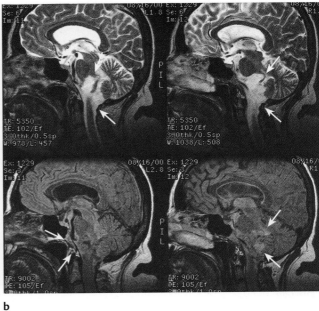

b

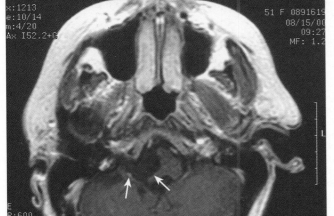

c

Fig. 1A.**114 Epidermoid. a** Axial T2WI shows a multilobulated extra-axial lesion with high signal located ventral to the anteromedial portion of the right cerebellar hemisphere (arrows). The lesion deforms the right side of the adjacent medulla. **b** Sagittal T2WI (upper) and sagittal FLAIR images show the lesion to have high signal that is not suppressed with the FLAIR method and therefore not consistent with CSF (arrows). **c** Postcontrast axial T1WI shows the epidermoid to have low signal and no associated enhancement (arrows).

Table 1A.**5** (Cont.) Extra-axial lesions in the posterior cranial fossa (infratentorial)

Disease	MRI Findings	Comments
Fibrous dysplasia (Fig. 1A.**115**)	Expansile process involving the skull base with mixed low to intermediate signal on T1WI and variable mixed low, intermediate, high signal on T2WI; usually heterogenous enhancement.	Usually seen in adolescents and young adults. Can result in narrowing of neuroforamina with cranial nerve compression, facial deformities. Mono-ostotic and poly-ostotic forms (endocrine abnormalities may be associated, such as with McCune-Albright syndrome, precocious puberty.)
Paget disease (Fig. 1A.**116**)	Expansile sclerotic/lytic process involving the skull with mixed low to intermediate signal on T1WI and variable mixed low, intermediate, high signal on T2WI; variable heterogenous enhancement. Irregular/indistinct borders between marrow and inner margins of the outer and inner tables of the skull.	Usually seen in older adults. Can result in narrowing of neuroforamina with cranial nerve compression, basilar impression. With or without compression of brainstem.
Inflammatory		
Subdural/epidural abscess–Empyema (Fig. 1A.**72**)	Epidural or subdural collections with low signal on T1WI and high signal on T2WI; thin, linear peripheral zones of Gd-contrast enhancement.	Often results from complications related to sinusitis (usually frontal), meningitis, otitis media, ventricular shunts, or surgery. Can be associated with venous sinus thrombosis and venous cerebral or cerebellar infarcts, cerebritis, brain abscess. Mortality 30%.
Leptomeningeal infection/inflammation (Fig. 1A.**117**)	Single or multiple nodular enhancing lesions and/or focal or diffuse abnormal subarachnoid enhancement. Low to intermediate signal on T1WI and intermediate to high signal on T2WI. Leptomeningeal inflammation often best seen on postcontrast images.	Gd-contrast enhancement in the intracranial subarachnoid space (leptomeninges) usually is associated with significant pathology (inflammation and/or infection versus neoplasm). Inflammation and/or infection of the leptomeninges can result from pyogenic, fungal, or parasitic diseases as well as tuberculosis. Neurosarcoidosis results in granulomatous disease in the leptomeninges producing similar patterns of subarachnoid enhancement.
Eosinophilic granuloma (Fig. 2B.**34**)	Single or mutiple circumscribed soft-tissue lesions in the marrow of the skull associated with focal bony destruction/erosion with extension extracranially, intracranially, or both. Lesions usually have low to intermediate signal on T1WI and mixed intermediate to slightly high signal on T2WI, with Gd-contrast enhancement. With or without enhancement of the adjacent dura.	*Single lesion:* Commonly seen in males more than females (below 20 years). Proliferation of histiocytes in medullary cavity with localized destruction of bone with extension in adjacent soft tissues. *Multiple lesions:* Associated with syndromes such as: Letterer-Siwe disease (lymphadenopathy hepatosplenomegaly), children below 2 years; Hand-Schüller-Christian disease (lymphadenopathy, exophthalmos, diabetes insipidus) children aged 5–10 years.
Other:		
Vascular		
AVM	Lesions with irregular margins that can be located in the brain parenchyma–pia, dura, or both locations. AVMs contain multiple tortuous tubular flow voids on T1WI and T2WI. The venous portions often show Gd-contrast enhancement. GRE MR images and MRA using TOF or phase contrast techniques show flow signal in patent portions of the vascular malformation. Usually not associated with mass effect except in the case of recent hemorrhage or venous occlusion.	Supratentorial AVMs occur more frequently (80–90%) than infratentorial AVMs (10–20%). Annual risk of hemorrhage. AVMs can be sporadic, congenital, or associated with a history of trauma.
Dural AVM (Fig. 1A.**78**)	Dural AVMs contain multiple tortuous tubular flow voids on T1WI and T2WI. The venous portions often show Gd-contrast enhancement. GRE MR images and MRA using TOF or phase contrast techniques show flow signal in patent portions of the vascular malformation and areas of venous sinus occlusion or recanalization. Usually not associated with mass effect except in cases of recent hemorrhage or venous occlusion.	Dural AVMs are usually acquired lesions resulting from thrombosis or occlusion of an intracranial venous sinus with subsequent recanalization, resulting in direct arterial to venous sinus communications. Location in order of decreasing frequency: transverse, sigmoid venous sinuses; cavernous sinus; straight, superior sagittal sinuses.

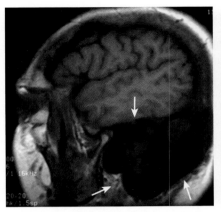

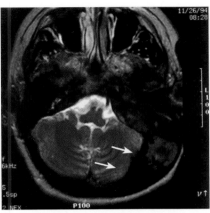

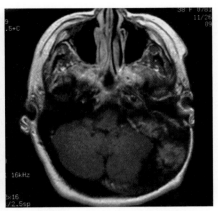

Fig. 1A.**115**   **Fibrous dysplasia.   a** Sagittal T1WI shows a well-circumscribed expansion of the skull with mixed low to intermediate signal (arrows).

Fig. 1A.**115 b**   Axial T2WI shows enlargement of the left petrous and occipital bones with delineated borders, containing mixed low and intermediate signal (arrows).

Fig. 1A.**115 c**   Postcontrast axial T1WI shows heterogeneous enhancement in portions of the fibrous dysplasia.

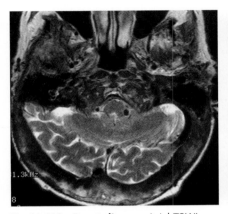

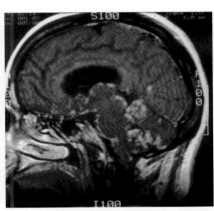

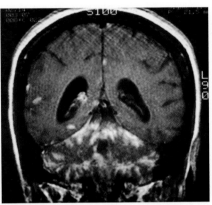

Fig. 1A.**116**   **Paget disease.** Axial T2WI shows an expansile sclerotic/lytic process involving the occipital bone with mixed low, intermediate, and high signal. Irregular/indistinct borders are seen between the marrow and outer and inner tables of the skull.

Fig. 1A.**117**   **a Neurosarcoidosis.** Postcontrast sagittal. T1WI show multiple nodular enhancing lesions in the leptoreninges.

Fig. 1A.**117 b**   Postcontrast coronal T1WI show multiple small nodular enhancing lesions in the supratentorial and infratentorial leptomeninges.

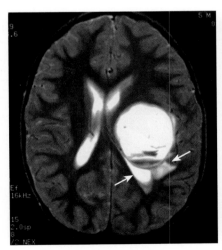

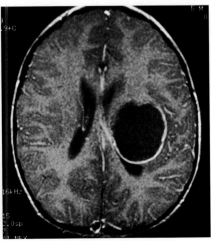

Fig. 1A.**118**   **Low-grade astrocytoma.   a** Axial T2WI shows a cystic lesion with predominantly high signal containing a small fluid level (low signal) (arrows) in the left cerebral hemisphere.

Fig. 1A.**118 b**   Postcontrast axial T1WI shows mild peripheral rim enhancement of the cystic lesion.

Table 1A.**5** (Cont.) Extra-axial lesions in the posterior cranial fossa (infratentorial)

Disease	MRI Findings	Comments
Hemorrhagic		
Epidural hematoma (Fig. 1A.**68)**	Biconvex extra-axial hematoma located between the skull and dura. Displaced dura has low signal on T2WI. The signal of the hematoma itself depends on its age, size, hematocrit, and oxygen tension. With or without associated edema. High signal on T2WI involving the displaced brain parenchyma. Subfalcine, uncal herniation may be associated. *Hyperacute:* intermediate signal on T1WI, intermediate to high signal on T2WI. *Acute:* low to intermediate signal on T1WI, high signal on T2WI. *Subacute:* high signal on T1WI and T2WI.	Epidural hematomas usually result from trauma/tearing of an epidural artery or dural venous sinus. Epidural hematomas do not cross cranial sutures. Skull fracture may be associated.
Subdural hematoma (Fig. 1A.**69–**1A.**71)**	Crescentic extra-axial hematoma located in the potential space between the inner margin of the dura and outer margin of the arachnoid membrane. The signal of the hematoma depends on its age, size, hematocrit, and oxygen tension. With or without associated edema. High signal on T2WI involving the displaced brain parenchyma. Subfalcine, uncal herniation may be associated. *Hyperacute:* intermediate signal on T1WI, intermediate to high signal on T2WI. *Acute:* low to intermediate signal on T1WI, low signal on T2WI. *Subacute:* high signal on T1WI and T2WI *Chronic:* Variable, often low to intermediate signal on T1WI, high signal on T2WI. With or without enhancement of collection and organizing neomembrane. Mixed MRI signal can result if rebleeding occurs into chronic collection.	Subdural hematomas usually result from trauma/stretching/tearing of cortical veins where they enter the subdural space to drain into dural venous sinuses. Subdural hematomas do cross sites of cranial sutures. Skull fracture may be associated.

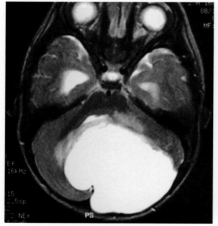

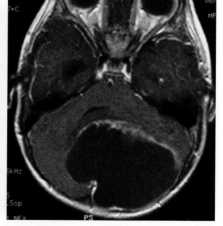

Fig. 1A.**119   Juvenile pilocytic astrocytoma, subtype.   a** Axial T2WI shows a large cystic lesion with high signal in the posterior cranial fossa, causing obstructive hydrocephalus.

Fig. 1A.**119 b**   Postcontrast axial T1WI shows the lesion to have irregular peripheral rim enhancement.

Table 1A.**6** Cystic, cyst-like, and cyst-containing intracranial lesions

Disease	MRI Findings	Comments
Intra-axial		
Astrocytoma	*Low-grade astrocytoma* (Fig. 1A.**118**): Focal or diffuse mass lesion usually located in white matter with low to intermediate signal on T1WI and high signal on T2WI, with or without mild Gd-contrast enhancement. Cysts may be associated. Minimal associated mass effect. *Juvenile pilocytic astrocytoma* (Fig. 1A.**119**): Subtype: solid/cystic focal lesion with low to intermediate signal on T1WI and high signal on T2WI, usually with prominent Gd-contrast enhancement. Lesions located in cerebellum, hypothalamus, adjacent to third or fourth ventricles, brainstem. *Anaplastic astrocytoma:* Often irregularly marginated lesion located in white matter with low to intermediate signal on T1WI and high signal on T2WI, with or without Gd-contrast enhancement. Cysts may be associated.	*Low-grade astrocytoma:* Often occur in children and adults (age 20–40 years). Tumors comprised of well-differentiated astrocytes. Association with neurofibromatosis type 1. Ten-year survival. May become malignant. *Juvenile pilocytic astrocytoma:* Subtype: common in children, usually favorable prognosis if totally resected. *Anaplastic astrocytoma:* Intermediate between low-grade astrocytoma and glioblastoma multiforme. Approximate 2-year survival.
Glioblastoma multiforme (Fig. 1A.**120**)	Irregularly marginated mass lesion with necrosis or cyst. Mixed signal on T1WI, heterogeneous high signal on T2WI. Hemorrhage may be associated. Prominent heterogeneous Gd-contrast enhancement. Peripheral edema. Can cross corpus callosum.	Most common primary CNS tumor. Highly malignant neoplasms with necrosis and vascular proliferation, usually in patients above 50 years. Extent of lesion underestimated by MRI. Survival less than 1 year.
Oligodendroglioma (Fig. 1A.**121**)	Circumscribed lesion with mixed low to intermediate signal on T1WI and mixed intermediate to high signal on T2WI; areas of signal void at sites of clump-like calcification; heterogenous Gd-contrast enhancement. Involves white matter and cerebral cortex. Cysts may be associated. Can cause chronic erosion of inner table of calvaria.	Uncommon slow-growing gliomas with usually mixed histologic patterns (e.g., astrocytoma). Usually in adults above 35 years of age, 85 % supratentorial. If low-grade 75 % 5-year survival; higher grade lesions have a worse prognosis.

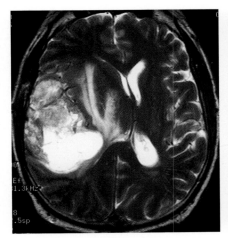

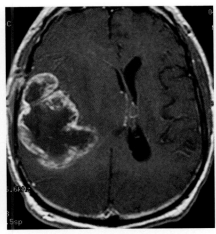

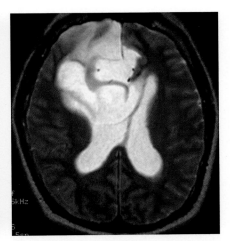

Fig. 1A.**120** **Glioblastoma multiforme.** **a** Axial T2WI shows a mixed solid and cystic(necrotic) tumor in the right cerebral hemisphere with heterogeneous high signal and associated mass effect with subfalcine herniation to the left.

Fig. 1A.**120 b** Postcontrast axial T1WI shows irregular peripheral enhancement at the lesion.

Fig. 1A.**121** **Oligodendroglioma.** Axial T2WI shows a mixed solid and cystic tumor in the right frontal lobe.

Table 1A.6 (Cont.) Cystic, cyst-like, and cyst-containing intracranial lesions

Disease	MRI Findings	Comments
Central neurocytoma (Fig. 1A.122)	Circumscribed lesion located at margin of lateral ventricle or septum pellucidum with intraventricular protrusion. Heterogeneous intermediate signal on T1WI; heterogeneous intermediate to high signal on T2WI. Calcifications and/or small cysts may be associated. Heterogeneous Gd-contrast enhancement.	Rare tumors that have neuronal differentiation. Imaging appearance similar to intraventricular oligodendrogliomas. Occur in young adults. Benign slow-growing lesions.
Ganglioglioma, ganglioneuroma, gangliocytoma (Fig. 1A.123)	Circumscribed tumor, usually supratentorial, often temporal or frontal lobes. Low to intermediate signal on T1WI; intermediate to high signal on T2WI. Cysts may be present. With or without Gd-contrast enhancement.	Ganglioglioma (contains glial and neuronal elements), ganglioneuroma (contains only ganglion cells). Uncommon tumors, below 30 years, seizure presentation, slow-growing neoplasms. Gangliocytoma (contains only neuronal elements, dysplastic brain tissue). Favorable prognosis if completely resected.
Dysembryoplastic neuroepithelial tumor (Fig. 1A.124)	Circumscribed lesions involving the cerebral cortex and subcortical white matter. Low signal on T1WI and high signal on T2WI. Small cysts may be present. Usually no Gd-contrast enhancement.	Benign superficial lesions commonly located in the temporal or frontal lobes.
Pleomorphic xanthoastrocytoma (Fig. 1A.125) (Fig. 1A.24)	Circumscribed supratentorial lesion involving cerebral cortex and white matter. Low to intermediate signal on T1WI and intermediate to high signal on T2WI. Cyst(s) may be present. Heterogeneous Gd-contrast enhancement. With or without enhancing mural nodule associated with cyst.	Rare type of astrocytoma occurring in young adults and children, associated with seizure history.
Primitive neuroectodermal tumor (Fig. 1A.126)	Circumscribed or invasive lesions with low to intermediate signal on T1WI and intermediate to high signal on T2WI; variable Gd-contrast enhancement. Cysts may be present. Frequent dissemination into the leptomeninges.	Highly malignant tumors that frequently disseminate along CSF pathways.

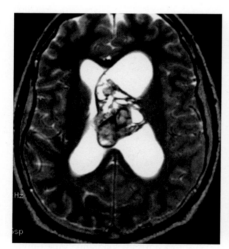

Fig. 1A.**122** **Central neurocytoma.** Axial T2WI shows a mixed solid and cystic tumor involving the septum pellucidum.

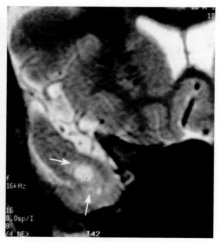

Fig. 1A.**123** **Ganglioglioma.** Coronal T2WI shows a mixed solid and cystic tumor in the anterior right temporal lobe (arrows).

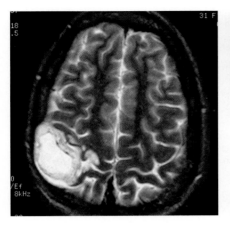
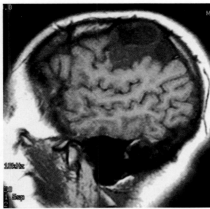

Fig. 1A.**124   Dysembryoplastic neuroepithelial tumor.   a** Axial T2WI shows a mixed solid and cystic tumor with heterogeneous high signal involving the right cerebral hemisphere.   **b** Sagittal T1WI shows the lesion with low and intermediate signal extending to the surface of the brain with chronic erosion of the adjacent inner table of the skull indicating a slow-growing neoplasm.

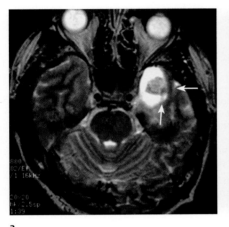

a

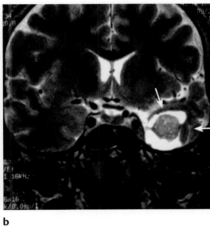

b

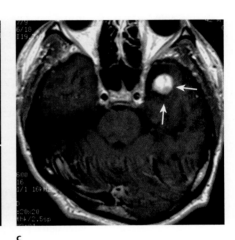

c

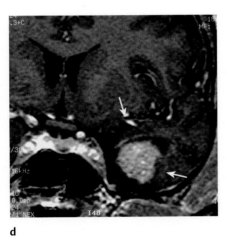

d

Fig. 1A.**125   Pleomorphic xanthoastrocytoma.** Axial (**a**) and coronal (**b**) T2WI show a cystic lesion with predominantly high signal containing a nodular zone with intermediate signal in the anterior left temporal lobe (arrows). Postcontrast axial (**c**) and coronal (**d**) T1WI show prominent enhancement at the nodular zone (arrows).

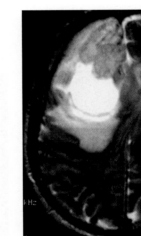

Fig. 1A.**126   Primitive neuroectodermal tumor.** Axial T2WI shows a mass lesion with mixed solid and cystic components located in the anterior right frontal lobe.

Table 1A.**6** (Cont.) Cystic, cyst-like, and cyst-containing intracranial lesions

Disease	MRI Findings	Comments
Ependymoma (Fig. 1A.**127**)	Circumscribed lobulated supratentorial lesion, often extra-ventricular. Cysts and/or calcifications may be associated. Low to intermediate signal on T1WI and intermediate to high signal on T2WI; variable Gd-contrast enhancement.	Occurs more commonly in children than adults. One-third supratentorial, two-thirds infratentorial. 45 % 5-year survival.
Hemangioblastoma (Fig. 1A.**128**)	Circumscribed tumors usually located in the cerebellum and/or brainstem. Small Gd-contrast-enhancing nodule with or without cyst, or larger lesion with prominent heterogeneous enhancement with or without flow voids within lesion or at the periphery. Intermediate signal on T1WI and intermediate to high signal on T2WI. Occasionally lesions have evidence of recent or remote hemorrhage.	Occurs in adolescents, young and middle-aged adults. Lesions are typically multiple in patients with von Hippel-Lindau disease.
Metastases (Fig. 1A.**129**)	Circumscribed spheroid lesions in brain that can have various intra-axial locations, often at gray-white matter junctions. Usually low to intermediate signal on T1WI and intermediate to high signal on T2WI. Hemorrhage, calcifications, cysts may be associated. Variable Gd-contrast enhancement. Often high signal on T2WI peripheral to nodular enhancing lesion representing axonal edema.	Represent approximately 33 % of intracranial tumors, usually from extracranial primary neoplasm in adults above 40 years.
Pyogenic brain abscess (Fig. 1A.**130**)	Circumscribed lesion with low signal on T1WI; central zone of high signal on T2WI (air-fluid level may be present) surrounded by a thin rim of low T2 signal; peripheral poorly defined zone of high signal on T2WI representing edema; ring-like Gd-contrast enhancement.	Formation of brain abscess occurs 2 weeks after cerebritis with liquefaction and necrosis centrally surrounded by a capsule and peripheral edema. Can be multiple. Complication from meningitis and/or sinusitis, septicemia, trauma, surgery, caridac shunt.
Fungal brain abscess (Fig. 1A.**37**)	Vary depending on organism. Lesions occur in meninges and brain parenchyma; solid or cystic lesions with low to intermediate signal on T2WI and high signal on T2WI. Nodular or ring enhancement. Peripheral high signal in brain lesions on T2WI (edema).	Occur in immunocompromised or diabetic patients with resultant granulomas in meninges and brain parenchyma. Abscess formation possible.

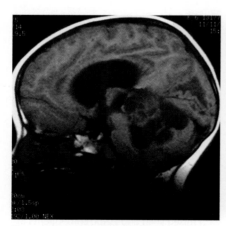

Fig. 1A.**127** **Ependymoma.** **a** Sagittal T1WI shows a mixed solid and cystic lesion in the upper fourth ventricle with involvement of the upper vermis and pineal recess.

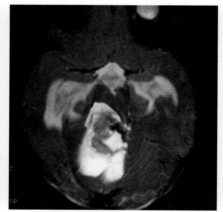

Fig. 1A.**127 b** Axial T2WI shows the cystic components with high signal and the solid portions with low and intermdediate signal.

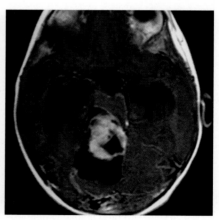

Fig. 1A.**127 c** Postcontrast axial T1WI shows enhancement at the solid portions of the lesion.

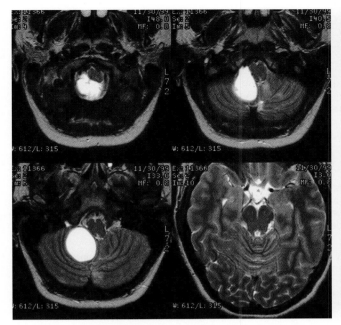

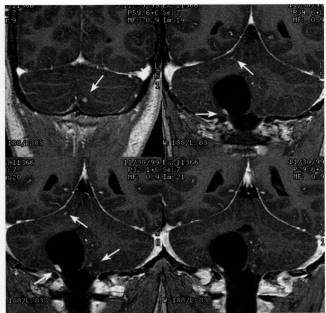

Fig. 1A.128 Hemangioblastomas/von Hippel-Lindau disease. **a** Axial T2WI show a cystic lesion at the inferior right cerebellar hemisphere.

Fig. 1A.128 b Postcontrast coronal (spoiled GRE) T1WI shows a small nodule of enhancement at the inferior margin of the cystic lesion as well as other small nodules of enhancement in the cerebellum representing additional hemangioblastomas (arrows).

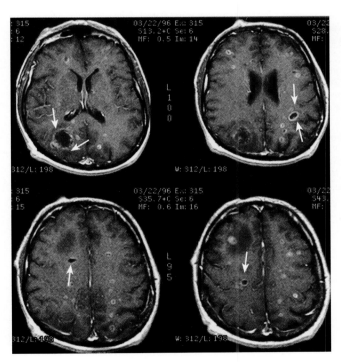

Fig. 1A.129 Metastases. Postcontrast axial T1WI shows multiple enhancing metastatic lesions in the brain as well as several ring-enhancing cystic-appearing metastases (arrows).

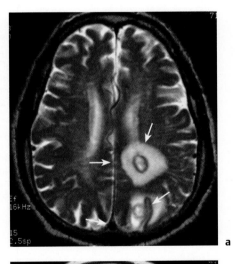

Fig. 1A.130 Pyogenic brain abscess. ▷
a Axial T2WI shows two pyogenic abscesses (arrows) in the left cerebral hemisphere surrounded by edematous zones with high signal. **b** Postcontrast axial T1WI shows thin rim enhancement patterns at the abscesses (arrows).

a

b

Table 1A.**6** (Cont.) Cystic, cyst-like, and cyst-containing intracranial lesions

Disease	MRI Findings	Comments
Parasitic		
Toxoplasmosis (Fig. 1A.131)	Single or multiple solid and/or cystic lesions located in basal ganglia and/or corticomedullary junctions in cerebral hemispheres. Low to intermediate signal on T1WI; high signal on T2WI. Nodular or rim pattern of Gd-contrast enhancement. With or without peripheral high T2 signal (edema).	Most common opportunistic CNS infection in AIDS patients, caused by ingestion of food contaminated with parasites (*Toxoplasma gondii*).
Cysticercosis (Fig. 1A.132)	Single or multiple cystic lesions in brain or meninges. *Acute/subacute phase:* Low to intermediate signal on T1WI and high signal on T2WI. Rim and possible nodular pattern of Gd-contrast enhancement, with or without peripheral high T2 signal (edema). *Chronic phase:* calcified granulomas.	Caused by ingestion of ova (*Taenia solium*) in contaminated food (undercooked pork). Involves in order of decreasing frequency: meninges, brain parenchyma, ventricles.
Hydatid cyst	*Echinococcus granulosus:* Single or rarely multiple cystic lesions with low signal on T1WI and high signal on T2WI with a thin wall with low signal on T2WI; typically no Gd-contrast enhancement or peripheral edema unless superinfected. Often located in vascular territory of the middle cerebral artery. *Echinococcus multilocularis:* Cystic (possibly multilocular) and/or solid lesions. Central zone of low to intermediate signal on T1WI and T2WI, surrounded by a slightly thickened rim of low signal on T2WI; Gd-contrast enhancement. Peripheral zone of high signal on T2WI (edema) and calcifications are common.	Caused by parasites: *Echinococcus granulosus* (South America, Middle East Australia, New Zealand) or *Echinococcus multilocularis* (North America, Europe, Turkey, China).CNS involvement in 2% of cases of hydatid infestation.
Demyelinating disease–ADEM, MS (Fig. 1A.133)	Demyelinating lesions rarely can have a cyst-like appearance. Lesions can be located in cerebral or cerebellar white matter, brainstem, basal ganglia. Gd-contrast enhancement can be ring-like, usually in acute/ early subacute phase of demyelination.	MS is the most common acquired demyelinating disease. Other demyelinating diseases include: ADEM–immune mediated demyelination after viral infection, toxins or metabolic disorders.
Radiation necrosis	Focal lesion with or without mass effect or poorly defined zone of low to intermediate signal on T1WI, intermediate to high signal on T2WI, with or without Gd-contrast enhancement involving tissue (gray matter and/or white matter) in field of treatment.	Usually occurs from 4–6 months to 10 years after radiation treatment. May be difficult to distinguish from neoplasm. PET and MRS might be helpful for evaluation.
Porencephalic cyst (Fig. 1A.52)	Irregular, relatively well-circumscribed zone with low signal on T1WI and high signal on T2WI similar to CSF. Surrounded by poorly defined thin zone of high T2 signal in adjacent brain tissue. No Gd-contrast enhancement or peripheral edema.	Represent remote sites of brain injury (trauma, infarct, infection, hemorrhage) with evolution into a cystic zone with CSF. MR signal characteristics surrounded by gliosis in adjacent brain parenchyma. Gliosis (high T2 signal) allows differentiation from schizencephaly.

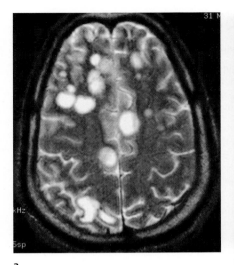

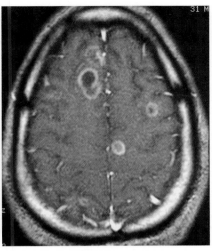

a **b**

Fig. 1A.**131** **Toxoplasmosis.** **a** Axial T2WI shows cystic lesions in both cerebral hemispheres from infection by toxoplasmosis. **b** Postcontrast axial T1WI shows thin rim enhancement patterns at the lesions.

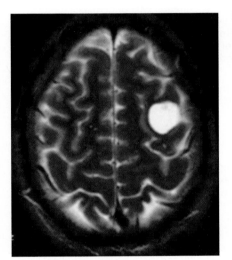

Fig. 1A.**132** **Cysticercosis.** Axial T2WI shows a single cystic lesion in the left cerebral hemisphere from acute/subacute phase of infection from Taenia solium.

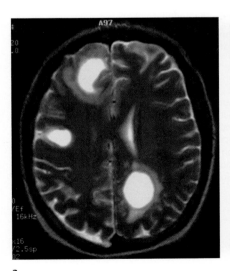

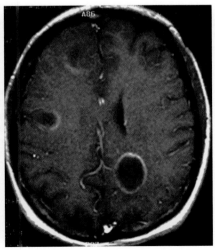

a **b**

Fig. 1A.**133** **Demyelinating disease–MS.** **a** Axial T2WI shows three cystic-appearing lesions in the cerebral white matter that had histologic patterns of active demyelination. **b** Postcontrast axial T1WI shows mild peripheral rim enhancement at the lesions.

Table 1A.6 (Cont.) Cystic, cyst-like, and cyst-containing intracranial lesions

Disease	MRI Findings	Comments
Neuroepithelial cyst (Fig. 1A.134)	Well-circumscribed cysts with low signal on T1WI and high signal on T2WI. Thin walls, no Gd-contrast enhancement or peripheral edema.	Cyst walls have histopathologic features similar to epithelium. Neuroepithelial cysts located in: choroid plexus, choroidal fissure, ventricles, brain parenchyma.
Extra-axial		
Craniopharyngioma (Fig. 1A.135)	Circumscribed lobulated lesions. Variable low, intermediate, and/or high signal on T1WI and T2WI; with or without nodular or rim Gd-contrast enhancement. May contain cysts, lipid components, and calcifications.	Usually histologically benign but locally aggressive lesions arising from squamous epithelial rests along Rathke's cleft. Occurs in children (10 years) and adults (above 40 years). Affects males and females equally.
Germinoma (Fig. 1A.59)	Circumscribed tumors with or without disseminated disease; pineal region, suprasellar region, third ventricle/basal ganglia. Low to intermediate signal on T1WI; occasionally high signal on T1WI; variable low, intermediate, high signal on T2WI. Gd-contrast enhancement of tumor and leptomeninges if disseminated.	Most common type of germ cell tumor; occurrence higher in males than females (10–30 years); usually midline neoplasms.
Teratoma (Fig. 1A.60)	Circumscribed lesions; pineal region, suprasellar region, third ventricle. Variable low, intermediate, and/or high signal on T1WI and T2WI; with or without Gd-contrast enhancement. May contain calcifications, cysts, as well as fatty components that can cause a chemical meningitis if ruptured.	Second most common type of germ cell tumors. Occurs in children, more common in males more than females. Benign or malignant types, composed of derivatives of ectoderm, mesoderm, and/or endoderm.
Pineal cyst (Fig. 1A.83)	Well-circumscribed extra-axial lesions with low signal on T1WI and high signal on T2WI similar to CSF. No central enhancement; thin linear peripheral Gd-contrast enhancement. Rarely atypical appearance with proteinaceous contents: intermediate, slightly high signal on T1WI.	Common usually incidental non-neoplastic cyst in pineal gland.
Arachnoid cyst (Figs. 1A.80, 1A.113)	Well-circumscribed extra-axial lesions with low signal on T1WI and high signal on T2WI similar to CSF; no Gd-contrast enhancement. Common locations in order of decreasing frequency: anterior middle cranial fossa, suprasellar/quadrigeminal, frontal convexities, posterior cranial fossa.	Non-neoplastic congenital, developmental or acquired extra-axial lesions filled with CSF. Usually mild mass effect on adjacent brain. More often supratentorial than infratentorial location. Affects males more than females. With or without related clinical symptoms.
Leptomeningeal cyst (Fig. 1A.82)	Well-circumscribed extra-axial lesions with low signal on T1WI and high signal on T2WI similar to CSF; no Gd-contrast enhancement. Associated with erosion of the adjacent skull.	Non-neoplastic extra-axial lesions filled with CSF thought to be secondary to trauma with dural tear/skull fracture. Usually mild mass effect on adjacent brain with progressive erosion of adjacent skull. Occasionally presents as a scalp lesion. More common in children than adults.
Colloid cyst (Fig. 1A.84)	Well-circumscribed spheroid lesions located at the anterior portion of the third ventricle. Variable signal (low, intermediate, or high) on T1WI and T2WI, often high signal on T1WI and low signal on T2WI, no Gd-contrast enhancement.	Common presentation of headaches and intermittent hydrocephalus. Removal leads to cure.
Epidermoid (Figs. 1A.85, 1A.114)	Well-circumscribed spheroid or multilobulated extra-axial ectodermal-inclusion cystic lesions with low to intermediate signal on T1WI and high signal on T2WI similar to CSF. Mixed low, intermediate, or high signal on FLAIR images; no Gd-contrast enhancement. Often insinuate along CSF pathways, chronic deformation of adjacent neural tissue (brainstem, brain parenchyma). Commonly located in posterior cranial fossa (cerebellopontine angle cistern), parasellar/middle cranial fossa.	Non-neoplastic, congenital or acquired extra-axial off-midline lesions filled with desquamated cells and keratinaceous debris. Usually mild mass effect on adjacent brain. Infratentorial locations more common than supratentorial locations. Affects male and female adults equally. With or without related clinical symptoms.

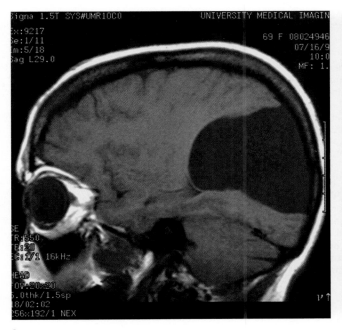

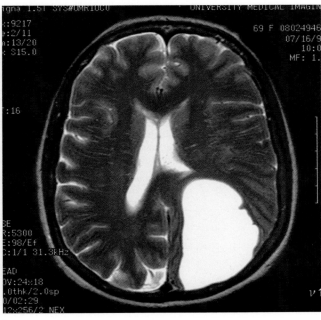

a

b

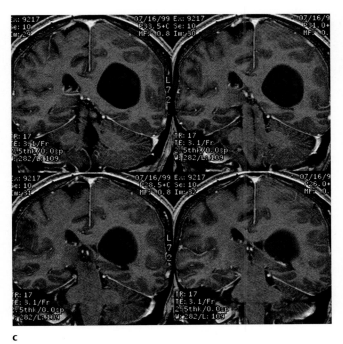

Fig. 1A.**134 Neuroepithelial cyst. a** Sagittal T1WI shows a large intra-axial cystic lesion involving the posterior left cerebral hemisphere. **b** Axial T2WI shows the cystic lesion to have homogeneous high signal without associated peripheral edema. **c** Postcontrast coronal (spoiled GRE) T1WI shows no enhancement at the cystic lesion.

c

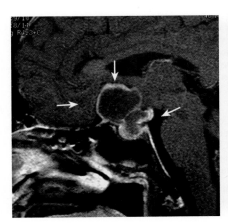

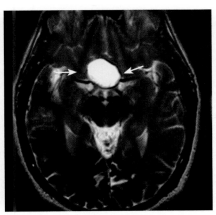

Fig. 1A.**135 Craniopharyngioma. a** Postcontrast sagittal T1WI with fat suppression shows a mixed solid and cystic lesion in the sella and suprasellar cistern with nodular and peripheral rim patterns of enhancement (arrows). **b** Axial T2WI shows the cystic component of the lesion with high signal (arrows).

a

b

Table 1A.**6** (Cont.) Cystic, cyst-like, and cyst-containing intracranial lesions

Disease	MRI Findings	Comments
Dermoid (Fig. 1A.136)	Well-circumscribed, spheroid or multilobulated extra-axial lesions, usually with high signal on T1WI and variable low, intermediate, and/or high signal on T2WI. No Gd-contrast enhancement. Fluid-fluid or fluid-debris levels may be present. Can cause chemical meningitis if dermoid cyst ruptures into the subarachnoid space. Commonly located at or near midline, supratentorial more common than infratentorial.	Non-neoplastic, congenital or acquired ectodermal-inclusion cystic lesions filled with lipid material, cholesterol, desquamated cells, and keratinaceous debris. Usually mild mass effect on adjacent brain. Slightly more common in adults males than adult females. With or without related clinical symptoms.
Rathke's cleft cyst (Fig. 1A.81)	Well-circumscribed lesion with variable low, inter-mediate, or high signal on T1WI and T2WI. On T1WI, two-thirds have high signal and one-third low signal; on T2WI, 50% have high signal, 25% low signal, and 25% intermediate signal. No Gd-contrast centrally, with or without thin peripheral enhancement. Lesion locations: 50% intrasellar, 25% suprasellar, 25% intrasellar and suprasellar.	Uncommon sellar/juxtasellar benign cystic lesion containing fluid with variable amounts of protein, mucopolysaccharide, and/or cholesterol; arise from epithelial rests of the craniopharyngeal duct.

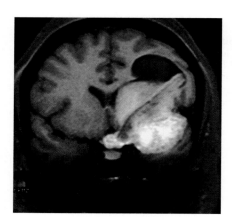

Fig. 1A.**136**   **Dermoid.** Coronal T1WI shows a complex solid and cystic extra-axial lesion on the left with zones of low and high signal.

Table 1A.**7** Lesions involving gray matter/cerebral cortex

Disease	MRI Findings	Comments
Congenital/developmental:		
Neuronal migration disorders		
Gray matter heterotopia (Figs. 1A.5–1A.7)	Laminar heterotopia appears as a band or bands of isointense gray matter within the cerebral white matter (Fig. 1A.**5**). Nodular heterotopia appears as one or more nodules of isointense gray matter along the ventricles or within the cerebral white matter (Figs. 1A.**6**, 1A.**7**).	Disorder of neuronal migration (7–22 weeks of gestation) where a collection or layer of neurons is located beween the ventricles and cerebral cortex. Can have a band-like (laminar) or nodular appearance isointense to gray matter. May be unilateral or bilateral. Associated with seizures, schizencephaly.
Schizencephaly (split brain) (Figs. 1A.8, 1A.9)	Cleft in brain extending from ventricle to cortical surface lined by heterotopic gray matter. Cleft may be narrow (closed lip, Fig. 1A.**8**) or wide (open lip, Fig. 1A.**9**).	Association with seizures, blindness, retardation, and other CNS anomalies (e.g., septo-optic dysplasia). Clinical manifestations related to severity of malformation. Ischemia or insult to portion or germinal matrix before hemisphere formation.
Unilateral hemi-megalencephaly (Fig. 1A.10)	Nodular or multinodular region of gray matter heterotopia involving all or part of a cerebral hemisphere with associated enlargement of the ipsilateral lateral ventricle and hemisphere.	Neuronal migration disorder associated with hamartomatous overgrowth of the involved hemisphere.

Table 1A.**7** (Cont.) Lesions involving gray matter/cerebral cortex

Disease	MRI Findings	Comments
Lissencephaly (Fig. 1A.3)	Absent or incomplete formation of gyri and sulci with shallow sylvian fissures and "figure 8" appearance of brain on axial images. Abnormally thick cortex, gray matter heterotopia with smooth gray-white matter interface.	Severe disorder of neuronal migration (7–16 weeks of gestation) with absent or incomplete formation of gyri, sulci, and sylvian fissures. Associated with severe mental retardation and seizures, early death. Other associated CNS anomalies include dysgenesis of corpus callosum, microcephaly, hypoplastic thalami, cephaloceles.
Pachygyria (nonlissencephalic cortical dysplasia) (Fig. 1A.4)	Thick gyri with shallow sulci involving all or portions of the brain. Thickened cortex with relatively smooth gray-white interface, may have areas of high T2 signal in the white matter (gliosis).	Severe disorder of neuronal migration. Clinical findings related to degree of extent of this malformation.
Neurocutaneous syndromes		
Hamartoma–Tuberous sclerosis (Fig. 1A.29)	*Cortical:* Subcortical lesion with high signal on T1WI and low signal on T2WI in neonates and infants; changes to low to intermediate signal on T1WI and high signal on T2WI in older children and adults. Calcifications in 50% in older children. Gd-contrast enhancement uncommon.	Cortical hamartomas are nonmalignant lesions associated with tuberous sclerosis.
Sturge-Weber (Fig. 1A.137)	Prominent localized unilateral leptomeningeal enhancement usually in parietal and/or occipital regions in children. With or without gyral enhancement. Slightly decreased signal on T2WI in adjacent gyri. Mild localized atrophic changes in brain adjacent to the pial angioma. Prominent medullary and/or subependymal veins and ipsilateral prominence of choroid plexus may be associated. Gyral calcifications above 2 years, progressive cerebral atrophy in region of pial angioma.	Also known as encephalotrigeminal angiomatosis, neurocutaneous syndrome associated with ipsilateral port wine cutaneous lesion and seizures. Results from persistence of primitive leptomeningeal venous drainage (pial angioma) and developmental lack of normal cortical veins, producing chronic venous congestion and ischemia.
Neurocutaneous melanosis	Extra-axial or intra-axial lesions usually less than 3 cm in diameter with irregular margins in the leptomeninges or brain parenchyma/brainstem (anterior temporal lobes, cerebellum, thalami, inferior frontal lobes) with intermediate to slightly high signal on T1WI secondary to increased melanin; Gd-contrast enhancement. Vermian hypoplasia, arachnoid cysts, Dandy-Walker malformation may be associated.	Neuroectodermal dysplasia with proliferation of melanocytes in leptomeninges associated with large and/or numerous cutaneous nevi. May change into CNS melanoma.

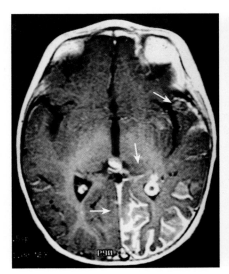

a

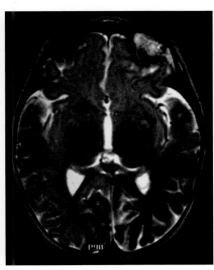

b

Fig. 1A.**137** **Sturge-Weber. a** Postcontrast axial T1WI shows abnormal unilateral leptomeningeal enhancement in the temporal and occipital regions representing the pial angioma (arrows). **b** Axial T2WI shows localized atrophic changes and decreased signal in the temporal and occipital lobes resulting from chronic venous congestion and calcium/mineral deposition.

Table 1A.**7** (Cont.) Lesions involving gray matter/cerebral cortex

Disease	MRI Findings	Comments
Neoplasms		
Astrocytoma (Fig. 1A.18–1A.21)	*Low-grade astrocytoma:* Focal or diffuse mass lesion usually located in white matter with occasional extension to the cortex. Low to intermediate signal on T1WI and high signal on T2WI; with or without mild Gd-contrast enhancement. Cysts may be present. Minimal associated mass effect. *Juvenile pilocytic astrocytoma:* Subtype: solid/cystic focal lesion with low to intermediate signal on T1WI and high signal on T2WI, usually with prominent Gd-contrast enhancement. Lesions located in cerebellum, hypothalamus, adjacent to third or fourth ventricles, brainstem. *Anaplastic astrocytoma:* Often irregularly marginated lesion located in white matter with extension to cortex late in disease. Low to intermediate signal on T1WI, high signal on T2WI; with or without Gd-contrast enhancement. Cysts may be present.	*Low-grade astrocytoma:* Often occur in children and adults (age 20–40 years). Tumors comprised of well-differentiated astrocytes. Association with neurofibromatosis type 1. Ten-year survival. May become malignant. *Juvenile pilocytic astrocytoma:* Subtype: common in children, usually favorable prognosis if totally resected. *Anaplastic astrocytoma:* Intermediate between low-grade astrocytoma and glioblastoma multiforme. Approximate 2-year survival.
Glioblastoma multiforme (Fig. 1A.22)	Irregularly marginated mass lesion with necrosis or cyst. Mixed signal on T1WI and heterogeneous high signal on T2WI. Hemorrhage may be associated. Prominent heterogeneous Gd-contrast enhancement. Peripheral edema. Can cross corpus callosum.	Most common primary CNS tumor, highly malignant neoplasms with necrosis and vascular proliferation, usually in patients older than 50 years. Extent of lesion underestimated by MRI. Survival less than 1 year.
Oligodendroglioma (Fig. 1A.25)	Circumscribed lesion with mixed low to intermediate signal on T1WI and mixed intermediate to high signal on T2WI; areas of signal void at sites of clump-like calcification; heterogenous Gd-contrast enhancement. Involves white matter and cerebral cortex. Cysts may be present. Can cause chronic erosion of inner table of calvaria.	Uncommon slow-growing gliomas with usually mixed histologic patterns (e.g., astrocytoma). Usually in adults older than 35 years of age, 85% supratentorial. If low-grade 75% 5-year survival; higher grade lesions have a worse prognosis.
Ganglioglioma, ganglioneuroma, gangliocytoma (Fig. 1A.27)	Circumscribed tumor. Usually supratentorial, often temporal or frontal lobes. Low to intermediate signal on T1WI and intermediate to high signal on T2WI. Cysts may be associated. With or without Gd-contrast enhancement.	Ganglioglioma (contains glial and neuronal elements), ganglioneuroma (contains only ganglion cells). Uncommon tumors, below 30 years, seizure presentation, slow-growing neoplasms. Gangliocytoma (contains only neuronal elements, dysplastic brain tissue). Favorable prognosis if completely resected.
Pleomorphic xanthoastrocytoma (Fig. 1A.24) (Fig. 1A.125)	Circumscribed supratentorial lesion involving cerebral cortex and white matter. Low to intermediate signal on T1WI, intermediate to high signal on T2WI. Cyst(s) may be associated. Heterogeneous Gd-contrast enhancement. With or without enhancing mural nodule associated with cyst.	Rare type of astrocytoma occurring in young adults and children, associated with seizure history.
Dysembryoplastic neuroepithelial tumor (Fig. 1A.32)	Circumscribed lesions involving the cerebral cortex and subcortical white matter. Low signal on T1WI, high signal on T2WI. Small cysts may be present. Usually no Gd-contrast enhancement.	Benign superficial lesions commonly located in the temporal or frontal lobes.
Metastatic tumor (Fig. 1A.34), (Fig. 1A.92), (Fig. 1A.104)	Single or multiple well-circumscribed or poorly defined lesions with initial common location at the corticomedullary junction with possible eventual extension to the cortex, or involving the leptomeninges with invasion of adjacent superficial brain parenchyma. Low to intermediate signal on T1WI and intermediate to high signal on T2WI, usually with Gd-contrast enhancement. Bone destruction and compression of neural tissue or vessels may be associated. Leptomeningeal tumor often best seen on postcontrast images.	Metastatic tumor or leptomeningeal lymphoma may have variable destructive or infiltrative changes involving single or multiple sites of involvement.

Table 1A.**7** (Cont.) Lesions involving gray matter/cerebral cortex

Disease	MRI Findings	Comments
Ischemic		
Cerebral infarct (Fig. 1A.**55**), (Fig. 1A.**102**), (Fig. 1A.**160**)	MRI features of cerebral and cerebellar infarcts depends on age of infarct relative to time of examination: *<12 hours:* Localized edema, usually isointense signal to normal brain on T1WI and T2WI. Diffusion weighted images can show positive findings related to decreased apparent diffusion coefficients secondary to cytotoxic edema, absence of arterial flow void or arterial enhancement in the vascular distribution of the infarct. *12–24 hours:* Intermediate signal on T1WI and high signal on T2WI. Localized edema. Signal abnormalities commonly involve the cerebral cortex and subcortical white matter and/or basal ganglia. *24 hours to 3 days:* Low to intermediate signal on T1WI and high signal on T2WI. Localized edema. Hemorrhage may be associated. With or without enhancement. *4 days to 2 weeks:* Low to intermediate signal on T1WI and high signal on T2WI. Edema/mass effect diminishing. Hemorrhage may be associated. With or without enhancement. *2 weeks to 2 months:* Low to intermediate signal on T1WI and high signal on T2WI. Edema resolves. Hemorrhage may be associated. Enhancement may eventually decline. *>2 months:* Low signal on T1WI and high signal on T2WI. Encephalomalacic changes. Calcification, hemosiderin may be present.	Cerebral infarcts usually result from occlusive vascular disease involving large, medium, or small arteries. Vascular occlusion may be secondary to atheromatous arterial disease, cardiogenic emboli, neoplastic encasement, hypercoagulable states, dissection, or congenital anomalies. Cerebral infarcts usually result from arterial occlusion involving specific vascular territories; occasionally result from metabolic disorders (e.g., mitochondrial encephalopathies) or intracranial venous occlusion (e.g., thrombophlebitis, hypercoagulable states, dehydration) that do not correspond to arterial distributions.
Trauma		
Cerebral contusions (Fig. 1A.**45**)	The MR appearance of contusions is initially one of focal hemorrhage involving the cerebral cortex and subcortical white matter. The MR signal of the contusion depends on its age and presence of oxyhemoglobin, deoxyhemoglobin, methemoglobin, hemosiderin, etc. Contusions eventually appear as focal superficial encephalomalacic zones with high signal on T2WI, with or without small zones of low signal on T2WI from hemosiderin.	Contusions are superficial brain injuries involving the cerebral cortex and subcortical white matter that result from skull fracture and/or acceleration/deceleration trauma to the inner table of the skull. Often involve the anterior portions of the temporal and frontal lobes and inferior portions of the frontal lobes.
Cerebral hemorrhage (Fig. 1A.**43**), (Fig. 1A.**44**)	The signal of the hematoma depends on its age, size, location, hematocrit, hemoglobin oxidation state, clot retraction, and extent of edema. *Hyperacute phase (4–6 hours):* Hemoglobin primarily as diamagnetic oxyhemoglobin (iron Fe^{+2} state), intermediate signal on T1WI and slightly high signal on T2WI. *Acute phase (12–48 hours):* Hemoglobin primarily as paramagnetic deoxyhemoglobin (iron, Fe^{+2} state), intermediate signal on T1WI and low signal on T2WI, surrounded by a peripheral zone of high T2 signal (edema). *Subacute phase (>2 days):* Hemoglobin becomes oxidized to the iron Fe^{+3} state, methemoglobin, which is strongly paramagnetic. When methemoglobin is initially intracellular: the hematoma has high signal on T1WI, progressing from peripheral to central, and low signal on T2WI, surrounded by a zone of high T2 signal (edema). When methemoglobin eventually becomes primarily extracellular: the hematoma has high signal on T1WI and T2WI. *Chronic phase:* Hemoglobin as extracellular methemoglobin is progressively degraded to hemosiderin. The hematoma progresses from a lesion with high signal on T1WI and T2WI with a peripheral rim of low signal on T2WI (hemosiderin) to predominant hemosiderin composition and low signal on T2WI.	

Table 1A.**7** (Cont.) Lesions involving gray matter/cerebral cortex

Disease	MRI Findings	Comments
Inflammatory		
Cerebritis (Fig. 1A.**35**)	Poorly defined zone or focal area of low to intermediate signal on T1WI and intermediate to high signal on T2WI; minimal or no Gd-contrast enhancement. Involves cerebral cortex and white matter for bacterial and fungal infections.	Focal infection/inflammation of brain tissue from bacteria or fungi, secondary to sinusitis, meningitis, surgery, hematogenous source (cardiac and other vascular shunts), and/or immunocompromised status. Can progress to abscess formation.
Pyogenic brain abscess (Fig. 1A.**36**)	Circumscribed lesion with low signal on T1WI; central zone of high signal on T2WI (air-fluid level may be present) surrounded by a thin rim of low T2 signal; peripheral poorly defined zone of high signal on T2WI representing edema. Ring-like Gd-contrast enhancement that is sometimes thicker laterally than medially.	Formation of brain abscess occurs 2 weeks after cerebritis with liquefaction and necrosis centrally surrounded by a capsule and peripheral edema. Can be multiple. Complication from meningitis and/or sinusitis, septicemia, trauma, surgery, caridac shunt.
Fungal brain abscess (Fig. 1A.**37**)	Vary depending on organism. Lesions occur in meninges and brain parenchyma; solid or cystic lesions with low to intermediate signal on T2WI and high signal on T2WI. Nodular or ring enhancement. Peripheral high signal in brain lesions on T2WI (edema).	Occur in immunocompromised or diabetic patients with resultant granulomas in meninges and brain parenchyma; Cryptococcus involves the basal meninges and extends along perivascular spaces into the basal ganglia. *Aspergillus* and *Mucor* spread via direct extension through paranasal sinuses or hematogenously invade blood vessels resulting in hemorrhagic lesions and/or cerebral infarcts. Coccidiomycosis usually involves the basal meninges.
Encephalitis (Fig. 1A.**38**)	Poorly defined zone(s) of low to intermediate signal on T1WI and intermediate to high signal on T2WI; minimal or no Gd-contrast enhancement. Involves cerebral cortex and/or white matter, minimal localized mass effect. Herpes simplex typically involves the temporal lobes/limbic system. Hemorrhage may be associated. CMV usually in periventricular/subependymal locations. HIV often involves periatrial white matter.	Encephalitis: infection/inflammation of brain tissue from viruses, often in immuncompromised patients (herpes simplex, CMV, HIV, progressive multifocal leukoencephalopathy) or immunocompetent (St Louis encephalitis, Eastern or Western equine encephalitis, Epstein-Barr virus).
Rasmussen's encephalitis (Fig. 1A.**138**)	Progressive atrophy of one cerebral hemisphere with poorly defined zones of high signal on T2WI involving the white matter, basal ganglia, and cortex. Usually no enhancement.	Usually seen in children below 10 years of age. Severe and progressive epilepsy and unilateral neurologic deficits–hemiplegia, psychomotor deterioration, chronic slow viral infectious process possibly caused by CMV or Epstein-Barr virus. Treatment: hemispherectomy.
Creutzfeld-Jakob disease (CJD)	Zones of high signal on T2WI in putamen and caudate nuclei bilaterally, with or without zones of high signal in white matter and cortex. Typically enhancement. Progressive cerebral atrophy.	Spongiform encephalopathy caused by slow infection from prion (proteinaceous infectious particle). Usually seen in adults aged 40–80 years. Progressive dementia. Les than 10% survive more than 2 years.
Tuberculoma (Fig. 1A.**39**)	Intra-axial lesions in cerebral hemispheres and basal ganglia (adults) and cerebellum (children). Low to intermediate signal on T1WI, central zone of high signal on T2WI with a thin peripheral rim of low signal, occasionally low signal on T2WI. Solid or rim Gd-contrast enhancement. With or without associated calcification. Meningeal lesions: nodular or cystic zones of basilar meningeal enhancement.	Occurs in immunocompromised patients and in developing countries. Caseating intracranial granulomas via hematogenous dissemination. Lesions more common in meninges than brain.
Parasitic brain lesions		
Toxoplasmosis (Fig. 1A.**40**)	Single or multiple solid and/or cystic lesions located in basal ganglia and/or corticomedullary junctions in cerebral hemispheres. Low to intermediate signal on T1WI; high signal on T2WI. Nodular or rim pattern of Gd-contrast enhancement, with or without peripheral high T2 signal (edema).	Most common opportunistic CNS infection in AIDS patients, caused by ingestion of food contaminated with parasites (*Toxoplasma gondii*).
Cysticercosis (Fig. 1A.**41**)	Single or multiple cystic lesions in brain or meninges. *Acute/subacute phase:* Low to intermediate signal on T1WI and high signal on T2WI. Rim and possible nodular pattern of Gd-contrast enhancement, with or without peripheral high T2 signal (edema). *Chronic Phase:* calcified granulomas.	Caused by ingestion of ova (*Taenia solium*) in contaminated food (undercooked pork). Involves in order of decreasing frequency: meninges, brain parenchyma, ventricles.

Table 1A.**7** (Cont.) Lesions involving gray matter/cerebral cortex

Disease	MRI Findings	Comments
Hydatid cyst	*Echinococcus granulosus:* Single or rarely multiple cystic lesions with low signal on T1WI and high signal on T2WI with a thin wall with low signal on T2WI; typically no Gd-contrast enhancement or peripheral edema unless superinfected. Often located in vascular territory of the middle cerebral artery. *Echinococcus multilocularis:* Cystic (possibly multilocular) and/or solid lesions. Central zone of low to intermediate signal on T1WI and T2WI, surrounded by a slightly thickened rim of low signal on T2WI; Gd-contrast enhancement. Peripheral zone of high signal on T2WI (edema) and calcifications are common.	Caused by parasites: *Echinococcus granulosus* (South America, Middle East Australia, New Zealand) or *Echinococcus multilocularis* (North America, Europe, Turkey, China). CNS involvement in 2% of cases of hydatid infestation.
Radiation injury/ necrosis (Fig. 1A.42), (Fig. 1A.97)	Focal lesion with or without mass effect, or poorly defined zone of low to intermediate signal on T1WI, intermediate to high signal on T2WI, with or without Gd-contrast enhancement involving tissue (gray matter and/or white matter) in field of treatment.	Usually occurs from 4–6 months to 10 years after radiation treatment. May be difficult to distinguish from neoplasm. PET and MRS might be helpful for evaluation.
Lysosomal enzyme defects (Fig. 1A.159)	*Tay-Sachs:* High signal on T2WI in caudate nuclei, putamen, and thalami, with or without high signal on T2WI in cerebral white matter. Progressive cerebral atrophy. *Neuronal ceroid–lipofuscinosis:* Progressive cerebral cortical atrophy. With or without low or high signal on T2WI in caudate, putamen, and thalami; with or without high signal on T2WI in white matter. Typically no Gd-contrast enhancement. *Mucopolysaccharidoses:* Foci or diffuse zones of high signal on T2WI in cerebral white matter; with or without foci of high signal on T2WI in corpus callosum and basal ganglia. Perivascular pits, cerebral cortical/subcortical infarcts, progressive cerebral atrophy. Macrocephaly, communicating hydrocephalus, meningeal thickening may be associated.	Lysosomal disorders result in axonal loss and demyelination related to toxic accumulation of abnormal metabolites within cells. These disorders are often autosomal recessive and include: Tay-Sachs disease from deficiency of functional hexosaminidase and neuronal ceroid lipofuscinosis with deposition of lipofuscin in cytosomes. Mucopolysaccharidoses represent another group of lysosomal disorders with abnormal metabolism of mucopolysaccharides and can be either autosomal recessive or X-linked. This group includes multiple types (Hurler, Hunter, Sanfilippo, Morquio syndromes).

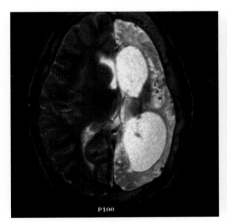

a

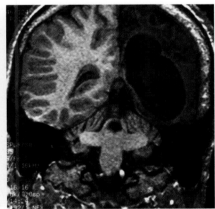

b

Fig. 1A.**138 Rasmussen's encephalitis. a** Axial T2WI shows severe atrophy of the left cerebral hemisphere with poorly defined zones of high signal involving the white matter, basal ganglia, and cerebral cortex. **b** Coronal (spoiled GRE) T1WI shows decreased signal involving the brain parenchyma with marked compensatory dilatation of the lateral ventricle.

Table 1A.**7** (Cont.) Lesions involving gray matter/cerebral cortex

Disease	MRI Findings	Comments
Other		
Mesial temporal sclerosis (Fig. 1A.139)	Signal abnormality involving the hippocampus (most easily seen involving the body more commonly than the head or tail). Low to intermediate signal on T1WI and high signal on T2WI; no abnormal Gd-contrast enhancement. With or without associated atrophy. Usually unilateral, bilateral in 15%.	Associated with temporal lobe epilepsy and used for surgical planning. High signal on T2WI associated with neuronal loss and gliosis.
Status epilepticus (Fig. 1A.140)	High signal on T2WI involving one or both hippocampi and amygdalae, temporal lobe cortex. With or without eventual reversal of high signal abnormality and eventual hippocampal atrophy and/or sclerosis.	Signal abnormality considered secondary to altered endogenous neurochemical reaction from seizure activity with cytoxic edema, and eventual neuronal necrosis
Alzheimer disease	Brain atrophy often most pronounced in temporal lobes. Sulcal and ventricular prominence. Cortical atrophic changes common.	Most common form of progressive dementia with neurofibrillary tangles, senile plaques, neuronal loss, amyloid angiopathy, gliosis.
Pick disease (Fig. 1A.141)	Brain atrophy often most pronounced in frontal and temporal lobes. Sulcal and ventricular prominence. Cortical atrophic changes common.	Acquired dementia much less common than Alzheimer disease. Histopathologic findings or neuronal loss and cytoplasmic inclusion bodies (Pick bodies).

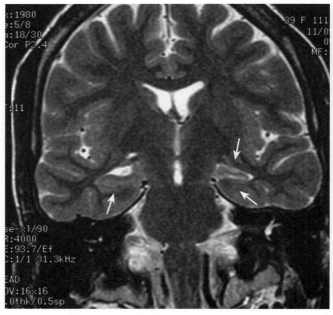 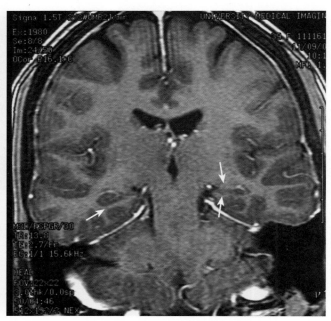

Fig. 1A.**139 Mesial temporal sclerosis. a** Coronal T2WI shows abnormal high signal at the left hippocampus (arrows). Note normal appearance of the right hippocampus (arrow).

Fig. 1A.**139 b** Coronal (spoiled GRE) T1WI shows prominent atrophy of the left hippocampus (arrows). Note normal size of the right hippocampus (arrow) for comparison.

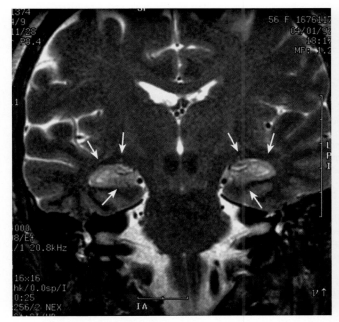 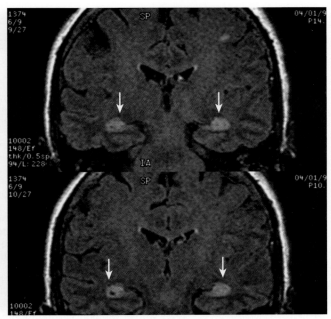

Fig. 1A.**140**   **Status epilepticus.   a** Coronal T2WI shows swelling and abnormal high signal at both hippocampi (arrows).

Fig. 1A.**140 b**   Coronal FLAIR images show symmetric abnormal high signal at both hippocampi (arrows).

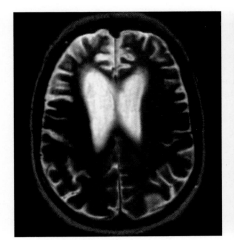 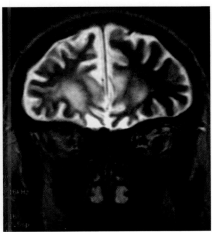

Fig. 1A.**141**   **Pick disease.** Axial (**a**) and coronal (**b**) T2WI show cerebral atrophy most pronounced involving the frontal lobes with cortical atrophy, sulcal and ventricular prominence.

Table 1A.8 Basal ganglia

Disease	MRI Findings	Comments
Neoplasms		
Astrocytoma (Fig. 1A.18–1A.21)	*Low-grade astrocytoma:* Focal or diffuse mass lesion usually located in white matter with low to intermediate signal on T1WI and high signal on T2WI, with or without mild Gd-contrast enhancement. Minimal associated mass effect. *Juvenile pilocytic astrocytoma:* Subtype: solid/cystic focal lesion with low to intermediate signal on T1WI and high signal on T2WI, usually with prominent Gd-contrast enhancement. Lesions located in cerebellum, hypothalamus, adjacent to third or fourth ventricles, brainstem. *Gliomatosis cerebri:* Infiltrative lesion with poorly defined margins with mass effect located in the white matter. Low to intermediate signal on T1WI and high signal on T2WI; usually no Gd-contrast enhancement until late in disease. *Anaplastic astrocytoma:* Often irregularly marginated lesion located in white matter with low to intermediate signal on T1WI and high signal on T2WI, with or without Gd-contrast enhancement.	*Low-grade astrocytoma:* Often occur in children and adults (age 20–40 years). Tumors comprised of well-differentiated astrocytes. Association with neurofibromatosis type 1. Ten-year survival. May become malignant. *Juvenile pilocytic astrocytoma:* Subtype: common in children, usually favorable prognosis if totally resected. *Gliomatosis cerebri:* Diffusely infiltrating astrocytoma with relative preservation of underlying brain architecture. Imaging appearance may be more prognostic than histologic grade. Approximate 2-year survival. *Anaplastic astrocytoma:* Intermediate between low-grade astrocytoma and glioblastoma multiforme. Approximate 2-year survival.
Glioblastoma multiforme (Fig. 1A.22)	Irregularly marginated mass lesion with necrosis or cyst. Mixed signal on T1WI and heterogeneous high signal on T2WI. Hemorrhage may be associated. Prominent heterogeneous Gd-contrast enhancement. Peripheral edema. Can cross corpus callosum.	Most common primary CNS tumor, highly malignant neoplasms with necrosis and vascular proliferation, usually in patients older than 50 years. Extent of lesion underestimated by MRI. Survival less than 1 year.
Giant cell astrocytoma-Tuberous sclerosis (Fig. 1A.23)	Circumscribed lesion located near the foramen of Monro with mixed low to intermediate signal on T1WI and mixed high signal on T2WI. Cysts and/or calcifications may be associated. Heterogenous Gd-contrast enhancement.	Subependymal hamartoma near foramen of Monro, occurs in 15 % of patients with tuberous sclerosis below 20 years of age. Slow-growing lesions that can progressively cause obstruction of CSF flow through the foramen of Monro. Long-term survival usual if resected.
Pleomorphic xanthoastrocytoma (Fig. 1A.24)	Circumscribed supratentorial lesion. Low to intermediate signal on T1WI and intermediate to high signal on T2WI. Cyst(s) may be associated. With or without heterogeneous Gd-contrast enhancement and enhancing mural nodule associated with cyst.	Rare type of astrocytoma occurring in young adults and children, associated with seizure history.
Oligodendroglioma (Fig. 1A.25)	Circumscribed lesion with mixed low to intermediate signal on T1WI and mixed intermediate to high signal on T2WI. Areas of signal void at sites of clump-like calcification. Heterogenous Gd-contrast enhancement.	Uncommon slow-growing gliomas with usually mixed histologic patterns (e.g., astrocytoma). Usually in adults older than 35 years of age, 85 % supratentorial. If low-grade 75 % 5-year survival; higher grade lesions have a worse prognosis.
Ganglioglioma, ganglioneuroma, gangliocytoma (Fig. 1A.27)	Circumscribed tumor. Usually supratentorial, often temporal or frontal lobes. Low to intermediate signal on T1WI and intermediate to high signal on T2WI. Cysts may be associated. With or without Gd-contrast enhancement.	Ganglioglioma (contains glial and neuronal elements), ganglioneuroma (contains only ganglion cells). Uncommon tumors, below 30 years, seizure presentation, slow-growing neoplasms. Gangliocytoma (contains only neuronal elements, dysplastic brain tissue). Favorable prognosis if completely resected.
Ependymoma (Fig. 1A.28)	Circumscribed lobulated supratentorial lesion, often extraventricular. Cysts and/or calcifications may be associated. Low to intermediate signal on T1WI; intermediate to high signal on T2WI. Variable Gd-contrast enhancement.	Occurs more commonly in children than adults. One-third supratentorial, two-thirds infratentorial. 45 % 5-year survival.
Lymphoma (Fig. 1A.28)	Primary CNS lymphoma: focal or infiltrating lesion located in the basal ganglia, periventricular regions, posterior fossa/brainstem. Low to intermediate signal on T1WI; intermediate to slightly high signal on T2WI. Hemorrhage/necrosis may be associated in immunocompromised patients. Usually Gd-contrast enhancement. Diffuse leptomeningeal enhancement is another pattern of intracranial lymphoma.	Primary CNS lymphoma more common than secondary, usually in adults above 40 years of age. B cell lymphoma more common than T cell lymphoma. Increasing incidence related to number of immunocompromised patients in population. MRI features of primary and secondary lymphoma of brain overlap. Intracranial lymphoma can involve the leptomeninges in secondary lymphoma more commonly than primary lymphoma.

Table 1A.**8** (Cont.) Basal ganglia

Disease	MRI Findings	Comments
Metastases (Fig. 1A.34), (Fig. 1A.92)	Circumscribed spheroid lesions in brain. Usually low to intermediate signal on T1WI and intermediate to high signal on T2WI. Hemorrhage, calcifications, cysts may be associated. Variable Gd-contrast enhancement. Often high signal on T2WI peripheral to nodular enhancing lesion representing axonal edema.	Represent approximately 33% of intracranial tumors, usually from extracranial primary neoplasm in adults older than 40 years. Primary tumor source in order of decreasing frequency: lung, breast, GI, GU, melanoma.
Neurofibromatosis type 1 (Fig. 1A.143)	Unilateral or bilateral circumscribed spheroid lesions with high signal on T2WI located in globus pallidus. Intermediate or slightly high signal on T1WI, typically no Gd-contrast enhancement. No associated edema or mass effect.	Neurofibromatosis type 1 is an autosomal dominant disorder (chromosome 17), the most common of the neurocutaneous syndromes (phakomatoses). Benign lesions seen in globus pallidus, sometimes referred to as "hamartomas," show histologic findings of spongiotic or vacuolar changes. May regress over time by serial MRI.

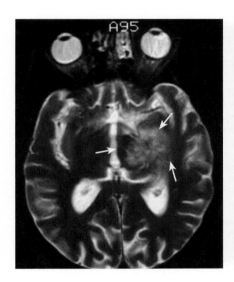
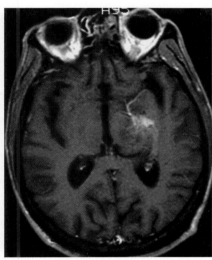

Fig. 1A.**142 Lymphoma. a** Axial T2WI shows a poorly defined lesion with high signal involving the left basal ganglia and thalamus (arrows).   **b** Postcontrast T1WI shows irregular enhancement at the lesion.

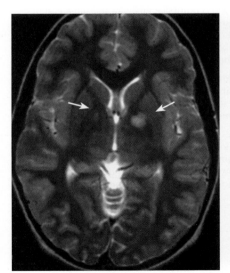
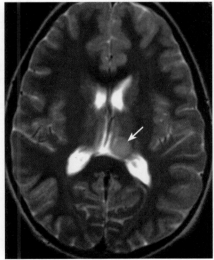
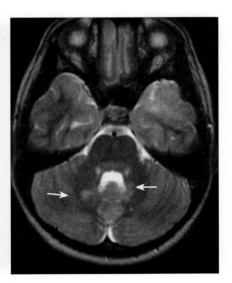

a   b   c

Fig. 1A.**143 Neurofibromatosis type 1.   a** Axial T2WI shows bilateral circumscribed spheroid lesions with high signal on T2WI located in each globus pallidus. Axial T2WI (**b, c**) show similar lesions (hamartomas) in the left thalamus and cerebellar white matter (arrows).

Table 1A.**8** (Cont.) Basal ganglia

Disease	MRI Findings	Comments
Neuroepithelial cyst (Fig. 1A.**134**)	Well-circumscribed cysts with low signal on T1WI and high signal on T2WI. Thin walls. No Gd-contrast enhancement or peripheral edema.	Cyst walls have histopathologic features similar to epithelium. Neuroepithelial cysts located in: choroid plexus, choroidal fissure, ventricles, brain parenchyma.
Perivascular spaces (Fig. 1A.**144**)	Focus or foci with signal similar to CSF with high signal on T2WI. Usually not apparent on proton density weighted images. Low signal on T1WI, no Gd-contrast enhancement. Located in the basal ganglia, high subcortical white matter/centrum semiovale.	Pial-lined spaces filled with CSF containing arteries supplying brain parenchyma, also referred to as Virchow-Robin spaces. Perivascular spaces increase in size and number with aging.
Infection/abscess		
Cerebritis (Fig. 1A.**35**)	Poorly defined zone or focal area of low to intermediate signal on T1WI and intermediate to high signal on T2WI; minimal or no Gd-contrast enhancement. Involves cerebral cortex and white matter for bacterial and fungal infections.	Focal infection/inflammation of brain tissue from bacteria or fungi, secondary to sinusitis, meningitis, surgery, hematogenous source (cardiac and other vascular shunts) and/or immunocompromised status. Can progress to abscess formation.
Pyogenic brain abscess (Fig. 1A.**36**)	Circumscribed lesion with low signal on T1WI; central zone of high signal on T2WI (air-fluid level may be present) surrounded by a thin rim of low T2 signal; peripheral poorly defined zone of high signal on T2WI representing edema. Ring-like Gd-contrast enhancement that is sometimes thicker laterally than medially.	Formation of brain abscess occurs 2 weeks after cerebritis with liquefaction and necrosis centrally surrounded by a capsule and peripheral edema. Can be multiple. Complication from meningitis and/or sinusitis, septicemia, trauma, surgery, cardiac shunt.
Fungal brain infection/abscess (Fig. 1A.**145**), (Fig. 1A.**37**)	Vary depending on organism. Lesions occur in meninges and brain parenchyma; solid or cystic lesions with low to intermediate signal on T2WI and high signal on T2WI. Nodular or ring enhancement. Peripheral high signal in brain lesions on T2WI (edema).	Occur in immunocompromised or diabetic patients with resultant granulomas in meninges and brain parenchyma; Cryptococcus involves the basal meninges and extends along perivascular spaces into the basal ganglia; *Aspergillus* and *Mucor* spread via direct extension through paranasal sinuses or hematogenously invade blood vessels resulting in hemorrhagic lesions and/or cerebral infarcts. Coccidiomycosis usually involves the basal meninges.
Encephalitis (Fig. 1A.**38**)	Poorly defined zone of low to intermediate signal on T1WI and intermediate to high signal on T2WI; minimal or no Gd-contrast enhancement. Involves cerebral cortex and/or white matter, minimal localized mass effect. Herpes simplex typically involves the temporal lobes/limbic system. Hemorrhage may be associated. CMV usually in periventricular location.	Encephalitis: infection/inflammation of brain tissue from viruses, often in immuncompromised patients (herpes simplex, CMV, progressive multifocal leukoencephalopathy) or immunocompetent (St Louis encephalitis, Eastern or Western equine encephalitis, Epstein-Barr virus).
Rasmussen's encephalitis (Fig. 1A.**138**)	Progressive atrophy of one cerebral hemisphere with poorly defined zones of high signal on T2WI involving the white matter, basal ganglia, and cortex. Usually no enhancement.	Usually seen in children below 10 years of age. Severe and progressive epilepsy and unilateral neurologic deficits–hemiplegia, psychomotor deterioration, chronic slow viral infectious process possibly caused by CMV or Epstein-Barr virus. Treatment: hemispherectomy.
Creutzfeldt-Jakob disease	Zones of high signal on T2WI in putamen and caudate nuclei bilaterally. With or without zones of high signal in white matter and cortex. Typically enhancement. Progressive cerebral atrophy.	Spongiform encephalopathy caused by slow infection from prion (proteinaceous infectious particle). Usually seen in adults aged 40–80 years. Progressive dementia. Les than 10% survive more than 2 years.
Tuberculoma (Fig. 1A.**39**)	Intra-axial lesions in cerebral hemispheres and basal ganglia (adults), cerebellum (children).Low to intermediate signal on T1WI, central zone of high signal on T2WI with a thin peripheral rim of low signal, occasionally low signal on T2WI. Solid or rim Gd-contrast enhancement. Calcification may be present. Meningeal lesions: nodular or cystic zones of basilar meningeal enhancement.	Occurs in immunocompromised patients and in developing countries. Caseating intracranial granulomas via hematogenous dissemination. Lesions more common in meninges than brain.

Table 1A.**8** (Cont.) Basal ganglia

Disease	MRI Findings	Comments
Parasitic brain lesions		
Toxoplasmosis (Fig. 1A.**40**)	Single or multiple solid and/or cystic lesions located in basal ganglia and/or corticomedullary junctions in cerebral hemispheres. Low to intermediate signal on T1WI; high signal on T2WI. Nodular or rim pattern of Gd-contrast enhancement, with or without peripheral high T2 signal (edema).	Most common opportunistic CNS infection in AIDS patients, caused by ingestion of food contaminated with parasites (*Toxoplasma gondii*).
Cysticercosis (Fig. 1A.**41**)	Single or multiple cystic lesions in brain or meninges. *Acute/subacute phase:* Low to intermediate signal on T1WI and high signal on T2WI. Rim and possible nodular pattern of Gd-contrast enhancement. With or without peripheral high T2 signal (edema). *Chronic phase:* calcified granulomas.	Caused by ingestion of ova (*Taenia solium*) in contaminated food (undercooked pork). Involves in order of decreasing frequency: meninges, brain parenchyma, ventricles.

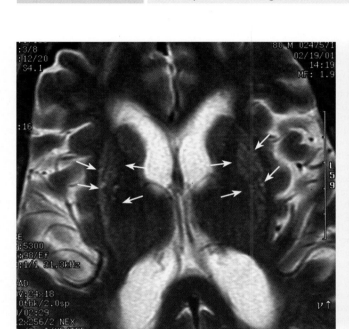

Fig. 1A.**144** **Perivascular spaces.** **a** Axial T2WI shows multiple small foci with signal similar to CSF in each putamen (arrows).

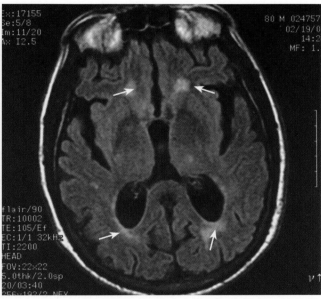

Fig. 1A.**144 b** Axial FLAIR image shows no foci of high signal within either putamen. Note zones of high signal in the periventricular white matter, consistent with small vessel ischemic disease (arrows).

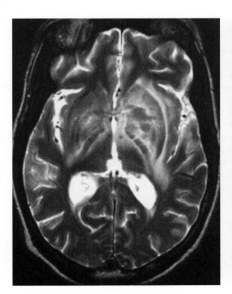

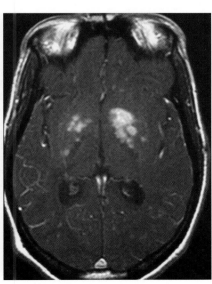

Fig. 1A.**145** **Cryptococcus infection.** **a** Axial T2WI shows poorly defined zones of high signal in the region of the basal ganglia bilaterally. **b** Postcontrast axial T1WI shows nodular and confluent zones of enhancement in the basal ganglia resulting from spread of infection along perivascular spaces.

Table 1A.**8** (Cont.) Basal ganglia

Disease	MRI Findings	Comments
Hydatid cyst	*Echinococcus granulosus:* Single or rarely multiple cystic lesions with low signal on T1WI and high signal on T2WI with a thin wall with low signal on T2WI; typically no Gd-contrast enhancement or peripheral edema unless superinfected. Often located in vascular territory of the middle cerebral artery. *Echinococcus multilocularis:* Cystic (possibly multilocular) and/or solid lesions. Central zone of low to intermediate signal on T1WI and T2WI, surrounded by a slightly thickened rim of low signal on T2WI; Gd-contrast enhancement. Peripheral zone of high signal on T2WI (edema) and calcifications are common.	Caused by parasites: *Echinococcus granulosus* (South America, Middle East Australia, New Zealand) or *Echinococcus multilocularis* (North America, Europe, Turkey, China).CNS involvement in 2% of cases of hydatid infestation.
Radiation necrosis (Fig. 1A.42), (Fig. 1A.91)	Focal lesion with or without mass effect, or poorly defined zone of low to intermediate signal on T1WI, intermediate to high signal on T2WI, with or without Gd-contrast enhancement involving tissue (gray matter and/or white matter) in field of treatment.	Usually occurs from 4–6 months to 10 years after radiation treatment. May be difficult to distinguish from neoplasm. PET and MRS might be helpful for evaluation.
Vascular		
AVM (Fig. 1A.47)	Lesions with irregular margins that can be located in the brain parenchyma–pia, dura, or both locations. AVMs contain multiple tortuous tubular flow voids on T1WI and T2WI secondary to patent arteries with high blood flow; as well as thrombosed vessels with variable signal. Areas of hemorrhage in various phases, calcifications, and gliosis. The venous portions often show Gd-contrast enhancement. GRE MRI shows flow-related enhancement (high signal) in patent arteries and veins of the AVM. MRA using TOF or phase contrast techniques can provide additional detailed information about the nidus, feeding arteries, and draining veins, and presence of associated aneurysms. Usually not associated with mass effect except in cases of recent hemorrhage or venous occlusion.	Infratentorial AVMs are much less common than supratentorial AVMs.
Cavernous hemangioma (Fig. 1A.48)	Single or multiple multilobulated intra-axial lesions that have a peripheral rim or irregular zone of low signal on T2WI secondary to hemosiderin, surrounding a central zone of variable signal (low, intermediate, high, or mixed) on T1WI and T2WI, depending on ages of hemorrhagic portions. GRE techniques useful for detecting multiple lesions.	Infratentorial lesions are less common than supratentorial lesions. Can be found in many different locations. Multiple lesions more than 50%. Association with venous angiomas and risk of hemorrhage.
Venous angioma (Fig. 1A.49)	On postcontrast T1WI, venous angiomas are seen as a Gd-contrast-enhancing transcortical vein draining a collection of small medullary veins (caput Medusa). The draining vein can be seen as a signal on T2WI.	Considered an anomalous venous formation, typically not associated with hemorrhage. Usually an incidental finding except when associated with cavernous hemangioma.
Moyamoya (Fig. 1A.146)	Multiple tortuous tubular flow voids seen in the basal ganglia and thalami on T1WI and T2WI secondary to dilated collateral arteries. Enhancement of these arteries related to slow flow within these collateral arteries versus normal-sized arteries. Often, Gd-contrast enhancement of the leptomeninges related to pial collateral vessels. Decreased or absent flow voids involving the supraclinoid portions of the internal carotid arteries and proximal middle and anterior cerebral arteries. MRA shows stenosis and occlusion of the distal internal carotid arteries with collateral arteries (lenticulostriate, thalamoperforate, and leptomeningeal) best seen after contrast administration, enabling detection of slow blood flow.	Progressive occlusive disease of the intracranial portions of the internal carotid arteries with resultant numerous dilated collateral arteries arising from the lenticulostriate and thalamoperforate arteries as well as other parenchymal, leptomeningeal, and transdural arterial anastomoses. Term translated as "puff of smoke," referring to the angiographic appearance of the collateral arteries (lenticulostriate, thalamoperforate). Usually nonspecific etiology but can be associated with neurofibromatosis, radiation angiopathy, atherosclerosis, sickle cell disease. In Asia, usually more common in children than adults.

Table 1A.**8** (Cont.) Basal ganglia

Disease	MRI Findings	Comments
Demyelinating disorders **Demyelinating disease– MS, ADEM (Fig. 1A.53), (Fig. 1A.54)**	Lesions located in cerebral or cerebellar white matter, brainstem, basal ganglia. Usually low to intermediate signal on T1WI and high signal on T2WI. With or without Gd-contrast enhancement. Enhancement can be ring-like or nodular, usually in acute/early subacute phase of demyelination. Lesions rarely can have associated mass effect simulating neoplasms.	MS is the most common acquired demyelinating disease usually affecting women (peak age 20–40 years). Other demyelinating diseases include: ADEM–immune mediated demyelination after viral infection; toxins (exogenous from environmental exposure or ingestion–alcohol, solvents etc.–or endogenous from metabolic disorder–leukodystrophies, mitochondrial encephalopathies, etc.), radiation injury, trauma, vascular disease.

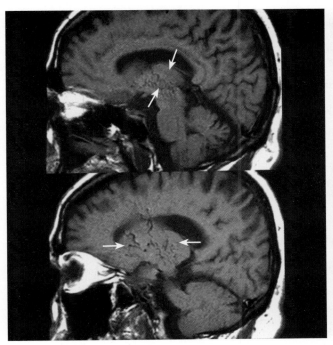

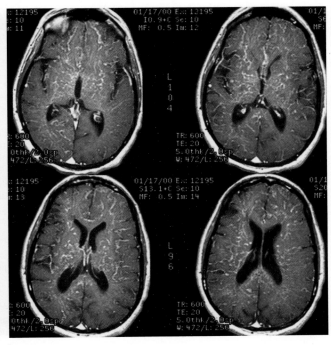

a

b

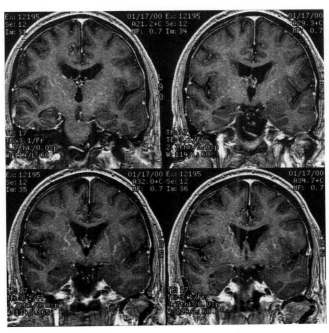

c

Fig. 1A.**146** **Moyamoya.** **a** Sagittal T1WI shows multiple tortuous tubular flow voids in the basal ganglia and thalami (arrows). **b** Postcontrast axial T1WI shows multiple small enhancing blood vessels in the lenticulostriate and thalamoperforate distributions, as well as leptomeningeal collateral vessels secondary to occlusion of the supraclinoid portions of the internal carotid arteries. **c** Postcontrast coronal (spoiled GRE) T1WI show the multiple small enhancing vessels in the basal ganglia.

Table 1A.8 (Cont.) Basal ganglia

Disease	MRI Findings	Comments
Cerebral infarct (Fig. 1A.**147**)		
Ischemic anoxic or lacunar infarcts	MRI features of cerebral infarcts depend on age of infarct relative to time of examination. *<12 hours:* Localized edema, usually isointense signal to normal brain on T1WI and T2WI. Diffusion weighted images can show positive findings related to decreased apparent diffusion coefficients secondary to cytotoxic edema. Absence of arterial flow void or arterial enhancement in the vascular distribution of the infarct. *12–24 hours:* Intermediate signal on T1WI and high signal on T2WI. Localized edema. Signal abnormalities commonly involve the cerebral cortex and subcortical white matter and/or basal ganglia. *24 hours to 3 days:* Low to intermediate signal on T1WI, high signal on T2WI. Localized edema. Hemorrhage may be associated. With or without enhancement. *4 days to 2 weeks:* Low to intermediate signal on T1WI, high signal on T2WI. Edema/mass effect diminishing. Hemorrhage may be associated. With or without enhancement. *2 weeks to 2 months:* Low to intermediate signal on T1WI, high signal on T2WI. Edema resolves. Hemorrhage may be associated. Enhancement may eventually decline. *>2 months:* Low signal on T1WI, high signal on T2WI. Encephalomalacic changes. Calcification, hemosiderin may be present.	Cerebral infarcts usually result from occlusive vascular disease involving large, medium, or small arteries. Vascular occlusion may be secondary to: atheromatous arterial disease, hypertension, cardiogenic emboli, neoplastic encasement, hypercoagulable states, dissection, or congenital anomalies or inherited disorders such as CADASIL. Cerebral infarcts usually result from arterial occlusion involving specific vascular territories; occasionally result from metabolic disorders (e.g., mitochondrial encephalopathies) or intracranial venous occlusion (e.g., thrombophlebitis, hypercoagulable states, dehydration) that do not correspond to arterial distributions.
Toxic		
Common monoxide poisoning	High signal on T2WI in putamen and globus pallidus bilaterally. No enhancement.	Toxic effects with selective necrosis of basal ganglia bilaterally.
Methanol intoxication *Metabolic/ Degenerative*	High signal on T2WI in putamen and globus pallidus bilaterally. No enhancement.	Toxic effects with selective necrosis of basal ganglia bilaterally.
MELAS and MERRF syndromes (Fig. 1A.**148**), (Fig. 1A.**160**)	High T2 signal in basal ganglia usually symmetric, high T2 signal in cerebral and cerebellar cortex and subcortical white matter not corresponding to a specific large arterial vascular territory. Signal abnormalities may resolve and reappear.	MELAS (Mitochondrial Encephalopathy, Lactic Acidosis, and Stroke-like events) is a maternally inherited disease affecting transfer RNA in mitochondria. MERRF (Myoclonic Epilepsy, Ragged Red Fibers) is a mitochondrial encephalopathy associated with muscle weakness and myoclonic epilepsy, short stature, ophthalmoplegia, cardiac disease.
Leigh disease (Fig. 1A.**149**)	Symmetric high signal on T2WI in globus pallidus, putamen, and caudate as well as high signal on T2WI in thalami, cerebral and cerebellar white matter, cerebellar cortex, brainstem, and spinal-cord gray matter. Typically no Gd-contrast enhancement.	Autosomal recessive disorder also referred to as subacute necrotizing encephalopathy, occurring in three forms (infantile, juvenile, and adult-onset type). Etiology related to abnormalities in oxidative metabolism in mitochondria from one of several defective enzymes, progressive neurodegenerative disease. Lesions in brainstem are associated with loss of respiratory control.
Kearns-Sayre syndrome (Fig. 1A.**161**)	Symmetric high signal on T2WI in globus pallidus, putamen, and caudate as well as high signal on T2WI in thalami, cerebral and cerebellar white matter, cerebellar cortex, and brainstem. Typically no Gd-contrast enhancement.	Mitochondrial disorder associated with external ophthalmoplegia, retinitis pigmentosa, and onset of clinical muscular and neurologic signs below 20 years.
Cockayne syndrome (Fig. 1A.**150**)	High signal on T2WI involving the periventricular white matter, basal ganglia, and dentate nuclei. Calcifications in basal ganglia and dentate nuclei, progressive cerebral and cerebellar atrophy, microcephaly.	Autosomal recessive disorder with deficient repair mechanisms for DNA. Presents in first decade with progressive neurologic dysfunction, cataracts, cutaneous photosensitivity, optic atrophy, and dwarfism.
Wilson disease (Fig. 1A.**151**)	High signal on T2WI in the putamen bilaterally as well as in the thalami, dentate nuclei, and brainstem (periaqueductal). Low signal on T2WI can also be seen in the caudate and putamen.	Autosomal recessive disease manifesting by decreased functional serum ceruloplasmin levels and altered copper metabolism with increased urinary excretion of copper. Usually presents in childhood with abnormal toxic copper deposition in tissues, resulting in cirrhosis, and degenerative changes in the basal ganglia (lentiform nuclei) and brainstem.

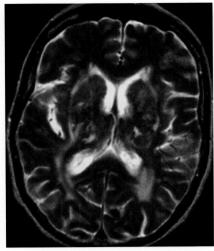

Fig. 1A.**147**   **Infarcts in the basal ganglia/ small vessel disease.** Axial T2WI shows multiple foci of high signal in the basal ganglia bilaterally as well as in the internal and extenal capsules, thalami, and periventricular white matter.

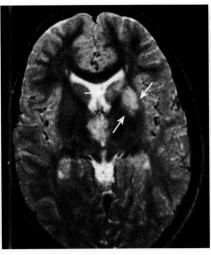

Fig. 1A.**148**   **MELAS.** Axial T2WI shows abormal high signal in the left caudate head and left putamen-corpus striatum (arrows).

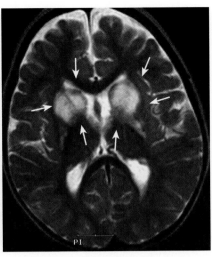

Fig. 1A.**149**   **Leigh disease.** Axial T2WI shows abnormal high signal involving the globus pallidus, putamen and caudate bilaterally, also localized edema (arrows).

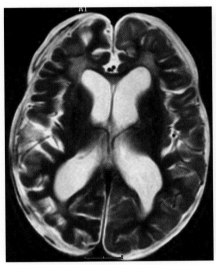

Fig. 1A.**150**   **Cockayne syndrome.   a** Axial T2WI shows mixed intermediate and low signal in the basal ganglia as well as zones of high signal in the cerebral white matter. Small subdural effusions are present bilaterally.

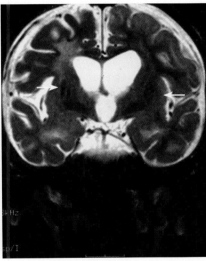

Fig. 1A.**150 b**   Coronal T2WI shows mixed intermediate and low signal (calcifications) in the basal ganglia (arrows).

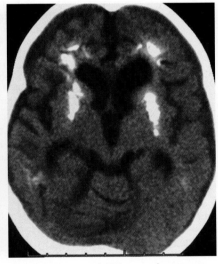

Fig. 1A.**150 c**   Axial CT image shows prominent calcifications in the basal ganglia and cerebral white matter as well as cerebral atrophy.

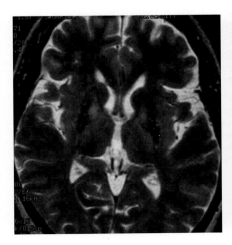

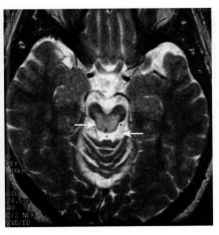

Fig. 1A.**151**   **Wilson disease.   a** Axial T2WI shows foci of high signal in the globus pallidus bilaterally and low signal in the putamina.   **b** Axial T2WI shows abnormal high signal in the periaqueductal portion of the midbrain (arrows).

Table 1A.8 (Cont.) Basal ganglia

Disease	MRI Findings	Comments
Shy-Drager syndrome	Low signal on T2WI in putamen, equal to or more pronounced than in the globus pallidus.	Autonomic dysfunction in adults with orthostatic hypotension, cerebellar and extrapyramidal clinical signs.
Hallervorden-Spatz disease (Fig. 1A.152)	Low signal with or without areas of high signal on T2WI in the globus pallidus bilaterally; no Gd-contrast enhancement.	Rare metabolic disorder with onset usually in childhood with progressive limb rigidity and gait dysfunction, dysarthria, and mental deterioration. Increased iron deposition and destruction of globus pallidus and substantia nigra bilaterally.
Pelizaeus-Merzbacher disease	Heterogeneneous or diffuse high signal on T2WI in cerebral white matter. May or may not involve cerebellum, brainstem. With or without low signal on T2WI in basal ganglia, thalami. No Gd-contrast enhancement. Progressive atrophy.	X-linked (type 1) or autosomal recessive (type 2) leukodystrophy. Five subtypes. Deficiency of proteolipid component of myelin. Presentation during neonatal period (type 2) and infancy (type 1) with abnormal eye movements, nystagmus, delayed psychomotor development, death in first decade; more common in males than females.
Lysosomal enzyme defects (Fig. 1A.159)	*Tay-Sachs:* High signal on T2WI in caudate nuclei, putamen, and thalami with or without high signal on T2WI in cerebral white matter. Progressive cerebral atrophy. *Neuronal ceroid–lipofuscinosis:* Progressive cerebral cortical atrophy. With or without low or high signal on T2WI in caudate, putamen, and thalami; with or without high signal on T2WI in white matter. Typically no Gd-contrast enhancement. *Mucopolysaccharidoses:* Foci or diffuse zones of high signal on T2WI in cerebral white matter; with or without foci of high signal on T2WI in corpus callosum and basal ganglia. Perivascular pits, cerebral cortical/subcortical infarcts, progressive cerebral atrophy. Macrocephaly, communicating hydrocephalus, and meningeal thickening may be associated.	Lysosomal disorders result in axonal loss and demyelination related to toxic accumulation of abnormal metabolites within cells. These disorders are often autosomal recessive and include: Tay-Sachs disease from deficiency of functional hexosaminidase and neuronal ceroid lipofuscinosis with deposition of lipofuscin in cytosomes. Mucopolysaccharidoses represent another group of lysosomal disorders with abnormal metabolism of mucopolysaccharides and can be either autosomal recessive or X-linked. This group includes multiple types (Hurler, Hunter, Sanfilippo, Morquio syndromes).
Disorders of amino acid metabolism (Phenylketonuria, propionic acidemia, methymalonic aciduria, homocystinuria, ornithine transcarbamoylase deficiency, leucinosis, maple syrup urine disease, glutaric acidemia, others)	High signal on T2WI in cerebral and/or cerebellar white matter, with or without high signal on T2WI in globus pallidi, putamen, caudate, thalami, brainstem.	Autosomal recessive disorders involving defective enzymes regulating amino acid metabolism and mitochodrial function. These enzymatic defects can cause significant alteration of myelin formation.
Idiopathic calcification	Low, intermediate, or high signal on T1WI and T2WI in basal ganglia. No enhancement.	Signal of calcium deposition can vary depending on size and configuration of deposits. Calcifications can also occur in basal ganglia secondary to endocrine abnormalities involving calcium (hypoparathyroidism) or iron metabolism, prior inflammatory disease (e.g., toxoplasmosis, tuberculosis, cystercerosis), prior ischemic disease or prior toxic exposure (e.g., lead intoxication, carbon monoxide).
Hepatocellular degeneration (Fig. 1A.153)	High signal on T1WI in basal ganglia. No enhancement.	Signal abnormality related to hepatic dysfunction possibly related to increased serum ammonia and manganese levels. The signal hyperintensity may reverse after liver transplantation.
Huntington disease (Fig. 1A.154)	Disproportionate atrophy of basal ganglia (in order of decreasing frequency: caudate, putamen, cerebellum/brainstem). Variable low or high signal changes on T2WI involving the putamen bilaterally. Usually no enhancement.	Autosomal dominant neurodegenerative disease usually presenting after 40 years with progressive movement disorders, behavioral and mental dysfunction.

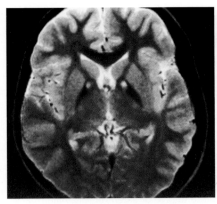

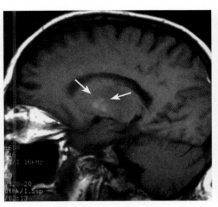

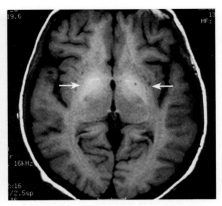

Fig. 1A.**152   Hallervorden-Spatz disease.** Axial T2WI shows foci of high signal in the globus pallidus bilaterally, surrounded by low signal.

Fig. 1A.**153   Hepatocellular degeneration.** Sagittal T1WI shows zones of high signal in the (**a**)

Fig. 1A.**153 b**   (**b**) basal ganglia (arrows).

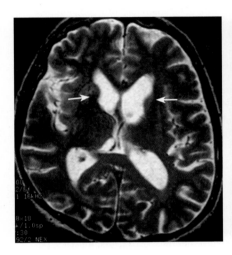

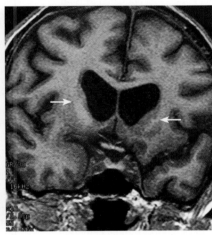

Fig. 1A.**154   Huntington disease.   a** Axial T2WI shows atrophy of the caudate nuclei (arrows) with enlargement of the frontal horns of the lateral ventricles. Atrophic changes are also seen involving the lentiform nuclei. Small zones of high signal are also seen in the caudate nuclei and putamina.   **b** Coronal (spoiled GRE) T1WI shows prominent atrophy of the caudate nuclei (arrows).

Table 1A.**9** Multiple or diffuse lesions involving white matter

Disease	MRI Findings	Comments
Congenital neuronal migration disorders		
Lissencephaly (Fig. 1A.**3**)	Absent or incomplete formation of gyri and sulci with shallow sylvian fissures and "figure 8" appearance of brain on axial images. Abnormally thick cortex, gray matter heterotopia with smooth gray-white matter interface.	Severe disorder of neuronal migration (7–16 weeks of gestation) with absent or incomplete formation of gyri, sulci, and sylvian fissures. Associated with severe mental retardation and seizures, early death. Other associated CNS anomalies include dysgenesis of corpus callosum, microcephaly, hypoplastic thalami, cephaloceles.
Pachygyria (non-lissencephalic cortical dysplasia) (Fig. 1A.**4**)	Thick gyri with shallow sulci involving all or portions of the brain. Thickened cortex with relatively smooth gray-white interface, may have areas of high T2 signal in the white matter (gliosis).	Severe disorder of neuronal migration. Clinical findings related to degree of extent of this malformation.
Gray matter heterotopia (Figs. 1A.**5**–1A.**7**)	*Laminar heterotopia:* appears as band(s) of isointense gray matter within the cerebral white matter (Fig. 1A.**5**). *Nodular heterotopia:* appears as nodule(s) of isointense gray matter along the ventricles (Fig. 1A.**6**) or within the cerebral white matter (Fig. 1A.**7**).	Disorder of neuronal migration (7–22 weeks of gestation) where a collection or layer of neurons is located beween the ventricles and cerebral cortex. Can have a band-like (laminar) or nodular appearance isointense to gray matter, may be unilateral or bilateral. Associated with seizures, schizencephaly.
Schizencephaly (split brain) (Figs. 1A.**8**, 1A.**9**)	Cleft in brain extending from ventricle to cortical surface lined by heterotopic gray matter. Cleft may be narrow (closed lip, Fig. 1A.**8**) or wide (open lip, Fig. 1A.**9**).	Association with seizures, blindness, retardation, and other CNS anomalies (e.g., septo-optic dysplasia). Clinical manifestations related to severity of malformation. Ischemia or insult to portion or germinal matrix before hemisphere formation.
Unilateral hemi-megalencephaly (Fig. 1A.**10**)	Nodular or multinodular region of gray matter heterotopia involving all or part of a cerebral hemisphere with associated enlargement of the ipsilateral lateral ventricle and hemisphere.	Neuronal migration disorder associated with hamartomatous overgrowth of the involved hemisphere.
Disorders of histogenesis		
Neurofibromatosis type 1 (Fig. 1A.**143**)	Poorly defined zones of high signal on T2WI located in cerebral and/or cerebellar white matter, globus pallidus. Intermediate or slightly high signal on T1WI; typically no Gd-contrast enhancement. No associated edema or mass effect.	Neurofibromatosis type 1 is an autosomal dominant disorder (chromosome 17), the most common of the neurocutaneous syndromes (phakomatoses). Lesions involve neurons, astrocytes, muscles, peripheral nerves (neurofibromas), dura (dural ectasia), bones. Benign lesions seen in cerebral or cerebellar white matter, sometimes referred to as "hamartomas," show histologic findings of spongiotic or vacuolar changes. May regress over time by serial MRI.
Tuberous sclerosis (Fig. 1A.**29**)	Foci and/or confluent zones of high signal on T2WI in cerebral white matter. Gd-contrast enhancement seen in approximately 10%.	Non-malignant lesions in white matter associated with tuberous sclerosis, consisting of areas of demyelination and/or dysplastic white matter along pathways of radial glial fibers during neuronal migration.
Congenital dysmyelinating disorders		
Alexander disease	High signal on T2WI involving the peripheral frontal white matter with progressive involvement of the white matter posteriorly and centrally (internal and external capsules). Typically no Gd-contrast enhancement. Associated with increases in size and weight of brain tissue.	Sporadic leukoencephalopathy, also referred to as fibrinoid leukoencephalopathy, presents in first year of life with macrocephaly, progressive psychomotor retardation. Often resulting in death during early childhood; also juvenile and adult forms.
Canavan-van Bogaert disease	High signal on T2WI involving the peripheral cerebral and cerebellar white matter diffusely with progressive involvement of the white matter centrally and subsequent atrophy. May or may not involve the globus pallidus. Typically no Gd-contrast enhancement. Associated with increases in size and weight of brain tissue. Enlarged NAA peak on H MR spectroscopy.	Autosomal recessive (common in Ashkenazi Jews). Spongy degeneration disorder of the brain caused by deficiency of aspartoacyclase resulting in N-acetyl aspartic aciduria and deposits in brain and plasma. Presents in infancy with macrocephaly, hypotonia, seizures, spasticity, optic atrophy. Death often occurs in second year.
Cockayne syndrome (Fig. 1A.**155**)	High signal on T2WI involving the periventricular white matter, basal ganglia, and dentate nuclei. Calcifications in basal ganglia and dentate nuclei, progressive cerebral and cerebellar atrophy, microcephaly.	Autosomal recessive disorder with deficient repair mechanisms for DNA. Presents in first decade with progressive neurologic dysfunction, cataracts, cutaneous photosensitivity, optic atrophy, and dwarfism.

Table 1A.**9** (Cont.) Multiple or diffuse lesions involving white matter

Disease	MRI Findings	Comments
Pelizaeus-Merzbacher disease	Heterogeneneous or diffuse high signal on T2WI in cerebral white matter. May or may not involve cerebellum, brainstem. With or without low signal on T2WI in basal ganglia, thalami. No Gd-contrast enhancement. Progressive atrophy.	X-linked (type 1) or autosomal recessive (type 2) leukodystrophy. Five subtypes. Deficiency of prote-olipid component of myelin. Presentation during neonatal period (type 2) and infancy (type 1) with abnormal eye movements, nystagmus, delayed psy-chomotor development, death in first decade; more common in males than females.
Metachromatic leukodystrophy (Fig. 1A.156)	Symmetric diffuse zones of low signal on T1WI and high signal on T2WI in deep cerebral/periventricular white matter with progression of abnormal signal peripherally to involve the subcortical white matter. High signal on T2WI involving the cerebellar white matter; with or without low signal on T2WI involv-ing the thalami; no Gd-contrast enhancement. Pro-gressive atrophy.	Autosomal recessive disease with deficiency of aryl-sulfatase in lysosomes resulting in toxic accumula-tion of ceramide sulfatide (myelin breakdown pro-duct) in macrophages and Schwann cells. Three subtypes depending on onset (late infantile form 80%, juvenile form, and adult form). Progressive neurologic deterioration with peripheral neu-ropathy, gait disorders, cognitive dysfunction lead-ing to death.

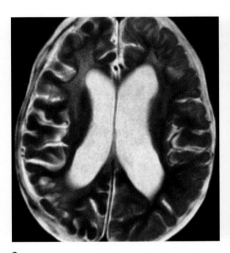

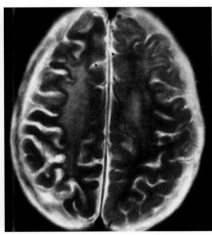

a **b**

**Fig. 1A.155 Cockayne syndrome.
a, b** Axial T2WI show poorly defined zones of high signal involving the periventricular and subcortical white matter associated with cerebral atrophy.

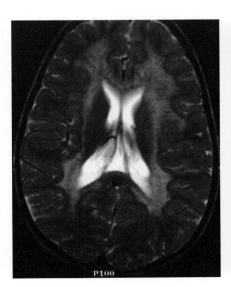

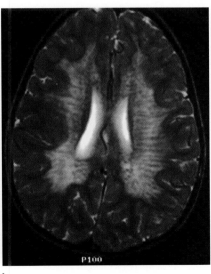

a **b**

Fig. 1A.156 Metachromatic leukodystro-phy. a, b Axial T2WI shows symmetric diffuse zones of high signal in the per-iventricular white matter, extending periph-erally toward the subcortical white matter.

Table 1A.**9** (Cont.) Multiple or diffuse lesions involving white matter

Disease	MRI Findings	Comments
Childhood adrenoleukodystrophy (Fig. 1A.157)	Diffuse abnormal high signal on T2WI usually with corresponding low signal on T1WI in parieto-occipital white matter and corpus callosum. Progression of signal abnormality to the remaining cerebral white matter. With or without enhancement at regions of active demyelination/inflammation. With or without high signal on T2WI in lateral geniculate bodies and corticospinal tracts.	X-linked recessive leukodystrophy (males) with functional deficiency of the peroxisomal enzyme acyl-CoA synthetase, resulting in abnormal metabolism and breakdown of very long chain fatty acids. These fatty acids accumulate in many tissues including the brain with resultant demyelination, inflammation, gliosis, and necrosis. Onset age 3–10 years with psychomotor retardation, seizures, hypotonia, facial dysmorphism, progressive deterioration. Also other subtypes (neonatal-onset, adult-onset).
Krabbe disease (Fig. 1A.158)	Symmetric confluent zones of high signal on T2WI involving the periventricular white matter with progressive involvement toward the subcortical white matter. More involvement of cerebral white matter than cerebellar white matter, No Gd-contrast enhancement. Progressive cerebral atrophy.	Also known as globoid cell leukodysrophy. Autosomal recessive disorder with deficiency of lysosomal enzyme galactocerebroside beta-galactosidase, resulting in destruction of oligodendrocytes/myelin production. Three subtypes (infantile [most common], late infantile, and adult-onset). Seizures, psychomotor dysfunction, optic atrophy, progressive neurologic deterioration leading to death.
Lysosomal enzyme defects (Fig. 1A.159)	*Tay-Sachs:* High signal on T2WI in caudate nuclei, putamen, and thalami with or without high signal on T2WI in cerebral white matter. Progressive cerebral atrophy. *Neuronal ceroid–lipofuscinosis:* Progressive cerebral cortical atrophy. With or without low or high signal on T2WI in caudate, putamen, and thalami; with or without high signal on T2WI in white matter. Typically no Gd-contrast enhancement. *Mucopolysaccharidoses:* Foci or diffuse zones of high signal on T2WI in cerebral white matter; with or without foci of high signal on T2WI in corpus callosum and basal ganglia. Perivascular pits, cerebral cortical/subcortical infarcts, progressive cerebral atrophy. Macrocephaly, communicating hydrocephalus, and meningeal thickening may be associated.	Lysosomal disorders result in axonal loss and demyelination related to toxic accumulation of abnormal metabolites within cells. These disorders are often autosomal recessive and include: Tay-Sachs disease from deficiency of functional hexosaminidase and neuronal ceroid lipofuscinosis with deposition of lipofuscin in cytosomes. Mucopolysaccharidoses represent another group of lysosomal disorders with abnormal metabolism of mucopolysaccharides and can be either autosomal recessive or X-linked. This group includes multiple types (Hurler, Hunter, Sanfilippo, Morquio syndromes).
Metabolic Disorders Disorders of amino acid metabolism (Phenylketonuria, propionic acidemia, methymalonic aciduria, homocystinuria, ornithine transcarbamyolase deficiency, leucinosis, maple syrup urine disease, glutaric acidemia, others)	High signal on T2WI in cerebral and/or cerebellar white matter, with or without high signal on T2WI in globus pallidi, putamen, caudate, thalami, brainstem.	Autosomal recessive disorders involving defective enzymes regulating amino acid metabolism and mitochodrial function. These enzymatic defects can cause significant alteration of myelin formation

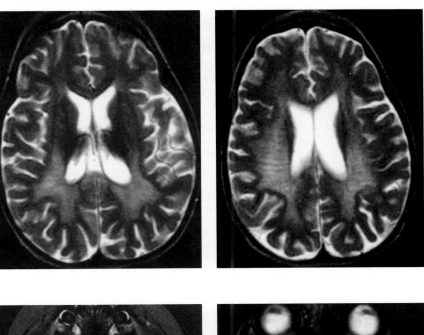

Fig. 1A.**157** **Childhood adrenoleukody-strophy. a, b** Axial T2WI shows symmetric zones of high signal in the periventricular parieto-occipital white matter, extending peripherally toward the subcortical white matter.

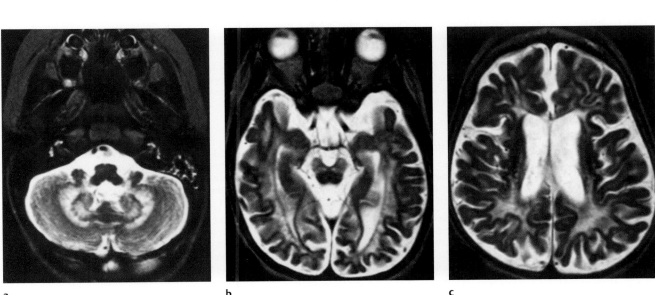

a   b   c

Fig. 1A.**158** **Krabbe disease. a, b, c** Axial T2WI shows symmetric confluent zones of high signal in the periventricular white matter, extending toward the subcortical white matter, with prominent cerebral and cerebellar atrophy.

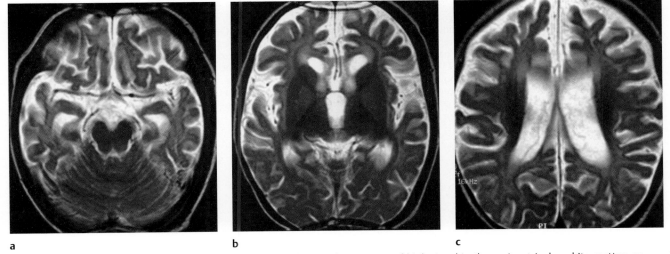

a   b   c

Fig. 1A.**159** **Neuronal ceroid–lipofuscinosis. a, b, c** Axial T2WI shows zones of high signal in the periventricular white matter, extending toward the subcortical white matter, with prominent cerebral atrophy.

Table 1A.**9** (Cont.) Multiple or diffuse lesions involving white matter

Disease	MRI Findings	Comments
Mitochondrial metabolic disorders (Fig. 1A.**160**) **MELAS and MERRF Syndromes**	High T2 signal in basal ganglia usually symmetric, high T2 signal in cerebral and cerebellar cortex and subcortical white matter not corresponding to a specific large arterial vascular territory. Signal abnormalities may resolve and reappear.	MELAS (Mitochondrial Encephalopathy, Lactic Acidosis, and Stroke-like events) is a maternally inherited disease affecting transfer of RNA in mitochodria. MERRF (Myoclonic Epilepsy, Ragged Red Fibers) is a mitochondrial encephalopathy associated with muscle weakness and myoclonic epilepsy, short stature, ophthalmoplegia, cardiac disease.
Leigh disease (Fig. 1A.**149**)	Symmetric high signal on T2WI in globus pallidus, putamen, and caudate as well as high signal on T2WI in thalami, cerebral and cerebellar white matter, cerebellar cortex, brainstem, and spinal cord gray matter. Typically no Gd-contrast enhancement.	Autosomal recessive disorder, also referred to as subacute necrotizing encephalopathy, occurs in three forms (infantile type, juvenile type, and adult-onset type). Etiology related to abnormalities in oxidative metabolism in mitochondria from one of several defective enzymes, progressive neurodegenerative disease. Lesions in brainstem are associated with loss of respiratory control.
Kearns-Sayre syndrome (Fig. 1A.**161**)	Symmetric high signal on T2WI in globus pallidus, putamen, and caudate as well as high signal on T2WI in thalami, cerebral and cerebellar white matter, cerebellar cortex, and brainstem. Typically no Gd-contrast enhancement.	Mitochondrial disorder associated with external ophthalmoplegia, retinitis pigmentosa, and onset of clinical muscular and neurologic signs below 20 years.
Cockayne syndrome (Figs. 1A.**150**, 1A.**155**)	High signal on T2WI involving the periventricular white matter, basal ganglia, and dentate nuclei. Calcifications in basal ganglia and dentate nuclei, progressive cerebral and cerebellar atrophy, microcephaly.	Autosomal recessive disorder with deficient repair mechanisms for DNA. Presents in first decade with progressive neurologic dysfunction, cataracts, cutaneous photosensitivity, optic atrophy, and dwarfism.
Toxic		
Marchiafava-Bignami disease	Variable mixed low, intermediate, and/or high signal on T1WI and T2WI. Involves corpus callosum, may involve other sites in cerebral white matter. With or without enhancement, depending on stage of demyelination (acute, subacute, chronic).	Acquired disorder associated with alcoholism with demyelination, necrosis, or hemorrhage involving the corpus callosum and other commissures and cerebral white matter.
Wernicke encephalopathy	Zones of intra-axial high signal on T2WI in the region of the cerebral acqueduct and adjacent to the third ventricle. With or without enhancement in the region of the cerebral acqueduct, adjacent to the third ventricle and mammillary bodies.	Acquired encephalopathy resulting from deficiency of thiamine, commonly seen in alcoholics. Associated clinical features include ophthalmoplegia, confusion, and ataxia. MRI findings and encephalopathy may resolve with vitamin replenishment.
Central pontine myelinolysis (osmotic myelinolysis) (Fig. 1A.**162**)	Poorly defined, usually large zone of high signal on T2WI involving the central portion of the pons. With or without high signal on T2WI involving midbrain, thalami, caudate nuclei, putamen, and subcortical white matter. With or without occasional enhancement.	Demyelinating disorder resulting form rapid correction of hyponatremia in chronically ill or alcoholic patients.
FK506 (Tacrolimus) (Fig. 1A.**163**)	Foci and/or confluent zones of high signal on T2WI in cerebral white matter, with or without high signal on T2WI in basal ganglia, pons; with or without high signal on T1WI and proton density weighted images involving the cerebral cortex. With or without enhancement. Signal abnormalities often reversible with correction of toxic levels of drug.	FK506 (Tacrolimus) is a drug used for immunosuppressive therapy in patients with organ transplantation. Toxic levels result in various neurologic symptoms including: confusion, headaches, seizures, dysarthria, coma. Cortical abnormalities may be related to cortical laminar necrosis secondary to hypoperfusion injury.

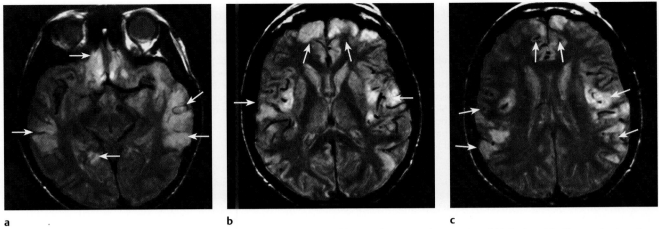

a   b   c

Fig. 1A.**160**   **MELAS. a, b, c** Axial proton density weighted (long TR/short TE) images show zones of high signal in the cerebral cortex and subcortical white matter not corresponding to a specific large arterial vascular territory (arrows).

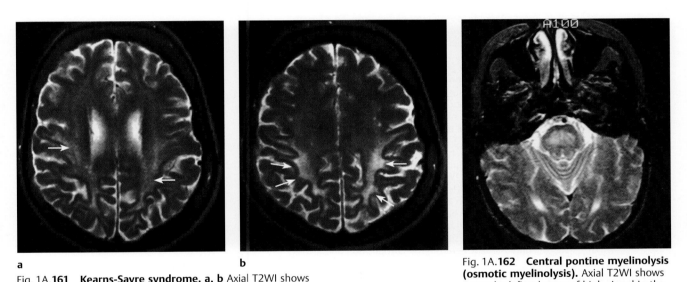

a   b

Fig. 1A.**161**   **Kearns-Sayre syndrome. a, b** Axial T2WI shows zones of high signal in the periventricular white matter, extending toward the subcortical white matter (arrows).

Fig. 1A.**162**   **Central pontine myelinolysis (osmotic myelinolysis).** Axial T2WI shows a poorly defined zone of high signal in the pons.

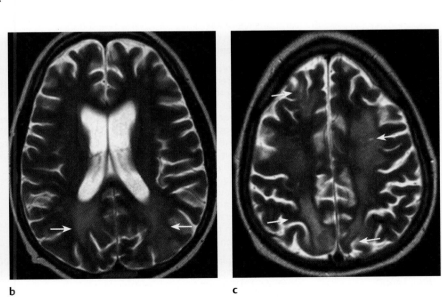

a   b   c

Fig. 1A.**163**   **FK506 (Tacrolimus). a, b, c** Axial T2WI shows poorly defined zones of high signal in the periventricular white matter bilaterally, extending toward the subcortical white matter (arrows).

Table 1A.**9** (Cont.) Multiple or diffuse lesions involving white matter

Disease	MRI Findings	Comments
Cyclosporin (Fig. 1A.**164**)	Foci and/or confluent zones of high T2 signal in cerebral white matter, with or without high signal on T1WI and proton density weighted images involving the cerebral cortex with or without cortical enhancement. Signal abnormalities can be reversible with correction of toxic levels of drug. Cortical abnormalities may be related cortical laminar necrosis related to hypoperfusion injury.	Cyclosporin A is a drug used for immunosuppressive therapy in patients with organ transplantation. Toxic levels result in various neurologic symptoms including: fever, seizures, altered mental status, cortical blindness, speech and motor dysfunction.
Hemorrhage		
Intracerebral hemorrhage (Fig. 1A.**43**), (Fig. 1A.**44**)	The signal of the hematoma depends on its age, size, location, hematocrit, hemoglobin oxidation state, clot retraction, and extent of edema. *Hyperacute phase (4–6 hours):* Hemoglobin primarily as diamagnetic oxyhemoglobin (iron Fe +2 state), intermediate signal on T1WI and slightly high signal on T2WI. *Acute phase (12–48 hours):* Hemoglobin primarily as paramagnetic deoxyhemoglobin (iron, Fe +2 state), intermediate signal on T1WI and low signal on T2WI, surrounded by a peripheral zone of high T2 signal (edema). *Subacute phase (>2 days):* Hemoglobin becomes oxidized to the iron Fe +3 state, methemoglobin, which is strongly paramagnetic. When methemoglobin is initially intracellular: the hematoma has high signal on T1WI, progressing from peripheral to central, and low signal on T2WI, surrounded by a zone of high T2 signal (edema). When methemoglobin eventually becomes primarily extracellular: the hematoma has high signal on T1WI and T2WI. *Chronic phase:* Hemoglobin as extracellular methemoglobin is progressively degraded to hemosiderin. The hematoma progresses from a lesion with high signal on T1WI and T2WI with a peripheral rim of low signal on T2WI (hemosiderin) to predominant hemosiderin composition and low signal on T2WI.	Can result from trauma, ruptured aneurysms or vascular malformations, coagulopathy, hypertension, adverse drug reaction, amyloid angiopathy, hemorrhagic transformation of cerebral infarct, metastases, abscesses, viral infections (herpes simplex, CMV).
Post-hemorrhagic lesions	Zone or zones with high signal on T2WI secondary to gliosis and encephalomalacia involving cerebral or cerebellar white matter, basal ganglia, thalami, and or cerebral or cerebellar cortex. With or without sites of low signal on T2WI where there is methemoglobin (also high signal on T1WI) and/or hemosiderin deposition. Typically no enhancement.	Sites of prior hemorrhage can have variable appearance depending on the relative ratios of gliosis, encephalomalacia, and blood breakdown products (e.g., methemoglobin, hemosiderin).
AVM (Fig. 1A.47)	Lesions with irregular margins that can be located in the brain parenchyma (white and/or gray matter), dura, or both locations. AVMs contain multiple tortuous tubular flow voids on T1WI and T2WI secondary to patent arteries with high blood flow, as well as thrombosed vessels with variable signal, areas of hemorrhage in various phases, calcifications, and gliosis. The venous portions often show Gd-contrast enhancement. MRA using TOF or phase contrast techniques can provide additional detailed information about the nidus, feeding arteries, and draining veins, and presence of associated aneurysms. Usually not associated with mass effect unless except in cases of recent hemorrhage or venous occlusion.	Supratentorial AVMs occur more frequently (80–90%) than infratentorial AVMs (10–20%). Annual risk of hemorrhage. AVMs can be sporadic, congenital, or associated with a history of trauma. Multiple AVMs can be seen in syndromes: Rendu-Osler-Weber, AVMs in brain and lungs, and mucosal capillary telangectasias; Wyburn-Mason, AVMs in brain and retina, and cutaneous nevi.
Cavernous hemangioma (Fig. 1A.**48**)	Single or multiple multilobulated intra-axial lesions that have a peripheral rim or irregular zone of low signal on T2WI secondary to hemosiderin, surrounding a central zone of variable signal (low, intermediate, high, or mixed) on T1WI and T2WI depending on ages of hemorrhagic portions. GRE techniques useful for detecting multiple lesions.	Supratentorial cavernous angiomas occur more frequently than infratentorial lesions. Can be found in many different locations. Multiple lesions more than 50%. Association with venous angiomas and risk of hemorrhage.

Table 1A.**9** (Cont.) Multiple or diffuse lesions involving white matter

Disease	MRI Findings	Comments
Venous angioma (Fig. 1A.**101**)	On postcontrast T1WI, venous angiomas are seen as a Gd-contrast-enhancing transcortical vein draining a collection of small medullary veins (caput Medusa). The draining vein can be seen as a signal void on T2WI.	Considered an anomalous venous formation typically not associated with hemorrhage. Usually an incidental finding except when associated with cavernous hemangioma.
Trauma shear injury	Foci and/or diffuse zones of high signal on T2WI in cerebral and/or cerebellar white matter (lobar white matter, corpus callosum) and/or brainstem. Usually no enhancement.	Traumatic injury from acceleration/deceleration or shaking, resulting in transection of axons. Often associated with other intracranial injuries such as traumatic subarachnoid or parenchymal hemorrhage, cerebral contusions.

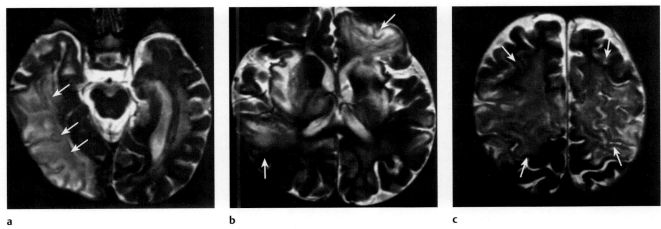

a   b   c

Fig. 1A.**164** **Cyclosporin.** **a, b, c** Axial T2WI shows poorly defined zones of high signal in the periventricular white matter bilaterally, extending to the subcortical white matter with involvement of the cerebral cortex (arrows).

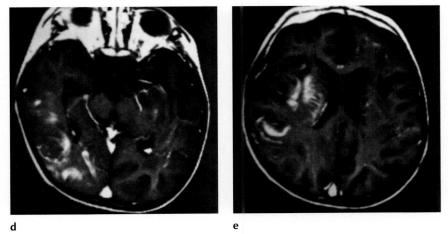

d   e

Fig. 1A.**164** **d, e** Postcontrast axial T1WI shows irregular zones of enhancement in brain parenchyma.

Table 1A.**9** (Cont.) Multiple or diffuse lesions involving white matter

Disease	MRI Findings	Comments
Ischemic–Small vessel (Fig. 1A.165)	Multiple foci and/or confluent zones of high signal on T2WI involving the subcortical and periventricular white matter, basal ganglia, brainstem. No associated mass effect, typically no enhancement. Chronic lesion may have low signal on T1WI.	Lesions in white matter and/or brainstem related to occlusive disease involving perforating arteries associated with hypertension, atherosclerosis, diabetes, vasculitis, and aging. Unlike MS, ischemic small vessel disease does not usually involve the corpus callosum because of its abundant blood supply from multiple branches arsing from the adjacent pericallosal arteries.
Periventricular leukomalacia (Fig. 1A.166)	Multiple foci and/or confluent zones of high signal onT2WI involving the subcortical and periventricular white matter, basal ganglia, brainstem. No associated mass effect, no enhancement. With or without low signal on T1WI. Irregular ventricular margins and ventricular enlargement related to cerebral volume loss.	Ischemic injury involving fetal brain/premature infants with gliosis and resultant encephalomalacic changes involving periventricular white matter (fetal watershed vascular zones). Associated with neurologic deficits depending on severity of injuries, cerebral palsy.
Demyelinating disease– Multiple Sclerosis, Acute Disseminated Encephalomyelitis (Fig. 1A.167)	Lesions located in cerebral or cerebellar white matter, brainstem, basal ganglia. Usually have low to intermediate signal on T1WI and high signal on T2WI. With or without Gd-contrast enhancement. Enhancement can be ring-like or nodular, usually in acute/early subacute phase of demyelination. Lesions rarely can have associated mass effect simulating neoplasms.	MS is the most common acquired demyelinating disease usually affecting women (peak age 20–40 years). Other demyelinating diseases include: ADEM–immune mediated demyelination after viral infection; toxins (exogenous from environmental exposure or ingestion–alcohol, solvents etc.–or endogenous from metabolic disorder–leukodystrophies, mitochondrial encephalopathies, etc.), radiation injury, trauma, vascular disease.
Amyotrophic lateral sclerosis (Fig. 1A.168)	Zones of abnormal high signal on T2WI in posterior limbs of internal capsules and cerebral peduncles in 25 %. Typically no enhancement.	Disorder affecting adults above age 55 years, with progressive muscle weakness and atrophy leading to death.

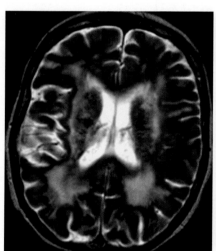
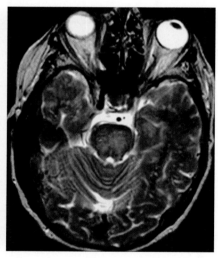

Fig. 1A.**165 Ischemic–small vessel. a, b** Axial T2WI shows foci and confluent zones of high signal in the subcortical and periventricular white matter bilaterally and pons.

a

b

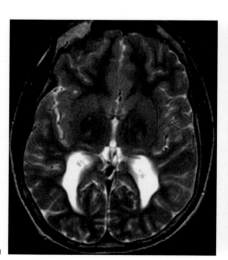
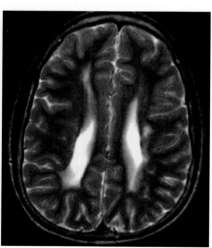

Fig. 1A.**166 Periventricular leukomalacia. a, b** Axial T2WI shows irregular ventricular margins and ventricular enlargement related to cerebral volume loss, as well as small zones of high signal in the periventricular white matter.

a

b

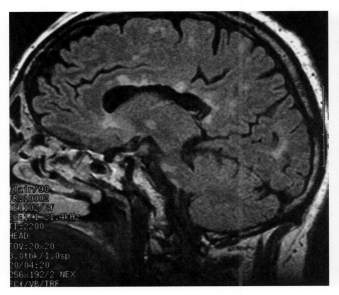

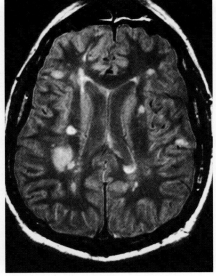

a

b

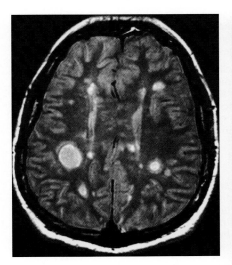

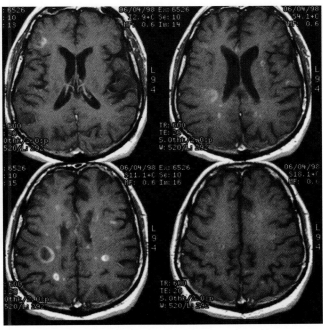

c

d

Fig. 1A.**167** **Multiple Sclerosis.**
a Sagittal FLAIR image shows multiple foci with high signal in the periventricular and subcortical white matter, corpus callosum, and middle cerebellar peduncle.
b, c Axial proton density weighted (long TR/short TE) images show multiple lesions with high signal in the cerebral white matter.
d Postcontrast axial T1WI shows enhancement associated with multiple lesions (active demyelination).

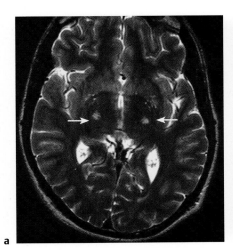

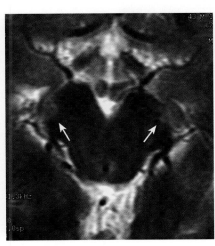

a

b

Fig. 1A.**168** **Amyotrophic lateral sclerosis.** **a** Axial T2WI shows bilateral foci of abnormal high signal in the posterior limbs of the internal capsules (arrows). **b** Axial T2WI shows small zones of high signal in the anterior portion of each cerebral peduncle (arrows).

Table 1A.**9** (Cont.) Multiple or diffuse lesions involving white matter

Disease	MRI Findings	Comments
Infection		
Cerebritis (Fig. 1A.35)	Poorly defined zone or focal area of low to intermediate signal on T1WI and intermediate to high signal on T2WI; minimal or no Gd-contrast enhancement. Involves cerebral cortex and white matter for bacterial and fungal infections.	Focal infection/inflammation of brain tissue from bacteria or fungi, secondary to sinusitis, meningitis, surgery, hematogenous source (cardiac and other vascular shunts), and/or immunocompromised status. Can progress to abscess formation.
Pyogenic brain abscess (Fig. 1A.36)	Circumscribed lesion with low signal on T1WI; central zone of high signal on T2WI (air-fluid level may be present) surrounded by a thin rim of low T2 signal; peripheral poorly defined zone of high signal on T2WI representing edema. Ring-like Gd-contrast enhancement that is sometimes thicker laterally than medially.	Formation of brain abscess occurs 2 weeks after cerebritis with liquefaction and necrosis centrally surrounded by a capsule and peripheral edema. Can be multiple. Complication from meningitis and/or sinusitis, septicemia, trauma, surgery, cardiac shunt.
Fungal brain abscess (Fig. 1A.37)	Vary depending on organism. Lesions occur in meninges and brain parenchyma; solid or cystic lesions with low to intermediate signal on T2WI and high signal on T2WI. Nodular or ring enhancement. Peripheral high signal in brain lesions on T2WI (edema).	Occur in immunocompromised or diabetic patients with resultant granulomas in meninges and brain parenchyma; *Cryptococcus* involves the basal meninges and extends along perivascular spaces into the basal ganglia. *Aspergillus* and *Mucor* spread via direct extension through paranasal sinuses or hematogenously invade blood vessels resulting in hemorrhagic lesions and/or cerebral infarcts. Coccidiomycosis usually involves the basal meninges.
Encephalitis (Figs. 1A.**169**, 1A.**170**) (Fig. 1A.38)	Poorly defined zone(s) of low to intermediate signal on T1WI and intermediate to high signal on T2WI; minimal or no Gd-contrast enhancement. Involves cerebral cortex and/or white matter. Minimal localized mass effect. Herpes simplex typically involves the temporal lobes/limbic system. Hemorrhage may be associated. CMV usually in periventricular/subependymal locations. HIV often involves periatrial white matter.	Encephalitis: infection/inflammation of brain tissue from viruses, often in immuncompromised patients (herpes simplex, CMV, HIV, progressive multifocal leukoencephalopathy) or immunocompetent (St Louis encephalitis, Eastern or Western equine encephalitis, Epstein-Barr virus).
Rasmussen's encephalitis (Fig. 1A.138)	Progressive atrophy of one cerebral hemisphere with poorly defined zones of high signal on T2WI involving the white matter, basal ganglia, and cortex. Usually no enhancement.	Usually seen in children below 10 years of age. Severe and progressive epilepsy and unilateral neurologic deficits–hemiplegia, psychomotor deterioration, chronic slow viral infectious process possibly caused by CMV or Epstein-Barr virus. Treatment: hemispherectomy.
Creutzfeld-Jakob disease	Zones of high signal on T2WI in putamen and caudate nuclei bilaterally, with or without zones of high signal in white matter and cortex. Typically no enhancement. Progressive cerebral atrophy.	Spongiform encephalopathy caused by slow infection from prion (proteinaceous infectious particle). Usually seen in adults age 40–80 years. Progressive dementia. Less than 10% survive more than 2 years.

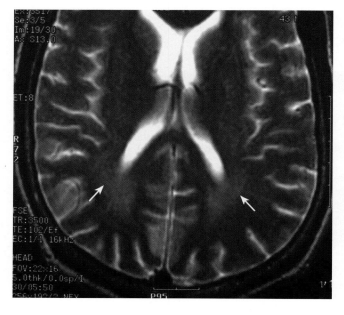

Fig. 1A.**169** **HIV encephalitis.** Axial T2WI shows poorly defined zones of intermediate to slightly high signal in the periatrial white matter bilaterally (arrows).

Table 1A.**9** (Cont.) Multiple or diffuse lesions involving white matter

Disease	MRI Findings	Comments
Reye syndrome	With or without diffuse edematous high signal on T2WI involving basal ganglia, white matter, and cortex bilaterally.	Disorder of unknown etiology occurring in children usually below age 16. Symptoms (vomiting, lethargy, seizures, sometimes coma leading to death) occur during recovery from viral-like illness. Mortality approximately 20%.
Lyme disease	Foci or confluent zones of high signal on T2WI in cerebral and/or cerebellar white matter. With or without enhancement.	CNS manifestations presumed to occur as a result of immune-related demyelination from Lyme disease (infection by spirochete–*Borrelia burgdorferi*) transmitted by ticks.
Tuberculoma (Fig. 1A.**39**)	Intra-axial lesions in cerebral hemispheres and basal ganglia (adults), cerebellum (children). Low to intermediate signal on T1WI, central zone of high signal on T2WI with a thin peripheral rim of low signal, occasionally low signal on T2WI. Solid or rim Gd-contrast enhancement. Calcification may be present. Meningeal lesions: nodular or cystic zones of basilar meningeal enhancement.	Occurs in immunocompromised patients and in developing countries. Caseating intracranial granulomas via hematogenous dissemination. Lesions more common in meninges than brain.
Parasitic brain lesions		
Toxoplasmosis (Fig. 1A.**40**)	Single or multiple solid and/or cystic lesions located in basal ganglia and/or corticomedullary junctions in cerebral hemispheres. Low to intermediate signal on T1WI; high signal on T2WI. Nodular or rim pattern of Gd-contrast enhancement, with or without peripheral high T2 signal (edema).	Most common opportunistic CNS infection in AIDS patients, caused by ingestion of food contaminated with parasites (*Toxoplasma gondii*).
Cysticercosis (Fig. 1A.**41**)	Single or multiple cystic lesions in brain or meninges. *Acute/subacute phase:* Low to intermediate signal on T1WI and high signal on T2WI. Rim and possible nodular pattern of Gd-contrast enhancement, with or without peripheral high T2 signal (edema). *Chronic phase:* calcified granulomas.	Caused by ingestion of ova (*Taenia solium*) in contaminated food (undercooked pork). Involves in order of decreasing frequency: meninges, brain parenchyma, ventricles.
Hydatid cyst	*Echinococcus granulosus:* Single or rarely multiple cystic lesions with low signal on T1WI and high signal on T2WI with a thin wall with low signal on T2WI; typically no Gd-contrast enhancement or peripheral edema unless superinfected. Often located in vascular territory of the middle cerebral artery. *Echinococcus multilocularis:* Cystic (possibly multilocular) and/or solid lesions. Central zone of low to intermediate signal on T1WI and T2WI, surrounded by a slightly thickened rim of low signal on T2WI; Gd-contrast enhancement. Peripheral zone of high signal on T2WI (edema) and calcifications are common.	Caused by parasites: *Echinococcus granulosus* (South America, Middle East Australia, New Zealand) or *Echinococcus multilocularis* (North America, Europe, Turkey, China).CNS involvement in 2% of cases of hydatid infestation.

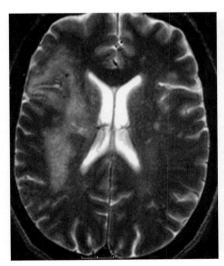

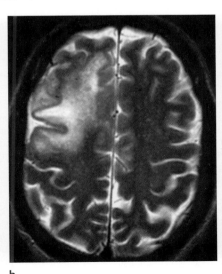

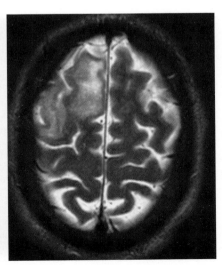

a   b   c

Fig. 1A.**170** **Progressive multifocal leukoencephalophy.** **a, b, c** Axial T2WI shows poorly defined zones of high signal in the right cerebral white matter with localized mass effect.

Table 1A.9 (Cont.) Multiple or diffuse lesions involving white matter

Disease	MRI Findings	Comments
Radiation injury/necrosis (Fig. 1A.42), (Fig. 1A.47)	Focal lesion with or without mass effect or poorly defined zone of low to intermediate signal on T1WI, intermediate to high signal on T2WI, with or without Gd-contrast enhancement involving tissue (gray matter and/or white matter) in field of treatment.	Usually occurs from 4–6 months to 10 years after radiation treatment. May be difficult to distinguish from neoplasm. PET and MRS might be helpful for evaluation. Radiation treatment in combination with intrathecal methotrexate may also result in necrotizing leukoencephalopathy.
Neoplastic		
Astrocytoma (Fig. 1A.18), (Fig. 1A.21)	*Low-grade astrocytoma:* Focal or diffuse mass lesion usually located in white matter with low to intermediate signal on T1WI and high signal on T2WI, with or without mild Gd-contrast enhancement. Minimal associated mass effect. *Juvenile pilocytic astrocytoma:* Subtype: solid/cystic focal lesion with low to intermediate signal on T1WI and high signal on T2WI, usually with prominent Gd-contrast enhancement. Lesions located in cerebellum, hypothalamus, adjacent to third or fourth ventricles, brainstem. *Gliomatosis cerebri:* Infiltrative lesion with poorly defined margins with mass effect located in the white matter. Low to intermediate signal on T1WI and high signal on T2WI; usually no Gd-contrast enhancement until late in disease. *Anaplastic astrocytoma:* Often irregularly marginated lesion located in white matter with low to intermediate signal on T1WI and high signal on T2WI, with or without Gd-contrast enhancement.	*Low-grade astrocytoma:* Often occur in children and adults (age 20–40 years). Tumors comprised of well-differentiated astrocytes. Association with neurofibromatosis type 1. Ten-year survival. May become malignant. *Juvenile pilocytic astrocytoma:* Subtype: common in children, usually favorable prognosis if totally resected. *Gliomatosis cerebri:* Diffusely infiltrating astrocytoma with relative preservation of underlying brain architecture. Imaging appearance may be more prognostic than histologic grade. Approximate 2-year survival. *Anaplastic astrocytoma:* Intermediate between low-grade astrocytoma and glioblastoma multiforme. Approximate 2-year survival.
Glioblastoma multiforme (Fig. 1A.22)	Irregularly marginated mass lesion with necrosis or cyst. Mixed signal on T1WI, heterogeneous high signal on T2WI. With or without associated hemorrhage. Prominent heterogeneous Gd-contrast enhancement, peripheral edema, can cross corpus callosum.	Most common primary CNS tumor. Highly malignant neoplasms with necrosis and vascular proliferation. Usually seen in patients above age 50. Extent of lesion underestimated by MRI. Survival less than 1 year.
Giant cell astrocytoma–Tuberous sclerosis (Fig. 1A.23)	Circumscribed lesion located near the foramen of Monro with mixed low to intermediate signal on T1WI and mixed high signal on T2WI. Cysts and/or calcifications may be associated. Heterogenous or homogenous Gd-contrast enhancement.	Subependymal hamartoma near foramen of Monro, occurs in 15% of patients with tuberous sclerosis below 20 years. Slow-growing lesions that can progressively cause obstruction of CSF flow through the foramen of Monro. Long-term survival usual if resected.
Pleomorphic xanthoastrocytoma (Fig. 1A.24)	Circumscribed supratentorial lesion involving cerebral cortex and white matter. Low to intermediate signal on T1WI and intermediate to high signal on T2WI. Cyst(s) may be present. Heterogeneous Gd-contrast enhancement. With or without enhancing mural nodule associated with cyst.	Rare type of astrocytoma occurring in young adults and children. Associated with seizure history.
Oligodendroglioma (Fig. 1A.25)	Circumscribed lesion with mixed low to intermediate signal on T1WI and mixed intermediate to high signal on T2WI; areas of signal void at sites of clump-like calcification; heterogenous Gd-contrast enhancement. Involves white matter and cerebral cortex. Can cause chronic erosion of inner table of calvaria.	Uncommon slow-growing gliomas with usually mixed histologic patterns (e.g., astrocytoma). Usually in adults older than 35 years, 85% supratentorial. If low-grade 75% 5-year survival, higher grade lesions have a worse prognosis.
Central neurocytoma (Fig. 1A.26)	Circumscribed lesion located at margin of lateral ventricle or septum pellucidum with intraventricular protrusion. Heterogeneous intermediate signal on T1WI, heterogeneous intermediate to high signal on T2WI; calcifications and/or small cysts may be associated; heterogeneous Gd-contrast enhancement.	Rare tumors that have neuronal differentiation. Imaging appearance similar to intraventricular oligodendrogliomas. Occur in young adults. Benign slow-growing lesions.
Ganglioglioma, ganglioneuroma, gangliocytoma (Fig. 1A.27)	Circumscribed tumor. Usually supratentorial, often temporal or frontal lobes. Low to intermediate signal on T1WI; intermediate to high signal on T2WI. Cysts may be present. With or without Gd-contrast enhancement.	Ganglioglioma (contains glial and neuronal elements), ganglioneuroma (contains only ganglion cells). Uncommon tumors, below 30 years, seizure presentation, slow-growing neoplasms. Gangliocytoma (contains only neuronal elements, dysplastic brain tissue). Favorable prognosis if completely resected.

Table 1A.**9** (Cont.) Multiple or diffuse lesions involving white matter

Disease	MRI Findings	Comments
Ependymoma (Fig. 1A.**28**)	Circumscribed lobulated supratentorial lesion, often extraventricular. Cysts and/or calcifications may be associated. Low to intermediate signal on T1WI, intermediate to high signal on T2WI; variable Gd-contrast enhancement.	Occurs more commonly in children than adults. One-third supratentorial, two-thirds infratentorial. 45 % 5-year survival.
Hamartoma–Tuberous sclerosis (Fig. 1A.**29**)	*Cortical:* Subcortical lesion with high signal on T1WI and low signal on T2WI in neonates and infants; changes to low to intermediate signal on T1WI and high signal on T2WI in older children and adults. Calcifications in 50 % in older children. Gd-contrast enhancement uncommon. *Subependymal hamartomas:* Small nodules located along and projecting into the lateral ventricles. Signal on T1WI and T2WI similar to cortical tubers. Calcification and Gd-contrast enhancement common.	Cortical and subependymal hamartomas are non-malignant lesions associated with tuberous sclerosis.
Primitive neuro-ectodermal tumor (Fig. 1A.**31**)	Circumscribed or invasive lesions with low to intermediate signal on T1WI and intermediate to high signal on T2WI; variable Gd-contrast enhancement. Frequent dissemination into the leptomeninges.	Highly malignant tumors located in the cerebrum, pineal gland, and cerebellum that frequently disseminate along CSF pathways.
Dysembryoplastic neuroepithelial tumor (Fig. 1A.**32**)	Circumscribed lesions involving the cerebral cortex and subcortical white matter. Low signal on T1WI, high signal on T2WI. Small cysts may be present. Usually no Gd-contrast enhancement.	Benign superficial lesions commonly located in the temporal or frontal lobes.
Lymphoma (Fig. 1A.**33**)	Primary CNS lymphoma: focal or infiltrating lesion located in the basal ganglia, periventricular regions, posterior fossa/brainstem. Low to intermediate signal on T1WI; intermediate to slightly high signal on T2WI. Hemorrhage/necrosis may be associated in immunocompromised patients. Usually Gd-contrast enhancement. Diffuse leptomeningeal enhancement is another pattern of intracranial lymphoma.	Primary CNS lymphoma more common than secondary, usually in adults above 40 years of age. B cell lymphoma more common than T cell lymphoma. Increasing incidence related to number of immunocompromised patients in population. MRI features of primary and secondary lymphoma of brain overlap. Intracranial lymphoma can involve the leptomeninges in secondary lymphoma more commonly than primary lymphoma.
Hemangioblastoma (Fig. 1A.**94**)	Circumscribed tumors usually located in the cerebellum and/or brainstem. Small Gd-contrast-enhancing nodule with or without cyst, or larger lesion with prominent heterogeneous enhancement with or without flow voids within lesion or at the periphery. Intermediate signal on T1WI; intermediate to high signal on T2WI. Occasionally lesions have evidence of recent or remote hemorrhage.	Rarely occur in cerebral hemispheres; occur in adolescents, young and middle-aged adults. Lesions are typically multiple in patients with von Hippel-Lindau disease.
Metastases (Fig. 1A.**34**)	Circumscribed spheroid lesions in brain that can have various intra-axial locations, often at gray-white matter junctions. Usually low to intermediate signal on T1WI; intermediate to high signal on T2WI. Hemorrhage, calcifications, cysts may be associated. Variable Gd-contrast enhancement, often high signal on T2WI peripheral to nodular enhancing lesion representing axonal edema.	Represent approximately 33 % of intracranial tumors, usually from extracranial primary neoplasm in adults above 40 years of age. Primary tumor source in order of decreasing frequency: lung, breast, GI, GU, melanoma.

Table 1A.**10** Cerebellopontine angle and/or internal auditory canal lesions

Disease	MRI Findings	Comments
Schwannoma (neurinoma)– acoustic, others (Figs. 1A.**171**–1A.**175**)	Circumscribed or lobulated extra-axial lesions with low to intermediate signal on T1WI and intermediate to high signal on T2WI; prominent Gd-contrast enhancement. High signal on T2WI and Gd-contrast enhancement can be heterogeneous in large lesions.	Acoustic (vestibular nerve) schwannoma account for 90 % of intracranial schwannomas and represent 75 % of lesions in the cerebellopontine angle cisterns. Trigeminal schwannomas are the next most common intracranial schwannoma, followed by facial nerve schwannomas, multiple schwannomas seen with neurofibromatosis type 2 (Figs. 1A.**174**, 1A.**175**).

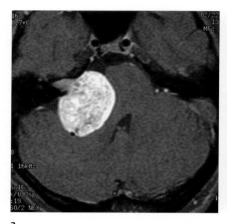
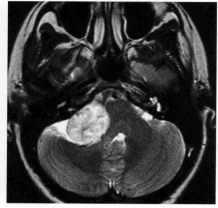

a   b

Fig. 1A.**171** **Acoustic schwannoma (neurinoma).** **a** Postcontrast axial FS T1WI shows a circumscribed enhancing lesion in the right cerebellopontine angle cistern, extending into the right internal auditory canal. **b** Axial T2WI shows the lesion to have heterogeneous high signal.

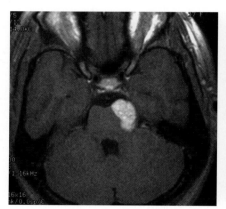
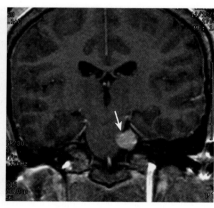

a   b

Fig. 1A.**172** **Trigeminal schwannoma(neurinoma).** **a** Postcontrast axial FS T1WI shows a circumscribed enhancing lesion in the left cerebellopontine angle cistern. **b** Postcontrast coronal (spoiled GRE) T1WI shows the enhancing lesion indenting the left side of the pons (arrow). The normal right trigeminal is also seen.

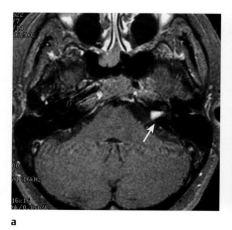
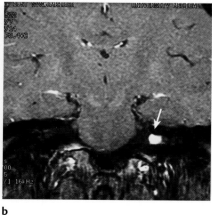
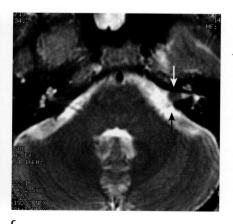

a   b   c

Fig. 1A.**173** **Facial nerve schwannoma.** Postcontrast axial (**a**) and coronal (**b**) FS T1WI shows a circumscribed enhancing lesion in the left internal auditory canal. **c** Axial T2WI shows the lesion to have intermediate signal (arrows).

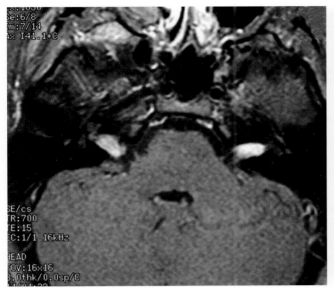

a

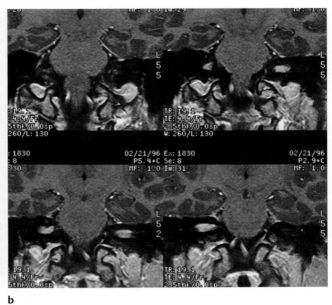

b

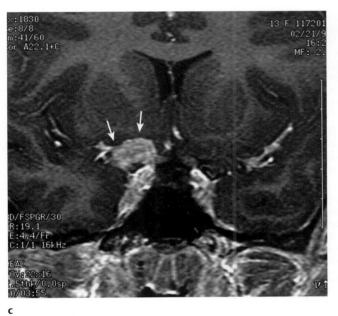

c

Fig. 1A.**174** **Bilateral acoustic schwannomas, neurofibromatosis type 2.** **a** Postcontrast axial FS T1WI shows circumscribed enhancing lesions in each internal auditory canal. **b** Postcontrast coronal (spoiled GRE) T1WI show the enhancing lesions in the internal auditory canals. **c** Postcontrast coronal (spoiled GRE) T1WI shows an enhancing meningioma above the right anterior clinoid process (arrows).

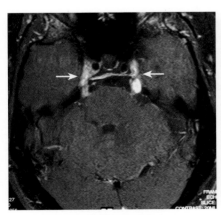

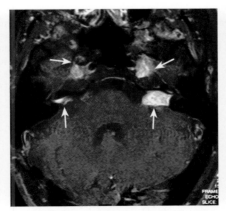

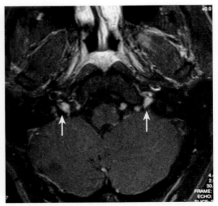

Fig. 1A.**175** **Multiple cranial nerve schwannomas, neurofibromatosis type 2.** **a** Postcontrast axial FS T1WI shows bilateral enhancing trigeminal schwannomas (arrows).

Fig. 1A.**175 b** Postcontrast axial FS T1WI shows enhancing lesions in each internal auditory canal (arrows) and in each trigeminal cistern (arrows).

Fig. 1A.**175 c** Postcontrast axial FS T1WI shows circumscribed enhancing lesions in each hypoglossal canal (arrows).

Table 1A.10 (Cont.) Cerebellopontine angle and/or internal auditory canal lesions

Disease	MRI Findings	Comments
Meningioma (Fig. 1A.176)	Extra-axial, well-circumscribed, dural-based lesions. Supratentorial location more common than infratentorial. Intermediate signal on T1WI and intermediate to slightly high signal on T2WI; usually prominent Gd-contrast enhancement. Calcifications may be associated.	Most common extra-axial tumor, usually benign neoplasms. Typically occurs in adults (above 40 years of age), more common in women than men. Multiple meningiomas seen with neurofibromatosis type 2, can result in compression of adjacent brain parenchyma, encasement of arteries, and compression of dural venous sinuses. Rarely invasive/malignant types.
Epidermoid (congenital cholesteatoma) (Fig. 1A.177)	Well-circumscribed, spheroid or multilobulated extra-axial ectodermal-inclusion cystic lesions with low to intermediate signal on T1WI and high signal on T2WI similar to CSF. Mixed low, intermediate, or high signal on FLAIR images; no Gd-contrast enhancement. Often insinuate along CSF pathways, chronic deformation of adjacent neural tissue (brainstem, brain parenchyma), although typically not associated with obstructive hydrocephalus. Commonly located in posterior cranial fossa (cerebellopontine angle cistern), parasellar/middle cranial fossa.	Non-neoplastic, congenital or acquired extra-axial off-midline lesions filled with desquamated cells and keratinaceous debris. Usually mild mass effect on adjacent brain. Infratentorial locations more common than supratentorial locations. Affects male and female adults equally. With or without related clinical symptoms.
Dermoid (Fig. 1A.86)	Well-circumscribed, spheroid or multilobulated extra-axial lesions, usually with high signal on T1WI and variable low, intermediate, and/or high signal on T2WI. No Gd-contrast enhancement. Fluid-fluid or fluid-debris levels may be present. Can cause chemical meningitis if dermoid cyst ruptures into the subarachnoid space. Commonly located at or near midline; supratentorial more common than infratentorial.	Non-neoplastic, congenital or acquired ectodermal-inclusion cystic lesions filled with lipid material, cholesterol, desquamated cells, and keratinaceous debris. Usually mild mass effect on adjacent brain. Slightly more common in adult males than adult females. With or without related clinical symptoms.
Lipoma (Fig. 1A.178)	Lipomas have MR signal isointense to subcutaneous fat on T1WI and T2WI. Signal suppression occurs with frequency-selective FS techniques or with a STIR method. Typically no Gd-contrast enhancement or peripheral edema.	Benign fatty lesions resulting from congenital malformation, often located in or near the midline. May contain calcifications and/or traversing blood vessels.
Arachnoid cyst (Fig. 1A.113)	Well-circumscribed extra-axial lesions with low signal on T1WI and high signal on T2WI similar to CSF; no Gd-contrast enhancement. Common locations in order of decreasing frequency: anterior middle cranial fossa, suprasellar/quadrigeminal, frontal convexities, posterior cranial fossa.	Non-neoplastic congenital, developmental or acquired extra-axial lesions filled with CSF. Usually mild mass effect on adjacent brain. More often supratentorial than infratentorial location. Affects males more than females. With or without related clinical symptoms.
Paraganglioma–Glomus jugulare (Fig. 1A.109)	Extra-axial mass lesions located in jugular foramen, often well-circumscribed. Intermediate signal on T1WI, often heterogeneous intermediate to slightly high signal on T2WI. With or without flow voids. Prominent Gd-contrast enhancement. Often associated erosive bone changes and expansion of jugular foramen.	Lesions, also referred to as chemodectomas, arise from paraganglia in multiple sites in the body and are named accordingly (e.g., glomus jugulare, tympanicum, vagale).
Vertebrobasilar dolichoectasia (Fig. 1A.179)	Elongated and ectatic vertebral and basilar arteries, variable intraluminal MR signal related to turbulent or slowed blood flow or partial/complete thrombosis.	Abnormal fusiform or focal dilatation of vertebrobasilar arteries secondary to: acquired/degenerative etiology, polycystic disease, connective-tissue disease, atherosclerosis, chronic hypertension, trauma, infection (mycotic), AVM, vasculitis, and drugs.

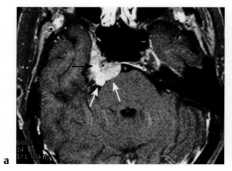
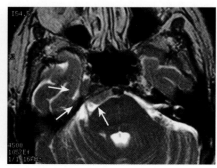

Fig. 1A.176 **Meningioma.** Postcontrast FS axial T1WI shows an enhancing extra-axial dural-based lesion indenting the right anterolateral margin of the pons (arrows). The lesion also extends into the right trigeminal cistern. **b** Axial T2WI shows the lesion to have intermediate signal (arrows).

a

b

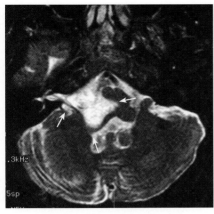

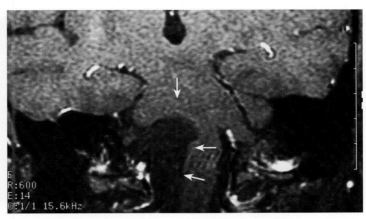

Fig. 1A.**177** **Epidermoid (congenital cholesteatoma).** **a** Axial FS T2WI shows a well-circumscribed multilobulated extra-axial lesion with high signal in the right cerebellopontine angle cistern (arrows).

Fig. 1A.**177 b** Postcontrast FS coronal T1WI shows no enhancement at the lesion. The lesion causes deformation of the right side of the pons and medulla (arrows).

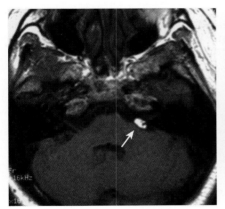

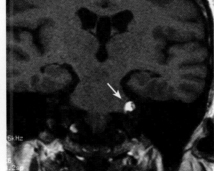

Fig. 1A.**178** **Lipoma.** Axial (**a**) and coronal (**b**) T1WI shows a small structure with high signal in the left cerebellopontine angle cistern (arrows).

a

b

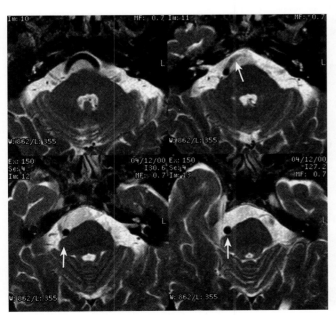

Fig. 1A.**179** **Vertebrobasilar dolichoectasia.** Axial T2WI show a tortuous and slightly dilated basilar artery seen as a flow void (arrows), which indents the right anterolateral aspect of the pons near the exit zone of the right trigeminal nerve.

Table 1A.**10** (Cont.) Cerebellopontine angle and/or internal auditory canal lesions

Disease	MRI Findings	Comments
Aneurysm		
Arterial aneurysm– Basilar artery/ branches, vertebral arteries (Fig. 1A.75)	*Saccular aneurysm:* Focal well-circumscribed zone of signal void on T1WI and T2WI. Variable mixed signal if thrombosed. *Giant aneurysm:* Focal well-circumscribed structure with layers of low, intermediate, and high signal on T2WI secondary to layers of thrombus of different ages, as well as a zone of signal void representing a patent lumen if present. On T1WI, layers of intermediate and high signal can be seen as well as a zone of signal void.	Abnormal focal dilatation of artery secondary to: acquired/degenerative etiology, polycystic disease, connective-tissue disease, atherosclerosis, trauma, infection (mycotic), AVM, vasculitis, and drugs.
Glioma of brainstem or cerebellum (Fig. 1A.180)	*Low-grade astrocytoma:* Focal or diffuse mass lesion usually located in cerebellar white matter or brainstem with low to intermediate signal on T1WI and high signal on T2WI; with or without mild Gd-contrast enhancement. Minimal associated mass effect. *Juvenile pilocytic astrocytoma:* Subtype: solid/cystic focal lesion with low to intermediate signal on T1WI and high signal on T2WI, usually with prominent Gd-contrast enhancement. Lesions located in cerebellum, brainstem. *Gliomatosis cerebri:* Infiltrative lesion with poorly defined margins with mass effect located in the white matter, with low to intermediate signal on T1WI and high signal on T2WI; usually no Gd-contrast enhancement until late in disease. *Anaplastic astrocytoma:* Often irregularly marginated lesion located in white matter with low to intermediate signal on T1WI and high signal on T2WI; with or without Gd-contrast enhancement.	*Low-grade astrocytoma:* Often occur in children and adults (age 20–40 years). Tumors comprised of well-differentiated astrocytes. Association with neurofibromatosis type 1. Ten-year survival. May become malignant. *Juvenile pilocytic astrocytoma:* Subtype: common in children, usually favorable prognosis if totally resected. *Gliomatosis cerebri:* Diffusely infiltrating astrocytoma with relative preservation of underlying brain architecture. Imaging appearance may be more prognostic than histologic grade. Approximate 2-year survival. *Anaplastic astrocytoma:* Intermediate between low-grade astrocytoma and glioblastoma multiforme. Approximate 2-year survival.
Hemangioblastoma (Fig. 1A.181)	Circumscribed tumors usually located in the cerebellum and/or brainstem. Small Gd-contrast-enhancing nodule with or without cyst, or larger lesion with prominent heterogeneous enhancement with or without flow voids within lesion or at the periphery. Intermediate signal on T1WI, intermediate to high signal on T2WI. Occasionally lesions have evidence of recent or remote hemorrhage.	Occurs in adolescents, young and middle-aged adults. Lesions are typically multiple in patients with von Hippel-Lindau disease.
Metastatic tumor (Figs. 1A.182, 1A.183)	Single or multiple well-circumscribed or poorly defined lesions involving the skull, dura, leptomeninges, and/or choroid plexus. Low to intermediate signal on T1WI, intermediate to high signal on T2WI; usually Gd-contrast enhancement. Bone destruction and compression of neural tissue or vessels may be associated. Leptomeningeal tumor often best seen on postcontrast images.	Metastatic tumor may have variable destructive or infiltrative changes involving single or multiple sites of involvement.

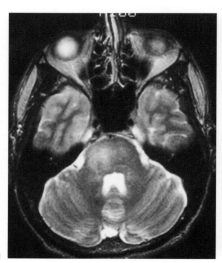

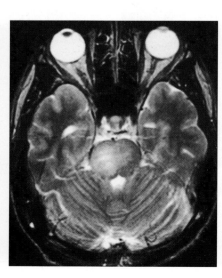

Fig. 1A.180 Astrocytoma of brainstem. Axial T2WI (**a, b**) shows a poorly defined zone of high signal in the right side of the pons with mild mass effect.

a
b

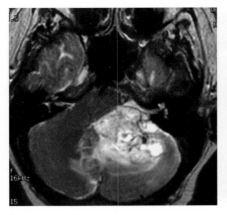 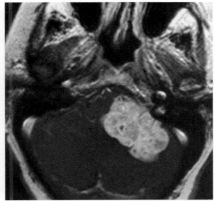

Fig. 1A.**181** **Hemangioblastoma.** **a** Axial T2WI shows a large lesion with heterogeneous high signal containing several flow voids located in the pons, left middle cerebellar peduncle, and left cerebellar hemisphere. **b** Postcontrast axial T1WI shows prominent enhancement at the lesion.

a   b

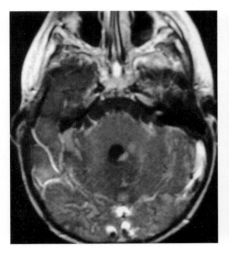 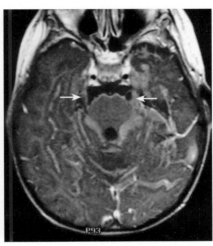

Fig. 1A.**182** **Disseminated medulloblastoma.** **a, b** Postcontrast axial T1WI shows extensive abnormal subarachnoid enhancement in the sulci surrounding the brainstem and along the trigeminal nerves (arrows).

a   b

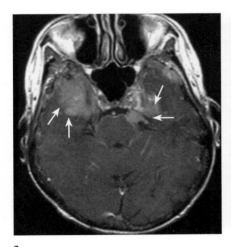 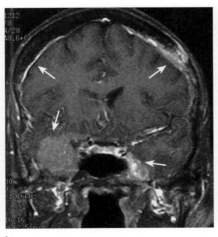 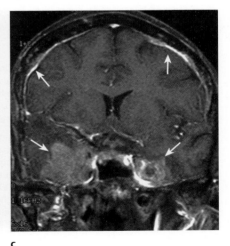

a   b   c

Fig. 1A.**183** **Metastatic breast carcinoma.** Postcontrast axial (**a**) and coronal FS (**b, c**) T1WI shows abnormal subarachnoid enhancement surrounding the brainstem and along the trigeminal nerves (arrows). Also shows dural carcinomatosis with intracranial extension of tumor into both middle cranial fossa from skull metastases (arrows).

Table 1A.**10** (Cont.) Cerebellopontine angle and/or internal auditory canal lesions

Disease	MRI Findings	Comments
Choroid plexus papilloma or carcinoma (Fig. 1A.63)	Circumscribed and/or lobulated lesions with papillary projections, intermediate signal on T1WI and mixed intermediate to high signal on T2WI. Usually prominent Gd-contrast enhancement. Calcifications may be associated. Locations: atrium of lateral ventricle (children) more common than fourth ventricle (adults); rarely other locations such as third ventricle. Associated with hydrocephalus.	Rare intracranial neoplasms. MR features of choroid plexus carcinoma and papilloma overlap; both histologic types can disseminate along CSF pathways and invade brain tissue.
Myeloma/ plasmacytoma (Fig. 1A.65)	Multiple (myeloma) or single (plasmacytoma) well-circumscribed or poorly defined lesions involving the skull and dura. Low to intermediate signal on T1WI, intermediate to high signal on T2WI; usually Gd-contrast enhancement. Associated bone destruction.	Myeloma may have variable destructive or infiltrative changes involving the axial and/or appendicular skeleton.
Lymphoma (Fig. 1A.64)	Single or multiple well-circumscribed or poorly defined lesions involving the skull, dura, and/or leptomeninges. Low to intermediate signal on T1WI, intermediate to high signal on T2WI; usually Gd-contrast enhancement. Bone destruction may be associated. Leptomeningeal tumor often best seen on postcontrast images.	Extra-axial lymphoma may have variable destructive or infiltrative changes involving single or multiple sites of involvement.
Chordoma (Fig. 1A.111)	Well-circumscribed lobulated lesions with low to intermediate signal on T1WI and high signal on T2WI; Gd-contrast enhancement (usually heterogeneous). Locally invasive associated with bone erosion/destruction, encasement of vessels and nerves. Skull base and clivus common location, usually in the midline.	Rare, slow-growing tumors. Detailed anatomic display of extension of chordomas by MRI is important for planning of surgical approaches.
Chondrosarcoma (Fig. 1A.112)	Lobulated lesions with low to intermediate signal on T1WI and high signal on T2WI. With or without matrix mineralization: low signal on T2WI. With Gd-contrast enhancement (usually heterogeneous). Locally invasive associated with bone erosion/destruction, encasement of vessels and nerves. Skull base and petro-occipital synchondrosis common location, usually off midline.	Rare, slow-growing tumors. Detailed anatomic display of extension of chondrosarcomas by MRI is important for planning of surgical approaches.
Osteogenic sarcoma (Fig. 1A.66)	Destructive lesions involving the skull base. Low to intermediate signal on T1WI and mixed low, intermediate, high signal on T2WI. Usually with matrix mineralization/ossification: low signal on T2WI. With Gd-contrast enhancement (usually heterogeneous).	Rare lesions involving the endochondral bone-forming portions of the skull base. More common than chodrosarcomas and Ewing sarcoma. Locally invasive, high metastatic potential. Occurs in children as primary tumors and adults (associated with Paget disease, irradiated bone, chronic osteomyelitis, osteoblastoma, giant cell tumor, fibrous dysplasia).
Ewing sarcoma	Destructive lesions involving the skull base with low to intermediate signal on T1WI and mixed low, intermediate, high signal on T2WI. With or without matrix mineralization: low signal on T2WI. Gd-contrast enhancement (usually heterogeneous).	Usually occurs between the ages of 5 and 30, affects males more than females. Rare lesions involving the skull base. Locally invasive, high metastatic potential.
Sinonasal squamous cell carcinoma	Destructive lesions in the nasal cavity, paranasal sinuses, nasopharynx. With or without intracranial extension via bone destruction or perineural spread through foramen ovale into trigeminal cistern/intracranially. Intermediate signal on T1WI and intermediate to slightly high signal on T2WI; mild Gd-contrast enhancement. Large lesions (necrosis and/or hemorrhage may be associated).	Occurs in adults, more common in males than females, usually above 55 years. Associated with occupational or other exposure to nickel, chromium, mustard gas, radium, manufacture of wood products.
Adenoid cystic carcinoma (Fig. 1A.67)	Destructive lesions in the paranasal sinuses, nasal cavity, nasopharynx. With or without intracranial extension via bone destruction or perineural spread through foramen ovale into trigeminal cistern/intracranially. Intermediate signal on T1WI, intermediate to high signal on T2WI; variable mild, moderate, or prominent Gd-contrast enhancement.	Account for 10% of sinonasal tumors. Arise in any location within sinonasal cavities. Usually occurs in adults above age 30.

Table 1A.**10** (Cont.) Cerebellopontine angle and/or internal auditory canal lesions

Disease	MRI Findings	Comments
Endolymphatic sac tumor (Fig. 1A.**184**)	Extra-axial retrolabyrinthine lesions involving the posterior petrous bone with extension into the cerebellopontine angle cistern, possibly middle ear. Homogeneous low to intermediate signal on T1WI, intermediate to high signal on T2WI, or heterogeneous mixed low, intermediate, and high signal on T1WI and T2WI; Gd-contrast enhancement.	Rare solid and/or cystic tumors (papillary adematous tumors arising from the endolymphatic sac) that are slow growing and rarely metastasize. Associated with localized bone destruction. Can be sporadic or associated with von Hippel-Lindau disease. Affects males and females (children and adults) equally. With or without hemorrhagic components.
Hemangiopericytoma (Fig. 1A.**108**)	Extra-axial mass lesions, often well-circumscribed, with intermediate signal on T1WI and intermediate to slightly high signal on T2WI; prominent Gd-contrast enhancement (may resemble meningiomas). With or without associated erosive bone changes.	Rare neoplasms in young adults (more common in males than females) sometimes referred to as angioblastic meningioma or meningeal hemangiopericytoma. Arise from vascular cells, pericytes. Frequency of metastases > meningiomas.
Neurocutaneous melanosis	Extra-axial or intra-axial lesions usually less than 3 cm in diameter with irregular margins in the leptomeninges or brain parenchyma/brainstem (anterior temporal lobes, cerebellum, thalami, inferior frontal lobes). Intermediate to slightly high signal on T1WI secondary to increased melanin; Gd-contrast enhancement. Vermian hypoplasia, arachnoid cysts, Dandy-Walker malformation may be associated.	Neuroectodermal dysplasia with proliferation of melanocytes in leptomeninges associated with large and/or numerous cutaneous nevi. May change into CNS melanoma.
Inflammatory: *Infectious (pyogenic, granulomatous [sarcoidosis, tuberculosis], parasitic)* *Noninfectious (e.g., sarcoidosis, Langerhans cell histiocytosis [LCH])* (Fig. 1A.**96**)		
Subdural/epidural abscess–Empyema (Fig. 1A.**72**)	Epidural or subdural collections with low signal on T1WI and high signal on T2WI; thin, linear peripheral zones of Gd-contrast enhancement.	Often results from complications related to sinusitis (usually frontal), meningitis, otitis media, ventricular shunts, or surgery. Can be associated with venous sinus thrombosis and venous cerebral or cerbellar infarcts, cerebritis, brain abscess. Mortality 30%.
Leptomeningeal infection/inflammation (Fig. 1A.**185**)	Single or multiple nodular enhancing lesions and/or focal or diffuse abnormal subarachnoid enhancement. Low to intermediate signal on T1WI, intermediate to high signal on T2WI. Leptomeningeal inflammation often best seen on postcontrast images.	Gd-contrast enhancement in the intracranial subarachnoid space (leptomeninges) usually is associated with significant pathology (inflammation and/or infection versus neoplasm). Inflammation and/or infection of the leptomeninges can result from pyogenic, fungal, or parasitic diseases as well as tuberculosis. Neurosarcoidosis and LCH can result in granulomatous disease in the leptomeninges, producing similar patterns of subarachnoid enhancement.

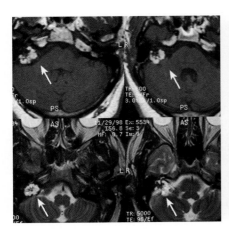

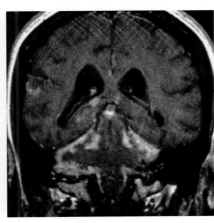

◁ ◁ Fig. 1A.**184 Endolymphatic sac tumor.** Axial T1WI (top figures) and axial T2WI (bottom figures) show a multilobulated extra-axial lesion with high signal involving the posterior right petrous bone extending into the cerebello-pontine angle cistern (arrows).

◁ Fig. 1A.**185 Leptomeningeal sarcoidosis.** Postcontrast coronal T1WI shows marked abnormal subarachnoid enhancement within the cerebellar sulci and surrounding the brainstem.

Table 1A.**10** (Cont.) Cerebellopontine angle and/or internal auditory canal lesions

Disease	MRI Findings	Comments
Eosinophilic granuloma (Fig. 1A.**74**)	Single or mutiple circumscribed soft-tissue lesions in the marrow of the skull associated with focal bony destruction/erosion with extension extracranially, intracranially, or both. Lesions usually have low to intermediate signal on T1WI and mixed intermediate to slightly high signal on T2WI; Gd-contrast enhancement. With or without enhancement of the adjacent dura.	*Single lesion:* Commonly seen in males more than females, below age 20. Proliferation of histiocytes in medullary cavity with localized destruction of bone with extension in adjacent soft tissues. *Multiple lesions:* Associated with syndromes such as: Letterer-Siwe disease (lymphadenopathy hepatosplenomegaly), children below 2 years of age; Hand-Schüller-Christian disease (lymphadenopathy, exophthalmos, diabetes insipidus), children age 5–10 years.
Other:		
Vascular		
AVM (Fig. 1A.**47**)	Lesions with irregular margins that can be located in the brain parenchyma–pia, dura, or both locations. AVMs contain multiple tortuous tubular flow voids on T1WI and T2WI secondary to patent arteries with high blood flow; as well as thrombosed vessels with variable signal, areas of hemorrhage in various phases, calcifications, and gliosis. The venous portions often show Gd-contrast enhancement. GRE MRI shows flow-related enhancement (high signal) in patent arteries and veins of the AVM. Usually not associated with mass effect except in the case of recent hemorrhage or venous occlusion.	Supratentorial AVMs occur more frequently than infratentorial AVMs. Annual risk of hemorrhage. AVMs can be sporadic, congenital, or associated with a history of trauma.
Hemorrhagic **Epidural hematoma** (Fig. 1A.**68**)	Biconvex extra-axial hematoma located between the skull and dura. Displaced dura has low signal on T2WI. The signal of the hematoma itself depends on its age, size, hematocrit, and oxygen tension. With or without associated edema. High signal on T2WI involving the displaced brain parenchyma. Subfalcine, uncal herniation may be associated. *Hyperacute:* intermediate signal on T1WI, intermediate to high signal on T2WI. *Acute:* low to intermediate signal on T1WI, high signal on T2WI. *Subacute:* high signal on T1WI and T2WI.	Epidural hematomas usually result from trauma/ tearing of an epidural artery or dural venous sinus. Epidural hematomas do not cross cranial sutures. Skull fracture may be associated.
Subdural hematoma (Fig. 1A.**69**), (Fig. 1A.**70**)	Crescentic extra-axial hematoma located in the potential space between the inner margin of the dura and outer margin of the arachnoid membrane. The signal of the hematoma depends on its age, size, hematocrit,and oxygen tension. With or without associated edema. High signal on T2WI involving the displaced brain parenchyma. Subfalcine, uncal herniation may be associated. *Hyperacute:* intermediate signal on T1WI, intermediate to high signal on T2WI. *Acute:* low to intermediate signal on T1WI, low signal on T2WI. *Subacute:* high signal on T1WI and T2WI. *Chronic:* Variable, often low to intermediate signal on T1WI, high signal on T2WI. With or without enhancement of collection and organizing neomembrane. Mixed MRI signal can result if rebleeding occurs into chronic collection.	Subdural hematomas usually result from trauma/ stretching/tearing of cortical veins where they enter the subdural space to drain into dural venous sinuses. Subdural hematomas do cross sites of cranial sutures. Skull fracture may be associated.
Fibrous dysplasia (Fig. 1A.**115**)	Expansile process involving the skull base with mixed low to intermediate signal on T1WI, variable mixed low, intermediate, high signal on T2WI; usually heterogenous enhancement.	Usually seen in adolescents and young adults. Can result in narrowing of neuroforamina with cranial nerve compression, facial deformities, mono-ostotic and poly-ostotic forms (endocrine abnormalities may be associated, such as with McCune-Albright syndrome, precocious puberty).
Paget disease (Fig. 1A.**186**)	Expansile sclerotic/lytic process involving the skull with mixed low to intermediate signal on T1WI, variable mixed low, intermediate, high signal on T2WI; variable heterogenous enhancement. Irregular/indistinct borders between marrow and inner margins of the outer and inner tables of the skull.	Usually seen in older adults. Can result in narrowing of neuroforamina with cranial nerve compression, basilar impression. With or without compression of brainstem.

Table 1A.**11** Sellar/juxtasellar lesions

Disease	MRI Findings	Comments
Developmental anomalies		
Ectopic posterior pituitary (Fig. 1A.187)	Posterior "bright spot" of pituitary gland (neurohypophysis) on T1WI is located at upper portion of infundibulum or undersuface of hypothalamus instead of dorsal portion of the sella.	Congenital anomaly with the aberrant position of the neurohypophysis (posterior pituitary) often seen located at undersurface of hypothalamus. Associated with pituitary dwarfism, delayed skeletal maturation. Males more commonly affected than females.

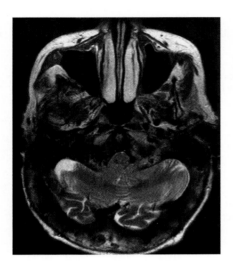

Fig. 1A.**186**   **Paget disease.** Axial T2WI shows an expansile process involving the skull with mixed low to intermediate signal. Irregular/indistinct borders are seen between marrow and inner margins of the outer and inner tables of the skull.

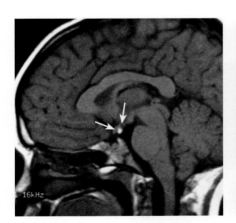

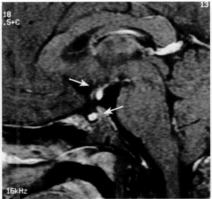

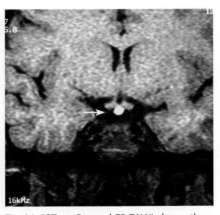

Fig. 1A.**187**   **Ectopic posterior pituitary.**   **a** Sagittal T1WI shows the posterior "bright spot" of the pituitary gland (neurohypophysis) located at the undersurface of the hypothalamus instead of dorsal portion of the sella (arrows).

Fig. 1A.**187 b**   Postcontrast sagittal FS T1WI shows normal enhancement of the anterior portion of the pituitary gland in the sella (arrow) and ectopic posterior pituitary tissue (arrow).

Fig. 1A.**187 c**   Coronal FS T1WI shows the ectopic posterior pituitary tissue with high signal in its location below the optic chiasm (arrow).

Table 1A.**11** (Cont.) Sellar/juxtasellar lesions

Disease	MRI Findings	Comments
Pituitary hypoplasia (Fig. 1A.188)	Absence or hypoplasia of portions or all of the pituitary gland and stalk.	Rare anomalies with absence or hypoplasia of anterior and/or posterior pituitary lobes, pituitary stalk. Associated with varying degrees of endocrine dysfunction including panhypopituitarism. Also associated with other congenital anomalies.
Cephaloceles (meningoceles or meningoencephaloceles) (Fig. 1A.189)	Defect in skull through which there is either herniation of meninges and CSF (meningocele) or meninges, CSF, and brain tissue (meningoencephaloceles).	Congenital malformation involving lack of separation of neuroectoderm from surface ectoderm with resultant localized failure of bone formation. Can involve the sphenoid with extension into the suprasellar cistern.
Lipoma of the sellar region (Fig. 1A.190)	Lipomas in the sellar region usually in suprasellar cistern, less commonly within the sella. MR signal isointense to subcutaneous fat on T1WI (high signal) and on T2WI. Signal suppression occurs with frequency-selective FS techniques or with a STIR method. Typically no Gd-contrast enhancement.	Benign fatty lesions resulting from congenital malformation, often located in or near the midline. May contain calcifications and/or traversing blood vessels. Usually asymptomatic unless cause mass effect.
Pituitary hypertrophy	Pituitary hypertrophy involves enlargement of the pituitary gland, usually without focal abnormalities in MRI signal characteristics or enhancement pattern. The normal pituitary gland in adults measures up to 10 mm in height. In the early postpartum period, the gland measures up to 12 mm in height and is referred to as physiologic hypertrophy. During late pregnancy and early postpartum period, the pituitary gland also has high signal on T1WI.	In addition to pregnancy, pituitary hypertrophy can be associated with endocrine end-organ failure and central precocious puberty.
Diabetes insipidus	The neurohypophysis or posterior pituitary lobe is seen as a zone of high signal (bright spot) on T1WI in almost all healthy patients. In patients with central diabetes insipidus this bright spot is usually absent.	Diabetes insipidus is a disorder of water balance with excretion of abnormally large volumes of dilute urine. Central diabetes insipidus results from inadequate secretion of antidiuretic hormone from hypothalamic/pituitary dysfunction that can result from trauma, surgery, neoplasms (germinomas, astrocytomas), inflammatory diseases such as LCH, sarcoidosis, etc.

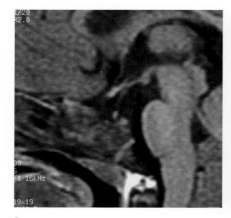

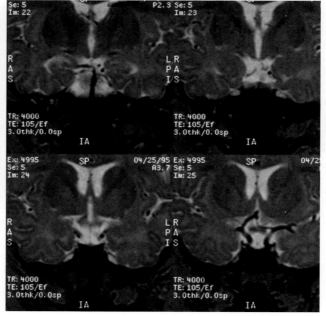

Fig. 1A.**188** **Pituitary hypoplasia.**
a Sagittal T1WI shows severe hypoplasia of the pituitary gland in this patient with panhypopituitary dysfunction since birth.
b Coronal T2WI show pituitary hypoplasia with normal midline position of the infundibulum.

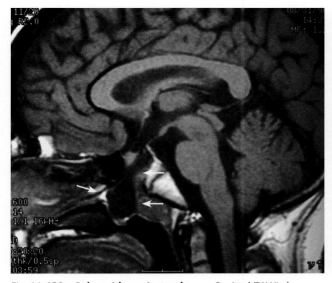

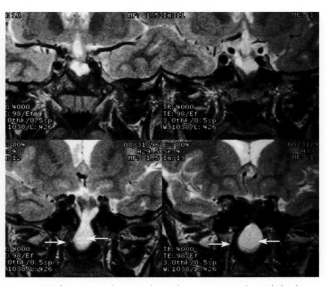

Fig. 1A.**189** **Sphenoid meningocele. a** Sagittal T1WI shows a defect in the sphenoid dorsal to the pituitary gland, through which there is herniation of meninges and CSF (arrows).

Fig. 1A.**189 b** Coronal T2WI show the meningocele with high signal extending into the nasopharynx (arrows).

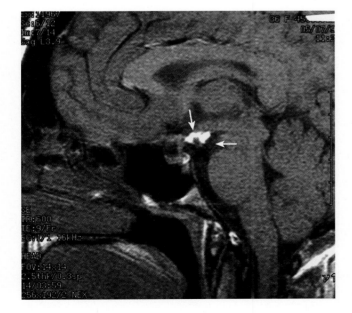

Fig. 1A.**190** **Lipoma of the sellar region.** Sagittal T1WI shows a lipoma with high signal at the undersurface of the hypothalamus and dorsal to the infundibulum (arrows).

Table 1A.11 (Cont.) Sellar/juxtasellar lesions

Disease	MRI Findings	Comments
Empty sella (Fig. 1A.191)	The pituitary gland is thinned and flattened along floor of sella, infundibulum is midline in position. The flattened pituitary gland itself has normal MR signal characteristics.	Usually represents a normal variant. A similar appearance may result from peripartum necrosis or injury from radiation/surgery. Can be associated with hydrocephalus and pseudotumor cerebrii.
Hypothalamic hamartoma (Fig. 1A.192)	Sessile or pedunculated lesions at the tuber cinereum of the hypothalamus. Often intermediate signal on T1WI and T2WI similar to gray matter, occasionally slightly high signal on T2WI; usually no enhancement. Rarely contain cystic and/or fatty portions.	Usually occur in children with isosexual precocious puberty (age 0–8 years) or seizures (gelastic or partial complex) in second decade. Congenital/developmental heterotopia/hamartoma (non-neoplastic lesions).
Rathke's cleft cyst (Fig. 1A.193)	Well-circumscribed lesion with variable low, intermediate, or high signal on T1WI and T2WI. On T1WI, two-thirds have high signal and one-third low signal; on T2WI, 50% have high signal, 25% low signal, and 25% intermediate signal. No Gd-contrast centrally, with or without thin peripheral enhancement. Lesion locations: 50% intrasellar, 25% suprasellar, 25% intrasellar and suprasellar.	Uncommon sellar/juxtasellar benign cystic lesion containing fluid with variable amounts of protein, mucopolysaccharide, and/or cholesterol; arise from epithelial rests of the craniopharyngeal duct.
Epidermoid (congenital cholesteatoma) (Fig. 1A.194)	Well-circumscribed, spheroid or multilobulated extra-axial ectodermal-inclusion cystic lesions with low to intermediate signal on T1WI and high signal on T2WI similar to CSF. Mixed low, intermediate, or high signal on FLAIR images; no Gd-contrast enhancement. Often insinuate along CSF pathways, chronic deformation of adjacent neural tissue (brainstem, brain parenchyma). Commonly located in posterior cranial fossa (cerebellopontine angle cistern), parasellar/middle cranial fossa.	Non-neoplastic, congenital or acquired extra-axial off-midline lesions filled with desquamated cells and keratinaceous debris. Usually mild mass effect on adjacent brain. Infratentorial locations more common than supratentorial locations. Affects male and female adults equally. With or without related clinical symptoms.

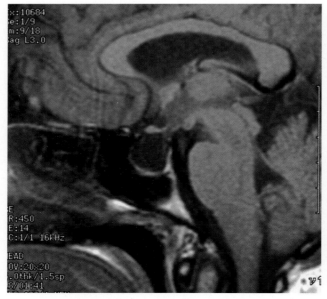

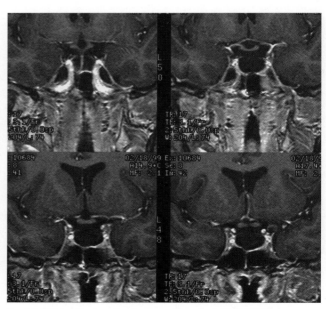

Fig. 1A.**191 Empty sella. a** Sagittal T1WI shows the pituitary gland thinned and flattened along floor of sella in this patient with normal pituitary function.

Fig. 1A.**191 b** Postcontrast coronal (spoiled GRE) T1WI shows enhancement of the flattened pituitary gland at the floor of sella with the infundibulum midline in position.

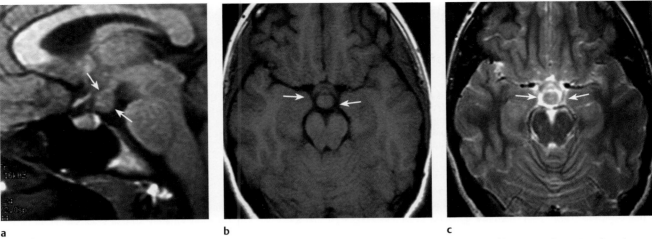

Fig. 1A.192   Hypothalamic hamartoma. Sagittal (**a**) and axial (**b**) T1WI shows a pedunculated lesion with intermediate signal at the undersurface of the tuber cinereum of the hypothalamus (arrows).   **c** Axial T2WI shows the lesion to have intermediate signal similar to gray matter (arrows).

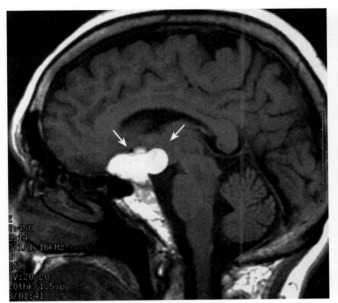

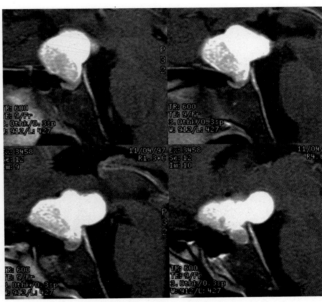

Fig. 1A.193   Rathke's cleft cyst.   a Sagittal T1WI shows a well-circumscribed lobulated lesion with high signal located in the sella, extending into the suprasellar cistern (arrows).

Fig. 1A.193 b   Postcontrast sagittal FS T1WI shows enhancement of the pituitary gland, which is flattened by the Rathke's cleft cyst.

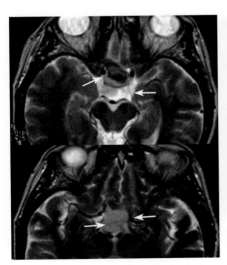

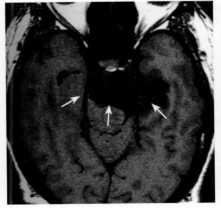

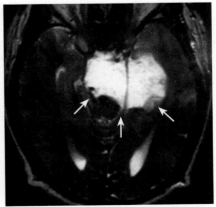

Fig. 1A.193 c   Axial T2WI shows the lesion to have low and slightly high signal zones (arrows).

Fig. 1A.194   Epidermoid (congenital cholesteatoma).   a Axial T1WI shows a multilobulated extra-axial lesion with low to intermediate signal located dorsal to the sella (arrows).

Fig. 1A.194 b   Axial T2WI shows the lesion to have high signal. The lesion extends upward into the suprasellar cistern (arrows).

Table 1A.**11** (Cont.) Sellar/juxtasellar lesions

Disease	MRI Findings	Comments
Dermoid **(Fig.** 1A.**86)**	Well-circumscribed, spheroid or multilobulated extra-axial lesions, usually with high signal on T1WI and variable low, intermediate, and/or high signal on T2WI. No Gd-contrast enhancement. Fluid-fluid or fluid-debris levels may be present. Can cause chemical meningitis if dermoid cyst ruptures into the subarachnoid space. Commonly located at or near midline; supratentorial more common than infratentorial.	Non-neoplastic, congenital or acquired ectodermal-inclusion cystic lesions filled with lipid material, cholesterol, desquamated cells, and keratinaceous debris. Usually mild mass effect on adjacent brain. Slightly more common in adult males than adult females. With or without related clinical symptoms.
Neoplasms		
Pituitary adenoma **(Figs.** 1A.**195–197)**	*Microadenomas (<10 mm):* Commonly have intermediate signal on T1WI and T2WI. Cyst, hemorrhage, necrosis may be associated. Typically enhance less than normal pituitary tissue. Often best seen with dynamic early-phase imaging. *Macroadenomas (>10 mm):* Commonly have intermediate signal on T1WI and T2WI similar to gray matter. Necrosis, cyst, hemorrhage may be associated. Usually prominent enhancement. Extension into suprasellar cistern with waist at diaphragma sella. With or without extension into cavernous sinus. Occasionally invades skull base.	Common benign slow-growing tumors representing approximately 50 % of sellar/parasellar neoplasms in adults. Can be associated with endocrine abnormalities related to oversecretion of hormones (prolactin, nonsecretory type, growth hormone, ACTH, others). Prolactinomas: more common in females than males; growth hormone tumors: more common in males than females. Rarely, extensive hemorrhage involving the adenoma resulting in pituitary apoplexy, Sheehan syndrome.
Granular cell tumor (choristoma) and glioma of the neurohypophysis (Fig. 1A.**198)**	Abnormal focal or diffuse enlargement of pituitary stalk, usually with enhancement.	These lesions represent the two rare primary neoplasms of neurohypophysis and pituitary stalk.

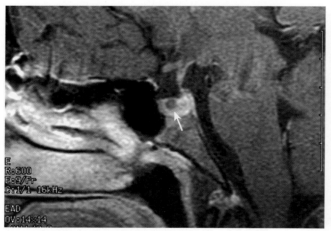

a

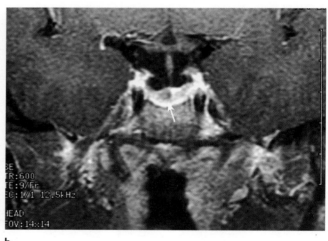

b

Fig. 1A.**195** **Pituitary microadenoma.** Postcontrast sagittal (**a**) and coronal (**b**) FS T1WI shows a 2-mm-diameter lesion in the right side of the pituitary gland (arrows) that enhances to a lesser degree than the adjacent normal pituitary tissue.

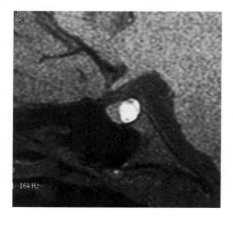

Fig. 1A.**196** **Pituitary microadenoma with hemorrhage.** Sagittal FS T1WI shows a 7-mm-diameter zone of high signal in the mid-posterior portion of the pituitary gland.

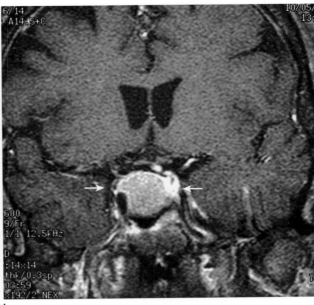

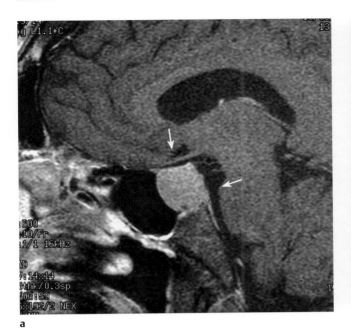

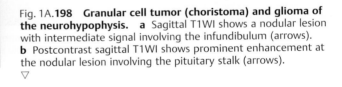

◁ Fig. 1A.**197** **Pituitary macroadenoma.** Postcontrast sagittal (**a**) and coronal (**b**) FS T1WI show a homogeneously enhancing lesion involving the pituitary gland measuring 20 mm in height (arrows). The lesion extends toward the right cavernous sinus. The infundibulum is also deviated to the left.   **c** Coronal T2WI shows the lesion to have intermediate signal.

Fig. 1A.**198** **Granular cell tumor (choristoma) and glioma of the neurohypophysis.**   **a** Sagittal T1WI shows a nodular lesion with intermediate signal involving the infundibulum (arrows). **b** Postcontrast sagittal T1WI shows prominent enhancement at the nodular lesion involving the pituitary stalk (arrows).
▽

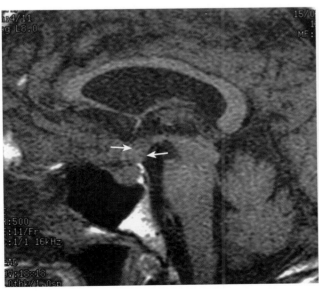

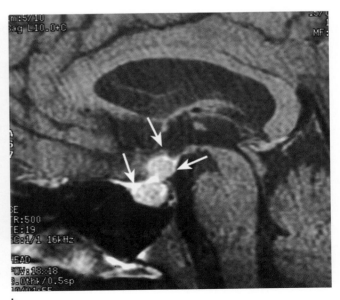

Table 1A.**11** (Cont.) Sellar/juxtasellar lesions

Disease	MRI Findings	Comments
Craniopharyngioma (Fig. 1A.199)	Circumscribed lobulated lesions; both suprasellar and intrasellar location, less commonly suprasellar or intrasellar only. Variable low, intermediate, and/or high signal on T1WI and T2WI. With or without nodular or rim Gd-contrast enhancement. May contain cysts, lipid components, and calcifications.	Usually histologically benign but locally aggressive lesions arising from squamous epithelial rests along Rathke's cleft. Occurs in children (10 years) and adults (above 40 years). Affects males and females equally.
Glioma (optic chiasm, hypothalamus) (Figs.1A.200, 1A.201)	Fusiform and/or nodular enlargement of optic chiasm and/or optic nerves. Usually low to intermediate signal on T1WI, intermediate to high signal on T2WI; variable enhancement. With or without cystic components with large lesions.	In children, usually associated with neurofibromatosis type 1 (approximately 10% of patients with neurofibromatosis type 1). Often slow-growing lesions. High signal abnormality on T2WI can extend along optic radiations.
Meningioma (Figs.1A.202, 1A.203)	Extra-axial well-circumscribed dural-based lesions. Supratentorial location more common than infratentorial. Intermediate signal on T1WI, intermediate to slightly high signal on T2WI; usually prominent Gd-contrast enhancement. Calcifications may be associated.	Most common extra-axial tumor. Usually benign neoplasms, typically occurring in adults above 40 years of age, more common in women than men. Multiple meningiomas seen with neurofibromatosis type 2. Can result in compression of adjacent brain parenchyma, encasement of arteries, and compression of dural venous sinuses. Rarely invasive/malignant types.

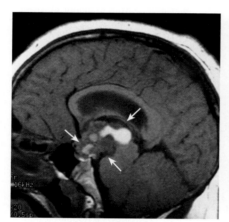

Fig. 1A.199   Craniopharyngioma.
a Sagittal T1WI shows a lobulated lesion with mixed intermediate and high signal located in the sella and suprasellar cistern (arrows).

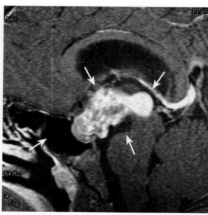

Fig. 1A.**199 b**   Postcontrast FS sagittal T1WI shows enhancement in portions of the lesion (arrows).

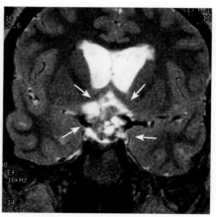

Fig. 1A.**199 c**   Coronal T2WI shows the lesion to contain zones with intermediate and high signal (arrows).

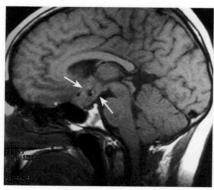

a

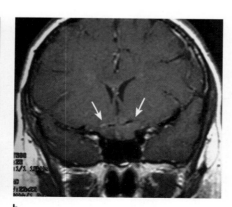

b

Fig. 1A.200   Glioma (optic chiasm).
a Sagittal T1WI shows fusiform enlargement of the optic chiasm and optic nerves (arrows). The lesion has predominantly intermediate signal containing several small zones of low signal.   **b** Postcontrast coronal T1WI shows minimal enhancement in a small portion of the lesion (arrows).

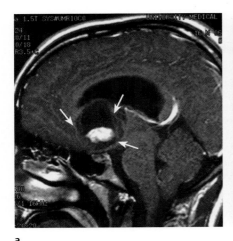

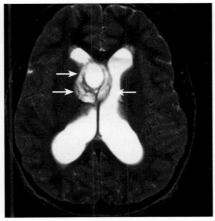

Fig. 1A.**201** **Pilocytic astrocytoma of the hypothalamus.** **a** Postcontrast sagittal T1WI shows a cystic lesion with an enhancing nodule at the hypothalamus (arrows). **b** Axial T2WI shows the lesion to have predomantly high signal with small zones of intermediate signal (arrows).

a

b

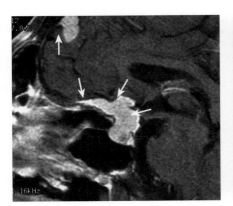

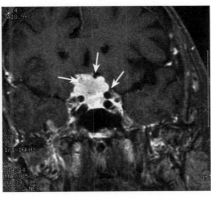

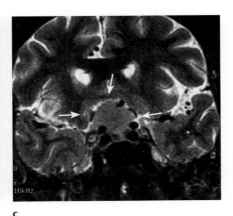

a

b

c

Fig. 1A.**202** **Meningioma.** Postcontrast sagittal (**a**) and coronal (**b**) FS T1WI show an enhancing extra-axial dural-based lesion

along the planum sphenoidale, extending dorsally into the suprasellar cistern (arrows). A small meningioma is also seen at the falx.

(curved arrow). **c** Coronal T2WI shows the lesion to have intermediate to slightly high signal similar to gray matter (arrows).

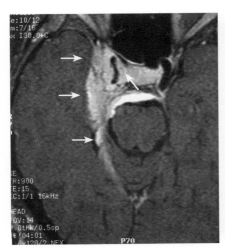

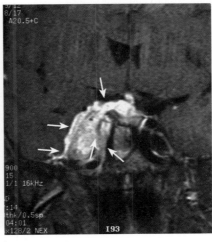

a

b

Fig. 1A.**203** **Meningioma.** Postcontrast axial (**a**) and coronal (**b**) FS T1WI shows an enhancing extra-axial lesion in the right parasellar region/middle cranial fossa, extending into the right side of the sella and displacing the pituitary gland and infundibulum to the left (arrows). The lesion extends into the right cavernous sinus, encasing and narrowing the flow void of the right internal carotid artery (arrows). The lesion also extends dorsally along the tentorial incisura.

Table 1A.**11** (Cont.) Sellar/juxtasellar lesions

Disease	MRI Findings	Comments
Paraganglioma	Lobulated lesion involving the pituitary gland and/or pituitary stalk. Intermediate signal on T1WI, high signal on T2WI with tubular zones of flow voids; prominent Gd-contrast enhancement.	Paragangliomas are neoplasms that arise from paraganglion cells of neural crest origin. Usually occur at carotid body, jugular foramen, middle ear, and along the vagus nerve. Rarely occur in suprasellar cistern or sella as well as pineal gland, cauda equina.
Germinoma (Fig. 1A.**204**)	Circumscribed tumors with or without disseminated disease. Location in order of decreasing frequency: pineal region, suprasellar region, third ventricle/basal ganglia. Low to intermediate signal on T1WI, occasionally high signal on T1WI, variable low, intermediate, high signal on T2WI; Gd-contrast enhancement of tumor and leptomeninges if disseminated.	Most common type of germ cell tumor. Occurs in males more commonly than females (age 10–30 years). Usually midline neoplasms.
Teratoma (Fig. 1A.**60**)	Circumscribed lesions. Location in order of decreasing frequency: pineal region, suprasellar region, third ventricle. Variable low, intermediate, and/or high signal on T1WI and T2WI; with or without Gd-contrast enhancement. May contain calcifications as well as fatty components that can cause a chemical meningitis if ruptured.	Second most common type of germ cell tumors; occurs in children, males more common than females. Benign or malignant types. Composed of derivatives of ectoderm, mesoderm, and/or endoderm.
Vascular		
Arterial aneurysm (Fig. 1A.**205**)	*Saccular aneurysm:* Focal well-circumscribed zone of signal void on T1WI and T2WI, variable mixed signal if thrombosed. *Giant aneurysm:* Focal well-circumscribed structure with layers of low, intermediate, and high signal on T2WI secondary to layers of thrombus of different ages, as well as a zone of signal void representing a patent lumen if present. On T1WI, layers of intermediate and high signal can be seen as well as a zone of signal void. *Fusiform aneurysm:* Elongated and ectatic arteries, variable intraluminal MR signal related to turbulent or slowed blood flow or partial/complete thrombosis. *Dissecting aneurysms:* The involved arterial wall is thickened and has intermediate to high signal on T1WI and T2WI; the signal void representing the patent lumen is narrowed.	Abnormal fusiform or focal dilatation of artery secondary to: acquired/degenerative etiology, polycystic disease, connective-tissue disease, atherosclerosis, trauma, infection (mycotic), AVM, vasculitis, and drugs.
AVM (Fig. 1A.47)	Lesions with irregular margins that can be located in the brain parenchyma–pia, dura, or both locations. AVMs contain multiple tortuous tubular flow voids on T1WI and T2WI secondary to patent arteries with high blood flow, as well as thrombosed vessels with variable signal, areas of hemorrhage in various phases, calcifications, and gliosis. The venous portions often show Gd-contrast enhancement. GRE MRI shows flow-related enhancement (high signal) in patent arteries and veins of the AVM. MRA using TOF or phase contrast techniques can provide additional detailed information about the nidus, feeding arteries, and draining veins, and presence of associated aneurysms. Usually not associated with mass effect except in cases of recent hemorrhage or venous occlusion.	Infratentorial AVMs are much less common than supratentorial AVMs.
Cavernous hemangioma (Fig. 1A.206)	Single or multiple multilobulated intra-axial lesions that have a peripheral rim or irregular zone of low signal on T2WI secondary to hemosiderin, surrounding a central zone of variable signal (low, intermediate, high, or mixed) on T1WI and T2WI depending on ages of hemorrhagic portions. GRE techniques useful for detecting multiple lesions.	Supratentorial cavernous angiomas occur more frequently than infratentorial lesions. Can be found in many different locations. Multiple lesions more than 50%. Association with venous angiomas and risk of hemorrhage.
Arachnoid cyst–Sellar/ suprasellar (Fig. 1A.**207**)	Well-circumscribed extra-axial lesions with low signal on T1WI and high signal on T2WI similar to CSF; no Gd-contrast enhancement.	Non-neoplastic congenital, developmental or acquired extra-axial lesions filled with CSF. Usually mild mass effect on adjacent brain. Location more commonly supratentorial than infratentorial. More common in males than females. With or without related clinical symptoms.

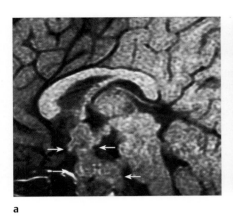

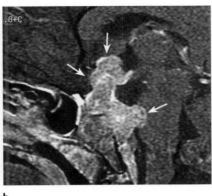

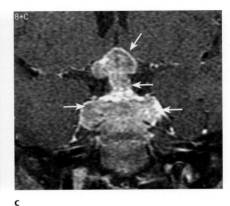

a   b   c

Fig. 1A.204 Germinoma. a Sagittal T1WI shows a large multilobulated lesion with intermediate signal in the suprasellar cistern, extending into the sella and posteriorly impressing the pons (arrows). Postcontrast sagittal (**b**) and coronal (**c**) FS T1WI shows prominent enhancement of the lesion (arrows). The lesion compresses the optic chiasm and displaces the optic nerves laterally.

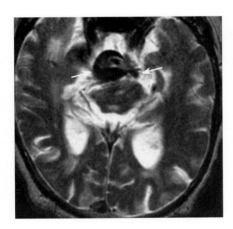

Fig. 1A.205 Giant aneurysm. Axial T2WI shows a focal well-circumscribed structure with layers of low, intermediate, and high signal in the dorsal lower portion of the suprasellar cistern.

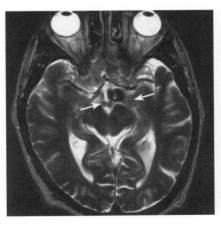

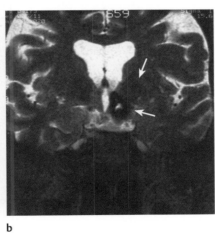

a   b

Fig. 1A.206 Cavernous hemangioma. Axial (**a**) and coronal (**b**) T2WI shows a lesion with predominantly low signal in the left hypothalamic region extending toward the supracellar cistern.

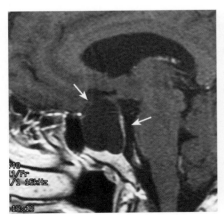

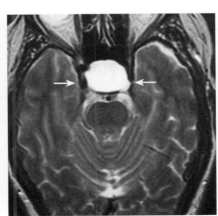

a   b

Fig. 1A.207 Arachnoid cyst–sella/suprasellar. a Postcontrast sagittal T1WI shows a large cystic structure with low signal similar to CSF located in the sella and suprasellar cistern (arrows). The cystic lesion uplifts the optic chiasm. **b** Axial T2WI shows the cyst to have high signal (arrows).

Table 1A.**11** (Cont.) Sellar/juxtasellar lesions

Disease	MRI Findings	Comments
Metastatic tumor (Figs. 1A.**208**, 1A.**209**)	Single or multiple well-circumscribed or poorly de-fined lesions involving the skull, dura, leptomen-inges, choroid plexus, or pituitary gland. Low to in-termediate signal on T1WI and intermediate to high signal on T2WI; usually Gd-contrast enhance-ment. Bone destruction and compression of neural tissue or vessels may be associated. Leptomening-eal tumor often best seen on postcontrast images.	Metastatic tumor may have variable destructive or infiltrative changes involving single or multiple sites of involvement.
Lymphoma (Fig. 1A.**210**)	Primary CNS lymphoma: focal or infiltrating lesion located in the basal ganglia, posterior fossa/brain-stem. Low to intermediate signal on T1WI, interme-diate to slightly high signal on T2WI. Hemorrhage/ necrosis may be associated in immunocom-promised patients. Usually Gd-contrast enhance-ment. Diffuse leptomeningeal enhancement is another pattern of intracranial lymphoma.	Primary CNS lymphoma more common than sec-ondary, usually seen in adults above 40 years of age. B cell lymphoma more common than T cell lymphoma. Increasing incidence related to number of immunocompromised patients in population. MRI features of primary and secondary lymphoma of brain overlap. Intracranial lymphoma can involve the leptomeninges in secondary lymphoma more commonly than primary lymphoma.
Myeloma/plasmacy-toma (Fig. 1A.**65**)	Multiple (myeloma) or single (plasmacytoma) well-circumscribed or poorly defined lesions involving the skull and dura. Low to intermediate signal on T1WI, intermediate to high signal on T2WI; usually Gd-contrast enhancement. Associated bone de-struction.	Myeloma may have variable destructive or infiltra-tive changes involving the axial and/or appendicular skeleton
Chordoma (Fig. 1A.**111**)	Well-circumscribed lobulated lesions with low to in-termediate signal on T1WI and high signal on T2WI; Gd-contrast enhancement (usually hetero-geneous). Locally invasive associated with bone erosion/destruction, encasement of vessels and nerves. Skull base and clivus common location, usually in the midline.	Rare, slow-growing tumors. Detailed anatomic dis-play of extension of chordomas by MRI is important for planning of surgical approaches.
Chondrosarcoma (Fig. 1A.**211**)	Lobulated lesions with low to intermediate signal on T1WI and high signal on T2WI. With or without matrix mineralization: low signal on T2WI. Gd-con-trast enhancement (usually heterogeneous). Locally invasive associated with bone erosion/destruction, encasement of vessels and nerves. Skull base and petrooccipital synchondrosis common location, usually off midline.	Rare, slow-growing tumors. Detailed anatomic dis-play of extension of chondrosarcomas by MRI is im-portant for planning of surgical approaches.
Osteogenic sarcoma (Fig. 1A.**66**)	Destructive lesions involving the skull base. Low to intermediate signal on T1WI, mixed low, interme-diate, high signal on T2WI. Usually with matrix mineralization/ossification: low signal on T2WI, Gd-contrast enhancement (usually heterogeneous).	Rare lesions involving the endochondral bone-form-ing portions of the skull base, more common than chodrosarcomas and Ewing sarcoma. Locally inva-sive, high metastatic potential. Occurs in children as primary tumors and adults (associated with Paget disease, irradiated bone, chronic osteomyeli-tis, osteoblastoma, giant cell tumor, fibrous dys-plasia).
Ewing sarcoma	Destructive lesions involving the skull base. Low to intermediate signal on T1WI, mixed low, interme-diate, high signal on T2WI. With or without matrix mineralization: low signal on T2WI. Gd-contrast en-hancement (usually heterogeneous).	Usually occurs between the ages of 5 and 30, more common in males than females. Rare lesions involv-ing the skull base. Locally invasive, high metastatic potential.
Sinonasal squamous cell carcinoma	Destructive lesions in the nasal cavity, paranasal sinuses, nasopharynx. With or without intracranial extension via bone destruction or perineural spread. Intermediate signal on T1WI, intermediate to slightly high signal on T2WI; mild Gd-contrast enhancement. Large lesions (necrosis and/or hemorrhage may be associated).	Occurs in adults usually below age 55, more com-mon in males than females. Associated with occu-pational or other exposure to: nickel, chromium, mustard gas, radium, manufacture of wood pro-ducts.

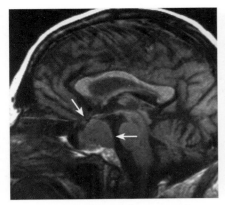

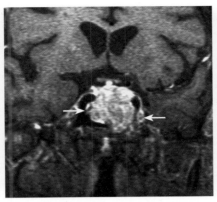

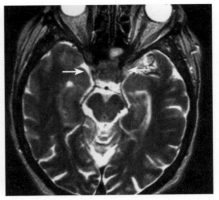

Fig. 1A.**208 Metastatic breast carcinoma. a** Sagittal T1WI shows a destructive lesion with intermediate signal involving the sphenoid "with extension into the sella and suprasellar cistern (arrows).

Fig. 1A.**208 b** Postcontrast coronal FS T1WI shows prominent enhancement of the metastatic lesion (arrows).

Fig. 1A.**208 c** Axial T2WI shows the lesion to have intermediate signal (arrows).

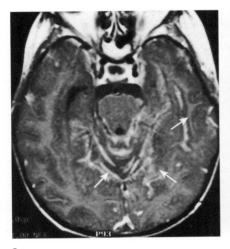

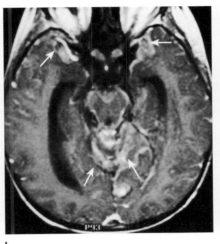

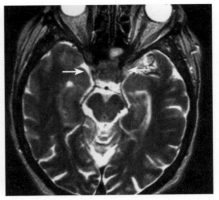

a

b

Fig. 1A.**210 Lymphoma.** Postcontrast axial T1WI shows abnormal enhancement in the leptomeninges, basal subarachnoid cisterns surrounding the brainstem, and suprasellar cistern.(arrows).

Fig. 1A.**209 Disseminated subarachnoid/leptomeningeal medulloblastoma.
a, b** Postcontrast axial T1WI shows abnormal enhancement in the supratentorial and infratentorial leptomeninges, basal subarachnoid cisterns, and suprasellar cistern surrounding the optic chiasm/ nerves (arrows).

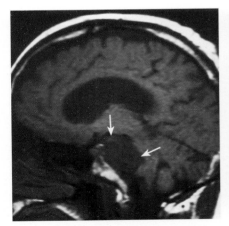

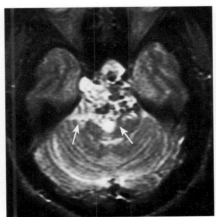

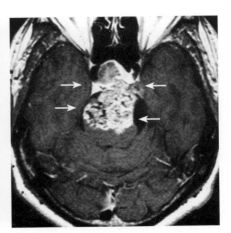

Fig. 1A.**211 Chondrosarcoma. a** Sagittal T1WI shows an extra-axial lesion with low to intermediate signal located within and along the endocranial surface of the clivus extending into the sella. The lesion deforms and displaces the brainstem dorsally (arrows).

Fig. 1A.**211 b** Axial T2WI shows the lesion to have predominantly high signal containing small zones of low signal (matrix mineralization) (arrows).

Fig. 1A.**211 c** Postcontrast axial T1WI shows heterogeneous enhancement of the lesion (arrows). The lesion is associated with bone erosion/destruction of the clivus and sphenoid.

Table 1A.**11** (Cont.) Sellar/juxtasellar lesions

Disease	MRI Findings	Comments
Adenoid cystic carcinoma (Fig. 1A.212)	Destructive lesions in the paranasal sinuses, nasal cavity, nasopharynx. With or without intracranial extension via bone destruction or perineural spread. Intermediate signal on T1WI, intermediate to high signal on T2WI; variable mild, moderate, or prominent Gd-contrast enhancement.	Account for 10 % of sinonasal tumors. Arise in any location within sinonasal cavities. Usually occurs in adults below age 30.
Esthesioneuroblastoma (Fig. 1A.213)	Locally destructive lesions with low to intermediate signal on T1WI and intermediate to high signal on T2WI; prominent Gd-contrast enhancement. Location: superior nasal cavity, ethmoid air cells with occasional extension into the other paranasal sinuses, orbits, anterior cranial fossa, cavernous sinuses.	Tumors also referred to as olfactory neuroblastoma. Arise from olfactory epithelium in the superior nasal cavity. Occurs in adolescents and adults, more common in males than females.
Leptomeningeal infection/inflammation (Figs. 1A.214, 1A.215)	Single or multiple nodular enhancing lesions and/or focal or diffuse abnormal subarachnoid enhancement in suprasellar cistern with or without intrasellar extension. Low to intermediate signal on T1WI, intermediate to high signal on T2WI. Leptomeningeal inflammation often best seen on postcontrast images.	Gd-contrast enhancement in the intracranial subarachnoid space (leptomeninges) usually is associated with significant pathology (inflammation and/or infection versus neoplasm). Inflammation and/or infection of the leptomeninges can result from pyogenic, fungal, or parasitic diseases as well as tuberculosis. Neurosarcoidosis results in granulomatous disease in the leptomeninges, producing similar patterns of subarachnoid enhancement.
Langerhans Cell Histiocytosis (Fig. 1A.216)	Fusiform or lobulated lesion with intermediate signal on T1WI and T2WI involving the pituitary stalk. Gd-contrast enhancement.	Disorder of reticuloendothelial system that rarely involves the CNS. Eosinophilic granulomas can be single or multiple in the skull, usually at the skull base. Intradural lesions occur at pituitary stalk and can present with diabetes insipidus. Lesions rarely occur in brain tissue.
Lymphocytic adenohypophysitis (Fig. 1A.217)	Slightly lobulated lesion with intermediate signal on T1WI and heterogeneous low to intermediate and high signal on T2WI, involving the anterior pituitary lobe. Prominent abnormal homogeneous or heterogeneous enhancement involving the pituitary gland and often the pituitary stalk and dura.	Rare autoimmune inflammatory process involving the pituitary gland confirmed by biopsy, showing varying degrees of lymphocytic infiltration and plasma cells with fibrotic changes without multinucleated giant cells. More common in women than men. Associated with pituitary hormonal dysfunction. Responds to steroid medication.

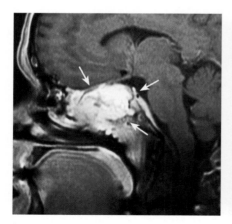

a

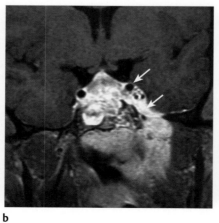

b

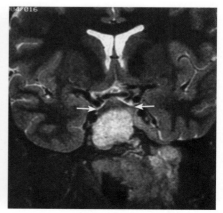

c

Fig. 1A.212 Adenoid cystic carcinoma.
Postcontrast sagittal (**a**) and coronal (**b**) FS T1WI shows a destructive enhancing lesion extending from the nasopharynx into the sphenoid and sella, as well as through a widened left foramen ovale into the left trigeminal cistern and cavernous sinus (arrows). **c** Coronal T2WI shows the lesion to have high signal. The lesion uplifts the pituitary gland (arrows).

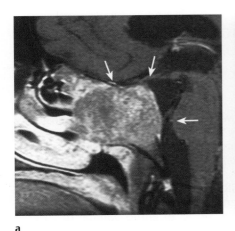
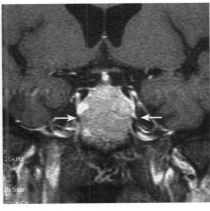
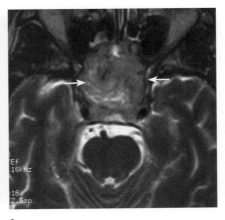

a

b

c

Fig. 1A.213 Esthesioneuroblastoma. Postcontrast sagittal (**a**) and coronal (**b**) FS T1WI shows a destructive enhancing lesion located in the nasopharynx, posterior ethmoid air cells, sphenoid sinus, and sella, extending from the nasopharynx into the sphenoid and sella(arrows). **c** Axial T2WI shows the lesion to have intermediate signal (arrows).

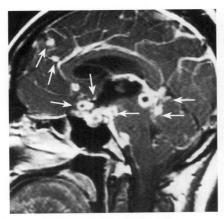
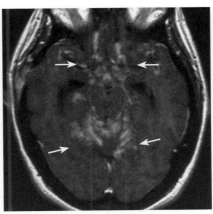
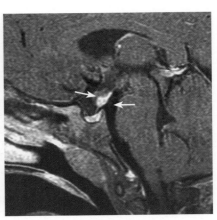

Fig. 1A.214 Leptomeningeal infection from tuberculosis. Postcontrast sagittal T1WI shows multiple nodular and ring-enhancing lesions in the suprasellar, superior cerebellar, and basilar cisterns (arrows). Additional lesions are also seen in the subarachnoid space surrounding the cerebrum and cerebellum.

Fig. 1A.215 Leptomeningeal inflammation from sarcoidosis. Postcontrast axial T1WI shows multiple small nodular enhancing lesions in the suprasellar, superior cerebellar, and basilar cisterns (arrows).

Fig. 1A.216 Langerhans Cell Histiocytosis. Postcontrast sagittal FS T1WI shows an enhancing nodular lesion at the upper pituitary stalk (arrows).

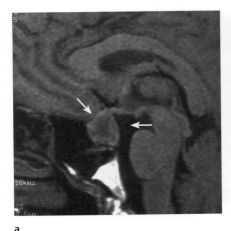
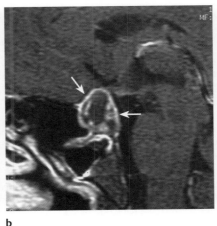
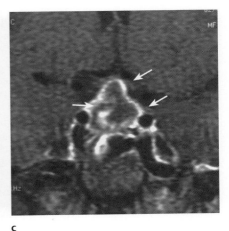

a

b

c

Fig. 1A.217 Lymphocytic adenohypophysitis. a Sagittal T1WI shows a lesion with low to intermediate signal involving the pituitary gland extending into the suprasellar cistern uplifting the optic chiasm (arrows). Postcontrast FS sagittal (**b**) and coronal (**c**) T1WI shows irregular, predominantly peripheral enhancement of the leion (arrows).

1B Cerebral Vasculature with Magnetic Resonance Angiography

Magnetic resonance imaging (MRI) is a powerful imaging modality for evaluating normal and abnormal blood vessels. The appearance of blood vessels on MRI depends on various factors such as: the type of MRI pulse sequence; pulsatility and range of velocities in the vessels of interest; and size, shape, and orientation of the vessels relative to the image plane. Useful anatomic information of blood vessels can be gained by using spin-echo (SE) pulse sequences, which can display patent vessels as zones of signal void (black-blood images), or gradient-recall-echo (GRE) pulse sequences, which displays the moving hydrogen atomic nuclei (protons) in blood as zones of high signal (bright-blood images).

The GRE technique is used to generate MR angiograms (MRA). The high signal from flowing blood on GRE images reflects movement patterns and velocities of hydrogen atomic nuclei rather than direct anatomic displays of the blood vessels. An operator of the MR equipment can choose parameters to optimize the imaging of various arteries and veins. There are two main types of GRE techniques used for MRA. One is based on hydrogen signal amplitude and is referred to as the time-of-flight (TOF) method. The other method is based on the phase differences of the moving protons (hydrogen) in blood compared with stationary tissue and is referred to as phase contrast MRA.

In TOF MRA, the GRE pulse sequence is optimized for demonstrating the inflow enhancement (high signal) of moving protons (hydrogen nuclei) in blood relative to the low signal of protons in stationary tissue. Phase contrast MRA is a technique that differentiates flowing and stationary protons through the use of bipolar flow-encoding gradients. If the flow velocity is known, the flow sensitivity of the sequence can be selected to emphasize the vessels of interest. Phase contrast MRA can be optimized for detecting slow flow in veins and at areas of high-grade arterial stenosis.

The individual GRE images can be acquired in a sequential mode, also referred to as two-dimensional (2D) TOF or phase contrast MRA, or as an entire volume of covered tissue, which is referred to as three-dimensional (3D) TOF or phase contrast MRA. The acquired image data from either of these two methods are post-processed with computer algorithms to generate the MRA images in a display format similar to conventional arteriograms. Two commercially available types of post-processing are the maximum-intensity-projection (MIP) technique and surface-rendering (SR). The former technique is more common, and the MIP MRA images can be displayed in any plane of obliquity on film or as a movie loop. SR is another post-processing method for MRA that shows 3D relationships by giving the displayed vessels shadowing and perspective. The MRA images are projected in a similar fashion to the MIP method. SR has been proven to be useful in showing spatial relationships between vessels on a single coronal image, allowing differentiation of adjacent and overlapping vessels.

MRA has proven to be clinically useful in the evaluation of the carotid arteries in the neck, intracranial arteries, veins, and dural venous sinuses. Disorders such as aneurysms, arteriovenous malformations (AVM), arterial occlusions, and dural venous sinus thrombosis can be seen with MRA.

Table 1B.1 Congenital/developmental vascular anomalies/variants

Disease	MRA Findings	Comments
Persistant fetal origin of posterior cerebral artery (Fig. 1B.1)	Large posterior communicating artery supplying the posterior cerebral artery, associated with hypoplasia or absence of connection between the basilar artery and the ipsilateral posterior cerebral artery.	Represents persistence of embryonic configuration, common vascular variant seen in approximately 20 % of arteriograms.
Hypoplasia of the A1 segment of anterior cerebral artery (Fig. 1B.2)	Hypoplasia or absent A1 segment associated with a patent communicating artery supplying blood to ipsilateral A2 segment.	Anatomic variant seen in approximately 10 % of arteriograms.
Persistent trigeminal artery (Fig. 1B.3)	Anomalous anastomosis connecting the internal carotid artery in cavernous sinus to the basilar artery at the level of the fifth cranial (trigeminal) nerve. Basilar artery below anatomosis and vertebral arteries are usually small.	Most common type of anomalous carotid-basilar anastomosis (0.5 % of cerebral arteriograms), failure of involution of persistent embryonic circulatory configuration. Associated with increased incidence of aneurysms and vascular malformations. Other less common types of anomalous carotid-basilar anastomosis include: persistent hypoglossal artery (adjacent to the twelfth cranial nerve), persistent otic artery, and proatlantal intersegment artery.

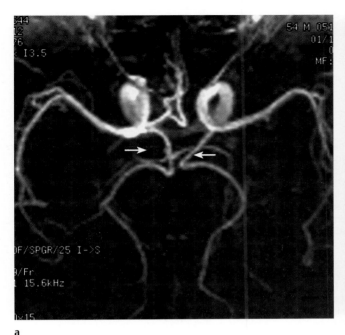

a

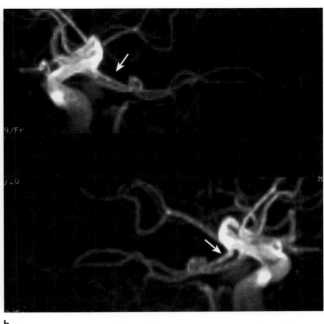

b

Fig. 1B.1   Persistant fetal origin of posterior cerebral artery.
Axial (**a**) and oblique sagittal (**b**) 3D TOF MRA images show bilateral posterior communicating arteries supplying the posterior cerebral arteries (arrows) associated with absence of connection between the basilar artery and the posterior cerebral arteries. Prominent hypoplasia of the A1 segment of the left anterior cerebral artery is also present.

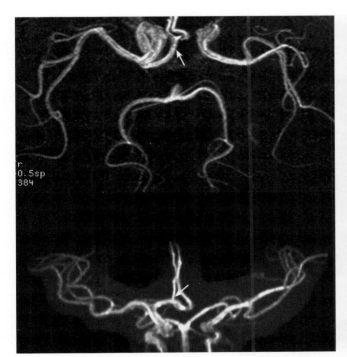

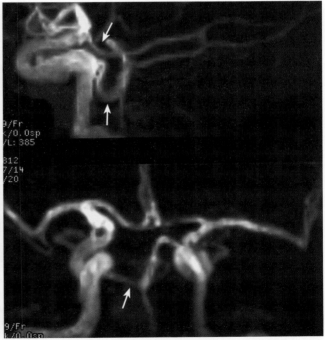

Fig. 1B.2   Hypoplasia of the A1 segment of anterior cerebral artery. Axial and coronal 3D TOF MRA images show an absent A1 segment of the left anterior cerebral artery associated with a patent anterior communicating artery supplying blood to both A2 segments (arrows).

Fig. 1B.3   Persistent trigeminal artery. Sagittal and coronal 3D TOF MRA images show an anomalous anastomosis connecting the internal carotid artery to the basilar artery at the level of the fifth cranial (trigeminal) nerve (arrows). Note the normal position of the posterior communicating artery (arrow). The basilar artery below the anastomosis is small.

Table 1B.**1** (Cont.) Congenital/developmental vascular anomalies/variants

Disease	MRA Findings	Comments
Duplicated middle cerebral artery (Fig. 1B.4)	Double middle cerebral artery pattern, may be bilateral	Duplication of the middle cerebral artery is an infrequent type of vascular variant compared with anomalies involving other intracranial arteries. Other less common types of variants include fenestrations and accessory arteries.
Sturge-Weber (Fig. 2B.9)	Prominent localized unilateral leptomeningeal enhancement, usually in parietal and/or occipital regions in children. With or without gyral enhancement, slightly decreased signal on T2WI in adjacent gyri. Mild localized atrophic changes in brain adjacent to the pial angioma. Prominent medullary and/or subependymal veins and ipsilateral prominence of choroid plexus may be associated. Gyral calcifications above 2 years. Progressive cerebral atrophy in region of pial angioma.	Also known as encephalotrigeminal angiomatosis, neurocutaneous syndrome associated with ipsilateral port wine cutaneous lesion and seizures. Results from persistence of primitive leptomeningeal venous drainage (pial angioma) and developmental lack of normal cortical veins, producing chronic venous congestion and ischemia.
Moyamoya (Fig. 1B.5)	Multiple tortuous tubular flow voids seen in the basal ganglia and thalami on T1WI and T2WI secondary to dilated collateral arteries; enhancement of these arteries related to slow flow within these collateral arteries versus normal-sized arteries. Often with Gd-contrast enhancement of the leptomeninges related to pial collateral vessels. Decreased or absent flow voids involving the supraclinoid portions of the internal carotid arteries and proximal middle and anterior cerebral arteries. MRA shows stenosis and occlusion of the distal internal carotid arteries with collateral arteries (lenticulostriate, thalamoperforate, and leptomeningeal), best seen after contrast administration enabling detection of slow blood flow.	Progressive occlusive disease of the intracranial portions of the internal carotid arteries with resultant numerous dilated collateral arteries arising from the lenticulostriate and thalamoperforate arteries as well as other parenchymal, leptomeningeal, and transdural arterial anastomoses. Term translated as "puff of smoke," referring to the angiographic appearance of the collateral arteries (lenticulostriate, thalamoperforate). Usually nonspecific etiology but can be associated with neurofibromatosis, radiation angiopathy, atherosclerosis, sickle cell disease. In Asia, usually more common in children than adults.

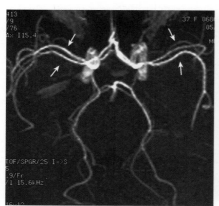

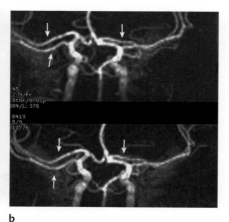

a   b

Fig. 1B.**4 Duplicated middle cerebral arteries.** Axial (**a**) and coronal (**b**) 3D TOF MRA image shows bilateral duplicated middle cerebral arteries (arrows).

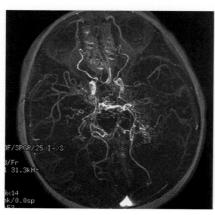

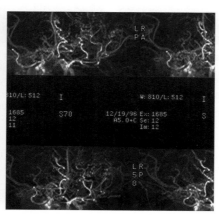

a   b

Fig. 1B.**5 Moyamoya.** Postcontrast axial (**a**) and coronal (**b**) 3D TOF MRA images show occlusion of the distal internal carotid arteries with multiple small enhancing collateral arteries (lenticulostriate, thalamoperforate, and leptomeningeal), supplying branches of the middle and anterior cerebral arteries distal to the zones of occlusion.

Table 1B.**2** Acquired vascular disease

Disease	MRA Findings	Comments
Stenosis/occlusive vascular disease		
Arterial stenosis/occlusion (Fig. 1B.6)	Focal narrowing (stenosis) or absence (occlusion) of flow signal on MRA in artery, with or without narrowing of flow signal distal to site of stenosis. Focal signal voids can be seen with stenosis greater than 70%. Newer MRA methods using Gd-contrast contrast may approximate results and images similar to conventional MRA.	Arterial stenosis or occlusion may result from atherosclerosis, emboli, fibromuscular disease/dysplasia, collagen vascular disease, coagulopathy, encasement by neoplasm, surgery, or radiation injury.

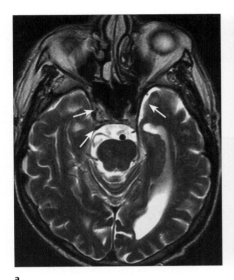

a

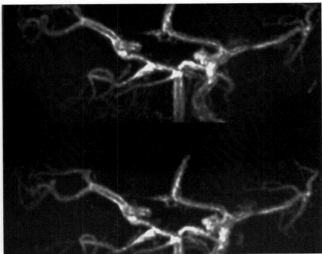

b

Fig. 1B.**6** **Occlusion of the right internal carotid artery.** **a** Axial T2WI shows intermediate to slightly high signal at the expected location of a flow void at the cavernous portion of the right internal carotid artery (arrows). Note the normal flow void at the left internal carotid artery (arrow). **b** Coronal 3D TOF MRA images show absence (occlusion) of flow signal of the right internal carotid artery. **c** Oblique coronal 2D TOF MRA images of the neck show flow signal in the patent right external carotid artery (arrows), but no flow signal in the proximal right internal carotid artery consistent with occlusion at its origin.

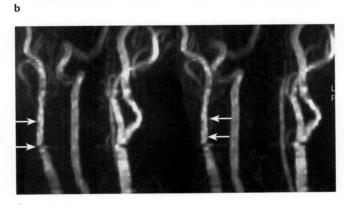

c

Table 1B.2 (Cont.) Acquired vascular disease

Disease	MRA Findings	Comments
Subclavian steal syndrome (Fig. 1B.7)	TOF MRA using superior saturation bans will suppress the flow signal of the vertebral artery on the side where there is stenosis or occlusion of the proximal subclavian artery. TOF MRA without saturation bands will show flow signal in the vertebral artery with reversed flow. Alternatively, phase contrast MRA will show flow in the affected vertebral artery regardless of direction.	Stenosis or occlusion of the proximal subclavian artery can cause reversal of blood flow of the ipsilateral vertebral artery to supply the subclavian artery distal to the stenosis. The reversed blood flow can result in signs of vertebrobasilar insufficiency (e.g., syncope, nausea, ataxia, vertigo, diplopia, headaches) elicited with exercise of the upper extremity on the same side where the stenosis/occlusion of the subclavian artery occurs.
Vasculitis (Fig. 1B.8)	Zones of arterial occlusion, and/or foci of stenosis and poststenotic dilatation. May involve large, medium, or small-sized intracranial and extracranial arteries. With or without associated cerebral and/or cerebellar infarcts.	Uncommon mixed group of inflammatory diseases/disorders involving the walls of cerebral blood vessels. Can result from noninfectious etiology (e.g., polyarteritis nodosa, Wegener granulomatosis, giant cell arteritis, Takayasu arteritis, sarcoidosis, drug-induced) or be related to infectious cause (bacteria, fungi, tuberculosis, syphilis, viral).

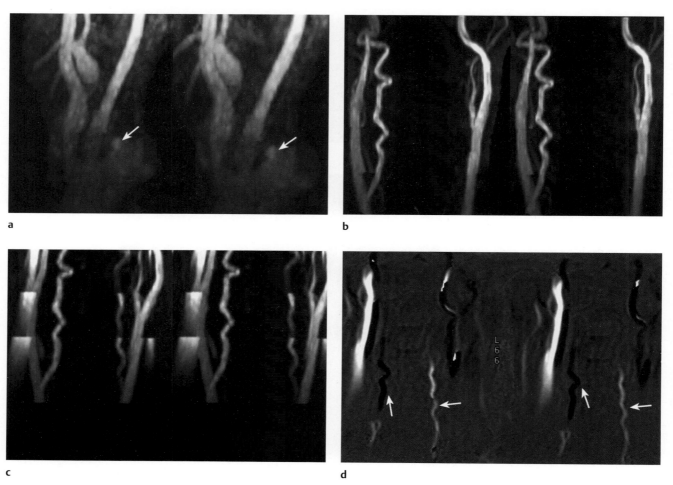

a

b

c

d

Fig. 1B.**7** **Subclavian steal syndrome.** **a** Oblique coronal 3D TOF MRA images show occlusion of the proximal left subclavian artery (arrows). **b** Coronal 3D TOF (MOTSA) MRA images using superior saturation bands show absence of flow signal in the left vertebral artery. **c** Coronal 3D TOF (MOTSA) MRA images without superior saturation bands show presence of flow signal in the left vertebral artery (arrows), indicating reversal of normal flow direction (inferior flow instead of normal upward flow cephalad). **d** Coronal cine phase contrast MRA images show opposite flow signal in the right (arrows: black signal) versus left vertebral artery (arrows: white signal).

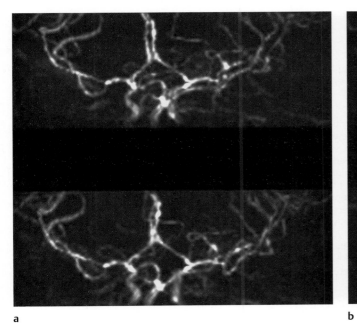

a

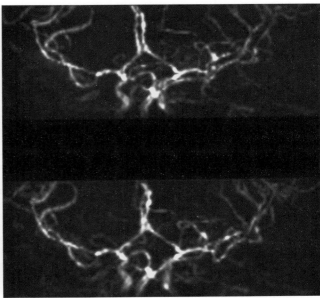

b

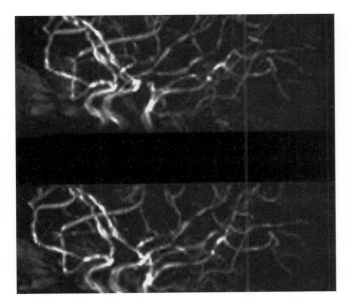

c

Fig. 1B.**8** **Vasculitis.** Axial (**a**), oblique coronal (**b**), and oblique sagittal (**c**) 3D TOF MRA images show multiple foci of stenosis and poststenotic dilatation involving the anterior, middle, and posterior cerebral arteries. Axial T2WI (**d**) and coronal FLAIR image (**e**) show multiple sites of cerebral infarction involving the cerebral cortex and subcortical white matter (arrows).

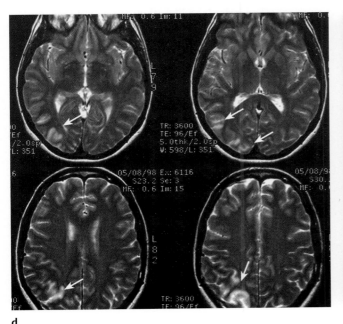

d

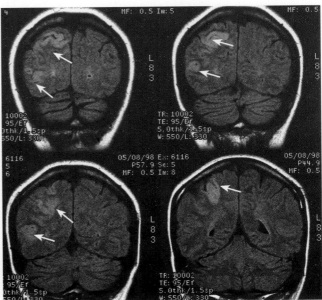

e

Table 1B.2 (Cont.) Acquired vascular disease

Disease	MRA Findings	Comments
Intracranial venous sinus thrombosis (Fig. 1B.9)	2D phase contrast or 2D TOF MR venography useful for determining patency of venous sinuses.	Venous sinus occlusion may result from coagulopathies, encasement or invasion by neoplasm, dehydration, adjacent infectious/inflammatory processes.
Arterial aneurysm (Figs. 1B.10–1B.12)	*Saccular aneurysm:* focal well-circumscribed zone of signal void on T1WI and T2WI, variable mixed signal if thrombosed. *Giant aneurysm:* Focal well-circumscribed structure with layers of low, intermediate, and high signal on T2WI secondary to layers of thrombus of different ages, as well as a zone of signal void representing a patent lumen if present. On T1WI, layers of intermediate and high signal can be seen as well as a zone of signal void. *Fusiform aneurysm:* Elongated and ectatic arteries. Variable intraluminal MR signal related to turbulent or slowed blood flow or partial/complete thrombosis. *Dissecting aneurysms:* The involved arterial wall is thickened and has intermediate to high signal on T1WI and T2WI; the signal void representing the patent lumen is narrowed.	Abnormal fusiform or focal dilatation of artery secondary to: acquired/degenerative etiology, polycystic disease, connective-tissue disease, atherosclerosis, trauma, infection (mycotic), AVM, vasculitis, and drugs. Focal aneurysms are also referred to as saccular aneurysms, which typically occur at arterial bifurcations and are multiple in 20 %. Saccular aneurysms greater than 2.5 cm in diameter are referred to as giant aneurysms. Fusiform aneurysms are often related to atherosclerosis or collagen vascular disease (e.g., Marfan syndrome, Ehlers-Danlos). Dissecting aneurysms: hemorrhage occurs in the arterial wall from incidental or significant trauma.

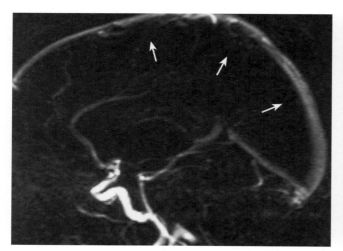

a

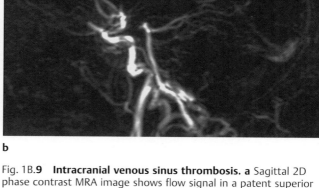

b

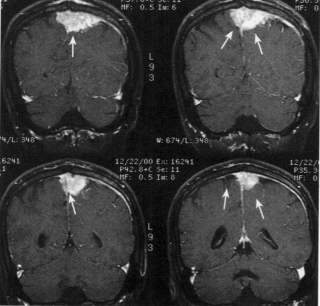

c

Fig. 1B.**9** **Intracranial venous sinus thrombosis. a** Sagittal 2D phase contrast MRA image shows flow signal in a patent superior sagittal sinus (arrows). **b** Sagittal 2D phase contrast MRA image of another patient shows absent flow signal in an occluded superior sagittal sinus. **c** Postcontrast fat-suppressed (FS) T1WI of same patient in (**b**) shows occlusion of the superior sagittal sinus by metastatic dural invasion (arrows).

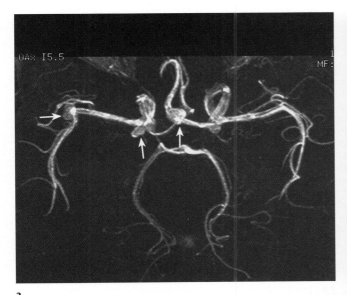

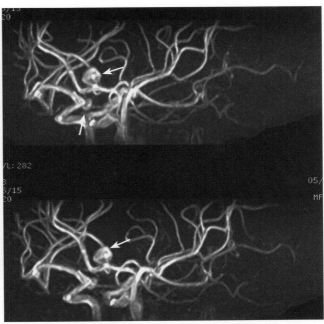

a

Fig. 1B.**10** **Saccular aneurysms.** Axial (**a**) and oblique sagittal (**b**) 3D TOF MRA images show three small saccular aneurysms. The aneursyms are located at the anterior communicating artery, right posterior communicating artery, and trifurcation of the right middle cerebral artery (arrows).

b

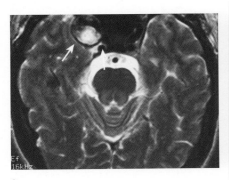

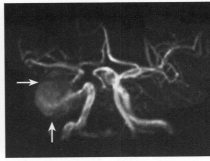

a

b

Fig. 1B.**11** **Giant aneurysm.** **a** Axial T2WI shows a partially thrombosed aneurysm of the cavernous portion of the right internal carotid artery with layers of low, intermediate, and high signal (arrows). **b** Coronal 3D TOF MRA image shows flow signal as well as high signal from thrombus at the aneurysm (arrows).

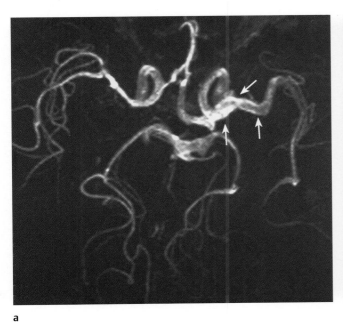

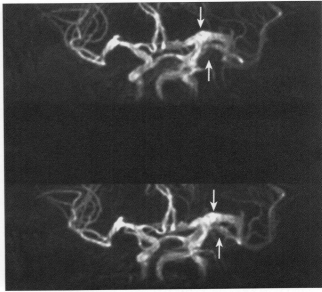

a

b

Fig. 1B.**12** **Fusiform aneurysm.** Axial (**a**) and coronal (**b**) 3D TOF MRA images show a fusiform aneurysm of the left middle cerebral artery (arrows).

Table 1B.2 (Cont.) Acquired vascular disease

Disease	MRA Findings	Comments
AVM (Fig. 1B.13)	Lesions with irregular margins that can be located in the brain parenchyma–pia, dura, or both locations. AVMs contain multiple tortuous tubular flow voids on T1WI and T2WI secondary to patent arteries with high blood flow, as well as thrombosed vessels with variable signal, areas of hemorrhage in various phases, calcifications, and gliosis. The venous portions often show Gd-contrast enhancement. GRE MRI shows flow-related enhancement (high signal) in patent arteries and veins of the AVM. MRA using TOF or phase contrast techniques can provide additional detailed information about the nidus, feeding arteries, and draining veins, and presence of associated aneurysms. Usually not associated with mass effect except in the case of recent hemorrhage or venous occlusion.	Supratentorial AVMs occur more frequently (80–90%) than infratentorial AVMs (10–20%). Annual risk of hemorrhage. AVMs can be sporadic, congenital, or associated with a history of trauma. Multiple AVMs can be seen in syndromes: Rendu-Osler-Weber, AVMs in brain and lungs, and mucosal capillary telangectasias; Wyburn-Mason, AVMs in brain and retina, with cutaneous nevi.

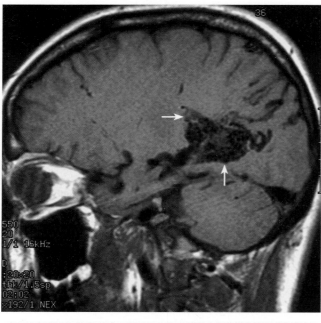

a

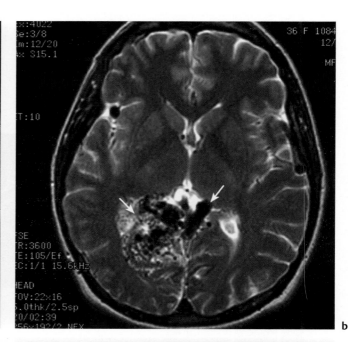

b

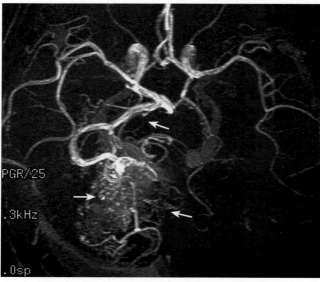

c

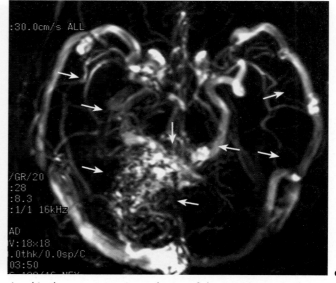

d

Fig. 1B.13 **AVM.** Sagittal T1WI (**a**) and axial T2WI (**b**) show a large collection of abnormal flow voids in the medial right temporal lobe and both occipital lobes (arrows). Axial 3D TOF MRA image (**c**) and axial 2D phase contrast MRA image (**d**) show flow signal in the patent arteries and veins of the AVM (arrows). The feeding arteries are optimally displayed on the 3D TOF image, and the draining veins on the 2D phase contrast image.

Table 1B.**3** Acquired vascular disease

Disease	MRA Findings	Comments
Vein of Galen aneursym (Figs. 1B.**14**,1A.**79**)	Multiple tortuous tubular flow voids on T1WI and T2WI involving choroidal and thalamoperforate arteries, internal cerebral veins, vein of Galen (aneurysmal formation), straight and transverse venous sinuses, and other adjacent veins and arteries. The venous portions often show Gd-contrast enhancement. GRE MR images and MRA using TOF or phase contrast techniques show flow signal in patent portions of the vascular malformation.	Heterogeneous group of vascular malformations with arteriovenous shunts and dilated deep venous structures draining into and from an enlarged vein of Galen. Hydrocephalus, hemorrhage, macrocephaly, parenchymal vascular malformation components, and seizures may be associated. High-output congestive heart failure in neonates.
Dural AVM (Figs.1B.**15**, 1A.**78**)	Dural AVMs contain multiple tortuous tubular flow voids on T1WI and T2WI. The venous portions often show Gd-contrast enhancement. GRE MR images and MRA using TOF or phase contrast techniques show flow signal in patent portions of the vascular malformation and areas of venous sinus occlusion or recanalization. Usually not associated with mass effect except in the case of recent hemorrhage or venous occlusion.	Dural AVMs are usually acquired lesions resulting from thrombosis or occlusion of an intracranial venous sinus with subsequent recanalization resulting in direct arterial to venous sinus communications. Location in order of decreasing frequency: transverse, sigmoid venous sinuses; cavernous sinus; straight, superior sagittal sinuses.

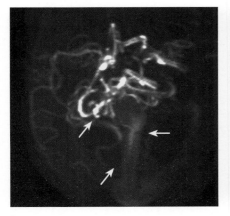
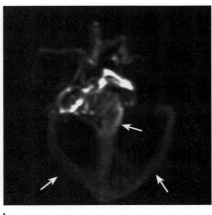
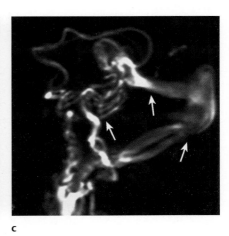

a b c

Fig. 1B.**14** **Vein of Galen aneursym.** Axial 3D TOF MRA image (**a**) and axial (**b**) and sagittal (**c**) 2D phase contrast MRA images show flow signal in the patent arteries and veins of the vein of Galen aneurysm (AVM/fistula) and enlarged venous sinuses (arrows).

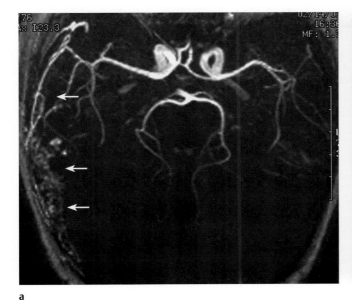
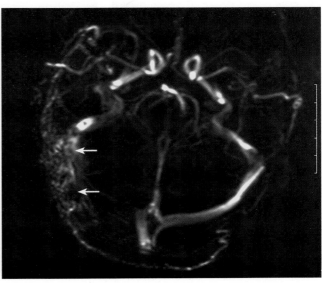

a b

Fig. 1B.**15** **Dural AVM.** Axial 3D TOF MRA image (**a**) and axial 2D phase contrast MRA image (**b**) show flow signal in the multiple small vessels at the site of right transverse venous sinus occlusion, representing recanalization with direct arterial to venous sinus communications. Note also dilated branches from the right middle cerebral artery.

Table 1B.3 (Cont.) Acquired vascular disease

Disease	MRA Findings	Comments
Carotid cavernous fistula (Fig. 1B.16)	MRA shows marked dilatation of the cavernous sinuses as well as the superior and inferior ophthalmic veins and facial veins.	Carotid artery to cavernous sinus fistulas usually occur as a result of blunt trauma, causing dissection or laceration of the cavernous portion of the internal carotid artery. Patients can present with pulsating exophthalmos.
Cavernous hemangioma (Fig. 1B.17)	Single or multiple multilobulated intra-axial lesions that have a peripheral rim or irregular zone of low signal on T2WI secondary to hemosiderin, surrounding a central zone of variable signal (low, intermediate, high, or mixed) on T1WI and T2WI depending on ages of hemorrhagic portions. GRE useful for detecting multiple lesions.	Supratentorial cavernous angiomas occur more frequently than infratentorial lesions. Can be found in many different locations. Multiple lesions in more than 50%. Association with venous angiomas and risk of hemorrhage.
Venous angioma (Fig. 1B.18)	On postcontrast T1WI, venous angiomas are seen as a Gd-contrast-enhancing transcortical vein draining a collection of small medullary veins (caput Medusa). The draining vein can be seen as a signal void on T2WI.	Considered an anomalous venous formation typically not associated with hemorrhage. Usually an incidental finding except when associated with cavernous hemangioma.
Capillary telangiectasia (Fig. 1B.19)	Small poorly defined zones with intermediate to slightly high signal on T2WI, with or without low signal on T1WI, with or without Gd-contrast enhancement. No abnormal mass effect	Small venous malformations located in pons more commonly than in other portions of brainstem, brain; typically show no enlargement over time.

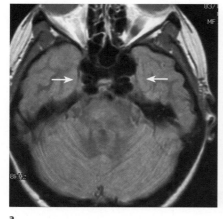
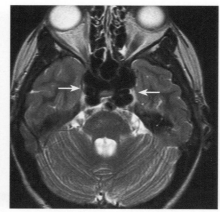
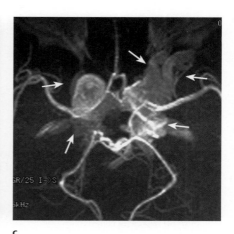

a

b

c

Fig. 1B.16 Carotid cavernous fistula.
Axial proton density weighted image (**a**) and axial T2WI (**b**) show prominent flow voids in the region of both cavernous sinuses (arrows). **c** Axial 3D TOF MRA image shows abnormally dilated flow signal at the cavernous sinuses as well as the markedly dilated orbital veins, particularly on the left (arrows).

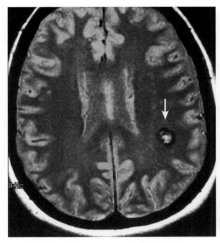

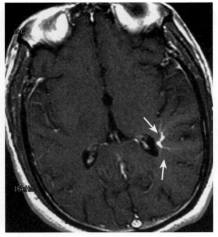

Fig. 1B.**17**   **Cavernous hemangioma.** Axial proton density weighted image shows a multilobulated intra-axial lesion that has a peripheral irregular zone of low signal surrounding a central zone of heterogeneous high signal (arrows).

Fig. 1B.**18**   **Venous angioma.** Post-contrast axial T1WI shows a GD-contrast-enhancing vein draining a collection of small medullary veins (arrows).

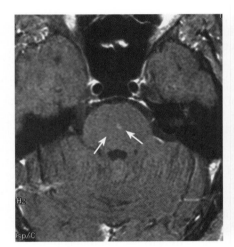

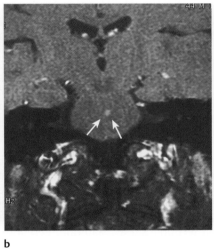

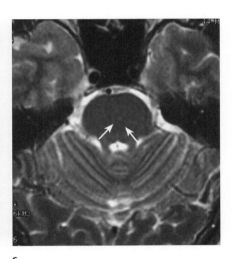

a

b

c

Fig. 1B.**19**   **Capillary telangiectasia.** Post-contrast FS axial (**a**) and coronal (**b**) T1WI shows a small poorly defined zone of Gd- contrast enhancement in the pons without abnormal mass effect (arrows).   **c** Axial T2WI shows minimal signal alteration in the pons at the site of the capillary telangiectasia (arrows).

2A Ventricles and Cisterns

The embryologic development of the ventricles begins with three expansions (primary vesicles) of the rostral neural tube (4–5 weeks of gestation), which are referred to as the forebrain (prosencephalon), midbrain (mesencephalon), and hindbrain (rhombencephalon). The primary vesicles subsequently expand and bend with localized constrictions to form the five secondary vesicles (approximately 7 weeks of gestation). The forebrain gives rise to the telencephalon (eventual cerebral hemispheres and lateral ventricles) and diencephalon (thalamus, hypothalamus, and third ventricle). The midbrain primary vesicle eventually forms the secondary vesicle, also referred to as the mesencephalon, which eventually forms the tectum, midbrain portion of the brainstem, and cerebral aqueduct. The hindbrain gives rise to the metencephalon (eventual pons, cerebellum, and upper portion of the fourth ventricle), and myelencephalon (eventual medulla and lower portion of the fourth ventricle).

Abnormalities in development of the cerebral vesicles results in congenital anomalies such as the holoprosencephalies, lissencephaly/pachygyria, Dandy-Walker malformations. Abnormalities in the closure of the caudal neural tube with altered internal pressure dynamics has been proposed as a mechanism in the malformation of the ventricles and other anomalies associated with Chiari II malformations.

The normal lateral ventricles are bilateral elongated C-shaped structures, each containing a contiguous frontal horn, body, atrium (trigone), occipital horn, and temporal horn. The lateral ventricles are often symmetric, but varying degrees of asymmetry are not uncommon. The anterior portions of the lateral ventricles are normally separated by the septum pellucidum.

The third ventricle appears as a slit-like compartment filled with cerebrospinal fluid (CSF) between the thalami. The inferior border of the third ventricle is the hypothalamus, and the upper border is the choroid tela (fusion of pia and ependymal lining of ventricle) and choroid plexus. The anterior border is the lamina terminalis and anterior commisure. The posterior border includes the pineal gland and recess and posterior commissure. The third ventricle communicates with the lateral ventricles via the foramina of Monro located anterolaterally. The third ventricle communicates with the fourth ventricle via the cerebral aqueduct posteroinferiorly.

The fourth ventricle has a pyramidal shape in the sagittal plane and an inverted C-shape/kidney-bean shape in the axial plane. The fourth ventricle is located dorsal to the pons with its roof comprised of the cerebellar vermis. The fourth ventricle communicates with the cerebral aqueduct at its upper margin, and inferiorly with the cisterna magna of the subarachnoid space via the foramen of Magendie and the paired foramina of Luschka.

CSF fills the ventricles and is produced by the choroid plexus located within the lateral, third and fourth ventricles, as well as the foramina of Luschka and Magendie. Choroid plexus typically enhances after intravenous Gd-DTPA contrast administration because of its lack of a blood-brain barrier. CSF from the ventricles communicates with the subarachnoid space adjacent to the brain and spinal cord through the foramina of Luschka and Magendie. CSF has a primary function of protecting the brain and spinal cord from trauma and rapid changes in venous pressure. CSF represents approximately 10% of the intracranial and intraspinal spaces. A total of approximately 150 ml of CSF is present within the ventricles and the intracranial and spinal subarachnoid spaces. The choroid plexus forms 500 ml of CSF daily, allowing turnover four to five times daily. More than 90% of the CSF is normally resorbed by arachnoid villi or granulations (grouping of villi) that penetrate the dura with resultant emptying of fluid into the intracranial venous sinuses. The remaining small amount of fluid is resorbed through the ependymal linings of the ventricles.

Obstruction of outflow of CSF from the ventricles results in dilatation of the ventricles proximal to the site of blockage. The obstruction can result from congenital malformations (e.g., Chiari II), neoplasms/other intracranial mass lesions (e.g., colloid cyst), inflammatory lesions, hemorrhage, brain edema/swelling (ischemia, trauma), etc. In addition to ventricular dilatation, transependymal leakage of fluid can be seen with MRI. Obstructive or noncommunicating hydrocephalus can result, if untreated, in abnormal increased intracranial pressure, intracranial herniation, and death.

Communicating hydrocephalus occurs with overproduction of CSF (choroid plexus papilloma/carcinoma), impaired resorption of CSF through the arachnoid villi, and/or obstruction of CSF flow through the cisterns and sulci). With communicating hydocephalus, the ventricles are disproportionately more prominent than the sulci. Subependymal edema may be seen with MRI due to the impaired resorption of CSF. Patients with communicating hydrocephalus (normal pressure hydrocephalus) may also have clinical features of gait disturbance, incontinence, and/or progressive impairment of mental function.

Ventricular enlargement can also result from cerebral infarction, cerebral atrophy, or various neurodegenerative diseases. With these disorders, sulcal prominence is usually evident with MRI.

Sulci normally vary in size, although typically increase in size with aging. Sulcal enlargement can also be seen in children with dehydration. Congenital malformations such as lissencephaly and pachygyria result in absence of sulci or few shallow sulci, respectively. Sulci may be asymmetrically prominent at sites of prior cerebral or cerebellar infarction, prior intra-axial hemorrhage, contusion, inflammation, or radiation injury.

The basal cisterns represent the subarachnoid compartment adjacent to the pial margins of the inferior portions of the brain and brainstem. The cisterns are named according to the adjacent neural structures. The larger of the cisterns include the cisterna magna (dorsal and inferior to the cerebellar vermis) and superior cerebellar cistern.

Approximately 10% of neoplasms in the central nervous system (CNS) extend into or are completely within the ventricles. The age of the patient and location of the tumor influence the differential diagnosis of lesions.

Table 2A.1 Common lateral ventricular masses

Patient age	Foramen of Monro	Trigone and atrium	Body of lateral ventricle
Adult	Colloid cyst Cysticercosis	Meningioma Choroid plexus cyst Neuroepithelial cyst Central neurocytoma Metastasis Neuroepithelial cyst Cysticercosis	Ependymoma Glioblastoma Metastasis Central neurocytoma Cysticercosis
Child older than 5 years	Giant cell astrocytoma Pilocytic astrocytoma Cysticercosis	Ependymoma Choroid plexus cyst Choroid plexus papilloma Choroid plexus carcinoma Hamartoma, tuberous sclerosis Gray matter heterotopia Cysticercosis	Ependymoma Pilocytic astrocytoma Hamartoma, tuberous sclerosis Gray matter heterotopia Cysticercosis
Child less than 5 years	Giant cell astrocytoma Pilocytic astrocytoma Cysticercosis	Choroid plexus papilloma Choroid plexus carcinoma Cysticercosis	Choroid plexus papilloma Choroid plexus carcinoma Primitive neuroectodermal tumor Teratoma Cysticercosis

Table 2A.2 Common third ventricular masses

Patient age	Foramen of Monro	Anterior recess	Body of the third ventricle	Posterior third ventricle
Adult	Colloid cyst Metastases Cysticercosis	Pituitary adenoma Meningioma Metastasis Aneurysm Craniopharyngioma Lymphoma Cysticercosis	Glioma Cysticercosis	Pineal tumor Glioma Vascular malformation Cysticercosis
Child	Giant cell astrocytoma Pilocytic astrocytoma Cysticercosis	Germ cell tumor LCH Glioma Craniopharyngioma Cysticercosis	Choroid plexus papilloma Glioma Cysticercosis	Pineal tumor Glioma Vascular malformation Cysticercosis

Table 2A.3 Fourth ventricular masses

Disease	MRI Findings	Comments
Child		
Astrocytoma (Figs. 2A.1, 2A.2)	*Low-grade astrocytoma:* Focal or diffuse mass lesion usually located in cerebellar white matter or brainstem with low to intermediate signal on T1WI and high signal on T2WI; with or without mild Gd-contrast enhancement. Minimal associated mass effect. May extend into ventricles. *Juvenile pilocytic astrocytoma:* Subtype: solid/cystic focal lesion with low to intermediate signal on T1WI and high signal on T2WI; usually with prominent Gd-contrast enhancement. Lesions located in cerebellum, brainstem. May extend into ventricles. *Gliomatosis cerebri:* Infiltrative lesion with poorly defined margins with mass effect located in the white matter. Low to intermediate signal on T1WI and high signal on T2WI; usually no Gd-contrast enhancement until late in disease. *Anaplastic astrocytoma:* Often irregularly marginated lesion located in white matter with low to intermediate signal on T1WI and high signal on T2WI, with or without Gd-contrast enhancement. May extend into ventricles.	*Low-grade astrocytoma:* Often occur in children and adults (age 20–40 years). Tumors comprised of well-differentiated astrocytes. Association with neurofibromatosis type 1. Ten-year survival. May become malignant. *Juvenile pilocytic astrocytoma:* Subtype: common in children, usually favorable prognosis if totally resected. *Gliomatosis cerebri:* Diffusely infiltrating astrocytoma with relative preservation of underlying brain architecture. Imaging appearance may be more prognostic than histologic grade. Approximate 2-year survival. *Anaplastic astrocytoma:* Intermediate between low-grade astrocytoma and glioblastoma multiforme. Approximate 2-year survival.
Medulloblastoma (primitive neuroectodermal tumor of the cerebellum) (Fig. 2A.3)	Circumscribed or invasive lesions with low to intermediate signal on T1WI and intermediate to high signal on T2WI; variable Gd-contrast enhancement. Frequent dissemination into the leptomeninges and/or ventricles.	Highly malignant tumors that frequently disseminate along CSF pathways.
Ependymoma (Fig. 2A.4)	Circumscribed spheroid or lobulated infratentorial lesion, usually in the fourth ventricle. Cysts and/or calcifications may be present. Low to intermediate signal on T1WI and intermediate to high signal on T2WI; variable Gd-contrast enhancement. With or without extension through the foramina of Luschka and Magendie.	Occurs more commonly in children than adults; two-thirds infratentorial, one-third supratentorial.
Metastatic tumor (Fig. 2A.5)	Single or multiple well-circumscribed or poorly defined lesions involving the skull, dura, leptomeninges, ventricles, choroid plexus, or pituitary gland. Low to intermediate signal on T1WI and intermediate to high signal on T2WI; usually Gd-contrast enhancement. Bone destruction, compression of neural tissue or vessels may be associated. Leptomeningeal tumor, drop metastasis often best seen on postcontrast images.	Metastatic tumor may have variable destructive or infiltrative changes involving single or multiple sites of involvement.

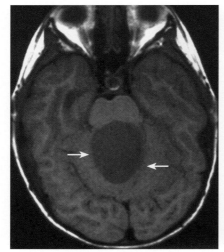

Fig. 2A.**1** **Low-grade astrocytoma. a** Axial T1WI shows a lesion with low to intermediate signal in the fourth ventricle (arrows).

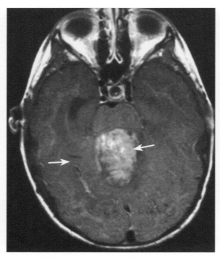

Fig. 2A.**1 b** Postcontrast axial T1WI shows moderate heterogeneous enhancement of the lesion (arrows).

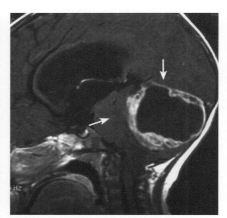

Fig. 2A.**2** **Juvenile pilocytic astrocytoma, subtype.** Postcontrast sagittal T1WI shows a cystic lesion with peripheral irregular enhancement located in the cerebellum. It extends into the fourth ventricle (arrows) causing obstructive hydrocephalus.

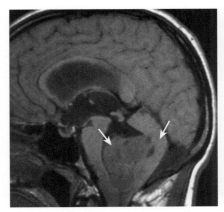

Fig. 2A.**3** **Medulloblastoma (primitive neuroectodermal tumor of the cerebellum).** **a** Sagittal T1WI shows a lesion with intermediate signal in the fourth ventricle resulting in obstructive hydrocephalus.

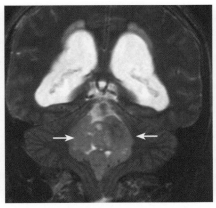

Fig. 2A.**3 b** Coronal T2WI shows the lesion to have intermediate to slightly high signal (arrows).

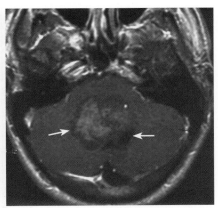

Fig. 2A.**3 c** Postcontrast axial T1WI shows heterogeneous enhancement of the lesion (arrows).

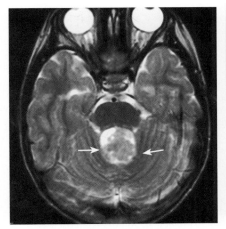

Fig. 2A.**4** **Ependymoma.** **a** Axial T2WI shows a lesion with intermediate and high signal located in the fourth ventricle (arrows).

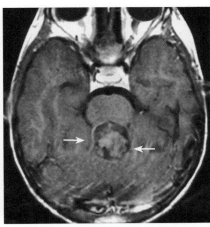

Fig. 2A.**4 b** Postcontrast axial T1WI shows equivocal minimal enhancement of portions of the lesion (arrows).

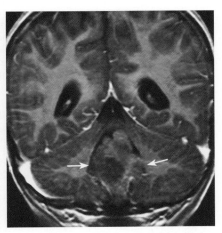

Fig. 2A.**4 c** Postcontrast coronal (spoiled GRE) T1WI shows the lesion filling the fourth ventricle (arrows).

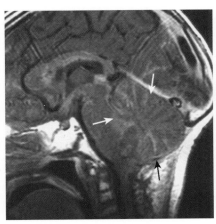

a

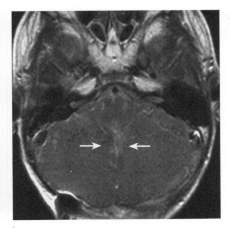

b

Fig. 2A.**5** **Disseminated medulloblastoma.** Postcontrast sagittal (**a**) and axial (**b**) T1WI shows abnormal enhancement in the fourth ventricle as well as in the basilar cisterns, infratentorial and supratentorial sulci (arrows).

Table 2A.**3** (Cont.) Fourth ventricular masses

Disease	MRI Findings	Comments
Hemangioblastoma (Fig. 2A.**6**)	Circumscribed tumors usually located in the cerebellum and/or brainstem. Small Gd-contrast-enhancing nodule with or without cyst, or larger lesion with prominent heterogeneous enhancement with or without flow voids within lesion or at the periphery. Intermediate signal on T1WI and intermediate to high signal on T2WI. Occasionally lesions have evidence of recent or remote hemorrhage. May extend into ventricles.	Multiple lesions occur in adolescents with von Hippel-Lindau disease.
Choroid plexus papilloma or carcinoma (Fig. 1A.**63**)	Circumscribed and/or lobulated lesions with papillary projections, intermediate signal on T1WI and mixed intermediate to high signal on T2WI. Usually prominent Gd-contrast enhancement. Calcifications may be associated. Locations: atrium of lateral ventricle (children) more common than fourth ventricle (adults); rarely other locations such as third ventricle. Associated with hydrocephalus.	Rare intracranial neoplasms. MR features of choroid plexus carcinoma and papilloma overlap; both histologic types can disseminate along CSF pathways and invade brain tissue.
Adult		
Metastatic tumor	Single or multiple well-circumscribed or poorly defined lesions involving the skull, dura, leptomeninges, brainstem, cerebellum, ventricles, choroid plexus, or pituitary gland. Low to intermediate signal on T1WI and intermediate to high signal on T2WI; usually Gd-contrast enhancement. Bone destruction and compression of neural tissue or vessels may be associated. Leptomeningeal tumor often best seen on postcontrast images.	Metastatic tumor may have variable destructive or infiltrative changes involving single or multiple sites of involvement.
Hemangioblastoma (Fig. 2A.**6**)	Circumscribed tumors usually located in the cerebellum and/or brainstem. Small Gd-contrast-enhancing nodule with or without cyst, or larger lesion with prominent heterogeneous enhancement with or without flow voids within lesion or at the periphery. Intermediate signal on T1WI; intermediate to high signal on T2WI. Occasionally lesions have evidence of recent or remote hemorrhage. May extend into ventricle.	Occurs in adolescents, young and middle-aged adults. Lesions are typically multiple in patients with von Hippel-Lindau disease.
Astrocytoma (Fig. 1A.**87**)	*Low-grade astrocytoma:* Focal or diffuse mass lesion usually located in cerebellum or brainstem with low to intermediate signal on T1WI and high signal on T2WI; with or without mild Gd-contrast enhancement. Minimal associated mass effect. May extend into ventricles. *Anaplastic astrocytoma:* Often irregularly marginated lesion located in cerebellum or brainstem with low to intermediate signal on T1WI and high signal on T2WI, with or without Gd-contrast enhancement. May extend into ventricles.	*Low-grade astrocytoma:* Often occur in children and adults (age 20–40 years). Tumors comprised of well-differentiated astrocytes. Association with neurofibromatosis type 1. Ten-year survival. May become malignant. *Anaplastic astrocytoma:* intermediate between low-grade astrocytoma and glioblastoma multiforme. Approximate 2-year survival.

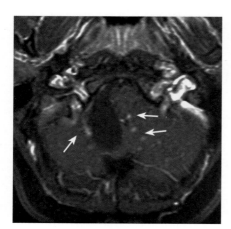

Fig. 2A.**6** **Hemangioblastoma (Von Hippel-Lindau disease).** Postcontrast axial T1WI shows multiple enhancing nodular lesions in the cerebellum (arrows). One lesion has an associated cystic component, and several are located near the inferior portion of the fourth ventricle.

Table 2A.**3** (Cont.) Fourth ventricular masses

Disease	MRI Findings	Comments
Ependymoma (Fig. 1A.**90**)	Circumscribed spheroid or lobulated infratentorial lesion, usually in the fourth ventricle.Cysts and/or calcifications may be present. Low to intermediate signal on T1WI and intermediate to high signal on T2WI; variable Gd-contrast enhancement. With or without extension through the foramina of Luschka and Magendie.	Occurs more commonly in children than adults; two-thirds infratentorial, one-third supratentorial.
Choroid plexus papilloma or carcinoma (Fig. 1A.**63**)	Circumscribed and/or lobulated lesions with papillary projections, intermediate signal on T1WI and mixed intermediate to high signal on T2WI. Usually prominent Gd-contrast enhancement. Calcifications may be associated. Locations: atrium of lateral ventricle (children) more common than fourth ventricle (adults); rarely other locations such as third ventricle. Associated with hydrocephalus.	Rare intracranial neoplasms. MR features of choroid plexus carcinoma and papilloma overlap; both histologic types can disseminate along CSF pathways and invade brain tissue.
Cysticercosis (Fig. 1A.**41**)	Single or multiple cystic lesions in brain, meninges, or ventricles. *Acute/subacute phase:* Low to intermediate signal on T1WI and high signal on T2WI. Rim and possible nodular pattern of Gd-contrast enhancement, with or without peripheral high T2 signal (edema). *Chronic phase:* calcified granulomas.	Caused by ingestion of ova (*Taenia solium*) in contaminated food (undercooked pork). Involves in order of decreasing frequency: meninges, brain parenchyma, ventricles.

Table 2A.**4** Excessively small ventricles

Disease	MRI Findings	Comments
Normal variant	Small ventricles with normal appearance of brain parenchyma and presence of CSF in subarachnoid spaces and cisterns.	Normal variation.
Postshunt	Small slit-like ventricles (with or without shunt tube present).	Small ventricular size can result form chronic overdrainage of ventricles with shunts.
Increased intracranial pressure	Small ventricles with effacement of subarachnoid spaces, with or without high signal on T2WI in brain parenchyma. Cerebral edema.	Ventricular size usually does not correlate well with intracranial pressure.
Pseudotumor cerebri (Fig. 2A.**7**)	Normal shaped but small ventricles, with or without mild prominence of intracranial subarachnoid spaces, with or without prominence of fluid in optic nerve sheath complex.	MRI with Gd-contrast contrast plays a role in excluding intracranial tumors involving the brain or leptomeninges.

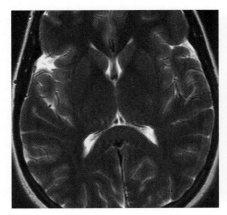
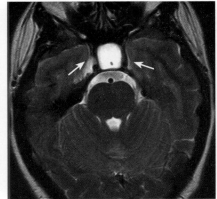
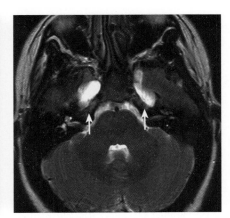

a   b   c

Fig. 2A.**7** **Pseudotumor cerebri.** Axial T2WI (**a-c**) shows small-sized lateral ventricles as well as an empty sella configuration and dilatation of the trigeminal cisterns (arrows).

Table 2A.5 Dilated ventricles

Disease	MRI Findings	Comments
Normal variant	Mild ventricular enlargement can occur without associated cerebral or cerebellar abnormality	Ventricular size usually increases with age, most pronounced after age 60.
Aqueductal stenosis (Fig. 2A.8)	Dilatation of lateral and third ventricles with normal-sized fourth ventricle, with or without dilatation of only the upper, not lower, portion of cerebral acqueduct. With or without discrete or poorly-defined lesion in midbrain.	Aqueductal stenosis can result from a small lesion/neoplasm in the midbrain, debris or adhesions from hemorrhage or inflammatory diseases. MRI can exclude other lesions causing obstructon of CSF flow through the aqueduct; such as lesions in the posterior third ventricle or posterior cranial fossa.
Chiari I malformation (Fig. 1A.11)	Cerebellar tonsils extend more than 5 mm below the foramen magnum in adults, 6 mm in children below 10 years. Syringohydromyelia in 20% to 40%. Hydrocephalus in 25%. Basilar impression in 25%. Less common association: Klippel-Feil, atlanto-occipital assimilation	Cerebellar tonsilar ectopia. Most common anomaly of CNS. Not associated with myelomeningocele.
Chiari II malformation (Arnold-Chiari) (Fig. 2A.9)	Small posterior cranial fossa with gaping foramen magnum through which there is an inferiorly positioned vermis associated with a cervicomedullary kink. Beaked dorsal margin of the tectal plate. Myelomeningoceles in nearly all patients. Hydrocephalus and syringomyelia common. Dilated lateral ventricles posteriorly (colpocephaly).	Complex anomaly involving the cerebrum, cerebellum, brainstem, spinal cord, ventricles, skull, and dura. Failure of fetal neural folds to develop properly results in altered development affecting multiple sites of the CNS.
Chiari III malformation	Features of Chiari II plus lower occipital or high cervical encephalocele.	Rare anomaly associated with high mortality.
Dandy-Walker malformation (Fig. 2A.10)	Vermian aplasia or severe hypoplasia, communication of fourth ventricle with retrocerebellar cyst, enlarged posterior fossa, high position of tentorium and transverse venous sinuses. Hydrocephalus common. Associated with other anomalies such as dysgenesis of the corpus callosum, gray matter heterotopia, schizencephaly, holoprosencephaly, and cephaloceles.	Abnormal formation of roof of fourth ventricle with absent or near incomplete formation of cerebellar vermis.
Dandy-Walker variant (Fig. 1A.16)	Mild vermian hypoplasia with communication of posteroinferior portion of the fourth ventricle with cisterna magna. No associated enlargement of the posterior cranial fossa.	Occasionally associated with hydrocephalus, dysgenesis of corpus callosum, gray matter heterotopia, other anomalies.
Colpocephaly (Fig. 2A.11)	Asymmetric enlargement of the occipital horns of the lateral ventricles.	Associated with Chiari II malformations and dysgenesis of corpus callosum.

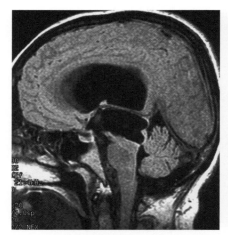 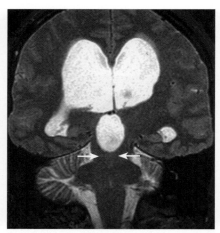 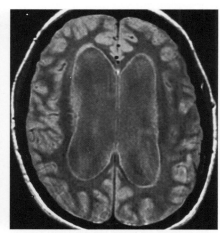

Fig. 2A.8 Aqueductal stenosis. a Sagittal T1WI shows dilatation of lateral ventricles, third ventricle, and upper portions of the cerebral acqueduct. The obstruction site is small and focal at the lower portion of the acqueduct. A normal-sized fourth ventricle is seen.

Fig. 2A.8 b   Coronal T2WI shows the level of obstruction without evidence of a discrete lesion in the lower midbrain (arrows).

Fig. 2A.8 c   Axial proton density weighted (long repetition-time [TR]/short echo-time[TE]) image shows hydrocephalus with dilatation of the lateral ventricles and subependymal edema.

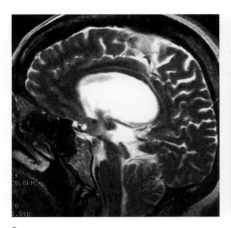

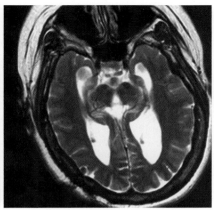

a   **b**

Fig. 2A.**9** **Chiari II malformation (Arnold-Chiari).** Sagittal (**a**) and axial (**b**) T2WI shows a small posterior cranial fossa with gaping foramen magnum through which there is an inferiorly positioned vermis. A beaked dorsal margin of the tectal plate is seen. Dilatation of the lateral ventricles is present.

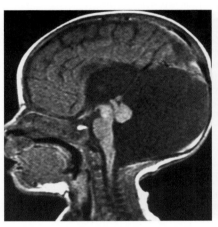
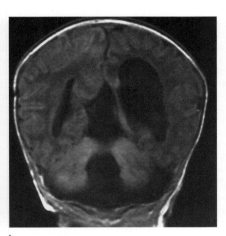

a   **b**

Fig. 2A.**10** **Dandy-Walker malformation.** **a** Sagittal T1WI shows severe vermian hypoplasia, communication of fourth ventricle with retrocerebellar cyst, and enlarged posterior fossa. **b** Coronal (spoiled GRE) T1WI shows dilatation of the lateral and third ventricles. The third ventricle has a high upper position related to agenesis of the corpus callosum.

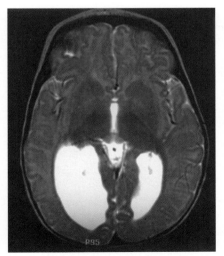

Fig. 2A.**11** **Colpocephaly.** Axial T2WI shows asymmetric enlargement of the occipital horns of the lateral ventricles.

Table 2A.5 (Cont.) Dilated ventricles

Disease	MRI Findings	Comments
Neoplasms causing obstructive hydrocephalus		
Metastatic tumor (Fig. 2A.5)	Single or multiple well-circumscribed or poorly defined lesions involving the skull, dura, leptomeninges, ventricles, choroid plexus or pituitary gland. Low to intermediate signal on T1WI and intermediate to high signal on T2WI; usually Gd-contrast enhancement. Bone destruction and compression of neural tissue or vessels may be present. Leptomeningeal tumor often best seen on postcontrast images.	Metastatic tumor may have variable destructive or infiltrative changes involving single or multiple sites of involvement.
Intra-axial primary tumors		
Astrocytoma (Fig. 2A.12)	*Low-grade astrocytoma:* Focal or diffuse mass lesion usually located in cerebellar white matter or brainstem with low to intermediate signal on T1WI and high signal on T2WI; with or without mild Gd-contrast enhancement. Minimal associated mass effect. *Juvenile pilocytic astrocytoma:* Subtype: solid/cystic focal lesion with low to intermediate signal on T1WI and high signal on T2WI; usually with prominent Gd-contrast enhancement. Lesions located in cerebellum, brainstem. *Gliomatosis cerebri:* Infiltrative lesion with poorly defined margins with mass effect located in the white matter. Low to intermediate signal on T1WI and high signal on T2WI; usually no Gd-contrast enhancement until late in disease. *Anaplastic astrocytoma:* Often irregularly marginated lesion located in white matter with low to intermediate signal on T1WI and high signal on T2WI, with or without Gd-contrast enhancement.	*Low-grade astrocytoma:* Often occur in children and adults (age 20–40 years). Tumors comprised of well-differentiated astrocytes. Association with neurofibromatosis type 1. Ten-year survival. May become malignant. *Juvenile pilocytic astrocytoma:* Subtype: common in children, usually favorable prognosis if totally resected. *Gliomatosis cerebri:* Diffusely infiltrating astrocytoma with relative preservation of underlying brain architecture. Imaging appearance may be more prognostic than histologic grade. Approximate 2-year survival. *Anaplastic astrocytoma:* Intermediate between low-grade astrocytoma and glioblastoma multiforme. Approximate 2-year survival.
Giant cell astrocytoma–Tuberous sclerosis (Fig. 1A.23)	Circumscribed lesion located near the foramen of Monro with mixed low to intermediate signal on T1WI and mixed high signal on T2WI. Cysts and/or calcifications may be associated. Heterogenous Gd-contrast enhancement.	Subependymal hamartoma near foramen of Monro, occurs in 15% of patients with tuberous sclerosis below 20 years of age. Slow-growing lesions that can progressively cause obstruction of CSF flow through the foramen of Monro. Long-term survival usual if resected.
Medulloblastoma (primitive neuroectodermal tumor of the cerebellum) (Fig. 1A.89)	Circumscribed or invasive lesions with low to intermediate signal on T1WI and intermediate to high signal on T2WI; variable Gd-contrast enhancement. Frequent dissemination into the leptomeninges.	Highly malignant tumors that frequently disseminate along CSF pathways.
Ependymoma (Fig. 2A.13)	Circumscribed lobulated supratentorial lesion, often extraventricular. Cysts and/or calcifications may be associated. Low to intermediate signal on T1WI, intermediate to high signal on T2WI; variable Gd-contrast enhancement. With or without extension through the foramina of Luschka and Magendie.	Occurs more commonly in children than adults. One-third supratentorial, two-thirds infratentorial.
Hemangioblastoma (Fig. 1A.94)	Circumscribed tumors usually located in the cerebellum and/or brainstem. Small Gd-contrast-enhancing nodule with or without cyst, or larger lesion with prominent heterogeneous enhancement with or without flow voids within lesion or at the periphery. Intermediate signal on T1WI; intermediate to high signal on T2WI. Occasionally lesions have evidence of recent or remote hemorrhage.	Multiple lesions occur in adolescents with von Hipple-Lindau disease.
Intraventricular tumors		
Choroid plexus papilloma or carcinoma (Fig. 1A.63)	Circumscribed and/or lobulated lesions with papillary projections, intermediate signal on T1WI and mixed intermediate to high signal on T2WI. Usually prominent Gd-contrast enhancement. Calcifications may be associated. Locations: atrium of lateral ventricle (children) more common than fourth ventricle (adults); rarely other locations such as third ventricle. Associated with hydrocephalus.	Rare intracranial neoplasms. MR features of choroid plexus carcinoma and papilloma overlap; both histologic types can disseminate along CSF pathways and invade brain tissue.

Table 2A.**5** (Cont.) Dilated ventricles

Disease	MRI Findings	Comments
Meningioma (Fig. 2A.**30**, 2A.**31**)	Well-circumscribed intraventricular lesions with intermediate signal on T1WI and intermediate to slightly high signal on T2WI. Usually prominent Gd-contrast enhancement. Calcifications may be present.	Usually benign neoplasms, typically occurring in adults above 40 years of age, in women more commonly than men. Multiple meningiomas seen with neurofibromatosis type 2. Can result in compression of adjacent brain parenchyma, encasement of arteries, and compression of dural venous sinuses. Rarely invasive/malignant types.
Hemangiopericytoma (Fig. 1A.**57**)	Extra-axial mass lesions, often well circumscribed with intermediate signal on T1WI and intermediate to slightly high signal on T2WI; prominent Gd-contrast enhancement (may resemble meningiomas). With or without associated erosive bone changes.	Rare neoplasms in young adults (more common in males than females), sometimes referred to as angioblastic meningioma or meningeal hemangiopericytoma. Arise from vascular cells, pericytes. Frequency of metastases > meningiomas
Central neurocytoma (Fig. 1A.**26**)	Circumscribed lesion located at margin of lateral ventricle or septum pellucidum with intraventricular protrusion. Heterogeneous intermediate signal on T1WI and heterogeneous intermediate to high signal on T2WI. Calcifications and/or small cysts may be present. Heterogeneous Gd-contrast enhancement.	Rare tumors that have neuronal differentiation. Imaging appearance similar to intraventricular oligodendrogliomas. Occur in young adults. Benign slow-growing lesions.
Rhabdoid tumors (Fig. 1A.**91**)	Circumscribed mass lesions with intermediate signal on T1WI, with or without zones of high signal from hemorrhage on T1WI; variable mixed low, intermediate, and/or high signal on T2WI, usually prominent Gd-contrast enhancement with or without heterogeneous pattern.	Rare malignant tumors involving the CNS usually occurring in the first decade. Histologically appear as solid tumors with or without necrotic areas, similar to malignant rhabdoid tumors of the kidney. Associated with a poor prognosis.

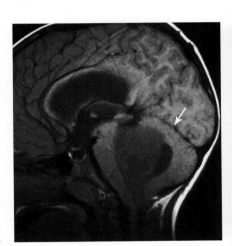

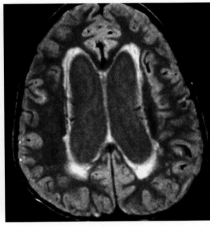

Fig. 2A.**12 Astrocytoma. a** Sagittal T1WI shows a lesion with low to intermediate signal in the fourth ventricle causing obstructive hydrocephalus (arrows). **b** Axial proton density weighted (long TR/short TE) axial image shows dilatation of the lateral ventricles with high supependymal signal representing transependymal egress of CSF.

a   b

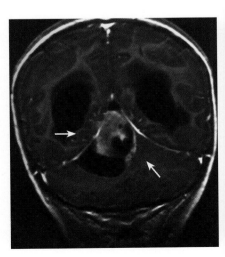

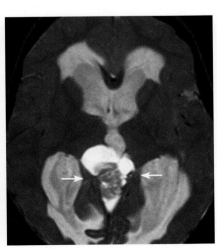

Fig. 2A.**13 Ependymoma. a** Postcontrast coronal (spoiled GRE) T1WI shows a mixed solid-enhancing and cystic lesion (arrows) causing obstructive hydrocephalus. **b** Axial T2WI shows the cystic/solid tumor (arrows) and dilatation of the third and lateral ventricles.

a   b

Table 2A.5 (Cont.) Dilated ventricles

Disease	MRI Findings	Comments
Intraventricular lesions		
Colloid cyst (Fig. 2A.14)	Well-circumscribed spheroid lesions located at the anterior portion of the third ventricle. Variable signal (low, intermediate, or high) on T1WI and T2WI, often high signal on T1WI and low signal on T2WI, no Gd-contrast enhancement.	Common presentation of headaches and intermittent hydrocephalus. Removal leads to cure
Neuroepithelial cyst (Fig. 1A.51)	Well-circumscribed cysts with low signal on T1WI and high signal on T2WI. Thin walls. No Gd-contrast enhancement or peripheral edema	Cyst walls have histopathologic features similar to epithelium. Neuroepithelial cysts located, in order of decreasing frequency, in: choroid plexus, choroidal fissure, ventricles, brain parenchyma.
Inflammation/infection		
Ependymitis/ventriculitis (Fig. 2A.15) (Fig. 1A.96)	Curvilinear and/or nodular Gd-contrast enhancement along ventricular/ependymal margins with resultant communicating or noncommunicating types of hydrocephalus.	Complications of intracranial inflammatory processes such as infections from bacteria, fungi, tuberculosis, viruses (cytomegalovirus [CMV]) and parasites. Noninfectious diseases, such as sarcoidosis, can result in a similar pattern.
Cysticercosis (Fig. 1A.41)	Single or multiple cystic lesions in brain or meninges. *Acute/subacute phase:* Low to intermediate signal on T1WI and high signal on T2WI; rim and possible nodular pattern of Gd-contrast enhancement, with or without peripheral high T2 signal (edema). *Chronic phase:* calcified granulomas.	Caused by ingestion of ova (*Taenia solium*) in contaminated food (undercooked pork). Involves in order of decreasing frequency: meninges, brain parenchyma, ventricles.
Hydatid cyst	*Echinococcus granulosus:* Single or rarely multiple cystic lesions with low signal on T1WI and high signal on T2WI with a thin wall with low signal on T2WI. Typically no Gd-contrast enhancement or peripheral edema unless superinfected. Often located in vascular territory of the middle cerebral artery. *Echinococcus multilocularis:* Cystic (possibly multilocular) and/or solid lesions. Central zone of low to intermediate signal on T1WI and T2WI, surrounded by a slightly thickened rim of low signal on T2WI; Gd-contrast enhancement. Peripheral zone of high signal on T2WI (edema) and calcifications are common.	Caused by parasites, *Echinococcus granulosus* (South America, Middle East Australia, New Zealand) or *Echinococcus multilocularis* (North America, Europe, Turkey, China). CNS involvement in 2% of cases of hydatid infestation.
Rasmussen's encephalitis (Fig. 2A.16)	Progressive atrophy of one cerebral hemisphere with poorly defined zones of high signal on T2WI involving the white matter, basal ganglia, and cortex. Usually no enhancement. Ipsilateral dilated lateral ventricle.	Usually seen in children below 10 years of age. Severe and progressive epilepsy and unilateral neurologic deficits–hemiplegia, psychomotor deterioration, chronic slow viral infectious process possibly caused by CMV or Epstein-Barr virus. Treatment: hemispherectomy.

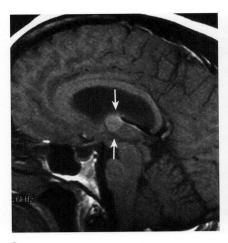

a

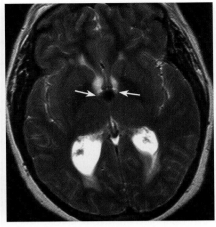

b

Fig. 2A.**14 Colloid cyst. a** Sagittal T1WI shows a spheroid lesion with slightly high signal located at the upper anterior portion of the third ventricle (arrows). **b** Axial T2WI shows the lesion to have low signal (arrows). Dilatation of the lateral ventricles is present with subependymal edema.

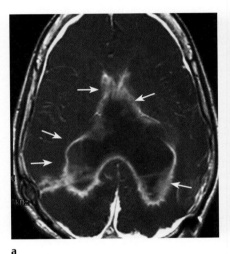

a

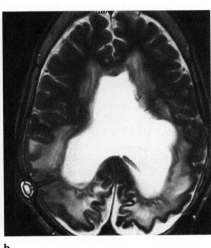

b

Fig. 2A.**15 Ependymitis/ventriculitis. a** Postcontrast axial T1WI shows abnormal irregular enhancement along dilated lateral ventricles (arrows) from pyogenic infection secondary to shunt tube placement. Dural enhancment is also present. **b** Axial T2WI shows ventricular dilatation and abnormal high signal in the periventricular brain parenchyma.

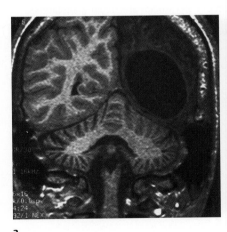

a

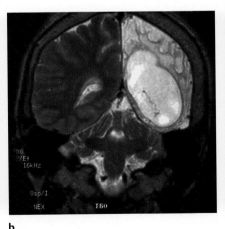

b

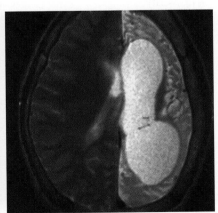

c

Fig. 2A.**16 Rasmussen's encephalitis. a** Coronal (spoiled GRE) T1WI shows severe atrophy of the left cerebral hemi-sphere with compensatory dilatation of the left lateral ventricle. Coronal (**b**) and axial (**c**) T2WI shows poorly defined zones of ab-normal high signal involving the white and gray matter of the left cerebral hemisphere associated with prominent atrophy.

Table 2A.5 (Cont.) Dilated ventricles

Disease	MRI Findings	Comments
Hydranencephaly (Fig. 2A.17)	Replacement of substantial portions of cerebral tissue with thin-walled sacs containing CSF. Inferomedial portions of frontal and temporal lobes often preserved. Cerebellum and thalami usually have a normal appearance.	In utero destruction of cerebral parenchyma from injury (e.g., vascular, infectious: CMV, toxoplamosis). Patients may be normocephalic, microcephalic, or macrocephalic. Children developmentally delayed.
Porencephalic cyst (Fig. 1A.52)	Irregular, relatively well-circumscribed zone with low signal on T1WI and high signal on T2WI similar to CSF, surrounded by poorly defined thin zone of high T2 signal in adjacent brain tissue; no Gd-contrast enhancement or peripheral edema.	Represent remote sites of brain injury (trauma, infarction, infection, hemorrhage) occurring in late second trimester with evolution by an encephaloclastic process into a cystic zone with CSF. MR signal characteristics surrounded by zones of gliosis in adjacent brain parenchyma. Gliosis (high T2 signal) allows differentiation from schizencephaly.
Encephalomalacia (Fig. 2A.18)	Poorly-defined zone of high signal on T2WI in brain tissue (gray and/or white matter) with localized volume loss and compensatory dilatation of adjacent ventricle.	Damaged residual brain tissue characterized by astrocytic proliferation related to prior infarct, hemorrhage, inflammation, infection, trauma; with compensatory ipsilateral ventricular dilatation resulting from localized volume loss. Encephalomalacia can occur during late gestation, the postnatal period, or with mature brain when an astrocytic proliferation response is possible.
Dyke-Davidoff-Mason syndrome (Fig. 2A.19)	Atrophy/encephalomalacia of one cerebral hemisphere with compensatory dilatation of ipsilateral lateral ventricle. Unilateral ipsilateral decrease in size of cranial fossa associated with thickened calvaria. Enlargement of ipsilateral paranasal sinuses may be associated.	Rare disorder in adolescents presenting with seizures, mental retardation, hemiparesis.
Alzheimer disease	Brain atrophy often most pronounced in temporal lobes; sulcal and ventricular prominence. Cortical atrophic changes common.	Most common form of progressive dementia with neurofibrillary tangles, senile plaques, neuronal loss, amyloid angiopathy, gliosis.
Pick disease (Fig. 1A.141)	Brain atrophy often most pronounced in frontal and temporal lobes; sulcal and ventricular prominence. Cortical atrophic changes common.	Acquired dementia much less common than Alzheimer Disease. Histopathologic findings or neuronal loss and cytoplasmic inclusion bodies (Pick bodies).
Huntington disease (Fig. 1A.154)	Disproportionate atrophy of basal ganglia (in order of decreasing frequency: caudate, putamen, cerebellum/brainstem). Variable low or high signal changes on T2WI involving the putamen bilaterally; usually no enhancement.	Autosomal dominant neurodegenerative disease usually presenting after age 40 with progressive movement disorders, behavioral and mental dysfunction.
Normal pressure hydrocephalus (Fig. 2A.20)	Disproportionately greater prominence of the ventricles relative to the sulci, with or without hyperdynamic flow void at the third ventricle, cerebral acqueduct, and fourth ventricle.	Dilatation of the ventricles with transependymal egress of CSF thought to be secondary to impaired resorption of CSF through arachnoid granulations. Associated with progressive memory impairment, urinary incontinence, and gait disorders.

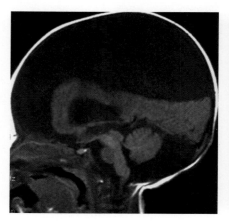
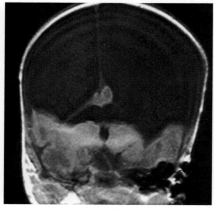
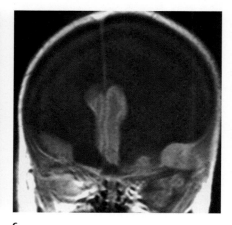

a   b   c

Fig. 2A.17   **Hydranencephaly.** Sagittal T1WI (**a**) and coronal (spoiled GRE) T1WI (**b, c**) show replacement of substantial portions of cerebral tissue with thin-walled sacs containing CSF. Inferomedial portions of frontal and temporal lobes are preserved.

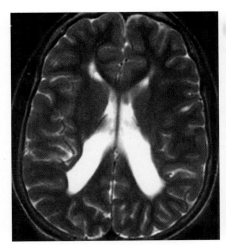

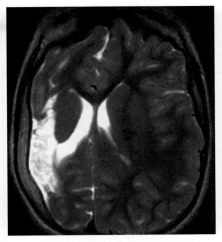

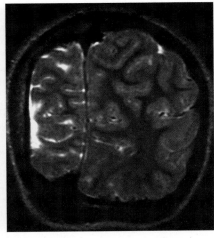

a, b

Fig. 2A.**18** **Periventricular leukomalacia.** Axial T2WI shows small, poorly defined zones of high signal in the periventricular white matter with localized volume loss and compensatory dilatation of adjacent ventricle.

Fig. 2A.**19** **Dyke-Davidoff-Mason syndrome.** Axial T2WI (**a, b**) shows atrophy/ encephalomalacia of the right cerebral hemisphere with compensatory dilatation

of ipsilateral lateral ventricle. Unilateral ipsilateral decrease in size of cranial fossa is associated with thickened calvaria.

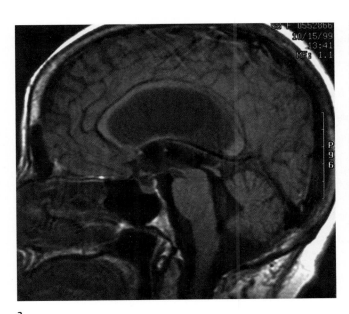

Fig. 2A.**20**
Normal pressure hydrocephalus.
a Sagittal T1WI shows ventricular dilatation without an obstructing mass lesion. Axial T2WI (**b-e**) show disproportionately greater prominence of the ventricles relative to the sulci, as well as hyperdynamic flow voids at the third ventricle, cerebral acqueduct, and fourth ventricle (arrows).

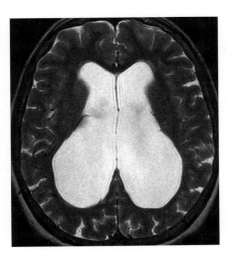

b

a

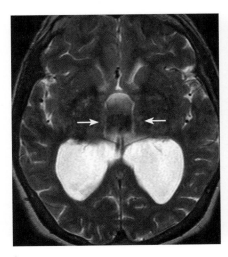

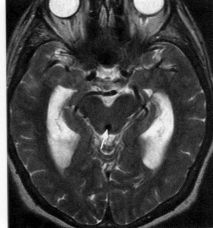

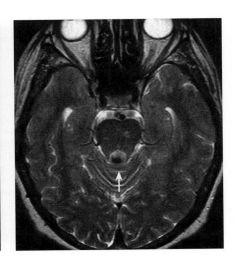

c

d

e

Table 2A.6 Abnormal or altered configuration of the ventricles

Disease	MRI Findings	Comments
Congenital, developmental, or acquired		
Holoprosencephaly (Fig. 1A.1) (Fig. 2A.21)	*Alobar:* Large monoventricle with posterior midline cyst, lack of hemisphere formation with absence of falx, corpus callosum, and septum pellucidum. Fused thalami. *Semilobar:* Monoventricle with partial formation of interhemispheric fissure, occipital and temporal horns, partially fused thalami. Absent corpus callosum and septum pellucidum. Associated with mild craniofacial anomalies. *Lobar:* Near complete formation of interhemispheric fissure and ventricles. Fused inferior portions of frontal lobes, dysgenesis of corpus callosum, absence of septum pellucidum, separate thalami, neuronal migration disorders. *Septo-optic dysplasia (de Morsier syndrome):* Mild form of lobar holoprosencephaly. Dysgenesis or agenesis of septum pellucidum, optic hypoplasia, squared frontal horns. Association with schizencephaly in 50%.	*Holoprosencephaly:* Disorders of diverticulation (4–6 weeks of gestation) characterized by absent or partial cleavage and differentiation of the embryonic cerebrum (prosenecephalon) into hemispheres and lobes.
Gray matter heterotopia (Fig. 2A.22)	*Nodular heterotopia* appears as one or more nodules of isointense gray matter along the ventricles or within the cerebral white matter.	Disorder of neuronal migration (7–22 weeks of gestation) where a collection or layer of neurons is located beween the ventricles and cerebral cortex. Can have a band-like (laminar) or nodular appearance isointense to gray matter, may be unilateral or bilateral. Associated with seizures, schizencephaly.
Schizencephaly (split brain) (Fig. 2A.23)	Cleft in brain extending from ventricle to cortical surface lined by heterotopic gray matter. The cleft may be narrow (closed lip) or wide (open lip).	Association with seizures, blindness, retardation, and other CNS anomalies (e.g., septo-optic dysplasia). Clinical manifestations related to severity of malformation. Ischemia or insult to portion or germinal matrix before hemisphere formation.
Unilateral hemimegalencephaly (Fig. 2A.24)	Nodular or multinodular region of gray matter heterotopia involving all or part of a cerebral hemisphere with associated enlargement of the ipsilateral lateral ventricle and hemisphere.	Neuronal migration disorder associated with hamartomatous overgrowth of the involved hemisphere.
Chiari II malformation (Arnold-Chiari) (Fig. 1A.12)	Small posterior cranial fossa with gaping foramen magnum through which there is an inferiorly positioned vermis associated with a cervicomedullary kink. Beaked dorsal margin of the tectal plate. Myelomeningoceles in nearly all patients. Hydrocephalus and syringomyelia common. Dilated lateral ventricles posteriorly (colpocephaly).	Complex anomaly involving the cerebrum, cerebellum, brainstem, spinal cord, ventricles, skull, and dura. Failure of fetal neural folds to develop properly, resulting in altered development affecting multiple sites of the CNS.
Dandy-Walker malformation (Fig. 1A.15)	Vermian aplasia or severe hypoplasia, communication of fourth ventricle with retrocerebellar cyst, enlarged posterior fossa, high position of tentorium and tranverse venous sinuses. Hydrocephalus common. Associated with other anomalies such as dysgenesis of the corpus callosum, gray matter heterotopia, schizencephaly, holoprosencephaly, cephaloceles.	Abnormal formation of roof of fourth ventricle with absent or near incomplete formation of cerebellar vermis.
Dysgenesis of the corpus callosum (Fig. 1A.14)	Spectrum of abnormalities ranging from complete to partial absence of the corpus callosum. Widely separated and parallel orientations of frontal horns and bodies of lateral ventricles, high position of third ventricle in relation to interhemispheric fissure, colpocephaly. Associated with interhemispheric cysts, lipomas, and anomalies such as Chiari II, gray matter heterotopia, Dandy-Walker malformations, holoprosencephaly, azygous anterior cerebral artery, cephaloceles.	Failure or incomplete formation of corpus callosum (7–18 weeks of gestation). Axons that normally cross from one hemisphere to the other are alligned parallel along the medial walls of lateral ventricles (bundles of Probst).

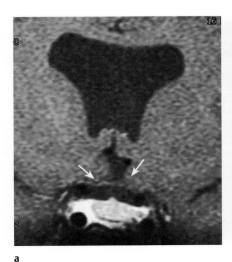

a

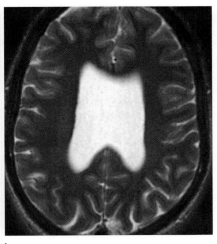

b

Fig. 2A.**21 Septo-optic dysplasia-(de Morsier syndrome). a** Postcontrast coronal fat-suppressed (FS) T1WI shows absence of the septum pellucidum and hypoplasia of the optic chiasm (arrows). **b** Axial T2WI shows agenesis of septum pellucidum.

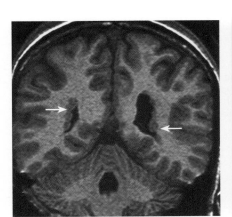

a

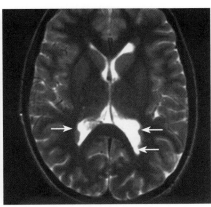

b

Fig. 2A.**22 Gray matter heterotopia.** Coronal (spoiled GRE) T1WI (**a**) and axial T2WI (**b**) show multiple nodules with signal isointense to gray matter along the ventricles (arrows).

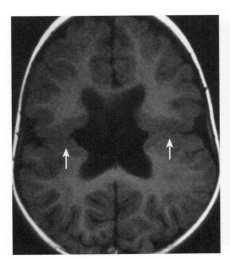

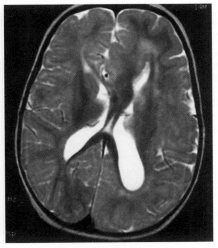

Fig. 2A.**23 Schizencephaly (closed-lip type).** Axial T1WI shows bilateral narrow clefts in the brain, extending from the lateral ventricles to the cortical surface, lined by heterotopic gray matter (arrows).

Fig. 2A.**24 Unilateral hemimegalencephaly.** Axial T2WI shows enlargement of the left cerebral hemisphere with associated enlargement of the ipsilateral lateral ventricle, pachygyria, gray matter heterotopia, and delayed myelination (high signal in white matter).

Table 2A.**6** Abnormal or altered configuration of the ventricles

Disease	MRI Findings	Comments
Porencephalic cyst (Fig. 1A.52)	Irregular, relatively well-circumscribed zone with low signal on T1WI and high signal on T2WI similar to CSF, surrounded by poorly defined thin zone of high T2 signal in adjacent brain tissue; no Gd-contrast enhancement or peripheral edema.	Represent remote sites of brain injury (trauma, infarction, infection, hemorrhage) with evolution into a cystic zone with CSF. MR signal characteristics surrounded by gliosis in adjacent brain parenchyma. Gliosis (high T2 signal) allows differentiation from schizencephaly.
Neuroepithelial cyst (Fig. 1A.51)	Well-circumscribed cysts with low signal on T1WI and high signal on T2WI. Thin walls. No Gd-contrast enhancement or peripheral edema.	Cyst walls have histopathologic features similar to epithelium. Neuroepithelial cysts located, in order of decreasing frequency, in: choroid plexus, choroidal fissure, ventricles, brain parenchyma.
Hamartoma–Tuberous sclerosis (Fig. 2A.25)	Subependymal hamartomas, small nodules located along and projecting into the lateral ventricles. Signal on T1WI and T2WI similar to cortical tubers. Calcification and Gd-contrast enhancement common.	Cortical and subependymal hamartomas are non-malignant lesions associated with tuberous sclerosis.
Subfalcine herniation	Compression and shift of the lateral and third ventricles under the falx cerebri to the other side, with or without dilatation of contralateral lateral ventricle because of CSF outflow obstruction from compression at contralateral foramen of Monro. With or without displacement of ipsilateral anterior cerebral artery and subependymal veins.	Most often occurs from primary or metastatic intra-axial tumor or hemorrhage.
Transtentorial herniation	*Ascending type:* Upward herniation of cerebellar vermis and hemispheres through the tentorial incisura, resulting in compression and displacement of the cerebral aqueduct and posterior portion of the third ventricle, effacement of superior vermian cistern, compression and anterior displacement of the fourth ventricle. Obstructive hydrocephalus may be associated. *Descending type:* Medial and inferior displacement of uncus and parahippocampal gyrus below the tentorium. Progressive effacement of suprasellar cistern and basal cisterns. Compression of ipsilateral portion of midbrain, which is displaced toward contralateral side, with or without Kernohan's notch. Duret hemorrhage may be associated, also inferior displacement and/or compression of anterior choroidal, posterior communicating, and posterior cerebral arteries, as well as perforating branches of the basilar artery resulting in cerebral, cerebellar, and/or brainstem infarcts. Often results in death.	Descending type more common than ascending type. Typically results from a focal mass lesion or hemorrhage causing displacement of brain tissue across tentorium.
Cavum septum pellucidum/cavum vergae (Figs. 2A.26, 2A.27)	*Cavum septum pellucidum:* CSF-containing zone between two septal leaves. *Cavum vergae:* same as cavum septum pellucidum with posterior extension of fluid-containing zone between septal leaves.	Developmental anomalies with lack of normal involution of fetal cavities separating the two septal leaves. Occurs in 3 % of normal adults. No clinical significance.

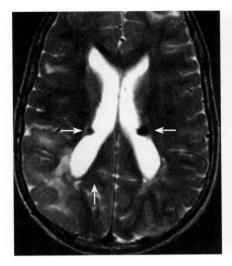

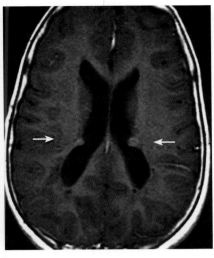

a

b

Fig. 2A.25 Hamartoma–tuberous sclerosis. a Axial T2WI shows small nodules with low signal located along and projecting into the lateral ventricles (arrows). Also present is a cortical hamartoma in the posterior right cerebral hemisphere (curved arrow). **b** Postcontrast axial T1WI shows minimal Gd-contrast enhancement of the ependymal hamartomas (arrows).

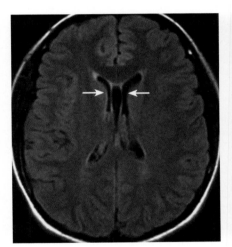

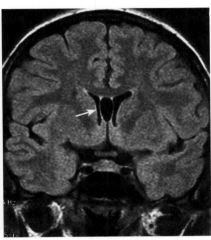

a

b

Fig. 2A.26 Cavum septum pellucidum. Axial (**a**) and coronal (**b**) FLAIR images show a CSF-containing zone between the two septal leaves (arrows).

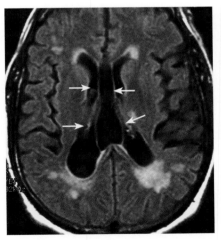

Fig. 2A.27 Cavum vergae. Axial FLAIR image shows a CSF-containing zone between the two septal leaves extending more posterior than a cavum septum pellucidum (arrows). Zones of high signal are seen in the periventricular and subcortical white matter secondary to small vessel ischemic disease.

Table 2A.**7** Intraventricular masses

Disease	MRI Findings	Comments
Congential or developmental		
Colloid cyst (Fig. 2A.28)	Well-circumscribed spheroid lesions located at the anterior portion of the third ventricle. Variable signal (low, intermediate, or high) on T1WI and T2WI, often high signal on T1WI and low signal on T2WI; no Gd-contrast enhancement.	Common presentation of headaches and intermittent hydrocephalus. Removal leads to cure.
Neuroepithelial cyst (Fig. 1A.51)	Well-circumscribed cysts with low signal on T1WI and high signal on T2WI. Thin walls. No Gd-contrast enhancement or peripheral edema.	Cyst walls have histopathologic features similar to epithelium. Neuroepithelial cysts located, in order of decreasing frequency, in: choroid plexus, choroidal fissure, ventricles, brain parenchyma.
Hamartoma–Tuberous sclerosis (Fig. 2A.25)	Subependymal hamartomas: small nodules located along and projecting into the lateral ventricles. Signal on T1WI and T2WI similar to cortical tubers. Calcification and Gd-contrast enhancement common.	Cortical and subependymal hamartomas are nonmalignant lesions associated with tuberous sclerosis.
Neoplastic		
Metastatic tumor (Fig. 2A.29)	Single or multiple well-circumscribed or poorly defined lesions involving the skull, dura, leptomeninges, choroid plexus/ventricles, or pituitary gland. Low to intermediate signal on T1WI and intermediate to high signal on T2WI; usually Gd-contrast enhancement. Bone destruction, compression of neural tissue or vessels may be associated. Leptomeningeal tumor often best seen on postcontrast images.	Metastatic tumor may have variable destructive or infiltrative changes involving single or multiple sites of involvement. Disseminated tumor within the ventricles can result from primary CNS tumors or extraneural primary neoplasms
Meningioma (Figs. 2A.30, 2A.31)	Extra-axial, well-circumscribed, dural-based lesions. Locations in order of decreasing frequency: supratentorial, infratentorial, parasagittal, convexity, sphenoid ridge, parasellar, posterior fossa, optic nerve sheath, intraventricular. Intermediate signal on T1WI and intermediate to slightly high signal on T2WI. Usually prominent Gd-contrast enhancement. Calcifications may be associated.	Most common extra-axial tumor. Usually benign neoplasms, typically occurring in adults above 40 years of age, in women more commonly than men. Multiple meningiomas seen with neurofibromatosis type 2. Can result in compression of adjacent brain parenchyma, encasement of arteries, and compression of dural venous sinuses. Rarely invasive/malignant types.

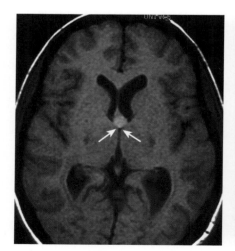

Fig. 2A.**28** **Colloid cyst. a** Axial T1WI shows a well-circumscribed spheroid lesion with slightly high signal located at the anterior portion of the third ventricle (arrows).

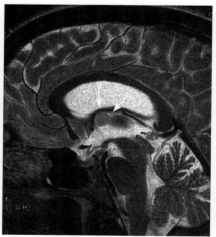

Fig. 2A.**28 b** Sagittal T2WI shows the lesion to have intermediate signal (arrows).

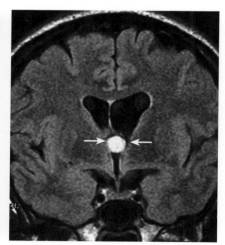

Fig. 2A.**28 c** Coronal FLAIR image shows the lesion to have high signal (arrows).

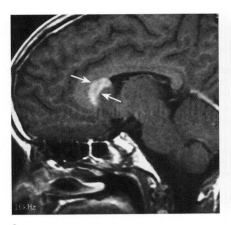

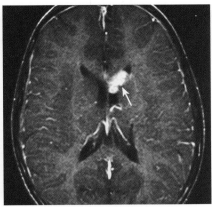

a

b

Fig. 2A.**29** **Metastatic medulloblastoma.** Postcontrast sagittal (**a**) and axial (**b**) T1WI shows an enhancing metastatic lesion in the frontal horn of the left lateral ventricle (arrows).

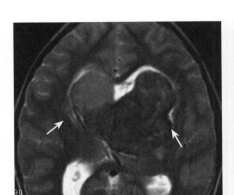

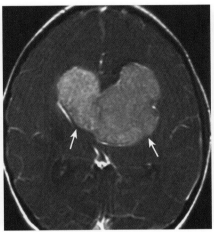

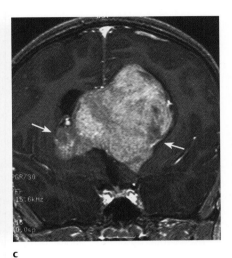

a

b

c

Fig. 2A.**30** **Meningioma.** **a** Axial T2WI shows a large lesion with heterogeneous intermediate signal in the frontal horns of

both lateral ventricles, foramina of Monro, and anterior third ventricle (arrows). Postcontrast axial (**b**) and coronal (spoiled GRE)

T1WI (**c**) show prominent enhancement of the intraventricular meningioma (arrows).

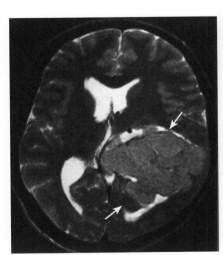

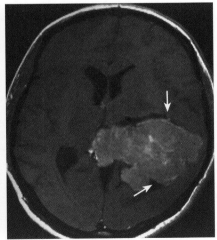

Fig. 2A.**31** **Meningioma.** **a** Axial T2WI shows a large lesion with heterogeneous intermediate signal in the atrium of the left lateral ventricle. (arrows).

Fig. 2A.**31 b** Postcontrast axial T1WI shows prominent enhancement of the in- traventricular meningioma (arrows).

Table 2A.**7** (Cont.) Intraventricular masses

Disease	MRI Findings	Comments
Hemangiopericytoma, (Fig. 2A.**32**), (Fig. 1A.**87**, 1A.**88**)	Extra-axial mass lesions, often well circumscribed, with intermediate signal on T1WI and intermediate to slightly high signal on T2WI; prominent Gd-contrast enhancement (may resemble meningiomas). With or without associated erosive bone changes.	Rare neoplasms in young adults (males more common than females), sometimes referred to as angioblastic meningioma or meningeal hemangiopericytoma. Arise from vascular cells, pericytes. Frequency of metastases > meningiomas.
Central neurocytoma (Fig. 2A.**33**)	Circumscribed lesion located at margin of lateral ventricle or septum pellucidum with intraventricular protrusion. Heterogeneous intermediate signal on T1WI, heterogeneous intermediate to high signal on T2WI. Calcifications and/or small cysts may be present. Heterogeneous Gd-contrast enhancement.	Rare tumors that have neuronal differentiation. Imaging appearance similar to intraventricular oligodendrogliomas. Occur in young adults. Benign slow-growing lesions.
Astrocytoma (Fig. 2A.**34**)	*Low-grade astrocytoma:* Focal or diffuse mass lesion usually located in cerebral or cerebellar white matter or brainstem with low to intermediate signal on T1WI and high signal on T2WI; with or without mild Gd-contrast enhancement. Minimal associated mass effect. May extend into ventricles. *Juvenile pilocytic astrocytoma:* Subtype: solid/cystic focal lesion with low to intermediate signal on T1WI and high signal on T2WI; usually with prominent Gd-contrast enhancement. Lesions located in cerebellum, brainstem. May extend into ventricles. *Gliomatosis cerebri:* Infiltrative lesion with poorly defined margins with mass effect located in the white matter. Low to intermediate signal on T1WI and high signal on T2WI; usually no Gd-contrast enhancement until late in disease. May extend into ventricles. *Anaplastic astrocytoma:* Often irregularly marginated lesion located in white matter with low to intermediate signal on T1WI and high signal on T2WI, with or without Gd-contrast enhancement. May extend into ventricles.	*Low-grade astrocytoma:* Often occur in children and adults (age 20–40 years). Tumors comprised of well-differentiated astrocytes. Association with neurofibromatosis type 1. Ten-year survival. May become malignant. *Juvenile pilocytic astrocytoma:* Subtype: common in children, usually favorable prognosis if totally resected. *Gliomatosis cerebri:* Diffusely infiltrating astrocytoma with relative preservation of underlying brain architecture. Imaging appearance may be more prognostic than histologic grade. Approximate 2-year survival. *Anaplastic astrocytoma:* Intermediate between low-grade astrocytoma and glioblastoma multiforme. Approximate 2-year survival.
Giant cell astrocytoma-Tuberous sclerosis (Fig. 1A.**23**)	Circumscribed lesion located near the foramen of Monro with mixed low to intermediate signal on T1WI and mixed high signal on T2WI. Cysts and/or calcifications may be present. With or without heterogenous Gd-contrast enhancement.	Subependymal hamartoma near foramen of Monro, occurs in 15% of patients with tuberous sclerosis below age 20. Slow-growing lesions that can progressively cause obstruction of CSF flow through the foramen of Monro. Long-term survival usual if resected.
Medulloblastoma (primitive neuroectodermal tumor of the cerebellum) (Fig. 1A.**89**)	Circumscribed or invasive lesions with low to intermediate signal on T1WI and intermediate to high signal on T2WI; variable Gd-contrast enhancement. Frequent dissemination into the leptomeninges.	Highly malignant tumors that frequently disseminate along CSF pathways.
Ependymoma (Fig. 1A.**28**), (Fig. 1A.**127**)	Circumscribed spheroid or lobulated infratentorial lesion, usually in the fourth ventricle. Cysts and/or calcifications may be present. Low to intermediate signal on T1WI, intermediate to high signal on T2WI; variable Gd-contrast enhancement. With or without extension through the foramina of Luschka and Magendie.	Occurs more commonly in children than adults. Two-thirds infratentorial, one-third supratentorial.
Oligodendroglioma (Fig. 1A.**25**)	Circumscribed lesion with mixed low to intermediate signal on T1WI and mixed intermediate to high signal on T2WI, areas of signal void at sites of clump-like calcification, heterogenous Gd-contrast enhancement. Involves white matter and cerebral cortex. Can cause chronic erosion of inner table of calvaria. Also occur within ventricles.	Uncommon slow-growing gliomas with usually mixed histologic patterns (e.g., astrocytoma). Usually in adults above age 35. 85% supratentorial. If low-grade 75% 5-year survival. Higher grade lesions have a worse prognosis.

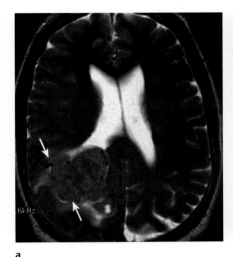

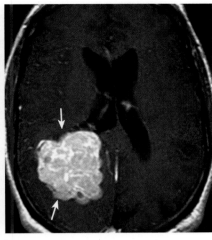

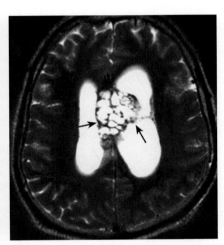

Fig. 2A.**32** **Hemangiopericytoma.** **a** Axial T2WI shows a lesion with heterogeneous intermediate signal in the region of the atrium of the right lateral ventricle (arrows). **b** Postcontrast axial T1WI shows prominent enhancement of the lesion (arrows).

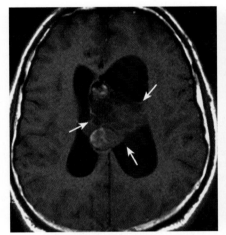

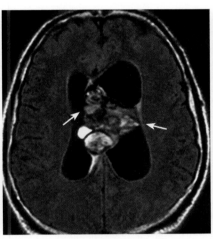

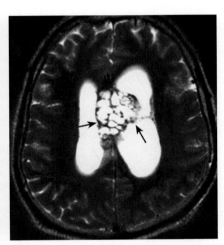

Fig. 2A.**33** **Central neurocytoma.** **a** Axial T1WI shows a slightly lobulated lesion with mixed low, intermediate, and slightly high signal at the septum pellucidum extending into the lateral ventricles (arrows). Dilatation of the lateral ventricles is present.

Fig. 2A.**33 b** Axial FLAIR image shows the lesion to have mixed low, intermediate, and high signal (arrows).

Fig. 2A.**33 c** Axial T2WI image shows the lesion to have predominanly high signal with thin low signal septations (arrows).

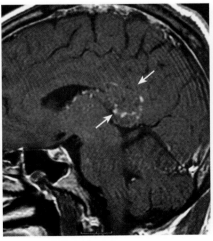

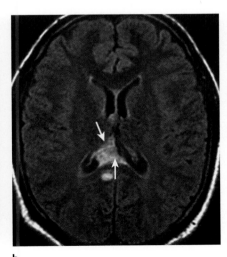

Fig. 2A.**34** **Astrocytoma.** **a** Postcontrast sagittal T1WI shows a lesion containing small foci of enhancement involving the splenium of the corpus callosum (arrows). **b** Axial FLAIR image shows the lesion to have high signal. The lesion deforms the atrium of the right lateral ventricle (arrows).

Table 2A.**7** (Cont.) Intraventricular masses

Disease	MRI Findings	Comments
Choroid plexus papilloma or carcinoma (Figs. 2A.**35**, 2A.**36**)	Circumscribed and/or lobulated lesions with papillary projections. Intermediate signal on T1WI and mixed intermediate to high signal on T2WI; usually prominent Gd-contrast enhancement. Calcifications may be present. Location: atrium of lateral ventricle (children) more common than fourth ventricle (adults), rarely other locations such as third ventricle. Associated with hydrocephalus.	Rare intracranial neoplasms. MR features of choroid plexus carcinoma and papilloma overlap; both histologic types can disseminate along CSF pathways and invade brain tissue.
Rhabdoid tumors (Figs. 1A.**91**, 2A.**37**)	Circumscribed mass lesions with intermediate signal on T1WI, with or without zones of high signal from hemorrhage on T1WI; variable mixed low, intermediate, and/or high signal on T2WI, usually prominent Gd-contrast enhancement with or without heterogeneous pattern.	Rare malignant tumors involving the CNS usually occurring in the first decade. Histologically appear as solid tumors with or without necrotic areas, similar to malignant rhabdoid tumors of the kidney. Associated with a poor prognosis.
Inflammatory		
Tuberculosis–Leptomeningeal/cisternal/intraventricular involvement (Fig. 1A.**96**)	Solid, linear, and/or ring-like Gd-contrast enhancement in basal cisterns, leptomeninges, and/or ventricles.	Occurs in immunocompromised patients and in developing countries. Caseating intracranial granulomas via hematogenous dissemination.
Parasitic brain lesions		
Toxoplasmosis (Fig. 1A.**40**)	Single or multiple solid and/or cystic lesions located in basal ganglia and/or corticomedullary junctions in cerebral hemispheres, rarely in ventricles. Low to intermediate signal on T1WI; high signal on T2WI. Nodular or rim pattern of Gd-contrast enhancement. With or without peripheral high T2 signal (edema).	Most common opportunistic CNS infection in AIDS patients, caused by ingestion of food contaminated with parasites (*Toxoplasma gondii*).
Cysticercosis (Fig. 1A.**41**)	Single or multiple cystic lesions in brain, meninges, and occasionally in ventricles. *Acute/subacute phase:* Low to intermediate signal on T1WI and high signal on T2WI. Rim and possible nodular pattern of Gd-contrast enhancement, with or without peripheral high T2 signal (edema). *Chronic phase:* calcified granulomas.	Caused by ingestion of ova (*Taenia solium*) in contaminated food (undercooked pork). Involves in order of decreasing frequency: meninges, brain parenchyma, ventricles.
Hydatid cyst	*Echinococcus granulosus:* Single or rarely multiple cystic lesions with low signal on T1WI and high signal on T2WI with a thin wall with low signal on T2WI; typically no Gd-contrast enhancement or peripheral edema unless superinfected. Often located in vascular territory of the middle cerebral artery. *Echinococcus multilocularis:* Cystic (possibly multilocular) and/or solid lesions. Central zone of low to intermediate signal on T1WI and T2WI, surrounded by a slightly thickened rim of low signal on T2WI; Gd-contrast enhancement. Peripheral zone of high signal on T2WI (edema) and calcifications are common.	Caused by parasites: *Echinococcus granulosus* (South America, Middle East Australia, New Zealand) or *Echinococcus multilocularis* (North America, Europe, Turkey, China). CNS involvement in 2% of cases of hydatid infestation.

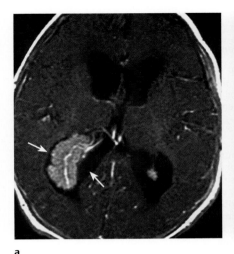

a

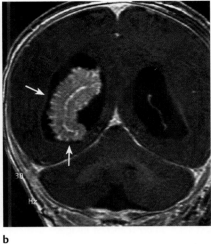

b

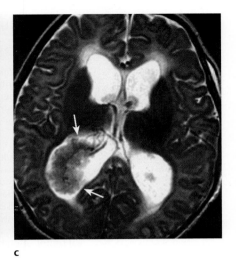

c

Fig. 2A.**35**   **Choroid plexus papilloma.** Postcontrast axial (**a**) and coronal (spoiled GRE) (**b**) T1WI shows prominent enhance- ment of the choroid plexus papilloma in the atrium of the right lateral ventricle (ar- rows). Dilatation of the lateral ventricles is also present.   **c** Axial T2WI shows the le- sion to have heterogeneous intermediate signal.

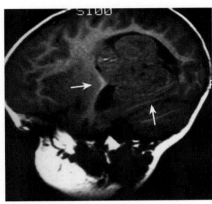

a

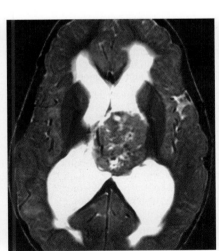

b

Fig. 2A.**36**   **Choroid plexus carcinoma.** **a** Sagittal T1WI shows a large lesion with intermediate signal in the atrium of the right lateral ventricle (arrows). **b** Axial T2WI shows the lesion to have het- erogeneous mixed intermediate and high signal with several peripheral flow voids (arrows). Dilatation of both lateral ven- tricles is evident.

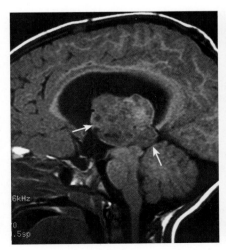

a

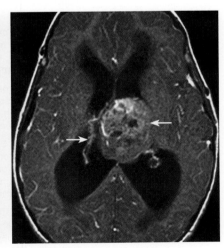

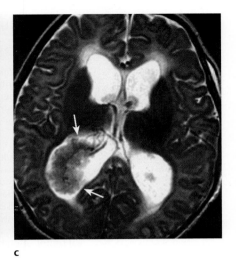

Fig. 2A.**37**   **Rhabdoid tumor. a** Sagittal T1WI shows a large lesion with predomi- nantly intermediate signal at the septum pellucidum resulting in obstructive hydro- cephalus (arrows).

Fig. 2A.**37 b**   Axial T2WI shows the lesion to have mixed intermediate and high signal zones. Prominent dilatation of the lateral ventricles is seen with evidence of transe- pendymal egress of CSF (subependymal high signal).

Fig. 2A.**37 c**   Postcontrast axial T1WI shows heterogeneous enhancement of the lesion (arrows).

Table 2A.8 Enhancing ventricular margins

Disease	MRI Findings	Comments
Normal vascular structures	Normal enhancing structures that can be seen after Gd-contrast contrast administration include ependymal/subependymal veins, which have a linear tubular configuration, and choroid plexus.	Vascular structures with slow flow (veins and venous sinuses) usually enhance because of T1 shortening effects of Gd-contrast contrast. Choroid plexus enhances because of lack of blood-brain barrier.
Neoplastic		
Metastatic tumor (Fig. 1A.103), (Fig. 1A.104)	Single or multiple well-circumscribed or poorly defined lesions involving the skull, dura, leptomeninges, and/or choroid plexus/ventricles. Low to intermediate signal on T1WI and intermediate to high signal on T2WI; usually Gd-contrast enhancement. Bone destruction, compression of neural tissue or vessels may be associated. Leptomeningeal tumor often best seen on postcontrast images.	Intraventricular metastatic tumor may appear as single or multiple sites of involvement. Metastatic neoplasms that can involve the ventricles include: glioblastoma, primitive neuroectodermal tumor, medulloblastoma, ependymoma, pinealblastoma, lymphoma, leukemia, choroid plexus papilloma/carcinoma, lung carcinoma, breast carcinoma, melanoma.
Astrocytoma (Fig. 1A.87)	*Low-grade astrocytoma:* Focal or diffuse mass lesion usually located in white matter with low to intermediate signal on T1WI and high signal on T2WI; with or without mild Gd-contrast enhancement. Minimal associated mass effect. *Juvenile pilocytic astrocytoma:* Subtype: solid/cystic focal lesion with low to intermediate signal on T1WI and high signal on T2WI; usually with prominent Gd-contrast enhancement. Lesions located in cerebellum, hypothalamus, adjacent to third or fourth ventricles, brainstem. *Anaplastic astrocytoma:* Often irregularly marginated lesion located in white matter with low to intermediate signal on T1WI and high signal on T2WI, with or without Gd-contrast enhancement.	*Low-grade astrocytoma:* Often occur in children and adults (age 20–40 years). Tumors comprised of well-differentiated astrocytes. Association with neurofibromatosis type 1. Ten-year survival. May become malignant. *Juvenile pilocytic astrocytoma:* Subtype: common in children, usually favorable prognosis if totally resected. *Anaplastic astrocytoma:* Intermediate between low-grade astrocytoma and glioblastoma multiforme. Approximate 2-year survival.
Glioblastoma multiforme (Fig. 1A.22)	Irregularly marginated mass lesion with necrosis or cyst. Mixed signal on T1WI and heterogeneous high signal on T2WI. Hemorrhage may be associated. Prominent heterogeneous Gd-contrast enhancement. Peripheral edema. Can cross corpus callosum.	Most common primary CNS tumor. Highly malignant neoplasms with necrosis and vascular proliferation, usually in patients above 50 years. Extent of lesion underestimated by MRI. Survival less than 1 year.
Giant cell astrocytoma–Tuberous sclerosis (Fig. 1A.23)	Circumscribed lesion located near the foramen of Monro with mixed low to intermediate or high signal on T1WI and T2WI. Cysts and/or calcifications may be associated. Heterogenous Gd-contrast enhancement.	Subependymal hamartoma near foramen of Monro, occurs in 15% of patients with tuberous sclerosis below 20 years of age. Slow-growing lesions that can progressively cause obstruction of CSF flow through the foramen of Monro. Long-term survival usual if resected.
Primitive neuroectodermal tumor (Fig. 1A.31)	Circumscribed or invasive lesions with low to intermediate signal on T1WI and intermediate to high signal on T2WI; variable Gd-contrast enhancement. Frequent dissemination into the leptomeninges.	Highly malignant tumors that frequently disseminate along CSF pathways.
Medulloblastoma (primitive neuroectodermal tumor of the cerebellum) (Fig. 1A.89)	Circumscribed or invasive unencapsulated lesions with low to intermediate signal on T1WI and intermediate to high signal on T2WI; variable Gd-contrast enhancement. Frequent dissemination into the leptomeninges.	Highly malignant tumors that frequently disseminate along CSF pathways.
Pineoblastoma (primitive neuroectodermal tumor of pineal gland)	Circumscribed or invasive lesions with low to intermediate signal on T1WI and intermediate to high signal on T2WI; variable Gd-contrast enhancement. Frequent dissemination into the leptomeninges.	Highly malignant tumors that frequently disseminate along CSF pathways.
Ependymoma (Fig. 1A.90)	Circumscribed spheroid or lobulated infratentorial lesion, usually in the fourth ventricle. Cysts and/or calcifications may be present. Low to intermediate signal on T1WI and intermediate to high signal on T2WI; variable Gd-contrast enhancement. With or without extension through the foramina of Luschka and Magendie.	Occurs more commonly in children than adults; two-thirds infratentorial, one-third supratentorial.

Table 2A.**8** (Cont.) Enhancing ventricular margins

Disease	MRI Findings	Comments
Oligodendroglioma (Fig. 1A.**25**)	Circumscribed lesion with mixed low to intermediate signal on T1WI and mixed intermediate to high signal on T2WI; areas of signal void at sites of clump-like calcification; heterogenous Gd-contrast enhancement. Involves white matter and cerebral cortex. Can cause chronic erosion of inner table of calvaria. Also occurs within ventricles.	Uncommon slow-growing gliomas with usually mixed histologic patterns (e.g., astrocytoma). Usually in adults older than 35 years of age, 85 % supratentorial. If low-grade 75 % 5-year survival; higher grade lesions have a worse prognosis.
Choroid plexus papilloma or carcinoma (Fig. 2A.**35**)	Circumscribed and/or lobulated lesions with papillary projections, intermediate signal on T1WI and mixed intermediate to high signal on T2WI. Usually prominent Gd-contrast enhancement. Calcifications may be associated. Locations: atrium of lateral ventricle (children) more common than fourth ventricle (adults); rarely other locations such as third ventricle. Associated with hydrocephalus.	Rare intracranial neoplasms. MR features of choroid plexus carcinoma and papilloma overlap; both histologic types can disseminate along CSF pathways and invade brain tissue.
Inflammatory		
Ependymitis/ventriculitis (Figs. 2A.**38**–2A.**40**)	Curvilinear and/or nodular Gd-contrast enhancement along ventricular/ependymal margins with resultant communicating or noncommunicating types of hydrocephalus.	Complications of intracranial inflammatory processes such as infections from bacteria, fungi, viruses (CMV), tuberculosis, and parasites. Noninfectious diseases such as sarcoidosis can result in a similar pattern.

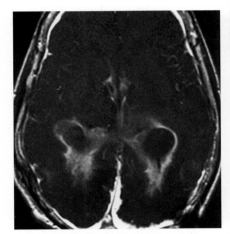

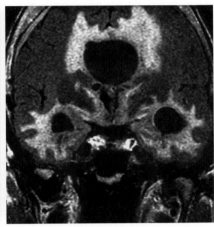

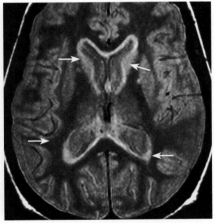

Fig. 2A.**38** **Pyogenic ependymitis/ventriculitis.** **a** Postcontrast axial T1WI shows irregular enhancement along the ventricular margins from pyogenic infection, resulting from a shunt tube complication. Dural enhancement along the inner calvaria margin is also present.

Fig. 2A.**38 b** Coronal FLAIR image shows abnormal high signal in the periventricular brain parenchyma resulting from the inflammatory/infectious process.

Fig. 2A.**39** **CMV ependymitis/ventriculitis.** Axial proton density weighted (long TR/short TE) image shows abnormal high signal along the ependymal margins of the lateral ventricles (arrows). Postcontrast T1WI (not shown) showed only minimal enhancement along the ventricles.

Fig. 2A.**40** **Sarcoidosis ependymitis/ventriculitis.** Postcontrast coronal (**a**) and axial (**b**) T1WI shows small nodular zones of enhancement along the lateral ventricles (arrows) as well as abnormal enhancement within the infratentorial and supratentorial sulci (leptomeninges).

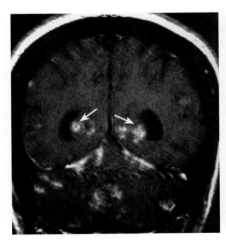

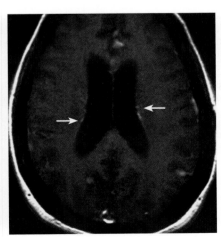

a

b

Table 2A.8 (Cont.) Enhancing ventricular margins

Disease	MRI Findings	Comments
Chemical ventriculitis	Curvilinear and/or nodular Gd-contrast enhancement along ventricular/ependymal margins with resultant communicating or noncommunicating types of hydrocephalus.	Complications relating to intrathecal administration of chemotherapeutic agents, rupture of intracranial dermoid into CSF spaces.
Radiation injury/ necrosis (Fig. 1A.42), (Fig. 1A.97)	Focal lesion with or without mass effect, or poorly defined zone of low to intermediate signal on T1WI, intermediate to high signal on T2WI. With or without Gd-contrast enhancement involving tissue (gray matter and/or white matter) in field of treatment. Can extend to and involve ventricular margins.	Usually occurs from 4–6 months to 10 years after radiation treatment. May be difficult to distinguish from neoplasm. Positron emission tomography (PET) and MR spectroscopy (MRS) might be helpful for evaluation.
Shunt placement	Transient curvilinear Gd-contrast enhancement along ventricular/ependymal margins.	Transient Gd-contrast enhancement related to recent placement of ventricular shunt, possibly related to mild hemorrhage.
Surgery	Transient curvilinear Gd-contrast enhancement along ventricular/ependymal margins as well as along encephalotomy margins.	Transient Gd-contrast enhancement related to recent surgery, usually resolves after 2–3 months.
Vascular		
Arteriovenous malformation (AVM) (Fig. 1A.47)	Lesions with irregular margins that can be located in the brain parenchyma–pia, dura, or both locations. AVMs contain multiple tortuous tubular flow voids on T1WI and T2WI secondary to patent arteries with high blood flow as well as thrombosed vessels with variable signal, areas of hemorrhage in various phases, calcifications, and gliosis. The venous portions often show Gd-contrast enhancement. Gradient echo (GRE) MRI shows flow-related enhancement (high signal) in patent arteries and veins of the AVM. MRA using time-of-flight (TOF) or phase contrast techniques can provide additional detailed information about the nidus, feeding arteries and draining veins, and presence of associated aneurysms. Usually not associated with mass effect except in the case of recent hemorrhage or venous occlusion.	Supratentorial AVMs occur more frequently (80–90%) than infratentorial AVMs (10–20%). Annual risk of hemorrhage. AVMs can be sporadic, congenital, or associated with a history of trauma. Multiple AVMs can be seen in syndromes: Rendu-Osler-Weber, AVMs in brain and lungs and mucosal capillary telangectasias; Wyburn-Mason, AVMs in brain and retina, cutaneous nevi.
Venous angioma (Fig. 1A.101), (Fig. 1A.49)	On postcontrast T1WI, venous angiomas are seen as a Gd-contrast-enhancing transcortical vein draining a collection of small medullary veins (caput Medusa). The draining vein can be seen as a signal void on T2WI.	Considered an anomalous venous formation typically not associated with hemorrhage. Usually an incidental finding except when associated with cavernous hemangioma.
Moyamoya (Fig. 1A.146)	Multiple tortuous tubular flow voids seen in the basal ganglia and thalami on T1WI and T2WI secondary to dilated collateral arteries. Enhancement of these arteries related to slow flow within these collateral arteries versus normal-sized arteries. Often, Gd-contrast enhancement of the leptomeninges related to pial collateral vessels. Decreased or absent flow voids involving the supraclinoid portions of the internal carotid arteries and proximal middle and anterior cerebral arteries. MRA shows stenosis and occlusion of the distal internal carotid arteries with collateral arteries (lenticulostriate, thalamoperforate, and leptomeningeal) best seen after contrast administration, enabling detection of slow blood flow.	Progressive occlusive disease of the intracranial portions of the internal carotid arteries with resultant numerous dilated collateral arteries arising from the lenticulostriate and thalamoperforate arteries as well as other parenchymal, leptomeningeal, and transdural arterial anastomoses. Term translated as "puff of smoke," referring to the angiographic appearance of the collateral arteries (lenticulostriate, thalamoperforate). Usually non-specific etiology but can be associated with neurofibromatosis, radiation angiopathy, atherosclerosis, sickle cell disease. In Asia, usually more common in children than adults.
Ependymal/sub-ependymal hamartomas–Tuberous sclerosis (Fig. 2A.25)	Ependymal/subependymal hamartomas: small nodules located along and projecting into the lateral ventricles. Signal on T1WI and T2WI similar to cortical tubers. Calcification and Gd-contrast enhancement common.	Cortical and subependymal hamartomas are nonmalignant lesions associated with tuberous sclerosis.

Table 2A.**8** (Cont.) Enhancing ventricular margins

Disease	MRI Findings	Comments
Sturge-Weber **(Fig.** 2A.**41)**	Prominent localized unilateral leptomeningeal enhancement usually in parietal and/or occipital regions in children. With or without gyral enhancement. Slightly decreased signal on T2WI in adjacent gyri. Mild localized atrophic changes in brain adjacent to the pial angioma. Prominent medullary and/or subependymal veins and ipsilateral prominence of choroid plexus may be associated. Gyral calcifications above 2 years, progressive cerebral atrophy in region of pial angioma.	Also known as encephalotrigeminal angiomatosis, neurocutaneous syndrome associated with ipsilateral port wine cutaneous lesion and seizures. Results from persistence of primitive leptomeningeal venous drainage (pial angioma) and developmental lack of normal cortical veins, producing chronic venous congestion and ischemia.

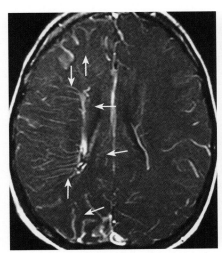

a

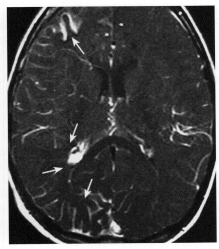

b

Fig. 2A.**41**   **Sturge-Weber.** Postcontrast axial T1WI (**a, b**) shows multiple medullary veins with centripetal flow to veins along the right lateral ventricle (arrows). Unilateral leptomeningeal enhancement is seen in the right frontal and occipital regions (arrows).

2B Lesions Involving the Meninges (Dura/Leptomeninges) and Skull

The cranial and spinal meninges represent three concentric contiguous membranes (dura mater, arachnoid, and pia mater) surrounding the central nervous system (CNS). The outer intracranial meningeal layer is the dura mater (pachymeninx). The outermost layer of the dura mater is a richly vascularized layer with elongated fibroblasts and large intercellular spaces, containing arteries and veins, that represents the periosteum of the inner table of the calvaria. The arteries and veins in this layer form impressions on the inner table of the skull. The outer layer of the dura mater terminates at the foramen magnum. An inner layer of the dura arises from the menix and consists of epithelial cells. This inner layer of the dura mater is contiguous with the spinal dura mater. The layers of the cranial dura separate at sites of large venous sinuses. Reflections of dura form the falx cerebri and tentorium cerebelli, which support the normal positions of the cerebrum and cerebellum.

The arachnoid and pia mater comprise the leptomeninges. The arachnoid membrane is immediately adjacent to the inner surface of the dura. A potential space exists between the dura and arachnoid, referred to as the subdural space. The arachnoid is thinner over the convexities than at the base of the skull. Deep to the arachnoid membrane is the subarachnoid space that contains cerebrospinal fluid (CSF). The inner boundary of the subarachnoid space is the cranial pia mater. The cranial pia mater is a thin layer adjacent to the surface of the brain, extending along the sulci. The cranial pia mater contains elastic fibers internally and collagenous fibers peripherally. Thin connective-tissue strands and cellular septae extend across the arachnoid membrane to the pia, except at the base of the brain where the arachnoid membrane and pia are widely separated. These regions are referred to as the basal subarachnoid cisterns. The spinal pia mater is thicker and more adherent to the nervous tissue than the cranial pia.

The meninges (dura, arachnoid, and pia) form the extra-axial compartments of the CNS. The epidural space exists when the dura is detached from the inner table, usually through trauma/fracture and injury to a meningeal artery/epidural hematoma or occasionally from neoplasms involving the skull. The subdural space forms when a pathologic process is present, such as subdural hematoma from trauma/skull fracture and injury of large veins, inflammatory/infectious disease, or neoplasm. Unlike the epidural and subdural compartment, the subarachnoid space exists without the presence of a pathologic process. The presence of extravascular blood in the subarachnoid space usually is associated with a ruptured intracranial aneurysm, vascular malformation, or trauma.

Gd-contrast enhancement of the dura can have various causes including: neoplasms (primary and metastatic); inflammation/infection; or benign dural fibrosis secondary to intracranial surgery, transient hypotension (secondary to lumbar puncture), or evolving subdural hematoma. The dural enhancement follows the inner contour of the calvaria without extension into the sulci.

Gd-contrast enhancement in the intracranial subarachnoid space (leptomeninges) is nearly always associated with significant pathology (inflammation and/or infection versus neoplasm). Inflammation and/or infection of the leptomeninges can result from pyogenic, fungal, or parasitic diseases as well as tuberculosis. Complications of infectious meningitis include cerebritis, intra-axial abscess, ventriculitis, hydrocephalus, and venous sinus thrombosis/venous cerebral infarction. Neurosarcoidosis results in granulomatous disease in the leptomeninges, producing similar patterns of subarachnoid enhancement. Disseminated or metatstatic disease involving the leptomeninges can result from CNS tumors or primary tumors outside of the CNS. Lymphoma and leukemia can also result in a similar pattern of leptomeningeal enhancement. Rarely, transient leptomeningeal enhancement can occur from chemical irritation resulting from subarachnoid blood.

Skull

The skull is comprised of two major components, the neurocranium and viscerocranium. The viscerocranium represents the facial bony structures. The neurocranium is the portion which encloses the brain and includes the skull base (chondrocranium: endochondral bone formation) and calvaria (membranous bone formation). Chondrocranial bones of the skull base include: the sphenoid, most of the occipital bone, petrous bones, and ethmoid. Sites where the chondrocranial bones of the skull base fuse are referred to as synchondroses. The calvaria originates from ossification centers derived from membranous bone. Growth of the calvaria is directly dependent on growth of the immediately subadjacent dura. The orientation of the dural fibers is related to the position of five chondrocranial structures of the skull base (both petrous crests, crista galli, and both lesser sphenoid wings). Calvarial bones include: two frontal bones, two parietal bones, small portion of occipital bone, and squamous portions of two temporal bones.

Membranous borders between calvarial bones are referred to as sutures. The coronal suture is located between the frontal and parietal bones, the sagittal suture between the parietal bones, the lambdoid suture between the parietal and occipital bones, and metopic suture between the frontal bones. The metopic suture normally closes approximately 7 months after birth. Junction regions where three or more calvarial bones meet are referred to as fontanelles. The largest is the anterior fontanelle, located between the frontal and parietal bones. The other fontanelles are considerably smaller and include the posterior, posterolateral (mastoid), and anterolateral (sphenoid) fontanelles. The size of the calvarial portion of the skull is dependent on growth of the intracranial contents (brain and ventricles). Patients with microcephalic brains have small-sized calvarial vaults, and those with enlarged brains (e.g., from neoplasms, Alexander disease, or Canavan disease) and/or ventricles have enlarged calvaria. Premature closure of one or more suture (craniosynostosis) results in various deformities of the calvaria depending on which suture is involved.

Growth of the chondrocranial bones of the skull base is

not dependent on brain growth as the calvaria. Disorders of skull base development are usually on a genetic basis (e.g., achondroplasia). Anomalies in brain formation can also affect development of the the skull base. Eaxamples include Chiari II malformations and cephaloceles. Chiari II malformations result in a small posterior cranial fossa and an enlarged foramen magnum. Cephaloceles are congenital defects in the skull through which there is either herniation of meninges and CSF or of meninges, CSF/ventricles, and brain tissue. The occipital cephalocele is the most common type in the western hemisphere, and the frontoethmoidal type is common in Southeast Asia. Other cephalocele locations include the parietal and sphenoid bones. Cephalo-

celes can also result from trauma or surgery.

Pathologic processes involving the skull can result from direct extension from adjacent anatomic structures (e.g., sinusitis resulting in osteomyelitis, intracranial neoplasm or inflammation eventually involving the skull), hematogenous seeding of infection or neoplasm into the diploic compartment, or systemic disorders (e.g., myeloma, thalassemia, sickle cell disease, hyperparathyrodism, renal osteodystrophy). Primary pathologic conditions involving the skull include: craniosynostosis, Paget disease, trauma/fracture, neoplasm, infection/inflammation, nonmalignant lesions (e.g., epidermoid, hemangioma), dermal sinus and vascular abnormalities (e.g., sinus pericranii).

Table 2B.**1** Abnormalities involving the meninges

Disease	MRI Findings	Comments
Developmental		
Cephaloceles (meningoceles or meningoencephaloceles) (Figs.2B.1, 2B.2)	Defect in skull through which there is either herniation of meninges and CSF (meningocele) or of meninges, CSF/ventricles, and brain tissue (meningoencephaloceles).	Congenital malformation involving lack of separation of neuroectoderm from surface ectoderm with resultant localized failure of bone formation. Occipital location most common in western hemisphere, frontoethmoidal location most common site in Southeast Asians. Other sites include parietal and sphenoid bones. Cephaloceles can also result from trauma or surgery.
Neurofibromatosis type 1–Meningeal dyplasia/ectasia	Neurofibromatosis type 1 associated with: focal ectasia of intracranial dura; widening of internal auditory canals from dural ectasia; dural and temporal lobe protusion into orbit through bony defect–bony hypoplasia of greater sphenoid wing.	Autosomal dominant disorder (1/2500 births) representing the most common type of neurocutaneous syndromes, associated with neoplasms of CNS and peripheral nervous system and skin. Also associated with meningeal and skull dysplasias.

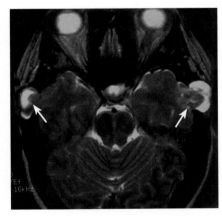

a

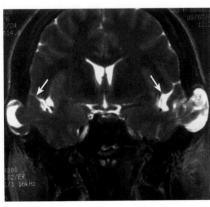

b

◁ Fig. 2B.**1** **Iatrogenic bilateral meningoencephaloceles.** Axial (**a**) and coronal (**b**) T2WI show bilateral meningoencephaloceles at burr holes secondary to placement of bilateral temporal subdural electrodes for epilepsy evaluation.

Fig. 2B.**2**

△
Fig. 2B.**2** **Meningocele.** Axial T2WI shows a meningocele anterior to the left middle cranial fossa (arrows).

Table 2B.**1** (Cont.) Abnormalities involving the meninges

Disease	MRI Findings	Comments
Neoplastic		
Meningioma (Fig. 2B.3)	Extra-axial, well-circumscribed, dural-based lesions. Locations in order of decreasing frequency: supratentorial, infratentorial, parasagittal, convexity, sphenoid ridge, parasellar, posterior fossa, optic nerve sheath, intraventricular. Intermediate signal on T1WI and intermediate to slightly high signal on T2WI. Usually prominent Gd-contrast enhancement. Calcifications may be associated.	Most common extra-axial tumor. Usually benign neoplasms, typically occurring in adults above 40 years of age, in women more commonly than men. Multiple meningiomas seen with neurofibromatosis type 2. Can result in compression of adjacent brain parenchyma, encasement of arteries, and compression of dural venous sinuses. Rarely invasive/malignant types.
Hemangiopericytoma (Fig. 2B.4)	Extra-axial mass lesions, often well-circumscribed. Intermediate signal on T1WI and intermediate to slightly high signal on T2WI; prominent Gd-contrast enhancement (may resemble meningiomas). With or without associated erosive bone changes.	Rare neoplasms in young adults (more common in males than females) sometimes referred to as angioblastic meningioma or meningeal hemangiopericytoma. Arise from vascular cells (pericytes). Frequency of metastases > meningiomas.
Metastatic tumor (Figs. 2B.5, 2B.6)	Single or multiple well-circumscribed or poorly defined lesions involving the skull, dura, leptomeninges, and/or choroid plexus. Low to intermediate signal on T1WI and intermediate to high signal on T2WI; usually Gd-contrast enhancement. Bone destruction and compression of neural tissue or vessels may be present. Leptomeningeal tumor often best seen on postcontrast images.	Metastatic tumor may have variable destructive or infiltrative changes involving single or multiple sites of involvement. Primary tumors can be within or outside of CNS. Metastatic disease can result from hematogenous dissemination, direct extension from bone lesions, or via the CSF pathways.
Lymphoma (Figs. 2B.7, 2B.8)	Single or multiple well-circumscribed or poorly defined lesions involving the skull, dura, and/or leptomeninges. Low to intermediate signal on T1WI and intermediate to high signal on T2WI, usually with Gd-contrast enhancement. Bone destruction may be present. Leptomeningeal tumor often best seen on postcontrast images.	Extra-axial lymphoma may have variable destructive or infiltrative changes involving single or multiple sites of involvement.

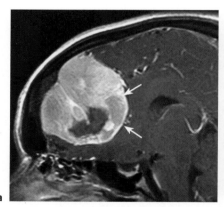
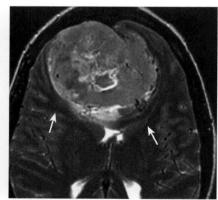

Fig. 2B.**3** **Meningioma. a** Postcontrast sagittal T1WI shows a large, heterogeneously enhancing extra-axial lesion anteriorly compressing the frontal lobes (arrows). **b** Axial T2WI shows the lesion to have mixed intermediate and high signal (arrows).

a

b

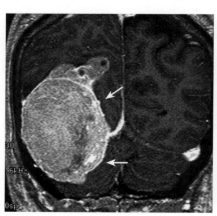
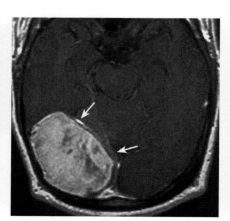
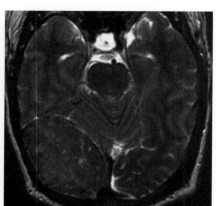

a, b

c

Fig. 2B.**4** **Hemangiopericytoma.** Postcontrast coronal (spoiled GRE) (**a**) and axial (**b**) T1WI show an enhancing extra-axial lesion involving the tentorium compressing the adjacent cerebrum and cerebellum (arrows). **c** Axial T2WI shows the lesion to have heterogeneous intermediate signal (arrows).

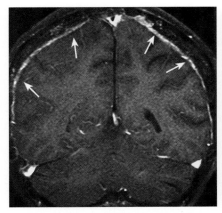

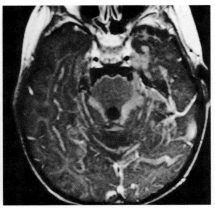

Fig. 2B.5 Metastatic breast carcinoma. Postcontrast FS T1WI shows abnormal enhancement and permeative destructive changes involving the skull with dural enhancement secondary to neoplastic involvement (arrows).

Fig. 2B.6 Disseminated medulloblastoma in the leptomeninges. Postcontrast axial T1WI shows abnormal enhancement in the sulci and cisterns representing extensive disseminated medulloblastoma in the leptomeninges.

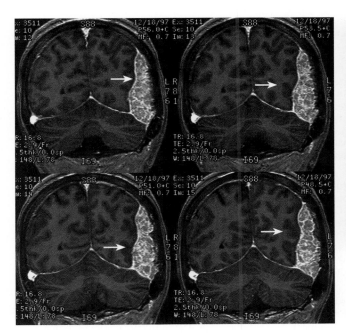

a

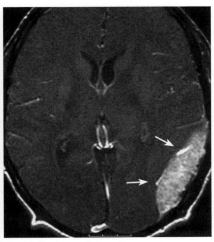

b

Fig. 2B.7 Lymphoma. Postcontrast coronal (**a**) (spoiled GRE) T1WI and axial (**b**) T1WI show a large enhancing lesion involving the dura (arrows).   **c** Axial T2WI shows the lesion to have heterogeneous signal (arrows).

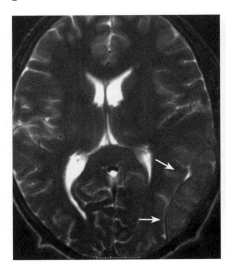

Fig. 2B.**7c**

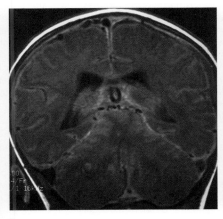

a

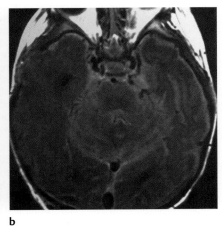

b

Fig. 2B.8 Lymphoma. Postcontrast coronal (**a**) and axial (**b**) T1WI show diffuse abnormal enhancement in the sulci and cisterns, representing extensive leptomeningeal lymphoma.

Table 2B.**1** (Cont.)　Abnormalities involving the meninges

Disease	MRI Findings	Comments
Vascular		
Arterial aneurysm (Fig. 1A.75)	*Saccular aneurysm:* Focal well-circumscribed zone of signal void on T1WI and T2WI; variable mixed signal if thrombosed. *Giant aneurysm:* Focal well-circumscribed structure with layers of low, intermediate, and high signal on T2WI secondary to layers of thrombus of different ages, as well as a zone of signal void representing a patent lumen if present. On T1WI, layers of intermediate and high signal can be seen as well as a zone of signal void. *Fusiform aneurysm:* elongated and ectatic arteries, variable intraluminal MR signal related to turbulent or slowed blood flow or partial/complete thrombosis. *Dissecting aneurysms:* The involved arterial wall is thickened and has intermediate to high signal on T1WI and T2WI; the signal void representing the patent lumen is narrowed.	Abnormal fusiform or focal dilatation of artery secondary to: acquired/degenerative etiology, polycystic disease, connective-tissue disease, atherosclerosis, trauma, infection (mycotic), arteriovenous malformation (AVM), vasculitis, and drugs. Focal aneurysms are also referred to as saccular aneurysms that typically occur at arterial bifurcations and are multiple in 20%. Saccular aneurysms greater than 2.5 cm in diameter are referred to as giant aneurysms. Fusiform aneurysms are often related to atherosclerosis or collagen vascular disease (e.g., Marfan syndrome, Ehlers-Danlos syndrome). Dissecting aneurysms: hemorrhage occurs in the arterial wall from incidental or significant trauma.
AVM (Fig. 1A.47)	Lesions with irregular margins that can be located in the brain parenchyma-pia, dura, or both locations. AVMs contain multiple tortuous tubular flow voids on T1WI and T2WI secondary to patent arteries with high blood flow; as well as thrombosed vessels with variable signal, areas of hemorrhage in various phases, calcifications, and gliosis. The venous portions often show Gd-contrast enhancement. Gradient-echo (GRE) MRI shows flow-related enhancement (high signal) in patent arteries and veins of the AVM. MR angiography (MRA) using time-of-flight (TOF) or phase contrast techniques can provide additional detailed information about the nidus, feeding arteries and draining veins, and presence of associated aneurysms. Usually not associated with mass effect except in cases of recent hemorrhage or venous occlusion.	Supratentorial AVMs occur more frequently (80–90%) than infratentorial AVMs (10–20%). Annual risk of hemorrhage. AVMs can be sporadic, congenital, or associated with a history of trauma. Multiple AVMs can be seen in syndromes: Rendu-Osler-Weber, AVMs in brain and lungs, and mucosal capillary telangectasias; Wyburn-Mason, AVMs in brain and retina, and cutaneous nevi.
Dural AVM (Fig. 1A.78)	Dural AVMs contain multiple tortuous tubular flow voids on T1WI and T2WI. The venous portions often show Gd-contrast enhancement. GRE MRI and MRA using TOF or phase contrast techniques show flow signal in patent portions of the vascular malformation and areas of venous sinus occlusion or recanalization. Usually not associated with mass effect except in cases of recent hemorrhage or venous occlusion.	Dural AVMs are usually acquired lesions resulting from thrombosis or occlusion of an intracranial venous sinus with subsequent recanalization resulting in direct arterial to venous sinus communications. Location in order of decreasing frequency: transverse, sigmoid venous sinuses; cavernous sinus; straight, superior sagittal sinuses.
Moyamoya (Fig. 1A.146)	Multiple tortuous tubular flow voids seen in the basal ganglia and thalami on T1WI and T2WI secondary to dilated collateral arteries. Enhancement of these arteries related to slow flow within these collateral arteries versus normal-sized arteries. Often, Gd-contrast enhancement of the leptomeninges related to pial collateral vessels. Decreased or absent flow voids involving the supraclinoid portions of the internal carotid arteries and proximal middle and anterior cerebral arteries. MRA shows stenosis and occlusion of the distal internal carotid arteries with collateral arteries (lenticulostriate, thalamoperforate, and leptomeningeal) best seen after contrast administration, enabling detection of slow blood flow.	Progressive occlusive disease of the intracranial portions of the internal carotid arteries with resultant numerous dilated collateral arteries arising from the lenticulostriate and thalamoperforate arteries as well as other parenchymal, leptomeningeal, and transdural arterial anastomoses. Term translated as "puff of smoke," referring to the angiographic appearance of the collateral arteries (lenticulostriate, thalamoperforate). Usually nonspecific etiology but can be associated with neurofibromatosis, radiation angiopathy, atherosclerosis, sickle cell disease. In Asia, usually more common in children than adults.
Sturge-Weber (Fig. 2B.9)	Prominent localized unilateral leptomeningeal enhancement usually in parietal and/or occipital regions in children. With or without gyral enhancement. Slightly decreased signal on T2WI in adjacent gyri. Mild localized atrophic changes in brain adjacent to the pial angioma. Prominent medullary and/or subependymal veins and ipsilateral prominence of choroid plexus may be associated. Gyral calcifications above 2 years, progressive cerebral atrophy in region of pial angioma.	Also known as encephalotrigeminal angiomatosis, neurocutaneous syndrome associated with ipsilateral port wine cutaneous lesion and seizures. Results from persistence of primitive leptomeningeal venous drainage (pial angioma) and developmental lack of normal cortical veins, producing chronic venous congestion and ischemia.

Table 2B.**1** (Cont.) Abnormalities involving the meninges

Disease	MRI Findings	Comments
Hemorrhagic (trauma, vascular malformation, or aneurysm)		
Epidural hematoma (Fig. 2B.10)	Biconvex extra-axial hematoma located between the skull and dura. Displaced dura has low signal on T2WI. The signal of the hematoma itself depends on its age, size, hematocrit, and oxygen tension. With or without associated edema. High signal on T2WI involving the displaced brain parenchyma. Subfalcine, uncal herniation may be associated. *Hyperacute:* intermediate signal on T1WI, intermediate to high signal on T2WI. *Acute:* low to intermediate signal on T1WI, high signal on T2WI. *Subacute:* high signal on T1WI and T2WI.	Epidural hematomas usually result from trauma/ tearing of an epidural artery or dural venous sinus. Epidural hematomas do not cross cranial sutures. Skull fracture may be associated.
Subdural hematoma (Fig. 2B.11)	Crescentic extra-axial hematoma located in the potential space between the inner margin of the dura and outer margin of the arachnoid membrane. The signal of the hematoma depends on its age, size, hematocrit, and oxygen tension. With or without associated edema. High signal on T2WI involving the displaced brain parenchyma. Subfalcine, uncal herniation may be associated. *Hyperacute:* intermediate signal on T1WI, intermediate to high signal on T2WI. *Acute:* low to intermediate signal on T1WI, low signal on T2WI. *Subacute:* high signal on T1WI and T2WI. *Chronic:* Variable, often low to intermediate signal on T1WI, high signal on T2WI. With or without enhancement of collection and organizing neomembrane. Mixed MRI signal can result if rebleeding occurs into chronic collection.	Subdural hematomas usually result from trauma/ stretching/tearing of cortical veins where they enter the subdural space to drain into dural venous sinuses. Subdural hematomas do cross sites of cranial sutures. Skull fracture may be associated.

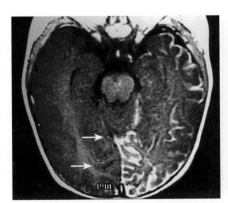

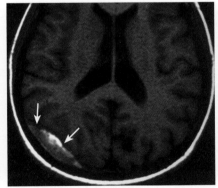

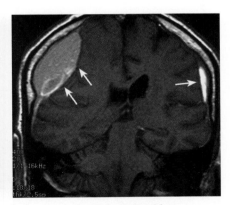

Fig. 2B.**9** **Sturge-Weber.** Postcontrast axial T1WI shows prominent localized unilateral leptomeningeal enhancement in the left temporal-occipital regions (arrows).

Fig. 2B.**10** **Epidural hematoma.** Axial T1WI shows a biconvex extra-axial hematoma with mixed intermediate and high signal located between the skull and dura (arrows).

Fig. 2B.**11** **Bilateral subdural hematomas.** Coronal T1WI shows bilateral subdural hematomas with high signal (arrows). The right subdural hematoma causes subfalcine herniation of the right cerebral hemisphere leftward.

Table 2B.1 (Cont.) Abnormalities involving the meninges

Disease	MRI Findings	Comments
Subarachnoid hemorrhage (Figs. 2B.**12**, 2B.**13**)	*Acute subarachnoid hemorrhage:* Subarachnoid hemorrhage is not usually seen on T1WI and T2WI, although it may be seen as intermediate to slightly high signal on proton density weighted or FLAIR images. CT is generally more reliable than MRI in the detection of acute subarachnoid hemorrhage. *Remote subarachnoid hemorrhage:* The results of remote episodes of subarachnoid hemorrhage can sometimes be seen with MRI as a thin rim of low signal on T2WI on the pial surface of the brain (superficial siderosis) secondary to deposition of hemosiderin.	Acute subarachnoid hemorrhage may not be seen with MRI because: extravasated blood in the subarachnoid space is diluted with CSF; intracranial CSF has a relatively high oxygen tension resulting in only a minority of extravasated hemoglobin being in the oxyhemoglobin state. Subarachnoid hemorrhage can result from ruptured aneurysm, vascular malformation, hypertensive hemorrhage, trauma, cerebral infarct, coagulopathy, etc.
Inflammatory		
Subdural/epidural abscess–Empyema (Fig. 2B.**14**)	Epidural or subdural collections with low signal on T1WI and high signal on T2WI; thin linear peripheral zones of Gd-contrast enhancement.	Often results from complications related to sinusitis (usually frontal), meningitis, otitis media, ventricular shunts, or surgery. Can be associated with venous sinus thrombosis and venous cerebral or cerebellar infarcts, cerebritis, brain abscess. Mortality 30%.
Leptomeningeal infection/inflammation (Figs. 2B.**15**, 2B.**16**)	Single or multiple nodular enhancing lesions and/or focal or diffuse abnormal subarachnoid enhancement. Low to intermediate signal on T1WI, intermediate to high signal on T2WI. Leptomeningeal inflammation is often best seen on postcontrast images.	Gd-contrast enhancement in the intracranial subarachnoid space (leptomeninges) usually is associated with significant pathology (inflammation and/or infection versus neoplasm). Inflammation and/or infection of the leptomeninges can result from pyogenic, fungal, or parasitic diseases as well as tuberculosis. Neurosarcoidosis results in granulomatous disease in the leptomeninges producing similar patterns of subarachnoid enhancement.
Postsurgical pseudo-meningocele (Fig. 2B.**17**)	CSF-filled collection contiguous with the subarachnoid space protruding through a surgical bony defect.	Usually are not clinically significant unless they become large or infected.

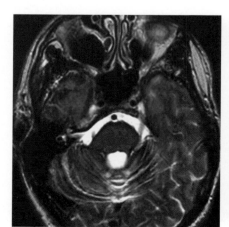

Fig. 2B.**12 a**

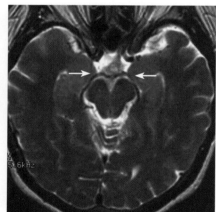

Fig. 2B.**12 b**

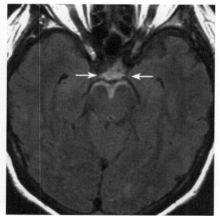

Fig. 2B.**12 c**

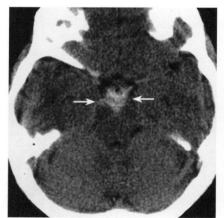

Fig. 2B.**13 a**

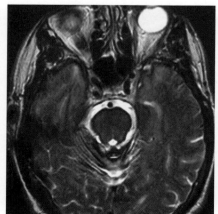

Fig. 2B.**13 b**

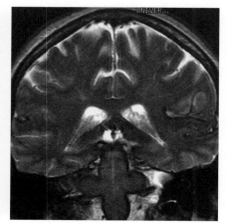

Fig. 2B.**13 c**

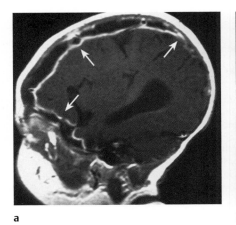

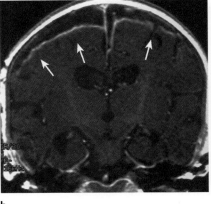

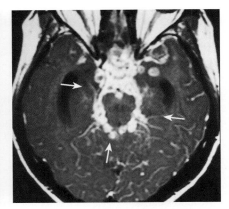

a   b   Fig. 2B.**15**   **Leptomeningeal infection/ tuberculosis.** Postcontrast axial T1WI shows multiple ring-shaped and poorly defined zones of enhancement in the basal cisterns (arrows).

Fig. 2B.**14**   **Subdural/epidural abscess–empyema.** Postcontrast sagittal (**a**) and coronal (**b**) T1WI show a subdural collection with low signal with thin irregular peripheral zones of enhancement (arrows).

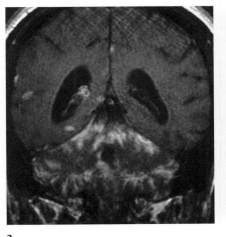

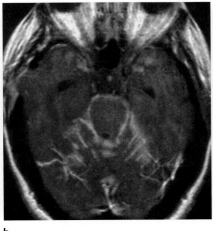

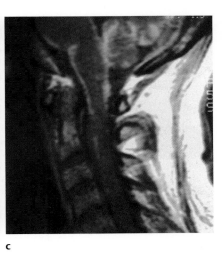

a   b   c

Fig. 2B.**16**   **Leptomeningeal inflammation/sarcoidosis.** Postcontrast coronal (**a**), axial (**b**), and sagittal (**c**) T1WI show poorly defined zones of enhancement along the pial margins of the cerebellar and cerebral gyri, also surrounding the brainstem and upper cervical spinal cord.

◁ Fig. 2B.**12**   **Subacute subarachnoid hemorrhage.**   **a** Axial CT image shows a poorly defined zone of high attenuation in the interpeduncular and suprasellar cisterns, representing recent subarachnoid hemorrhage (arrows).   **b** Axial T2WI shows a poorly defined zone of intermediate signal in the interpeduncular and suprasellar cisterns (arrows).   **c** Axial FLAIR image shows corresponding abnormal high signal in the cisterns (arrows).

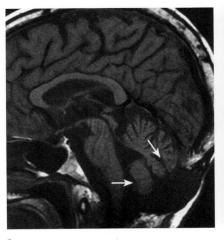

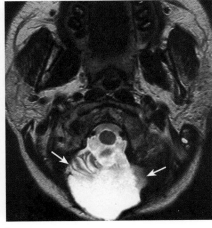

a   b

◁ Fig. 2B.**13**   **Remote subarachnoid hemorrhage (superficial siderosis).** Axial T2WI (**a, b**) show thin rims of low signal on the pial surface of the brainstem and cerebellar gyri.   **c** Coronal T2WI of another patient with similar findings along the brainstem and several cerebral gyri.

Fig. 2B.**17**   **Postsurgical pseudomeningocele.** Sagittal T1WI (**a**) and axial T2WI (**b**) show a CSF-filled collection contiguous with the subarachnoid space protruding through a surgical bony defect at the inferior occipital region (arrows).

Table 2B.2 Abnormalities involving the skull

Disease	MRI Findings	Comments
Developmental abnormalities		
Cephaloceles (meningoceles or meningoencephaloceles) (Fig. 2B.18)	Defect in skull through which there is either herniation of meninges and CSF (meningocele) or of meninges, CSF/ventricles, and brain tissue (meningoencephaloceles).	Congenital malformation involving lack of separation of neuroectoderm from surface ectoderm with resultant localized failure of bone formation. Occipital location most common in western hemisphere, frontoethmoidal location most common site in Southeast Asians. Other sites include parietal and sphenoid bones. Cephaloceles can also result from trauma or surgery.
Achondroplasia	Small foramen magnum, skull base shortened, brachycephaly, large calvaria, frontal bossing.	Autosomal dominant: sporadic disorder with defective endochondral bone formation. Mental and motor function typically within normal limits.
Chiari II malformation (Arnold-Chiari) (Fig. 1A.12)	Large foramen magnum through which there is an inferiorly positioned vermis associated with a cervicomedullary kink. Myelomeningoceles in nearly all patients. Hydrocephalus and syringomyelia common. Dilated lateral ventricles posteriorly (colpocephaly).	Complex anomaly involving the cerebrum, cerebellum, brainstem, spinal cord, ventricles, skull, and dura. Failure of fetal neural folds to develop properly resulting in altered development affecting multiple sites of the CNS.
Neurofibromatosis type 1 (Fig. 2B.19)	Neurofibromatosis type 1 associated with: focal ectasia of intracranial dura; widening of internal auditory canals from dural ectasia; dural and temporal lobe protusion into orbit through bony defect–bony hypoplasia of greater sphenoid wing, bone malformation or erosion from plexiform neurofibromas.	Autosomal dominant disorder (1/2500 births) representing the most common type of neurocutaneous syndromes. Associated with neoplasms of CNS and peripheral nervous system and skin. Also associated with meningeal and skull dysplasias.
Craniosynostosis	*Isolated synostosis:* Involves single suture. Usually sporadic. Abnormal head shape depending on which suture is prematurely closed. *Sagittal suture:* Premature closure. Most common type (approximately 50%). Results in a long-shaped skull (dolichocephaly or scaphocephaly). *Metopic suture:* Premature closure. Results in a wedge-shaped skull with apex anteriorly (trigonocephaly). *Coronal or lambdoid suture:* Premature closure. Approximately 10%. Results in a vertically elongated skull that is aymmetric from the anterior to posterior portions of the skull. *Unilateral coronal or lambdoid suture:* Premature closure. Cranial asymmetry from left to right sides (plagiocephaly).	Premature closure of cranial suture resulting from developmental anomaly (primary synostosis) or from extraneous causes such as intrauterine or postnatal trauma, toxins, metabolic disorders (e.g., hyperthyroidism, hypercalcemia, hypophosphatasia, rickets), lack of brain growth/microcephaly.
Multiple synostosis syndromes	*Premature synostosis* involving more than one suture with various deformities of skull shape. Associations with underlying anomalies of brain, ventriculomegaly.	Usually associated with various genetic disorders such as: Apert, Apert-Crouzon, Crouzon.
Dyke-Davidoff-Mason syndrome (Fig. 2B.20)	Hypoplasia/atrophy or encephalomalacia of one cerebral hemisphere with compensatory dilatation of ipsilateral lateral ventricle. Unilateral ipsilateral decrease in size of cranial fossa associated with thickened calvaria. Enlargement of ipsilateral paranasal sinuses may be associated.	Rare disorder in adolescents presenting with seizures, mental retardation, hemiparesis.

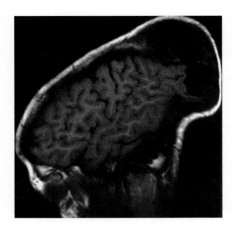

Fig. 2B.**18** **Meningoencephalocele.** Sagittal T1WI shows a defect in the skull through which there is herniation of meninges, CSF, and brain tissue.

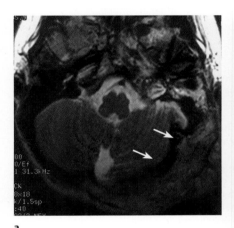

a

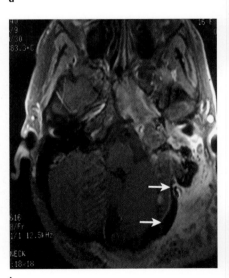

b

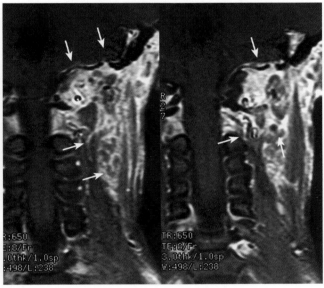

c

Fig. 2B.**19** **Plexiform neurofibroma/neurofibromatosis type 1.**
a Axial T2WI shows altered configuration of the left occipital bone related to a plexiform neurofibroma involving the posterior left scalp (arrows). Postcontrast FS axial (**b**) and coronal (**c**) T1WI show irregular zones of enhancement associated with the plexiform neurofibroma (arrows).

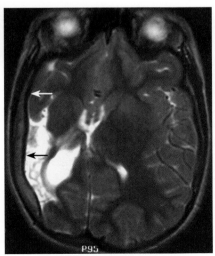

Fig. 2B.**20** **Dyke-Davidoff-Mason syndrome.** Axial T2WI shows encephalomalacia of the right cerebral hemisphere with compensatory dilatation of ipsilateral lateral ventricle. Ipsilateral decrease in size of cranial fossa associated with thickened calvaria (arrows).

Table 2B.**2** (Cont.) Abnormalities involving the skull

Disease	MRI Findings	Comments
Acquired		
Paget disease (Fig. 2B.**21**)	Expansile sclerotic/lytic process involving the skull with mixed low to intermediate signal on T1WI and variable mixed low, intermediate, high signal on T2WI; variable heterogenous enhancement. Irregular/indistinct borders between marrow and inner margins of the outer and inner tables of the skull.	Usually seen in older adults. Can result in narrowing of neuroforamina with cranial nerve compression, basilar impression with or without compression of brainstem.
Fibrous dysplasia (Fig. 2B.**22**)	Expansile process involving the skull base with mixed low to intermediate signal on T1WI and variable mixed low, intermediate, high signal on T2WI; usually heterogenous enhancement.	Usually seen in adolescents and young adults. Can result in narrowing of neuroforamina with cranial nerve compression, facial deformities. Mono-ostotic and polyostotic forms (endocrine abnormalities may present, such as with McCune-Albright syndrome, precocious puberty).
Hyperostosis frontalis (Fig. 2B.**23**)	Thickening of inner table of frontal bones, distinct interface between cortical margin of inner table and marrow within diploic space. Indentations within the zones of bony thickening result from the process sparing large dural veins and dural venous sinuses.	Idiopathic thickening of inner table of frontal bones, usually occurring in women.
Hematopoetic disorders	Enlargement of the diploic space with thinning of the inner and outer tables.	Thickening of diploic space related to erythroid hyperplasia from sickle cell disease, thalasemia major.
Trauma		
Cephalohematoma	Hematoma located beneath periosteum of outer table, does not cross suture lines. Skull fracture and subdural hematoma may be associated.	Results from birth trauma (complication of forceps delivery), associated with 1 % of births
Fracture	*Nondisplaced/nondepressed skull fractures:* Abnormal low signal on T1WI and high signal on T2WI in marrow at the site of fracture. Possible associated subgaleal hematoma, epidural hematoma, subdural hematoma, subarachnoid hemorrhage. *Depressed skull fracture:* Angulation and internal displacement of fractured skull. Abnormal low signal on T1WI and high signal on T2WI in marrow at the site of fracture. Possible associated subgaleal hematoma, epidural hematoma, subdural hematoma, subarachnoid hemorrhage.	Traumatic fractures of the skull can involve the calvaria or skull base, and significant complications that can result include: epidural hematoma, subdural hematoma, subarachnoid hemorrhage, CSF leakage/rhinorrhea, otorrhea.

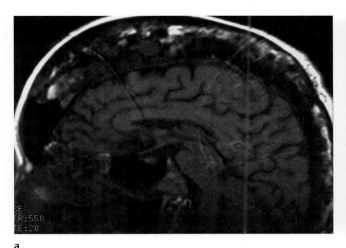

a

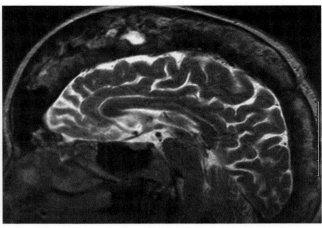

b

Fig. 2B.**21**   **Paget disease.** Sagittal T1WI (**a**) and T2WI (**b**) show expansile sclerotic/lytic process involving the skull with mixed heterogeneous signal in the diploic/marrow compartment. Irregular/ indistinct borders are seen between the marrow and inner margins of the outer and inner tables of the skull. Basilar impression is also present.

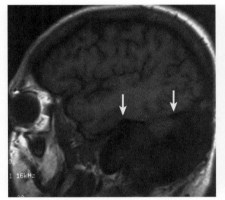

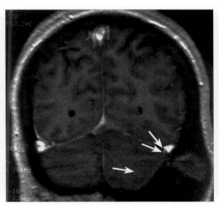

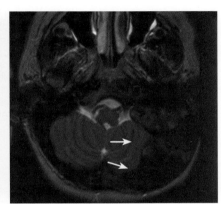

Fig. 2B.**22   Fibrous dysplasia.   a** Sagittal T1WI shows an expansile process involving the skull base with mixed low to intermediate signal (arrows).

Fig. 2B.**22 b** Postcontrast coronal (spoiled GRE) T1WI shows irregular mild enhancement in portions of the abnormality (arrows).

Fig. 2B.**22 c** Axial T2WI shows mixed low and intermediate signal at the abnormality (arrows).

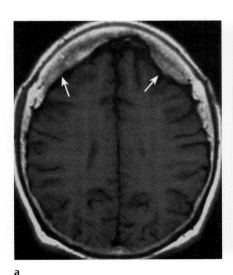

a

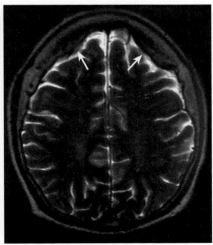

b

Fig. 2B.**23   Hyperostosis frontalis.** Axial T1WI (**a**) and T2WI (**b**) show expansion of the marrow space of the frontal bones with distinct interfaces between cortical margins of inner and outer tables and marrow within diploic space (arrows).

Table 2B.**2** (Cont.) Abnormalities involving the skull

Disease	MRI Findings	Comments
Neoplastic disease		
Metastatic tumor (Fig. 2B.24)	Single or multiple well-circumscribed or poorly defined lesions involving the skull, dura, leptomeninges, and/or choroid plexus. Low to intermediate signal on T1WI and intermediate to high signal on T2WI, usually with Gd-contrast enhancement. Bone destruction, compression of neural tissue or vessels may be associated. Leptomeningeal tumor often best seen on postcontrast images.	Metastatic tumor may have variable destructive or infiltrative changes involving single or multiple sites of involvement. Primary tumors are usually from outside of CNS.
Lymphoma	Single or multiple well-circumscribed or poorly defined lesions involving the skull, dura, and/or leptomeninges. Low to intermediate signal on T1WI and intermediate to high signal on T2WI; usually with Gd-contrast enhancement. Bone destruction may be associated. Leptomeningeal tumor often best seen on postcontrast images.	Extra-axial lymphoma may have variable destructive or infiltrative changes involving single or multiple sites of involvement.
Myeloma/plasmacytoma (Figs. 2B.25, 2B.26)	Multiple (myeloma) or single (plasmacytoma) well-circumscribed or poorly defined lesions involving the skull and dura. Low to intermediate signal on T1WI and intermediate to high signal on T2WI; usually with Gd-contrast enhancement. Bone destruction may be associated.	Myeloma may have variable destructive or infiltrative changes involving the axial and/or appendicular skeleton.
Chordoma (Fig. 2B.27)	Well-circumscibed lobulated lesions with low to intermediate signal on T1WI and high signal on T2WI. Gd-contrast enhancement (usually heterogeneous). Locally invasive associated with bone erosion/destruction, encasement of vessels and nerves. Skull base and clivus common location, usually in the midline.	Rare, slow-growing tumors at the skull base. Detailed anatomic display of extension of chordomas by MRI is important for planning of surgical approaches.

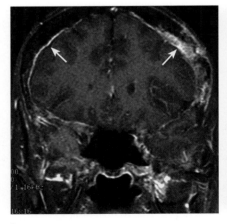
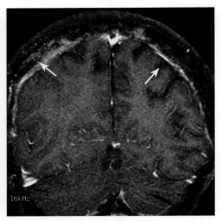

a   b

Fig. 2B.**24 Metastatic breast carcinoma.** Postcontrast FS coronal T1WI (**a, b**) shows permeative destructive changes involving the skull where there are irregular zones of abnormal enhancement (arrows). Abnormal dural enhancement is also present secondary to neoplastic involvement (arrows).

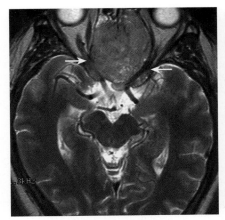

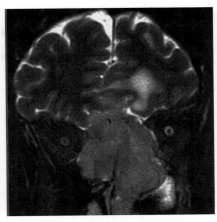

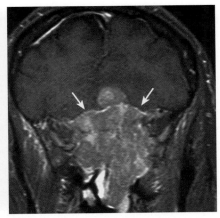

Fig. 2B.25 Plasmacytoma. a Axial T2WI shows a lesion with intermediate signal involving the ethmoid air cells extending through the skull base (arrows).

Fig. 2B.25 b Coronal inversion recovery (IR) image shows the lesion to have intermediate to high signal.

Fig. 2B.25 c Postcontrast coronal FS T1WI shows the lesion to have moderate heterogeneous enhancement. The lesion compresses the inferior portions of the frontal lobes (arrows).

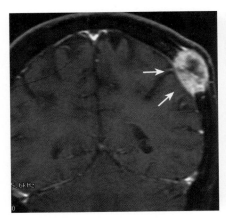

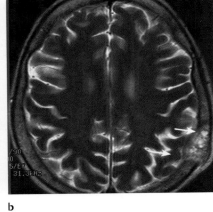

Fig. 2B.26 Myeloma. a Postcontrast coronal FS T1WI shows an enhancing lesion destroying the adjacent skull with extension intracranially and into the subcutaneous soft tissues (arrows). **b** Axial T2WI shows the lesion to have heterogeneous intermediate to slightly high signal (arrows).

a

b

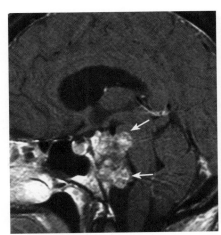

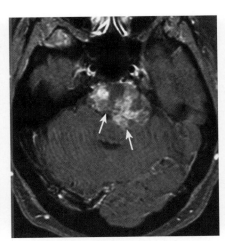

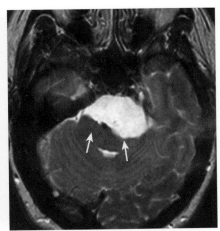

Fig. 2B.27 Chordoma. a Postcontrast sagittal T1WI shows a well-circumscribed lobulated lesion with heterogeneous enhancement along the endocranial surface of the clivus compressing the brainstem (arrows).

Fig. 2B.27 b Postcontrast FS axial T1WI shows the lesion to be slightly lobulated (arrows).

Fig. 2B.27 c Axial T2WI shows the lesion to have high signal (arrows).

Table 2B.**2** (Cont.) Abnormalities involving the skull

Disease	MRI Findings	Comments
Chondrosarcoma (Fig. 2B.28)	Lobulated lesions. Low to intermediate signal on T1WI, high signal on T2WI. With or without matrix mineralization: low signal on T2WI. Gd-contrast enhancement (usually heterogeneous). Locally invasive associated with bone erosion/destruction, encasement of vessels and nerves. Skull base and petrooccipital synchondrosis common location, usually off midline.	Rare, slow-growing tumors. Detailed anatomic display of extension of chondrosarcomas by MRI is important for planning of surgical approaches.
Osteogenic sarcoma (Fig. 2B.29)	Destructive lesions involving the skull base. Low to intermediate signal on T1WI; mixed low, intermediate, high signal on T2WI. Usually with matrix mineralization/ossification: low signal on T2WI. Gd-contrast enhancement (usually heterogeneous).	Rare lesions involving the endochondral bone-forming portions of the skull base, more common than chodrosarcomas and Ewing sarcoma. Locally invasive, high metastatic potential. Occurs in children as primary tumors and adults (associated with Paget disease, irradiated bone, chronic osteomyelitis, osteoblastoma, giant cell tumor, fibrous dysplasia).
Ewing sarcoma	Destructive lesions involving the skull base. Low to intermediate signal on T1WI; mixed low, intermediate, high signal on T2WI. With or without matrix mineralization: low signal on T2WI. Gd-contrast enhancement (usually heterogeneous).	Usually occurs between the ages of 5 and 30, more common in males than females. Rare lesions involving the skull base. Locally invasive, high metastatic potential.
Sinonasal squamous cell carcinoma	Destructive lesions in the nasal cavity, paranasal sinuses, nasopharynx. With or without intracranial extension via bone destruction or perineural spread. Intermediate signal on T1WI, intermediate to slightly high signal on T2WI; mild Gd-contrast enhancement. Large lesions (necrosis and/or hemorrhage may be associated).	Occurs in adults usually above age 55, more common in males than females. Associated with occupational or other exposure to: nickel, chromium, mustard gas, radium, manufacture of wood products.
Adenoid cystic carcinoma (Fig. 2B.30)	Destructive lesions in the paranasal sinuses, nasal cavity, nasopharynx, with or without intracranial extension via bone destruction or perineural spread. Intermediate signal on T1WI and intermediate to high signal on T2WI; variable mild, moderate, or prominent Gd-contrast enhancement.	Account for 10 % of sinonasal tumors. Arise in any location within sinonasal cavities. Usually occurs in adults above 30 years of age.
Esthesioneuroblastoma (Fig. 2B.31)	Locally destructive lesions with low to intermediate signal on T1WI and intermediate to high signal on T2WI; prominent Gd-contrast enhancement. Location: superior nasal cavity, ethmoid air cells with occasional extension into the other paranasal sinuses, orbits, anterior cranial fossa, cavernous sinuses.	Tumors also referred to as olfactory neuroblastoma. Arise from olfactory epithelium in the superior nasal cavity. Occurs in adolescents and adults, more common in males than females.

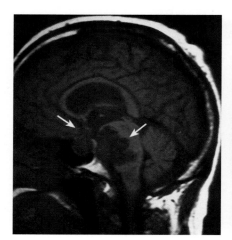
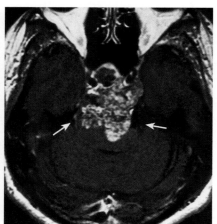

a

b

Fig. 2B.**28 Chondrosarcoma. a** Sagittal image shows a lobulated lesion with low to intermediate signal in the sella and along the endocranial surface of the clivus compressing the brainstem (arrows). **b** Postcontrast axial T1WI shows the lesion to have heterogeneous enhancement (arrows).

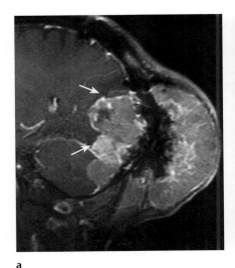

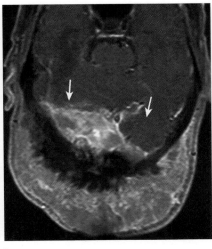

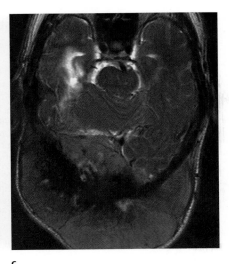

a

Fig. 2B.29 **Osteogenic sarcoma.** Postcontrast FS sagittal (**a**) and axial (**b**) T1WI show a large enhancing lesion involving the posterior skull–associated with bone de-

b

struction, intracranial and extracranial extension, and intratumoral ossification (low signal) (arrows)–with heterogeneous enhancement along the endocranial surface

c

of the clivus compressing the brainstem (arrows). **c** Axial T2WI shows the lesion to have heterogeneous low to intermediate signal.

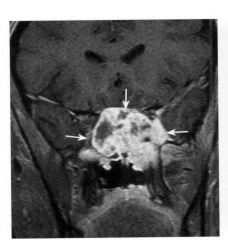

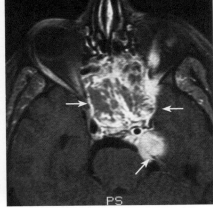

Fig. 2B.30 **Adenoid cystic carcinoma.** Postcontrast FS coronal (**a**) and axial (**b**) T1WI show a large heterogeneously enhancing lesion involving the ethmoidal and sphenoidal sinuses extending intracranially into the anterior cranial fossae, left middle cranial fossa, left cavernous sinus (encasing the left internal carotid artery), and left trigeminal cistern.

a

b

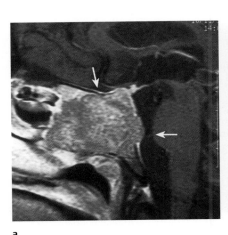

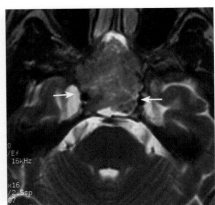

Fig. 2B.31 **Esthesioneuroblastoma.** **a** Postcontrast sagittal T1WI shows an enhancing lesion involving the nasopharynx, ethmoidal and sphenoidal sinuses, sella, and prepontine cistern (arrows). **b** Axial T2WI shows the lesion to have low to intermediate signal (arrows).

a

b

Table 2B.2 (Cont.) Abnormalities involving the skull

Disease	MRI Findings	Comments
Meningioma (Fig. 1A.107)	Extra-axial, well-circumscribed, dural-based lesions. Locations in order of decreasing frequency: supratentorial, infratentorial, parasagittal, convexity, sphenoid ridge, parasellar, posterior fossa, optic nerve sheath, intraventricular. Intermediate signal on T1WI and intermediate to slightly high signal on T2WI. Usually prominent Gd-contrast enhancement. Calcifications may be associated.	Most common extra-axial tumor. Usually benign neoplasms, typically occurring in adults above 40 years of age, in women more commonly than men. Multiple meningiomas seen with neurofibromatosis type 2. Can result in compression of adjacent brain parenchyma, encasement of arteries, and compression of dural venous sinuses. Rarely invasive/malignant types.
Hemangiopericytoma (Fig. 1A.108)	Extra-axial mass lesions, often well-circumscribed. Intermediate signal on T1WI and intermediate to slightly high signal on T2WI; prominent Gd-contrast enhancement (may resemble meningiomas). With or without associated erosive bone changes.	Rare neoplasms in young adults (more common in males than females), sometimes referred to as angioblastic meningioma or meningeal hemangiopericytoma. Arise from vascular cells (pericytes). Frequency of metastases > meningiomas.
Pituitary adenoma (Fig. 1A.197)	*Macroadenomas (>10 mm):* Commonly have intermediate signal on T1WI and T2WI similar to gray matter. Necrosis, cyst, hemorrhage may be associated. Usually prominent enhancement. Extension into suprasellar cistern with waist at diaphragma sella, with or without extension into cavernous sinus. Occasionally invades skull base.	Common benign slow-growing tumors representing approximately 50% of sellar/parasellar neoplasms in adults. Can be associated with endocrine abnormalities related to oversecretion of hormones (prolactin, nonsecretory type, growth hormone, ACTH, and others). Prolactinomas: more common in females than males; growth hormone tumors: more common in males than females.
Other lesions involving the skull		
Osteoma (Fig. 2B.32)	Well-circumscribed lesions involving the skull with low to intermediate signal on T1WI and T2WI; no Gd-contrast enhancement.	Benign proliferation of bone located in the skull or paranasal sinuses (in order of decreasing frequency: frontal, ethmoidal, maxillary, sphenoidal).
Epidermoid (Fig. 1A.194)	Well-circumscribed spheroid ectodermal-inclusion cystic lesions in the skull associated with chronic bone erosion. Low to intermediate signal on T1WI, high signal on T2WI; no Gd-contrast enhancement.	Non-neoplastic lesions filled with desquamated cells and keratinaceous debris involving the skull.
Dermoid (Fig. 1A.86)	Well-circumscribed spheroid lesions in the skull associated with chronic bone erosion. Usually with high signal on T1WI and variable low, intermediate, and/or high signal on T2WI. No Gd-contrast enhancement. Fluid-fluid or fluid-debris levels may be present.	Non-neoplastic ectodermal-inclusion cystic lesions involving the skull, filled with lipid material, cholesterol, desquamated cells, and keratinaceous debris.
Hemangioma	Circumscribed or poorly marginated structures (less than 4 cm in diameter) in marrow of skull (often frontal bone). Intermediate to high signal on T1WI (often isointense to marrow fat), high signal on T2WI, usually high signal on T2WI with fat suppression (FS); Gd-contrast enhancement. Widening of diploë may be associated.	Benign skull lesions, occurring in adults over 30 years of age.
Inflammatory lesions		
Pyogenic osteomyelitis (Fig. 2B.33)	Abnormal low signal on T1WI and high signal on T2WI in marrow, Gd-contrast enhancement, focal sites of bone destruction. With or without associated complications including: subgaleal empyema, epidural empyema, subdural empyema, meningitis, cerebritis, intra-axial abscess, venous sinus thrombosis.	Osteomyelitis of the skull can result from surgery, trauma, hematogenous dissemination from another source of infection, or direct extension of infection from an adjacent site such as the paranasal sinuses.
Eosinophilic granuloma (Fig. 2B.34)	Single or mutiple circumscibed soft-tissue lesions in the marrow of the skull associated with focal bony destruction/erosion with extension extracranially, intracranially, or both. Lesions usually have low to intermediate signal on T1WI, mixed intermediate to slightly high signal on T2WI; with Gd-contrast enhancement. With or without enhancement of the adjacent dura.	*Single lesion:* Commonly seen in males more than females (below 20 years). Proliferation of histiocytes in medullary cavity with localized destruction of bone with extension in adjacent soft tissues. *Multiple lesions:* Associated with syndromes such as: Letterer-Siwe disease (lymphadenopathy hepatosplenomegaly), children below 2 years; Hand-Schüller-Christian disease (lymphadenopathy, exophthalmos, diabetes insipidus) children aged 5–10 years.

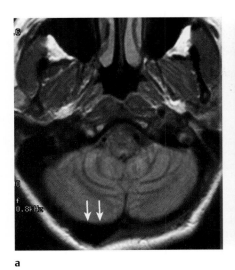

a

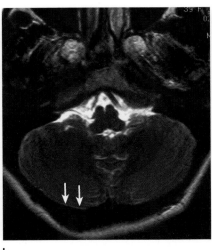

b

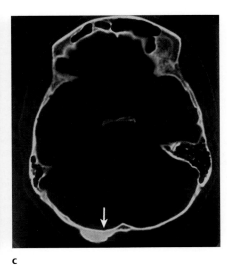

c

Fig. 2B.**32** **Osteoma.** Axial proton density weighted (long repetition-time [TR]/short echo-time [TE]) axial image (**a**) and axial

T2WI (**b**) show a well-circumscribed lesion involving the skull with low signal (arrows). **c** Axial CT image shows a well-circum-

scribed ossified structure at the posterior left skull (arrow).

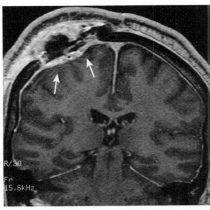

a

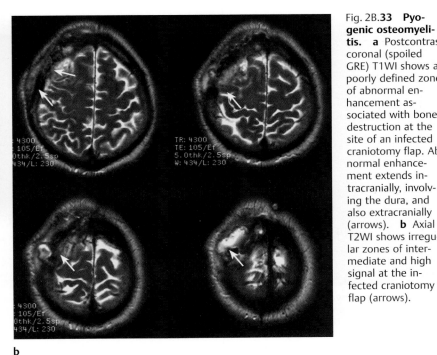

b

Fig. 2B.**33** **Pyogenic osteomyelitis.** **a** Postcontrast coronal (spoiled GRE) T1WI shows a poorly defined zone of abnormal enhancement associated with bone destruction at the site of an infected craniotomy flap. Abnormal enhancement extends intracranially, involving the dura, and also extracranially (arrows). **b** Axial T2WI shows irregular zones of intermediate and high signal at the infected craniotomy flap (arrows).

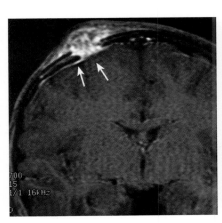

a

b

Fig. 2B.**34** **Eosinophilic granuloma.** **a** Postcontrast coronal FS T1WI shows an enhancing lesion associated with bone erosion with intracranial extension and mild dural enhancement. The lesion also extends into the subcutaneous soft tissues (arrows). **b** Coronal FS T2WI shows the lesion to have intermediate to slightly high signal (arrows).

Table 2B.2 (Cont.) Abnormalities involving the skull

Disease	MRI Findings	Comments
Bone infarcts	Focal ring-like lesion or poorly defined zone in marrow with low to intermediate signal on T1WI and intermediate to high signal on T2WI centrally. With or without Gd-contrast enhancement.	Bone infarcts can occur after radiation treatment, surgery, chemotherapy, or trauma.
Basilar invagination (Fig. 2B.35)	Position of the vertebral cervical spine is abnormally high (above 5 mm) in relation to the Chamberlain line (line extending from the hard palate dorsally to the opisthion, or posterior margin of the foramen magnum) secondary to a developmental anomaly.	Developmental anomalies associated with basilar invagination include basioccipital hypoplasia, atlanto-occipital assimilation, and occipital condyle hypoplasia.
Basilar impression– Secondary basilar invagination (Fig. 2B.36)	Position of the vertebral cervical spine is abnormally high (above 5 mm) in relation to the Chamberlain line (line extending from the hard palate dorsally to the opisthion, or posterior margin of the foramen magnum) secondary to acquired disorders.	Acquired conditions resulting in basilar impression (secondary basilar invagination) include Paget disease, hyperparathyroidism, rickets, osteomyelitis, osteogenesis imperfecta.

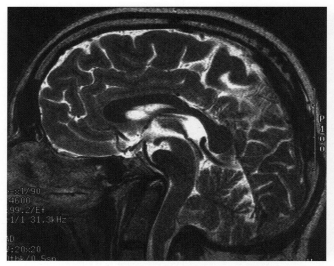

Fig. 2B.**35** **Basilar invagination from bassiocciput hypoplasia.** Sagittal T2WI shows prominent hypoplasia of the clivus and basilar invagination with the tip of the dens more than 2 cm above the Chamberlain line. Note deformity of the brainstem (pons) related to the anomaly.

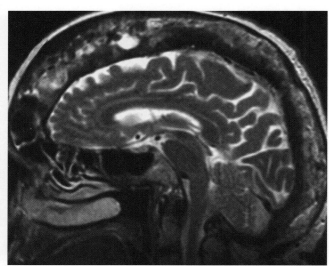

Fig. 2B.**36** **Basilar impression from Paget disease.** Sagittal T2WI shows Paget disease involving the skull associated with basilar impression with the tip of the dens more than 2 cm above the Chamberlain line. Note deformity of the brainstem (pons) related to the basilar impression.

Section II

Head and Neck

3   Skull Base and Temporal Bone

The skull base consists of five bones: the frontal, ethmoid, sphenoid, temporal, and occipital. An anterior, middle, and posterior cranial fossa can be differentiated. The anterior skull base is composed laterally and anteriorly by the paired frontal bones. They form the roof of both orbits and ethmoidal sinuses. The medial floor of the anterior fossa is formed by the ethmoid comprising the cribriform plate, through which the fibers of the olfactory nerve pass, and the crista galli, which serves as the anterior anchor for the falx cerebri. The foramen cecum, located at the anterior aspect of the crista galli, is occasionally the starting point of cephaloceles. The sphenoid, comprising the basisphenoid and the greater and lesser wings, forms the midsection of the skull base and the anterior wall of the middle cranial fossa, respectively. The basisphenoid, comprising the dorsum sella, posterior clinoids, sella turcica, tuberculum sella, and sphenoid sinus, is connected in the adult to the clivus by the fused spheno-occipital synchondrosis. Important sphenoid openings include the foramen ovale, foramen spinosum, foramen rotundum, optic canal, superior orbital fissure, precavernous carotid canal, and foramen lacerum. The temporal bone, consisting of petrous pyramid and mastoid process, forms most of the skull base between middle and posterior cranial fossae. The apex of the petrous pyramid joins the anterolateral margin of the clivus and the posteromedial margin of the greater wing of the sphenoid along the basisphenoid synchondrosis. Important temporal bone apertures include the jugular foramen, facial nerve canal, internal auditory canal, eustachian tube, and petrous carotid canal. The occipital bone, comprising the basiocciput (clivus and jugular tubercles), condylar (lateral) and squamous (posterior) portions, forms the floor of the posterior fossa. It contains the foramen magnum and posterior condylar and hypoglossal canals. Cranial nerve skull base apertures and skull base apertures and their contents are summarized in Tables 3.**1** and 3.**2**, respectively.

Lesions of the skull base can be divided into three categories: 1) intracranial lesions that involve the skull base from above; 2) lesions originating in the skull base, including fractures (intrinsic lesions); and 3) extracranial lesions involving the skull base from below. All these lesions are covered in other sections of this text: intracranial lesions are discussed in Section I (Brain), intrinsic bone lesions in Section IV (Musculoskeletal System), and extracranial lesions in Chapter 5 (Paranasal Sinuses and Nasal Cavity) and Chapter 6 (Upper Neck) of this section. All major lesions involving the skull base, with emphasis on intrinsic lesions, are summarized in Table 3.**3**.

The temporal bone consists of five bony parts: the squamous, mastoid, petrous, tympanic, and styloid portions. Since compact bone and air are signal void on MRI, the normal mastoid, external auditory canal, and middle ear cavity all appear as dark, structureless areas. In the petrous bone the internal auditory canal containing cerebrospinal fluid (CSF) and the membranous labyrinth containing endolymph and perilymph are well demonstrated on T2WI. The petrous apex is pneumatized in 30% of the population depicting a signal void or contains bone marrow or fat within its diploë emitting strong signals.

The *inner ear* contains the membranous labyrinth set within the bony labyrinth (otic capsule), which forms the cochlea, vestibule, semicircular canals, and vestibular and cochlear aqueducts. The *cochlea* has two and three-quarter turns encircling a central bony axis, the modiolus. The basal first turn opens posteriorly into the round window (fenestra cochleae). The *vestibule*, containing the utricle and saccule, is the central part of the labyrinth and is separated laterally from the middle ear by the oval window (fenestra vestibuli). The *semicircular canals* project off the superior, posterior, and lateral aspects of the vestibule. The superior semicircular canal forms the convexity of the arcuate eminence. The posterior semicircular canal points posteriorly along the line of the petrous ridge. The lateral (horizontal) semicircular canal juts into the epitympanum of the middle ear. The *cochlear aqueduct* contains the perilymphatic duct. It is about 8 mm long and extends from the basal turn of the cochlea to the lateral border of the jugular foramen paralleling the internal auditory canal. The *vestibular aqueduct* contains the endolymphatic duct and extends from the vestibule to the endolymphatic sac.

The *internal auditory canal* enters the petrous pyramid from the posteromedial surface. The porus acusticus internus is shaped much like the beveled tip of a needle, with the maximum diameter in the same axis as the petrous pyramid. Normally, the two internal auditory canals of the same patient are symmetric, but their shape varies considerably from one individual to the next. In 50% of cases the canals are cylindrical, in 25% they have an oval shape, and in the remaining 25% the canals taper either medially or laterally. The canal's vertical diameter varies from 2–12 mm (mean: 5 mm) and its length from 4–15 mm (mean: 8 mm). In 95% of normal individuals, the difference between the two internal auditory canals does not exceed 1 mm in diameter and 2 mm in length.

Thin gradient-echo (GRE) pulse sequences permit separate visualization of the facial nerve located anterosuperiorly in the internal auditory canal, the cochlear nerve located anteroinferiorly, the superior vestibular branch of the vestibulocochlear nerve located posterosuperiorly, and the inferior vestibular branch located posteroinferiorly.

The *facial nerve canal* originates at the porus acusticus internus and terminates in the foramen stylomastoideum. The following six segments of the facial nerve can be distinguished: 1) intracranial (from brainstem to porus acusticus internus); 2) internal auditory canal (in anterosuperior portion of canal); 4) labyrinthine (curling anteriorly over the top of the cochlea to the geniculate ganglion in the anterior genu); 4) tympanic (from anterior to posterior genu just underneath the lateral semicircular canal); 5) mastoid (from posterior genu to stylomastoid foramen); and 6) extracranial (between superficial and deep lobe of the parotid gland).

The *foramen jugulare* is situated below and slightly posterior to the internal auditory canal. It is bounded anterolaterally by the petrous bone and posteromedially by the occipital bone. The foramen is divided into the smaller pars nervosa anteromedially and the larger pars vascularis posterolaterally. The pars nervosa contains the glossopharyngeal nerve (cranial nerve IX), Jacobson's nerve (inferior tympanic branch of the cranial nerve IX), and inferior petrosal sinus (connecting the cavernous sinus with the internal jugular vein). The pars vascularis contains the vagus nerve (cranial nerve X), the spinal accessory nerve (cranial nerve IX), Arnold's nerve (auricular branch of cranial nerve X), the bulb of the internal jugular vein, and small meningeal arterial branches. On the endocranial site of the jugular foramen a dural septum separates the glossopharyngeal nerve from the vagus and accessory nerves. The bony carotid canal containing the vertical segment of the petrous internal carotid artery lies immediately anterior to the jugular foramen and is separated from the latter by the carotid spine. The genu of the petrous internal carotid artery that connects the vertical and horizontal segments is at the level of the hypotympanum.

Sixty percent of *congenital ear anomalies* occur in the external auditory canal, middle ear, or both. Inner ear anomalies account for 30% of congenital defects and, because of a different embryogenesis of the inner ear, are not associated with external and middle ear deformities. Combined anomalies involving all three compartments make up the remaining 10% and are associated with craniofacial dysplasias and trisomies 13, 18, and 21.

Congenital inner ear anomalies resulting in sensorineural deafness are caused by abnormal development of the membranous labyrinth. Thin GRE pulse sequences allow excellent visualization of the intralabyrinthine fluid spaces, thus enabling the diagnosis of membranous labyrinthine pathology even in the absence of bony labyrinth abnormalities.

Otosclerosis (otospongiosis) is a primary focal disease of the otic capsule usually presenting in young adults with gradually progressing hearing loss. The otoscopic examination is initially normal, but tinnitus may be present. The disease is commonly bilateral. Pathologically enchondral bone is replaced initially by foci of spongy bone that with time calcifies into dense ossific plaques. Computed tomography (CT) is the imaging modality of choice for diagnosis of the different stages of otosclerosis and the differentiation between fenestral (80–90%) and cochlear (retrofenestral) otosclerosis. In early (spongiotic) cochlear otosclerosis MRI may, however, reveal focal areas of punctate enhancement in the otic capsule after intravenous administration of Gd-DTPA.

A variety of dysplasias may involve the temporal bone and present with hearing loss. These conditions are diagnosed by their clinical presentation, plain film radiography, and CT. Otic capsule involvement by *osteogenesis imperfecta* cannot be differentiated with any imaging modality from (primary) otosclerosis. *Paget disease* may cause either demineralization or sclerosis of the otic capsule, but other parts of the temporal bone are similarly affected and depict bony expansion, a heterogeneous and increased signal intensity on T2WI, and usually marked contrast enhancement on MRI. Expansion and sclerosis of the temporal bone is also seen with *fibrous dysplasia*, but the signal intensity on MRI tends to be homogeneous and low on both T1WI and T2WI and the contrast enhancement is variable. Bilateral diffuse sclerosis of the temporal bone, presenting on MRI as signal void on all pulse sequences without appreciable contrast enhancement, is found with *osteopetrosis, progressive diaphyseal dysplasia (Camurati-Engelmann disease), generalized cortical hyperostosis (van Buchem disease)*, and *craniotubular dysplasias,* among others. In these conditions diffuse sclerosis of the skull base and various other parts of the skeleton are always associated.

The normal external auditory canal, middle ear, and mastoid appear on MRI as black structureless areas since they consist of compact bone and air that are devoid of signal. For this reason CT is recognized as the imaging modality of choice to evaluate those structures. However, in chronic otomastoiditis CT is frequently unable to differentiate between *inflammatory granulation tissue, acquired cholesteatoma*, and *cholesterol granuloma*, all of which may complicate chronic otomastoiditis and require a different treatment approach. On MRI, both inflammatory granulation tissue and cholesteatoma (either acquired or congenital) are hypointense on T1WI and hyperintense on T2WI. However, inflammatory granulation tissue depicts marked enhancement after intravenous Gd-DTPA, whereas cholesteatomas do not enhance. Cholesterol granulomas in the middle ear and mastoid can be differentiated from the other two conditions by their high signal intensity on T1WI due to their high content of both cholesterol and methemoglobin.

Interpretation of MRI of the temporal bone is greatly aided by clinical and otoscopic findings. *Pulsatile tinnitus* is caused by an aberrant internal carotid artery, dehiscent or high jugular bulb, arteriovenous malformation (AVM) in the temporal bone region, aneurysm in the temporal bone region, high-grade stenosis of the internal or external carotid artery, glomus tumor, hemangioma and meningioma in the temporal bone region. A *vascular mass behind the eardrum* (often referred to as "*vascular tympanic membrane*") is associated with an aberrant internal carotid artery, dehiscent jugular bulb, inflammatory granulation with hemorrhage, cholesterol granuloma, glomus tympanicum or jugulotympanicum tumors, hemangioma, and meningioma (angioblastic).

The differential diagnosis of petrous bone lesions are discussed in Table 3.**4** and vascular variants and lesions involving the jugular foramen in Table 3.**5**.

Table 3.1 Cranial nerve skull base apertures

Cranial nerve	Number	Skull base passage
Olfactory	I	Cribriform plate
Optic	II	Optic canal
Oculomotor	III	Superior orbital fissure
Trochlear	IV	Superior orbital fissure
Trigeminal	V	
Ophthalmic division	V_1	Superior orbital fissure
Maxillary division	V_2	Foramen rotundum
Mandibular division	V_3	Foramen ovale
Abducens	VI	Superior orbital fissure
Facial	VII	Stylomastoid foramen
Vestibulocochlear	VIII	Internal auditory canal
Cochlear		Modiolus
Vestibular		Superior and inferior vestibular apertures
Glossopharyngeal	IX	Jugular foramen
		Pars nervosa
Vagus	X	Jugular foramen
		Pars vascularis
Spinal accessory	XI	Jugular foramen
		Pars vascularis
Hypoglossal	XII	Hypoglossal canal

Table 3.2 Skull base apertures and their contents

Aperture	Location	Content
Cribriform plate	Medial floor of the anterior cranial fossa	Olfactory nerve (I) Ethmoid arteries
Optic canal	Lesser wing of sphenoid bone	Optic nerve (II) Ophthalmic artery
Superior orbital fissure	Between lesser and greater sphenoid wings	Cranial nerves III, IV, V_1, VI Superior ophthalmic vein
Foramen rotundum	Medial cranial fossa floor inferior to roof of pterygopalatine fossa	Maxillary division of V (V_2) Emissary veins Artery of foramen rotundum
Foramen ovale	Floor of middle cranial fossa lateral to sella	Mandibular division of V (V_3) Emissary veins from cavernous sinus to pterygoid plexus Accessory meningeal branch of maxillary artery
Foramen spinosum	Posterolateral to foramen ovale	Middle meningeal artery Recurrent (meningeal) branch, mandibular nerve
Foramen lacerum	Base of medial pterygoid plate at petrous apex	Meningeal branches of ascending pharyngeal artery
Pterygoid (vidian) canal	In sphenoid bone inferomedial to foramen rotundum	Vidian artery Vidian nerve
Carotid canal	Within petrous temporal bone	Internal carotid artery Sympathetic plexus

Jugular foramen	Posterolateral to carotid canal, between petrous temporal bone and the occipital bone	Pars nervosa
		    Inferior petrosal sinus
		    Glossopharyngeal nerve (IX)
		    Jacobson's nerve
		Pars vascularis
		    Internal jugular vein
		    Cranial nerves X, XI
		    Arnold's nerve
		    Small meningeal branches of ascending pharyngeal and occipital arteries

Stylomastoid foramen	Behind styloid process	Facial nerve (VII)
Hypoglossal canal	Base of occipital condyles	Hypoglossal nerve (XII)
Foramen magnum	Floor of posterior fossa	Medulla Spinal segment of cranial nerve XI Vertebral arteries and veins Anterior and posterior spinal arteries

Table 3.3 Skull base lesions

Disease	MRI Findings	Comments
Temporal bone lesions	See Table 3.4	
Cephalocele	Extracranial herniation of meninges (meningocele) or brain parenchyma and meninges (encephalocele) through a cranial defect. *Congenital cephaloceles* occur in 25 % in the anterior cranial fossa and in 75 % in the occipital bone. MRI determines the composition of the cephalocele, visualizes the route of herniation, and diagnoses frequently associated brain anomalies such as dysgenesis of the corpus callosum, intracranial lipomas, and dermoids.	Congenital cephaloceles involving the anterior cranial fossa may be visible (sincipital) or not visible (basal) from the outside. Sincipital encephaloceles (15 %) present as an external mass along the nose or orbital margin of the forehead and usually originate from a bony defect near the foramen cecum. Basal or nasopharyngeal cephaloceles (10 %) are divided into transethmoidal, sphenoethmoidal, transsphenoidal, and sphenomaxillary subtypes and are frequently clinically occult. Occipital cephaloceles consist of cervico-occipital, low occipital (involving the foramen magnum), and high occipital lesions (above the intact foramen magnum). *Acquired cephaloceles* occur secondary to surgery or trauma.
Skull base dysplasia (Figs. 3.1–3.3)	Fibrous dysplasia is the most common cause producing expansion of the skull base with variable but usually low to intermediate signal intensity on both T1WI and T2WI and variable contrast enhancement after intravenous Gd-DTPA administration. Involvement of facial bones is frequently associated.	Other skeletal dysplasias affecting the skull base include neurofibromatosis type 1, achondroplasia, osteogenesis imperfecta, and craniotubular dysplasia. Diffuse skull base involvement also occurs with mucopolysaccharidosis, histiocytosis X, Paget disease, and severe anemias.
Esthesioneuroblastoma (olfactory neuroblastoma) (Fig. 3.4)	Originates in the high nasal vault near the cribriform plate, which is usually destroyed, and frequently extends into the ethmoidal and sphenoidal sinuses, anterior cranial fossa, or orbits causing destruction of the intervening bony walls. The tumor is of low signal intensity on T1WI, mixed intermediate to high signal intensity on T2WI, and moderate contrast enhancement after intravenous Gd-DTPA administration.	Slow-growing malignant tumor occurring at any age but with predilection for the second and sixth decade of life. Clinically it may present with nasal obstruction, episodic epistaxis, hyposmia, headache, and/or visual disturbance.

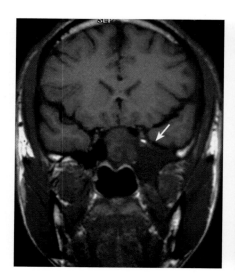

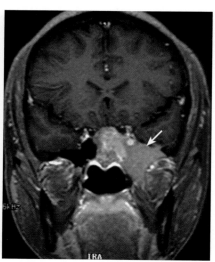

a   b

Fig. 3.**1** **Fibrous dysplasia. a** Homogeneous low-density lesion (arrow) is seen (T1WI, coronal). **b** After intravenous Gd-DTPA administration, marked contrast enhancement occurs (arrow) (T1WI, FS, +C, coronal).

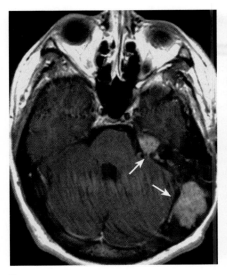

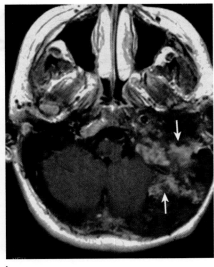

a   b

Fig. 3.**2** **Fibrous dysplasia.** Widening of the temporal and occipital bone bilaterally is present, but much more pronounced on the left side. After intravenous Gd-DTPA administration only two foci (arrows) enhance (T1WI, +C) (**a**), whereas an inhomogeneous patchy enhancement (arrows) of part of the bone involved with fibrous dysplasia is seen in (**b**) (T1WI, +C).

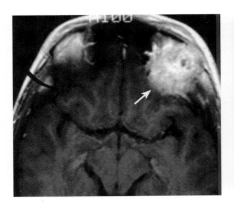

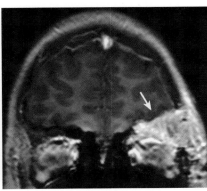

a   b

Fig. 3.**3** **Histiocytosis X (Langerhans cell histiocytosis).** After intravenous Gd-DTPA administration a marked, somewhat inhomogeneous contrast enhancement occurs in the lesion (arrow) involving the left orbital roof (T1WI, +C, axial [**a**] and coronal [**b**]).

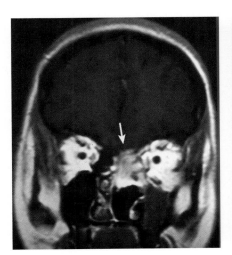

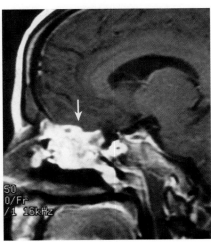

a   b

Fig. 3.**4** **Esthesioneuroblastoma.** After intravenous administration of Gd-DTPA, considerable enhancement of an inhomogeneous lesion (arrow) originating in the nasal vault is seen (T1WI, +C, coronal [**a**] and sagittal [**b**]).

Table 3.3 (Cont.) Skull base lesions

Disease	MRI Findings	Comments
Schwannoma and neurofibroma (Figs. 3.5, 3.6)	Fusiform mass with low signal intensity on T1WI, high signal intensity on T2WI, and considerable contrast enhancement causing smooth, scalloped enlargement of the affected passage in the skull base. Larger lesions depict internal heterogeneity on T2WI.	Any of the cranial nerves exiting the skull base may be involved with either tumor, but outside the temporal bone, including the jugular foramen. The trigeminal nerve is most frequently involved.
Meningioma (Fig. 3.7)	Dura-based, well-circumscribed mass displacing the brain, slightly hypointense to brain on T1WI and slightly hyperintense to brain on T2WI. When associated with calcifications and/or hyperostosis focal or diffuse signal loss may be found on all pulse sequences. Intense contrast enhancement is seen after intravenous Gd-DTPA administration.	Common sites in the skull base include sphenoid wing, cavernous sinus region, planum sphenoidale, and olfactory groove. Because of the relatively slow tumor growth, the symptoms are often minimal and may include headache, visual disturbance, anosmia, or other cranial nerve palsies.
Pituitary adenoma (Fig. 3.8)	Sellar or parasellar mass, isointense to the gray matter on T1WI and slightly hyperintense on T2WI. Larger lesions may undergo internal hemorrhage and cystic degeneration. Suprasellar extension, invasion of the cavernous sinus, bone erosion, and destruction of the sellar floor may be associated. Marked contrast enhancement is seen after intravenous Gd-DTPA administration.	Benign tumor arising from the anterior pituitary lobe/adenohypophysis. May present with a variety of endocrinopathies or visual disturbance. DD: simple pituitary cyst (*Rathke pouch cyst*).
Craniopharyngioma (Fig. 3.9)	Suprasellar lesion with frequent sellar involvement and, when large, erosion of the skull base. Heterogeneous lesion with cystic component that is hypointense or hyperintense on T1WI. Tumor is hyperintense on T2WI and moderate contrast enhancement is limited to the solid component.	Nodular or curvilinear tumor calcifications are radiographically evident in 75% of cases. Majority of cases are diagnosed in the first and second decade of life, but a second peak occurs in the fifth decade of life.

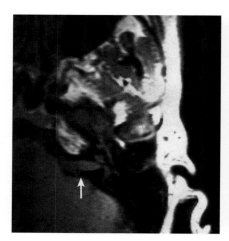

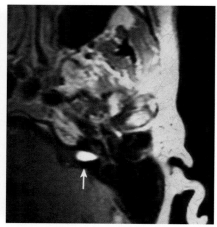

a

b

Fig. 3.5 **Acoustic neuroma (schwannoma).** A small lesion (arrow) is seen that demonstrates low signal intensity (T1WI) (**a**) and marked enhancement (T1WI, +C) after intravenous Gd-DTPA administration (**b**).

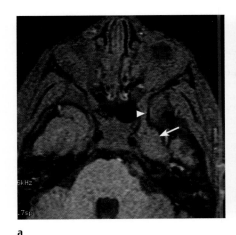

a

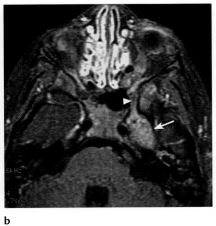

b

Fig. 3.**6** **Neurofibroma.** An ovoid lesion (arrow) is seen, originating from the trigeminal ganglion and extending along the maxillary nerve (arrowhead) through the foramen rotundum. The lesion is hypointense to the cerebellum (**a**) (GRE) and enhances in (**b**) (T1WI, FS, +C) after intravenous Gd-DTPA administration.

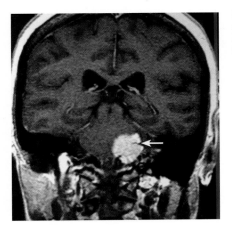

Fig. 3.**7** **Meningioma.** After intravenous Gd-DTPA administration an intensely enhanced lesion (arrow) is seen in the cerebellopontine angle (T1WI, +C).

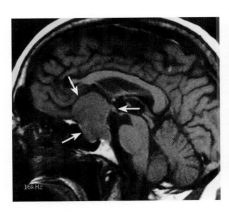

a

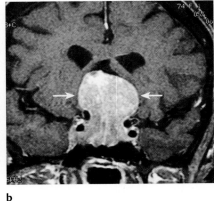

b

Fig. 3.**8** **Pituitary adenoma.** **a** A large sellar lesion (arrows) is seen with suprasellar extension and destruction of the sellar floor and adjacent clivus. The lesion appears isointense to the gray matter (T1WI, sagittal). **b** After intravenous Gd-DTPA administration marked uniform contrast enhancement in the lesion (arrows) occurs (T1WI, FS, +C, coronal).

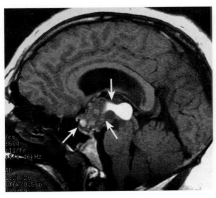

a

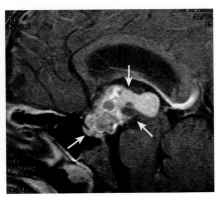

b

Fig. 3.**9** **Craniopharyngioma.** **a** A heterogeneous suprasellar lesion (arrows) with intrasellar extension is seen. The cystic components of the lesion appear hypointense or hyperintense with methemoglobin formation (T1WI, sagittal). **b** After intravenous Gd-DTPA administration enhancement of the noncystic components of the lesion (arrows) is seen (T1WI, FS, +C, sagittal).

Table 3.3 Skull base lesions

Disease	MRI Findings	Comments
Chordoma (Fig. 3.10)	Heterogeneous midline lesion arising near the spheno-occipital synchondrosis with variable signal intensity that tends to be low to intermediate on T1WI and high on T2WI. Areas of hemorrhage and calcifications are frequently present within the tumor and affect the signal intensity accordingly. Bone destruction, especially of the clivus and dorsum sellae, is present in 90% of cases. Contrast enhancement is considerable and inhomogeneous.	Spheno-occipital chordomas (20%) are the second most common tumor location (after sacrococcygeal chordomas) and occur most frequently in patients of 20–40 years of age, presenting frequently with orbitofrontal headache, visual disturbances, ptosis, and abducens palsy. *Chondroid chordomas* contain cartilaginous foci within the tumor matrix.
Chondrosarcoma (Fig.3.11)	Most common sites in the skull base are the petro-occipital synchondrosis and the sphenoethmoid junction. The expansile, destructive bone lesion with matrix calcifications tends to originate off midline and demonstrates a low to intermediate signal intensity on T1WI and a high signal intensity on T2WI. Contrast enhancement is considerable but usually inhomogeneous. The tumor may extend above and/or below the skull base.	Occurs most frequently in the fifth and sixth decade of life. *Osteosarcomas* (Fig. 3.12), Ewing sarcoma (Fig. 3.13), and *benign bone tumors* such as chondromas, giant cell tumors, osteoblastomas, and hemangiomas originate infrequently in the skull base.
Metastases and multiple myeloma (Fig. 3.14)	Focal, multifocal, or diffuse involvement of the skull base with or without extraosseous extension. Signal intensity is variable, but usually low on T1WI and high on T2WI. Osteoblastic lesions are hypointense on T2WI.	Metastases are the most common malignancy of the skull base resulting from local extension or hematogenous spread (e.g., carcinoma of lung, breast, and prostate). On MRI, multiple myeloma presents similarly to hematogenous metastases.

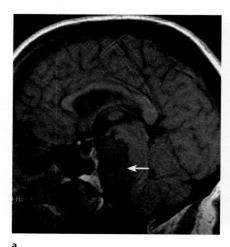
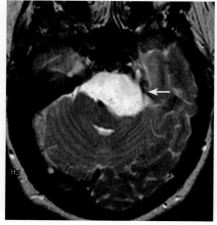
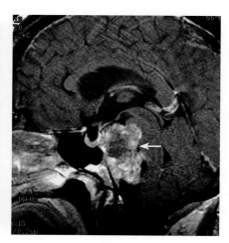

a   b   c

Fig. 3.10   Chordoma. A heterogeneous midline lesion (arrow) with partial destruction of the clivus is seen with (**a**) low signal intensity (T1WI, sagittal) and (**b**) high signal intensity (T2WI, axial). **c** After intravenous Gd-DTPA administration, inhomogeneous contrast enhancement occurs (T1WI, +C, sagittal).

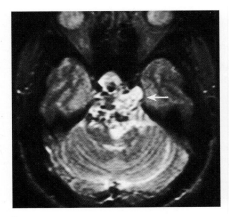

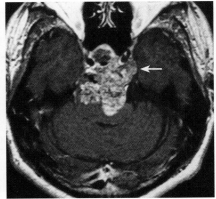

a

b

Fig. 3.**11** **Chondrosarcoma of the clivus.** **a** A heterogeneous lesion (arrow) with high signal intensity is seen (T2WI). **b** After intravenous Gd-DTPA considerable inhomogeneous contrast enhancement is seen in the lesion (arrow) reflecting the chondroid matrix calcification (T1WI, +C).

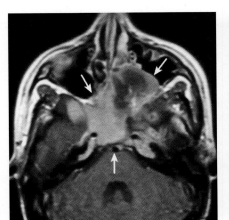

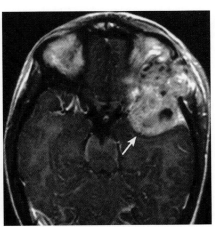

Fig. 3.**12** **Osteosarcoma.** After intravenous Gd-DTPA administration the extensive skull base lesion (arrows) demonstrates variable contrast enhancement ranging from moderate to intense (T1WI, +C).

Fig. 3.**13** **Ewing sarcoma.** A markedly enhancing, inhomogeneous lesion (arrow) is seen originating from the left orbital roof (T1WI, +C).

Fig. 3.**14** **Breast carcinoma metastases.** A heterogeneous mass (arrows) of intermediate signal intensity is seen involving C1, C2, and the right skull base around the foramen magnum (**a**: PDWI, axial. **b**: T1WI, sagittal).

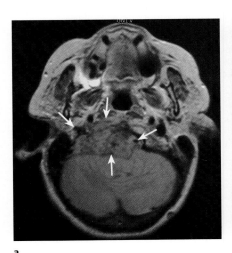

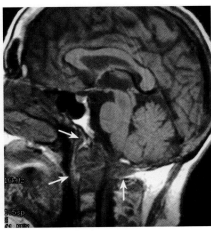

a

b

Table 3.3 (Cont.) Skull base lesions

Disease	MRI Findings	Comments
Lymphoma (Fig. 3.15)	Homogeneous, poorly defined mass with signal intensity similar to gray matter on both T1WI and T2WI and variable but uniform contrast enhancement ranging from poor to intense. Lack of frank bone destruction even with tumor present on both sides of the skull base is suggestive of lymphoma.	Occurs usually in patients with systemic non-Hodgkin lymphoma or AIDS patients.
Nasopharyngeal and sinonasal carcinoma (Fig. 3.16)	Heterogeneous, poorly defined mass with direct extension and destruction of the adjacent skull base. Normal apertures in the skull base may serve as a conduit for tumor spread, including perineural tumor extension. The lesions tend to be hypointense on T1WI and hyperintense on T2WI and depict considerable contrast enhancement after intravenous Gd-DTPA administration.	Squamous cell carcinoma of the nasopharynx is the most common carcinoma to involve the skull base. Approximately one-third of all sinonasal carcinomas arise in the vicinity of the skull base and have the potential for direct invasion and destruction of the skull base.
Rhabdomyosarcoma	Heterogeneous, poorly defined mass with low signal intensity on T1WI, high signal intensity on T2WI and variable contrast enhancement. Lesions originate most commonly in the nasopharynx and orbit, but also from the paranasal sinuses and middle ear. They frequently invade and destroy the adjacent skull base with subsequent intracranial tumor spread.	Most common sarcoma in the head and neck with the vast majority occurring in children, with a peak age between 2 and 5 years of age.
Juvenile nasopharyngeal angiofibroma (Fig. 3.17)	Invasive mass originating from the roof of the posterior nasal cavity or anterior nasopharynx with extension into the pterygopalatine fossa and from there into the orbit through the infraorbital fissure and subsequently through the superior orbital fissure into the cavernous sinus region. Direct intracranial extension from the sphenoid or ethmoidal sinuses is uncommon. The tumor depicts intermediate signal intensity on T1WI and relatively high signal intensity on T2WI interspersed with flow voids due to large tumor vessels. Intense contrast enhancement is seen after intravenous Gd-DTPA administration.	Benign, but locally aggressive, highly vascular tumor that can grow to an enormous size. It is exclusively found in adolescent and young males with a mean age of 15 years at the time of diagnosis. Patients present with nasal obstruction and severe recurrent epistaxis.
Mucocele	Well-defined, expansile cystic mass with low or high signal intensity on T1WI (depending on viscosity and protein content) and high signal intensity on T2WI. Mucoceles containing inspissated secretions may depict low signal intensity or even signal void on both T1WI and T2WI. After intravenous Gd-DTPA administration, rim enhancement is evident.	Mucoceles develop from obstruction of a sinus ostium or a compartment of a septated sinus. They arise usually as a complication of chronic sinus inflammation or occasionally secondary to trauma or tumor. They occur most frequently in the frontal sinus followed in order of decreasing frequency, by ethmoidal, maxillary, and sphenoid sinuses.
Osteomyelitis (Fig. 3.18)	Heterogeneous skull base infiltrate of variable signal intensity, typically low on T1WI and high on T2WI with inhomogeneous contrast enhancement. The signal intensity is decreased in the presence of sclerosis. Intracranial extension may lead to cavernous sinus thrombosis, meningitis, and cerebral abscess formation.	Usually secondary to a sinus or ear infection or in immunocompromised hosts (e.g., AIDS patients) or diabetics. Bacterial, tuberculous, and fungal infections occur.

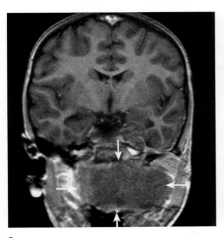
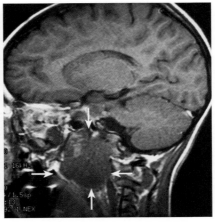

a   b

Fig. 3.**15** **Lymphoma.** A large mass (arrows) is seen originating from the nasopharynx and demonstrating only moderate contrast enhancement (**a**: T1WI, +C, coronal, and **b**: T1WI, +C, sagittal).

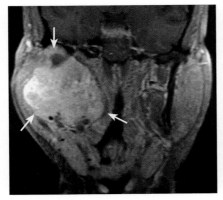
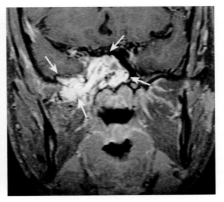

Fig. 3.**16** **Parotid carcinoma.** Direct extension of a large, inhomogeneously enhanced parotid mass (arrows) into the skull base is seen (T1WI, FS, +C).

Fig. 3.**17** **Juvenile nasopharyngeal angiofibroma.** An intensely enhanced, inhomogeneous mass (arrows) is seen extending into the middle cranial fossa (T1WI, FS, +C).

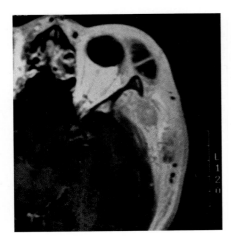

Fig. 3.**18** **Osteomyelitis secondary to chronic frontal sinusitis.** An inhomogeneous enhancing lesion is seen in the left frontal bone with extension into the anterior cranial fossa (T1WI, +C).

Table 3.4 Petrous bone lesions

Disease	MRI findings	Comments
Complete labyrinthine aplasia (Michel's deformity)	In place of normal inner ear structures, either a single small cystic cavity or several small cavities are seen in a hypoplastic petrous pyramid.	Rare congenital anomaly with total sensorineural hearing loss that is usually bilateral and occasionally associated with Klippel-Feil syndrome.
Mondini malformation	Instead of the normal $2^2/_3$ turns of the cochlea, only $1^1/_2$ turns are present, since the basal cochlear duct terminates in a common cavity, where the middle and apical ducts would otherwise be. Other associated findings frequently include dilatation and malformation of the saccule, utricle, and ampullar ends of the horizontal and superior semicircular ducts, and shortening and dilatation of both the perilymphatic and endolymphatic ducts within the cochlear and vestibular aqueducts, respectively.	Present with unilateral or bilateral, severe or complete hearing loss discovered in early childhood. With CT a usually hypoplastic cochlea with absent bony partition between its coils produces the "empty cochlea" appearance. The vestibule appears larger and more globular than normal. Mondini malformation is sometimes defined as any dysplasia of the inner ear.
Vestibular aqueduct anomaly	MRI visualizes the endolymphatic duct contained within the aqueduct and the endolymphatic sac lying on the posterior surface of the petrous bone. A normal endolymphatic duct measures between 0.5 and 1.5 mm at midpoint and is usually smaller than the diameter of the adjacent fluid-filled posterior semicircular duct.	Congenital anomalies range from total obliteration of the endolymphatic duct and sac, which may be unilateral or, more often, bilateral, and result in hearing loss. A narrowed endolymphatic may also be associated with Ménière-like disturbances and appears to be a predisposing factor for Ménière disease.
Obliterative labyrinthitis	Unilateral or bilateral obliteration of the lumen of one or more inner ear structures by fibrosis and eventual ossification.	May be congenital or acquired (infectious or posttraumatic). Infection may be tympanogenic, meningogenic, or hematogenic (e.g., mumps or measles).
Internal auditory canal stenosis or atresia	Absence of CSF between cerebellopontine angle and intralabyrinthine fluid is diagnostic for atresia; a decreased amount of CSF reduced to a thin layer indicates stenosis. Aplasia of the cochlear or vestibular nerve may be associated and can be accurately diagnosed.	Rarely the internal auditory canal is abnormally dilated and shortened bilaterally in cases of chronic hydrocephalus secondary to increased intracranial pressure.
Facial nerve agenesis	Partial or complete absence of the facial nerve is seen. Variations in the course of the facial nerve occur and the absence of the nerve from its normal location should not be mistaken for agenesis. May be an isolated finding, or, more frequently, is associated with atresia of the external auditory canal.	Facial nerve agenesis presents with total paralysis. Hypoplasia and/or stenosis of the facial nerve canal seen on CT may lead to intermittent episodes of facial paresis.
Arachnoid cyst	Well-defined, homogenous, cystic lesion, often with angular margins, in the cerebellopontine angle with signal intensity equal to cerebrospinal fluid (low on T1WI and high on T2WI). After intravenous Gd-DTPA administration no contrast enhancement is seen, including the margins of the cyst.	Congenital arachnoid cysts result from CSF accumulation in a split or duplication of the arachnoid membrane. Arachnoid cysts located in the cerebellopontine angle may produce smooth erosions on the adjacent bone. Hearing loss is usually not associated with this lesion.
Cholesterol granuloma (cholesterol cyst) (Fig. 3.19)	Most common primary petrous bone lesion, measuring 2–4 cm in diameter and depicting very high signal intensity on both T1WI and T2WI. Occasionally the lesion contains hemosiderin presenting as small nonhomogeneous foci of low signal intensity. A hypointense rim is sometimes seen representing a fibrous lining with or without hemosiderin deposition. After intravenous Gd-DTPA administration there is no contrast enhancement, except for a thin peripheral rim in some cases.	Acquired inflammatory lesion originating in the petrous apex or middle ear cavity consisting of cholesterol crystals and blood products, especially methemoglobin ("chocolate cyst"). Petrous apex cholesterol granulomas may be an incidental finding or, when larger, may present with a long history of hearing loss, tinnitus, and/or hemifacial spasm, and occasionally with deficits of cranial nerves V, VI, IX, X, XI, and XII. *Lipomas* (Fig. **3.19***) occur occasionally in these locations and may present in similar fashion.

Table 3.**4** (Cont.) Petrous bone lesions

Disease	MRI Findings	Comments
Epidermoid (congenital cholesteatoma) (Fig. 3.20)	Slightly inhomogeneous lesion, usually isointense or slightly hyperintense to CSF on T1WI and hyperintense on T2WI. After intravenous Gd-DTPA administration no contrast enhancement occurs generally, but rarely rim enhancement is seen. Lesions may originate in the temporal bone, frequently in the petrous apex, and the cerebellopontine angle. In the latter location the lesions have a variable configuration, since they conform to the shape of the space of origin and burrow into the brainstem or the crevices of the brain. Rarely epidermoids consisting predominantly of cholesterol may appear hyperintense on T1WI.	Epidermoids contain keratin debris shed from a lining of squamous epithelium and solid cholesterin. The proportions of these two components determines the signal intensity on MRI. Epidermoids of the petrous apex are slow-growing lesions eroding into the internal auditory canal, facial nerve canal, otic capsule, and eventually middle ear. Besides the petrous apex the lesion may also originate in the middle ear, mastoid, external auditory canal, and squamous portion of the temporal bone.

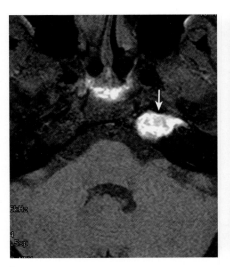

a

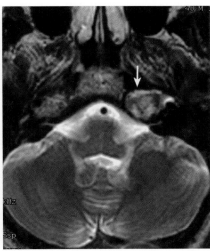

b

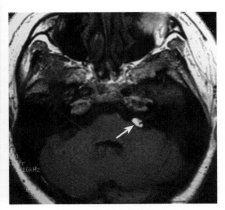

Fig. 3.**19** **Cholesterol granuloma.** An inhomogeneous lesion is seen in the petrous apex demonstrating (**a**) very high signal intensity (T1WI) and (**b**) intermediate signal intensity (T2WI).

Fig. 3.**19*** **Lipoma.** A small hyperintense focus (arrow) is seen in the right cerebellopontine angle (T1WI).

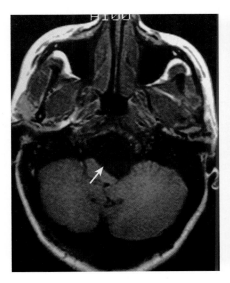

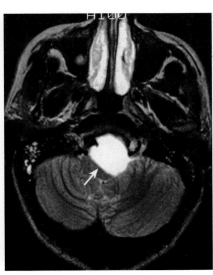

Fig. 3.**20** **Epidermoid (congenital cholesteatoma).** A cystic lesion (arrow) that appears to adapt its shape to the confinements of its place of origin resulting in a nonglobular configuration demonstrates (**a**) low signal intensity (T1WI) and (**b**) high signal intensity (T2WI).

Table 3.4 (Cont.) Petrous bone lesions

Disease	MRI Findings	Comments
Meningioma (Fig. 3.21)	Second most common cerebellopontine angle mass that tends to be more or less isointense to gray matter on both T1WI and T2WI. When densely fibrous or calcified it may be hypointense on T2WI. A dural tail of thickened meninges in continuity with the mass is seen in 60% of cases. The lesion typically has the shape of a mushroom cap, is eccentric to the porus acusticus internus, and does not extend into the internal auditory canal. After intravenous Gd-DTPA administration intense contrast enhancement is seen in 85% of cases.	Clinical presentation depends on location and size of lesion. May be found incidentally or is associated with deficiencies of cranial nerves VI, VII, and VIII. On CT a densely enhancing mass forming an obtuse angle with the adjacent temporal bone which may be hyperostotic is seen. Tumoral calcifications may be present.
Acoustic neuroma (schwannoma) (Fig. 3.22)	Most common mass in the internal auditory canal and cerebellopontine angle approximating the signal intensity of gray matter on T1WI and T2WI. Smaller tumors appear homogeneous before and after contrast enhancement. Larger lesions with tumor necrosis and/or hemorrhage may depict a heterogeneous signal intensity on precontrast images and are inhomogeneous after contrast enhancement. Small tumors (> 2 cm) assume the shape of the internal auditory canal and may remain intracanalicular. Larger tumors consist of an intracanalicular (internal auditory canal) and an extracanalicular (cerebellopontine angle) component which is centered over the porus acusticus producing an "ice cream in a cone" appearance. An arachnoid cyst is associated in 5% of cases.	Patients are usually between 40 and 70 years of age and present with sensorineural hearing loss, tinnitus, dizziness, gait disturbance, and headaches. When bilateral, the patient has neurofibromatosis type 2. On CT a homogeneous, uniformly enhancing mass in the internal auditory canal and cerebellopontine angle is seen forming an acute angle with the temporal bone. Erosions of the internal auditory canal are usually evident, but neither tumor calcifications nor hyperostosis of the adjacent bone occur.
Facial neuroma (schwannoma) (Fig. 3.23)	Signal intensity and enhancement characteristics identical to acoustic neuroma. Tumor may occur anywhere along the facial nerve course in the temporal bone, but the labyrinthine segment, including geniculate ganglion and the mastoid segment, are the most common locations. Involvement of multiple segments is not unusual. Tumors limited to the internal auditory canal are rare.	*Bell palsy* accounts for 80% of peripheral facial nerve paralysis. Diffuse intense enhancement of the facial nerve with or without discernable swelling is seen from the porus acusticus internus to the stylomastoid foramen. The enhancement is particularly visible in the labyrinthine segment that normally never enhances. Infectious processes presenting in a similar fashion include the *Ramsay-Hunt syndrome* caused by herpes zoster and *Lyme disease.* A nodular enhancement pattern of the facial nerve is neoplastic and includes *perineural metastases*.
Hemangioma	Poorly defined, heterogeneous mass of intermediate signal intensity on T1WI and high signal intensity on T2WI with intense, inhomogeneous enhancement after intravenous Gd-DTPA administration. Most common locations in the petrous bone are the geniculate fossa, from where they may extend along the facial nerve canal (especially the labyrinthine segment) and the internal auditory canal. At time of presentation the tumor frequently measures less than 1 cm in diameter.	Since nerve deficits are caused rather by invasion than compression, symptoms such as facial spasm and palsy or sensorineural hearing loss occur with small lesions which may escape detection. On CT a diffuse mottled demineralization of the petrous pyramid may be seen often producing a reticular or "honeycomb" appearance.
Chondrosarcoma	Well or poorly marginated mass with low to intermediate signal intensity on T1WI and high signal intensity on T2WI. Typically the tumor is homogeneous on T2WI. Contrast enhancement is marked but inhomogeneous. The tumor originates from the petrosphenoidal or petro-occipital fissure rather than the petrous apex itself.	Most common primary malignant neoplasm in the region of the petrous apex. On CT tumor calcifications and bone destruction are evident. Rare benign cartilaginous neoplasm such as *chondroma* and *chondroblastoma* cannot be differentiated from a low-grade chondrosarcoma.
Endolymphatic sac tumor	Heterogeneous mass originating from the posterior wall of the petrous pyramid in the expected location of the endolymphatic sac. Its signal intensity is mixed, but predominantly high on both T1WI and T2WI due to the presence of methemoglobin and proteinaceous cystic components. Marked inhomogeneous contrast enhancement is seen after intravenous Gd-DTPA administration.	Rare, locally invasive papillary cystadenomatous tumor causing sensorineural hearing loss and at times facial palsy. May be bilateral when associated with von Hippel-Lindau disease. On CT erosion of the adjacent temporal bone and intratumoral stippled or spiculated bony fragments may be seen.

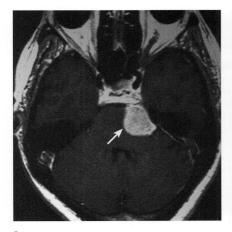

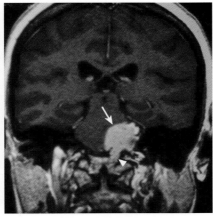

a

b

Fig. 3.**21** **Meningioma.** After intravenous Gd-DTPA administration an intensely enhanced lesion (arrow) shaped like a mushroom cap is seen in the cerebellopontine angle in (**a**) (T1WI, +C, axial) and with a dural tail (arrowhead) in (**b**) (T1WI, +C, coronal).

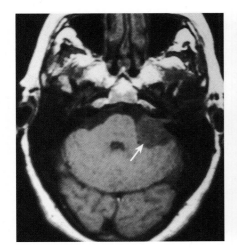

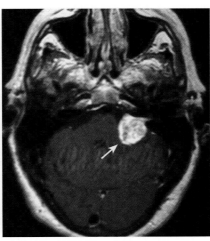

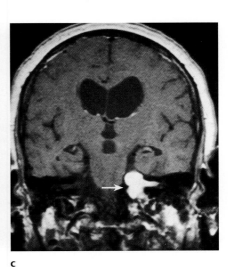

a

b

c

Fig. 3.**22** **Acoustic neuroma (schwannoma). a** Slightly heterogeneous lesion of intermediate signal intensity is seen in the cerebellopontine angle (T1WI). **b, c** After intravenous Gd-DTPA administration considerable enhancement occurs in the lesion with the appearance of an "ice cream in a cone" (axial and coronal T1WI, +C). A hydrocephalus is also evident in **c**.

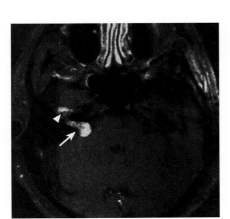

Fig. 3.**23** **Facial neuroma (schwannoma).** A considerably enhanced lesion (arrow) is seen in the temporal bone involving the labyrinthine segment and geniculate ganglion (arrowhead) after intravenous Gd-DTPA administration (T1WI, FS, +C).

Table 3.4 (Cont.) Petrous bone lesions

Disease	MRI Findings	Comments
Metastases, multiple myeloma, and lymphoma	Findings are nonspecific and depend on tumor size and histology. Small osteolytic lesions tend to be homogeneous, hypointense on T1WI, mildly hyperintense on T2WI, and tend to enhance only moderately and uniformly after intravenous Gd-DTPA administration.	Usually in patients with known primary tumor depicting similar signal characteristics and contrast enhancement pattern as metastatic deposits in temporal bone and elsewhere. When the cerebellopontine angle is also involved, bilateral involvement and other leptomeningeal or intra-axial deposits may be present.
Histiocytosis X (Langerhans cell histiocytosis [LCH])	Single or multiple, often bilateral foci of low signal intensity on T1WI and high and often inhomogeneous signal intensity on T2WI with moderate contrast enhancement. Temporal bone involvement is common, but usually not an isolated manifestation of the disease.	Occurs usually in children under 10 years of age presenting with unilateral and bilateral intractable otitis media with a chronically draining ear. Frequent unilateral or bilateral mastoid and inner ear invasion may simulate cholesteatomas both clinically and radiographically.
Petrous apicitis	Irregularly defined, somewhat inhomogeneous lesion in the petrous apex with low to intermediate signal intensity on T1WI and high signal intensity on T2WI. After intravenous administration of Gd-DTPA inhomogeneous enhancement of the lesion and surrounding inflamed structures including dura is seen. Petrous apicitis may be part of a more widespread skull base osteomyelitis.	Infection of a pneumatized petrous apex (30% of normal population). Usually a complication of otitis media and mastoiditis, or, less commonly, of sinonasal infection or *malignant external otitis* (pseudomonas infection in diabetics or immunocompromised patients originating at the bony-cartilagineous junction of the external auditory canal and spreading into the upper neck and skull base). *Gradenigo syndrome*: otomastoiditis, sixth nerve palsy, and pain in distribution of fifth nerve in conjunction with petrous apicitis.
Vascular lesions	Aneurysm of the intrapetrous horizontal carotid artery are very rare and present as well-defined ovoid expanding mass with signal void on spin echo sequences when not thrombosed. AVMs in the cerebellopontine angle present as multiple serpiginous flow voids and may be associated with hemorrhages of varying stages.	Other vascular abnormalities in the cerebellopontine angle include aneurysm of the anterior inferior cerebellar artery (very rare) and vertebrobasilar dolichoectasia (ectatic and tortuous basilar and/or vertebral arteries which may swing into the cerebellopontine angle causing significant displacement of the facial and/or vestibulocochlear nerves).

Table 3.5 Vascular variants and lesions involving the jugular foramen

Disease	MRI Findings	Comments
Aberrant internal carotid artery	The aberrant artery presents as a tubular structure that enters the middle ear cavity posterolateral to the cochlea, crosses the middle ear at the level of the cochlear promontory, and reenters the petrous internal carotid artery at its posterior horizontal margin. Nonenhancing spin-echo sequences do not visualize the anomaly. Contrast enhancement or flow-sensitive GRE techniques are required. On magnetic resonance angiography (MRA), lateral looping of the internal carotid artery in the middle ear is characteristic.	May be an incidental finding or present with tinnitus or conductive hearing loss. Otoscopically a retrotympanic pulsatile mass is seen. On CT a soft-tissue mass in the hypotympanon extending toward the oval window area, indenting the promontory or displacing the tympanic membrane laterally is diagnostic. Two rare carotid anomalies associated with dehiscence of the carotid plate have to be differentiated: a laterally displaced internal carotid artery herniating into the middle ear, and an aneurysm of the junction between its horizontal and vertical segments protruding into the middle ear.
High jugular bulb (jugular megabulb deformity)	The high-riding jugular bulb ascends above the level of the external auditory canal with preservation of the bony plate (not visualized by MRI) separating the bulb from the middle ear cavity.	Asymptomatic anatomic variation without clinical implications, unless inadvertently entered by surgeons. Size of jugular bulb is greatly variable, even from side to side in the same individual.
Dehiscent jugular bulb	Protrusion of the bulb into the middle ear through defect in bony plate separating the bulb from the posteroinferior middle ear. Visualization of the bulb requires flow-sensitive imaging techniques or contrast enhancement.	May be asymptomatic or present with pulsatile tinnitus or conductive hearing loss. Otoscopically a retrotympanic bluish mass is seen. Unequivocal demonstration of dehiscence requires CT.
Jugular diverticulum	Compared to a high jugular bulb this outpouching of the jugular bulb lies more medial and posterior in the petrous bone, does not invade the middle ear, but may erode into the internal auditory canal with encroachment of the acoustic nerve, or obliterate the endolymphatic duct.	May present with nonpulsatile tinnitus, sensorineural hearing loss, or symptoms mimicking Ménière disease. Otoscopic examination is negative.

Table 3.5 (Cont.) Vascular variants and lesions involving the jugular foramen

Disease	MRI Findings	Comments
Glomus tumor (paraganglioma) (Figs. 3.24, 3.25, 3.25*)	Poorly defined heterogeneous mass with low to intermediate signal intensity on T1WI (isointense to cerebellum) and relatively high signal intensity on T2WI (hyperintense to cerebellum). Characteristic are serpiginous flow voids due to tumor vessels and a "salt-and-pepper" pattern reflecting tumor hypervascularity. Intense contrast enhancement is seen after intravenous Gd-DTPA. At peak gadolinium concentration in the tumor a temporary decrease in signal intensity may be observed ("drop-out effect"). *Glomus jugulare tumors* originate from the jugular foramen; *Glomus jugulotympanicum tumors* extend into the middle ear cavity; *Glomus tympanicum tumors* arise in the middle ear cavity along the cochlear promontory; *Glomus vagale tumors* originate near the ganglion nodosum at the skull base close to the jugular foramen and tend to grow inferiorly along the carotid sheath.	Tumors arise from nonchromaffin paraganglion cells of neuroectodermal origin. They occur at any age, but have a predilection for middle-aged women. Multicentricity is present in 10% and malignant transformation with regional lymph node metastases in 4% of the cases. Glomus jugulare tumors present with deficiencies of cranial nerves IX, X, and XI. Glomus jugulotympanicum and glomus tympanicum tumors present with pulsatile tinnitus, conductive hearing loss, and vascular retrotympanic mass. Tumor response to radiation therapy is evident on MRI by reduction in size, decrease in T2WI signal intensity, decreased intratumoral flow voids, and decreased contrast enhancement.
Schwannoma (neuroma)	Well-defined, fusiform, homogeneous mass in the jugular foramen with signal intensity similar to the cerebellum (low to intermediate on T1WI and moderately high on T2WI). Uniform contrast enhancement occurs after intravenous Gd-DTPA administration. Extension of the tumor into the middle ear is rare. Larger schwannomas with extracranial components may appear heterogeneous or cystic.	Schwannomas of the jugular foramen originate from cranial nerves IX, X, or XI and present with corresponding neurologic deficits. CT may be useful to differentiate schwannomas presenting with symmetric expansion of the jugular foramen from a small glomus tumor presenting with an irregularly eroded or destroyed jugular foramen. *Hypoglossal schwannomas* depict the same signal characteristics and contrast enhancement pattern. They may be intracranial, extracranial, or both ("dumbbell-shaped"). *Neurofibromas* may present in similar fashion.

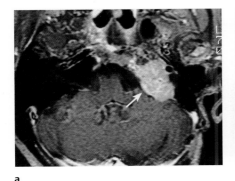
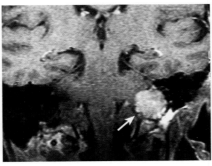
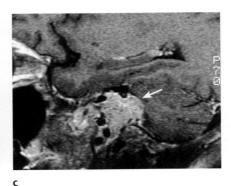

a   b   c

Fig. 3.**24** **Glomus jugulare tumor.** After intravenous administration of Gd-DTPA, a markedly enhancing, heterogeneous lesion (arrow) is seen in the jugular foramen with intracranial extension (axial, coronal, and sagittal T1WI, FS, +C).

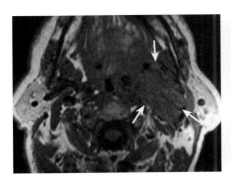
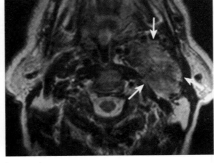
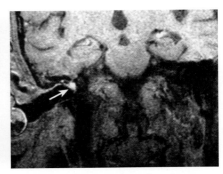

a   b

Fig. 3.**25** **Glomus vagale tumor.** A heterogeneous, poorly defined lesion (arrows) is seen demonstrating (**a**) low signal intensity (T1WI) and (**b**) intermediate signal intensity (T2WI).

Fig. 3.**25*** **Glomus tympanium tumor.** After intravenous Gd-DTPA administration, a small, markedly enhanced focus (arrow) is found in the petrous bone (T1WI, FS, +C).

Table 3.**5** (Cont.) Vascular variants and lesions involving the jugular foramen

Disease	MRI Findings	Comments
Meningioma	Relatively well-defined, intrinsic appearing mass in the jugular foramen that is slightly hypointense to the cerebellum on T1WI and hyperintense on T2WI. Associated intratumoral calcifications and hyperostosis of adjacent bone may decrease the signal intensity. Invasion into the middle ear and/or extension along the jugular vein are not unusual. Marked, uniform contrast enhancement after intravenous administration of Gd-DTPA is seen.	Occurs usually in patients between 35 and 70 years of age with predilection for women. Presents with lower cranial neuropathy. On plain radiography or CT tumor calcifications and hyperostosis of the adjacent bone may be evident.
Metastases (Fig. 3.26)	Destruction of the jugular foramen by usually poorly defined mass with variable signal intensity. Nasopharyngeal carcinomas and chondrosarcomas originating from the petro-occipital fissure tend to invade the medial aspect of the jugular foramen and appear hyperintense and heterogeneous on T2WI.	Hematogenous metastases, multiple myeloma, and lymphoma involving the jugular fossa, including the foramen, depict homogeneous signal intensity on MRI and usually only moderate contrast enhancement.

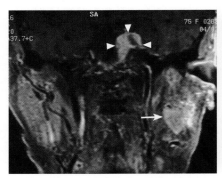 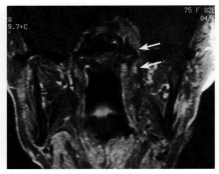

a   b

Fig. 3.**26 Intracranial perineural tumor extension from parotid carcinoma.**
a A poorly defined enhanced mass in the left parotid gland (arrow) and an intracranial metastasis (arrowheads) is seen (T1WI, FS, +C, coronal). **b** The perineural intracranial tumor spread occurred along the mandibular nerve (arrows) (T1WI, FS, +C, coronal).

4 Orbit and Eye

The contents of the orbit can be divided into four major anatomic compartments: 1) the globe, 2) the optic nerve and sheath, 3) the intraconal area, and 4) the extraconal area (Fig. 4.1).

The *optic nerve* is approximately 4.5 cm long and consists of the orbital, canalicular, and intracranial segments. The orbital segment follows a tortuous course from the optic canal to its insertion onto the back of the globe. It is a round collection of axons surrounded by the same meningeal sheaths as the brain itself.

The *orbital conus* is formed by the four rectus muscles and a fenestrated interconnecting fascia (Fig. 4.2). The *intraconal space* is filled with orbital fat and contains, in addition to the optic nerve sheath complex, the ophthalmic artery, superior ophthalmic vein, and cranial nerves I, III, IV, V$_1$, and VI. Embedded in fat in the *extraconal space* are the lacrimal gland and sac, as well as a portion of the superior ophthalmic vein.

The eye consists of three primary layers: 1) the *sclera* or outer layer, extending from the *cornea* to the optic nerve, where it becomes continuous with the dural sheath; 2) the *uvea* or middle layer consisting of the *iris*, *ciliary body*, and *choroid*; and 3) the *retina* or inner layer. The sclera is covered by *Tenon's capsule*, a fibroelastic membrane that envelops the eyeball from the optic nerve to the level of ciliary muscle. *Bruch's membrane* is a tough, acellular, bimalleolar structure situated between the retina and the choroid. The *choriocapillaris* is the capillary layer of the choroid lying immediately external to Bruch's membrane. The different layers of the wall of the globe normally cannot be differentiated by MRI. The *vitreous body chamber*, which occupies the space between the *lens* and the *retina*, represents about two-thirds of the volume of the eye, amounting to approximately 4 ml. Its water content (99%) is bound with a fibrillar collagen meshwork and hyaluronic acid. Any insult to the vitreous body may result in a fibroproliferation reaction, which subsequently can result in fractional retinal detachment.

On T1WI the eye is depicted as a more or less uniform low signal intensity with the exception of the lens capsule, which is moderately hyperintense. On T2WI the eye has an overall high signal intensity, except for the nucleus of the lens which appears hypointense. Thus any pathologic process within the globe appears hyperintense to the vitreous on T1WI and hypointense on T2WI. Intraocular lesions which do enhance are almost always best delineated after the intravenous administration of Gd-DTPA.

Detachment of various layers of the globe occurs in three potential spaces. The *posterior hyaloid (subhyaloid) space* lies between the posterior hyaloid membrane of the vitreous and the retina (*posterior hyaloid detachment*). The *subretinal space* is located between the two retinal layers, the inner sensory retina, and the outer retinal pigment epithelium (*retinal detachment*). The *suprachoroidal space* lies between choroid and sclera (*choroidal detachment*).

Differentiation between the various forms of detachment is not always possible with MRI. Both a rapidly changing appearance of the fluid accumulation with a change in body position and the formation of fluid-fluid levels are associated with posterior hyaloid or retinal detachment. Blood or fluid in the vitreous body chamber and suprachoroidal space shift only slowly. Consequently fluid-fluid levels are not found with either vitreous hemorrhage or choroidal detachment. When the detached coats of the globe are visualized, their appearance may suggest the diagnosis. In choroidal detachment the detached leaves of the choroid are separated posteriorly and assume a U-shape with the intervening posterior wall of the globe. In a more advanced stage, the detached leaves may become convex, producing the "kissing choroid" sign. The leaves of a detached retina converge toward the optic disk, producing a characteristic V-shaped configuration (Fig. 4.3).

A *posterior hyaloid detachment* commonly occurs in the elderly with liquefaction of the vitreous, but may also be present in children with persistent hyperplastic primary vitreous (PHPV). *Retinal detachment* may result from retraction associated with a fibroproliferative disease in the vitreous, from endophthalmitis, or from retinal vascular leakage and hemorrhage. *Choroidal detachment* frequently occurs after intraocular surgery, penetrating ocular trauma, and inflammatory choroidal disorders.

Leukokoria is an abnormal white, pinkish, or yellowish pupillary light reflex commonly associated with retinoblastoma and PHPV. Other causes of leukokoria in children include retinopathy of prematurity, congenital cataracts, coloboma, Coats disease, and toxocariasis.

Microphthalmia is a congenital underdevelopment or acquired diminution of the globe. Bilateral microphthalmia and cataracts are seen with congenital rubella, PHPV, retinopathy of prematurity, Norrie disease, and Warburg syndrome. Unilateral acquired microphthalmia, usually associated with dystrophic calcifications, is termed phthisis bulbi and found after trauma, infection, surgery, or radiation therapy. A small globe is also found in optic nerve atrophy.

Macrophthalmia (enlargement of the globe) is most commonly the result of juvenile glaucoma or myopia. Its most severe form, buphthalmos, is caused by juvenile-onset glaucoma. Macrophthalmia has to be differentiated from *exophthalmos* (*proptosis*) indicating the anterior protrusion of a normal-sized globe.

Intraocular calcifications are an important differential diagnostic criterion, but compared to plain film radiography and computed tomography (CT) are difficult to appreciate by MRI. Intraocular calcifications are associated with cataracts, drusen (usually bilateral, discrete round calcifications of the optic nerve disk), colobomas, phthysis bulbi, radiation therapy, chronic retinal detachment, retinopathy of prematurity, toxoplasmosis, and hypercalcemic states (corneal, conjunctival, or scleral calcifications). Tumor calcifications in the globe are characteristic of retinoblastomas and the rare astrocytic hamartoma (retinal astrocytoma) that is commonly associated with tuberous sclerosis or neurofibromatosis, and choroidal osteoma typically occurring in young women. Meningiomas of the nerve sheath infiltrating the posterior globe and vascular lesions associated with Sturge-Weber syndrome and von Hippel-Lindau disease may also produce intraglobal calcifications.

Extraglobal calcifications are most often of vascular origin (arteriosclerosis, phleboliths, hemangiomas, and arteriovenous malformations [AVMs]). Calcified hematomas, granulomas, and abscesses occur also. The most common calcified tumor is a meningioma of the optic nerve sheath. Other calcified tumors include optic glioma, neurofibroma, neuroblastoma, lacrimal gland neoplasm, and dermoid. Lesions from the orbital wall and retinoblastomas may occasionally also extend into the extraglobal space.

The differential diagnosis of ocular lesions is discussed in Table 4.1, optic nerve sheath lesions in Table 4.2, and extraocular (intraconal and extraconal) lesions in Table 4.3.

Table 4.1 Ocular lesions

Disease	MRI Findings	Comments
Microphthalmia (Fig. 4.4)	*Congenital*: small globe associated with small, poorly developed orbit. Usually bilateral and associated with cataracts. *Acquired*: shrunken, calcified globe (*phthisis bulbi*) in normal-sized orbit.	*Congenital*: coloboma, congenital rubella, persistent hyperplastic primary vitreous, retinopathy of prematurity (PHPV), Norrie disease, and Warburg syndrome. *Acquired*: optic nerve atrophy and sequelae of trauma, infection, surgery, and radiation therapy.
Macrophthalmia (Fig. 4.5)	Enlarged globe with thinned sclera. *Buphthalmos* is the most severe form. *Staphyloma* is a focal bulge of the globe involving either its posterior pole or the cornea (berry-like corneal protrusion). May be associated with a diffusely enlarged globe.	In axial myopia and juvenile glaucoma with or without Sturge-Weber syndrome. An intraocular tumor may rarely mimic macrophthalmia. Occasionally connective tissue disorders, such as Marfan syndrome, Ehlers-Danlos syndrome, and homocystinuria, are associated with macrophthalmia.
Exophthalmos (proptosis) (Fig. 4.6)	Anterior protrusion of a normal-sized globe. Secondary to a variety of orbital disorders which can usually be identified by MRI.	Associated with thyroid ophthalmopathy, fracture, histiocytosis X, fibrous dysplasia, neurofibromatosis, and orbital mass lesions including abscess, hematomas, pseudotumor, mucoceles, and benign or malignant neoplasms.
Coloboma	Posterior cystic, often funnel-shaped outpouching of the vitreous in the area of the optic disk is characteristic. A retroglobal (colobomatous) cyst and microphthalmia are typically associated. Occasionally retinal detachment or other congenital abnormalities are also evident.	Congenital (rarely acquired) defect in the globe, usually at the insertion of the optic nerve. Vision ranges from normal to complete blindness. Ophthalmoscopically an enlarged and excavated disk with central core of white gliotic tissue is diagnostic ("morning glory anomaly"). Calcification of the central core is occasionally evident radiographically.
Posterior hyaloid detachment	Fluid or blood accumulates in the retrohyaloid space between the posterior hyaloid membrane of the gel-like vitreous and the retina. Fluid or blood in the retrohyaloid space is usually mobile, tends to accumulate in the most dependent portion and may depict fluid-fluid levels or layering. The signal intensity varies depending on the presence and age of the blood.	Occurs usually in adults over 50 years of age, or in children with PHPV. In adults it is usually caused by liquefaction of the vitreous and is frequently associated with macular degeneration.
Retinal detachment (Fig. 4.7)	Accumulation of fluid or blood in the subretinal space, which is located between the two retinal layers, the inner sensory retina and the outer retinal pigment epithelium. Subretinal fluid or blood is mobile and tends to accumulate in the most dependent portions. Subretinal fluid usually appears homogeneous and slightly hyperintense to the vitreous on T1WI, whereas nonacute subretinal blood usually appears bright on T1WI and is often layered. The detached retina is only visualized when outlined by a significant contrast difference between the intensity of the subretinal fluid and vitreous cavity. Retinal detachment characteristically has a crescent-shaped or V-shaped appearance on axial images with the apex of the V (representing the leaves of the detached retina) at the optic disk and the extremities of the V near the ciliary body.	Retinal detachment resulting from a tear in the retina usually occurs in the adult and is referred to as rhegmatogenous retinal detachment. Nonrhegmatogenous retinal detachments are secondary to other ocular diseases, such as tumors of the retina or choroidea, retinopathy of prematurity, vitreoretinopathy of diabetes, toxocariasis, and Coats disease. Subretinal hemorrhage commonly occurs with trauma, senile macular degeneration, and PHPV.

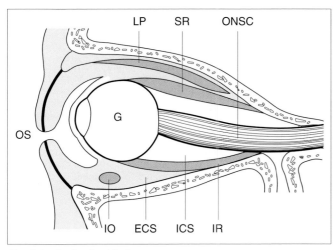

Fig. 4.**1**   **Sagittal orbital anatomy.**
ECS: extraconal space; G: globe; ICS: intraconal space; IO: inferior oblique muscle; IR: inferior rectus muscle; LP: levator palpebrae muscle; ONSC: optic nerve sheath complex; OS: orbital septum; SR: superior rectus muscle.

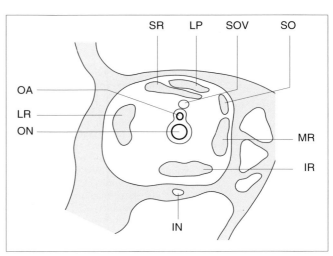

Fig. 4.**2**   **Coronal orbital anatomy.**
IN: infraorbital nerve; IR: inferior rectus muscle; LP: levator palpebrae muscle; LR: lateral rectus muscle; MR: medial rectus muscle; OA: ophthalmic artery; ON: optic nerve; SO: superior oblique muscle; SOV: superior ophthalmic vein; SR: superior rectus muscle.

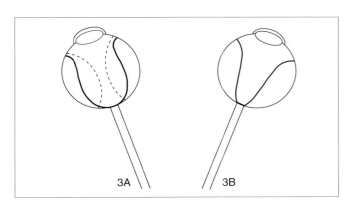

Fig. 4.**3**   **Choroidal versus retinal detachment.   a** Choroidal detachment. The detached leaves form a "U" (solid lines) or, in a more advanced stage, the "kissing choroid" sign (dashed lines).   **b** Retinal detachment. The leaves of the detached retina converge toward the optic disk, thereby producing a characteristic V-shaped configuration.

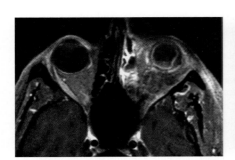

Fig. 4.**4**   **Microphthalmia.** A shrunken left globe with extensive bulbar and postbulbar traumatic changes is seen (T1WI, +C).

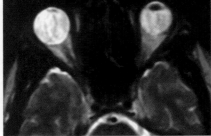

Fig. 4.**5**   **Macrophthalmia.** An enlarged right globe is seen (T2WI).

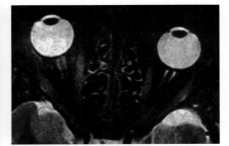

Fig. 4.**6**   **Exophthalmos (proptosis).** Anterior protrusion of the right globe is caused by thyroid ophthalmopathy (Graves disease of the orbit) (T2WI).

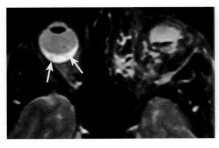

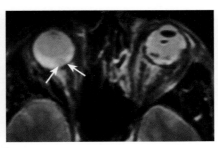

Fig. 4.**7**   **Retinal detachment (posttraumatic).   a** Retinal detachment with subretinal hemorrhage (arrows) is seen in the right globe. Sequelae from penetrating trauma are seen in the left globe (T2WI).   **b** At the level of the optic disk the leaves (arrows) of the detached retina remain attached (T2WI).

a

b

Table 4.1 (Cont.) Ocular lesions

Disease	MRI Findings	Comments
Choroidal detachment (Fig. 4.8)	Accumulation of blood or fluid in the supra-choroidal space confined by the choroid on the inside and sclera on the outside. A choroidal hematoma presents as a focal, well demarcated, lenticular mass in the wall of the eyeball. The signal intensity depends on its age. It is initially hypointense to the vitreous on T1WI and, especially T2WI, and markedly hyperintense to the vitreous on T1WI and variable on T2WI by 2 weeks. Fluid accumulation involving the entire circumference of the supra-choroidal space may have a semilunar or ring-shaped appearance or, if more extensive, bulges from the periphery towards the center of the globe so that the leaves of the detached choroid may produce the "kissing choroid" sign. Posteriorly the choroidal detachment is restricted by the anchoring effect of the short posterior ciliary arteries and nerves, thus preventing the convergence of the detached choroidal leaves to a single point (see Fig. 4.**3**). This finding and a fluid accumulation that only shifts slowly at best favor the diagnosis of choroidal rather than retinal detachment.	Hemorrhagic choroidal detachment often occurs after contusion, penetrating trauma, or as a complication of intraocular surgery. Serous or exudative choroidal detachment is associated with inflammatory choroidal disease or may be a sequela of noncomplicated eye surgery or glaucoma therapy. The detachment may be secondary to choroidal swelling and edema, often referred to as choroidal effusion. Choroidal edema and small amounts of fluid in the suprachoroidal space cannot be differentiated by MRI.
Coats disease	Normal-sized globe without calcification demonstrating usually complete retinal detachment with a subretinal exudate of relatively high signal intensity on both T1WI and T2WI. After intravenous Gd-DTPA administration, the detached leaves of the retina show enhancement due to the intraretinal telangiectasia.	Idiopathic retinal telangiectasia with secondary retinal detachment due to lipoproteinaceous and hemorrhagic exudation. In children (peak age: 6 to 8 years), mostly males, presenting usually with unilateral leukokoria and loss of central vision. May rarely occur also in adults.
Norrie disease (retinal dysplasia)	Bilateral microphthalmia with hyperintense (hemorrhagic) vitreous, partial, or complete retinal detachment with subretinal hemorrhage, optic nerve atrophy, small lens with retrolental bulge (pear-shaped), and shallow anterior chamber. PHPV may be associated.	Rare X-linked recessive syndrome in males presenting with retinal dysplasia, sensorineural deafness, and mental retardation. Ophthalmologically partial or complete retinal detachment, vitreoretinal hemorrhage, and glaucoma leading to bilateral blindness are seen.
Warburg syndrome	Bilateral microphthalmia with complete retinal detachment, subretinal, and vitreous hemorrhage, sometimes with layered blood levels. PHPV may be associated.	Rare congenital syndrome consists of hydrocephaly, agyria, and congenital retinal nonattachment with or without encephalocele. Death occurs usually in infancy.
Persistent hyperplastic primary vitreous (PHPV)	Unilateral or bilateral microphthalmia with increased signal intensity in the vitreous chamber on T1WI and hemorrhagic retinal or posterior hyaloid detachment. A tubular structure extending from the posterior surface of the lens through the vitreous canal to the posterior and inner surface of the globe is occasionally seen and thought to represent either embryonic tissue remnants along Cloquet's canal or the leaves of the retina that are congenitally unattached.	Rare condition with persistence and subsequent hyperplasia of the embryonic hyaloid vascular system of the primary vitreous (Cloquet's canal). Presents in infancy with leukokoria, microphthalmos, cataract, retinal detachment, and vitreous hemorrhage. May be associated with other ocular malformations (e.g., Norrie disease or Warburg syndrome).
Retinopathy of prematurity (retrolental fibroplasia)	Bilateral, but often asymmetric microphthalmia with increased signal intensity in the vitreous body on T1WI due to hemorrhage. Partial or complete retinal detachment is frequently associated. A persistent hyaloid vascular system may be present.	History of premature baby requiring long-term ventilator support with high concentration of oxygen is characteristic. Lenticular and/or choroidal calcifications are rare, but may occur in an advanced late stage.
Scleritis	Unilateral or bilateral edematous and swollen sclera with considerable contrast enhancement after intravenous Gd-DTPA administration.	Idiopathic or associated with connective tissue disease with female predilection. Posterior scleritis or Tenon's fasciitis produces semicircular distension of the Tenon's capsule and may mimic a uveal melanoma.
Endophthalmitis (infectious)	Unilateral, usually diffuse edematous swelling of the uvea and sclera that cannot be differentiated from early choroidal detachment. Localized mounding of the choroid is rare, unless there is a choroidal abscess.	Infections inside the eye are secondary to accidental or surgical perforation of the globe. *Infectious chorioretinitis* is caused by *cytomegalovirus (CMV)* (in AIDS and immunosuppression) or found in *congenital toxoplasmosis, syphilis, tuberculosis*, and *cryptococcosis*.

Table 4.1 (Cont.) Ocular lesions

Disease	MRI Findings	Comments
Toxocariasis (sclerosing endophthalmitis)	Unilateral or bilateral, single or multiple lesions caused by proteinaceous subretinal exudate secondary to the inflammatory response to larval infiltration with increased signal intensity (hyperintense to the vitreous) on T1WI and isointensity to the vitreous on T2WI. Lesions may be well or poorly defined and demonstrate contrast enhancement after intravenous Gd-DTPA administration.	Presents usually in young children with a history of playing in soil contaminated by the eggs of the nematode Toxocara canis. ELISA (immunoassay for Toxocara) is positive. Imaging findings of toxocariasis may mimic noncalcified retinoblastoma.
Retinoblastoma	Retinoblastomas have relatively short T1 and T2 relaxation times presenting slightly to moderately hyperintense to the normal vitreous on T1WI and moderately to markedly hypointense to the vitreous on T2WI. Tumor calcifications presenting as signal void are frequently not appreciated. Moderate to marked contrast enhancement is seen after intravenous Gd-DTPA administration. Retinal detachment is frequently associated and may occasionally be the only manifestation. Extraocular extension along the optic nerve to the orbital apex and intracranial space occurs in 25% of cases.	Round or lobulated, smoothly marginated mass with punctate, clumped, or complete calcifications seen on CT in over 90% of cases. Most common intraocular malignancy in childhood, bilateral in 30%. Presents in 90% under the age of 2 years with leukokoria, loss of vision, and pain. Radiation-induced sarcomas (especially osteosarcomas) subsequently develop in 20% of cases. *Trilateral retinoblastoma* refers to the association of bilateral retinoblastoma with a pinealoblastoma.
Uveal melanoma (Fig. 4.9)	Ill-defined thickening of the wall of the globe to a well-defined round or mushroom-shaped mass protruding into the vitreous. Lesions are homogeneous and depict moderately high signal intensity on T1WI (hyperintense to vitreous) and moderately low signal intensity on T2WI (hypointense to vitreous). Occasionally necrotic or hemorrhagic foci are present, causing tumor heterogeneity. Contrast enhancement is moderate. Exudative retinal detachment may be associated and depict moderate to high signal intensity in the most dependent location. Tumor invasion of sclera, optic disk, Tenon's capsule, and extraocular orbit may be seen.	Most common primary intraocular malignancy in adults (50–70 years of age) presenting with unilateral ocular complaint. The tumor arises from the choroid in 85%, the ciliary body in 9%, and the iris in 6%.
Ocular metastases	Often bilateral and usually multiple small areas of wall thickening with similar signal characteristic as uveal melanomas (hyperintense to the vitreous on T1WI and hypointense to the vitreous on T2WI). Widespread retinal detachment is frequently associated and may produce a mottled appearance of the metastases. Most common location is the posterior temporal portion of the uvea near the macula (an area of rich vascular supply). Contrast enhancement is variable, ranging from minimal to moderate.	A primary tumor is known in only about 50% of patients. Metastases originate most often from breast and lung carcinomas. In children ocular metastases occur with neuroblastoma, Ewing sarcoma, Wilms tumor, and leukemia. *Vitreous lymphoma* presents as an ill-defined mass that is hyperintense to the vitreous on T1WI and hypointense on T2WI.

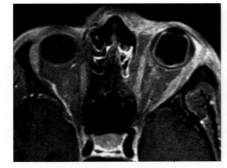

Fig. 4.**8** **Choroidal detachment (post-traumatic).** After intravenous Gd-DTPA administration the enhanced detached leaves are seen as thin lines paralleling the entire inner wall of the left globe with the exception of the lens (T1WI, +C).

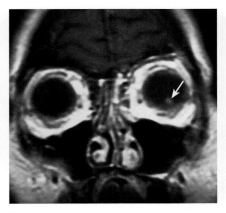

a

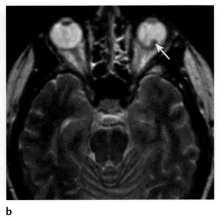

b

Fig. 4.**9** **Uveal melanoma.** A small nodule (arrow) is seen that is hyperintense to the vitreous in (**a**) (T1WI, coronal) and hypointense to the vitreous in (**b**) (T2WI, axial).

Table 4.1 (Cont.) Ocular lesions

Disease	MRI Findings	Comments
Choroidal hemangioma	Usually a flat mass of low signal intensity on T1WI and high signal intensity on T2WI in the wall of the globe that may be difficult to appreciate on pre-contrast images. After intravenous administration of Gd-DTPA, intense contrast enhancement is seen.	Isolated finding or in association with Sturge-Weber syndrome.
Retinal angioma	Similar to choroidal hemangiomas, but because of their small size (1–2 mm), they are frequently not identified.	Usually associated with von Hippel-Lindau disease (bilateral involvement).
Astrocytic hamartoma (retinal astrocytoma)	Single or multiple often calcified nodules, simulating retinoblastomas. Besides the retina, they may also originate from the optic nerve.	Usually associated with tuberous sclerosis or neurofibromatosis type 1, but they may occasionally precede their clinical manifestations. Sporadic in one-third of the cases.
Medulloepithelioma	Tumor originating from the ciliary body and spreading forward along the surface of the iris or backward along the surface of the retina. Signal characteristics and enhancement pattern similar to retinoblastoma.	Usually seen in young children, but occurs rarely also in adults. *Leiomyoma* is an extremely rare smooth muscle tumor of the ciliary body.
Choroidal osteoma	Flat intraocular lesion with curvilinear calcifications causing signal void on all pulse sequences.	Rare choroidal lesion consisting of mature bone, occurring in young women.
Choroidal cyst	Unilateral or, less commonly, bilateral lesion that may cause retinal detachment.	Very rare lesion which may be mistaken for a choroidal tumor.
Choroidal nevus	Small flat or minimally elevated lesion located most often in the posterior third of the choroid. Lesion cannot be differentiated from a small uveal melanoma, but is usually too little to be visualized.	Benign congenital lesion, usually diagnosed in the first decade of life. Most commonly misdiagnosed lesion to be enucleated under the presumption of malignant melanoma.
Macular degeneration	Localized wall thickening or small mass in the area of the macula of variable signal intensity, sometimes similar to a uveal melanoma. Compared with the latter the contrast enhancement is, however, much more pronounced. The disease is frequently complicated by hemorrhagic retinal detachment and eventually scar formation or liquefaction of the vitreous with posterior hyaloid detachment.	Leading cause of legal blindness in the elderly. The earliest changes in the macula include hyalinization and thickening of Bruch's membrane followed by ingrowth of choroidal neovascularization.
Ocular hemorrhage (Figs. 4.10, 4.11)	Vitreous hemorrhage presents as poorly defined lesion with variable signal intensity, depending on the age of the blood, and subsequently may induce a fibroproliferative reaction leading eventually to tractional retinal detachment or even phthisis bulbi.	Intraocular hemorrhage may be spontaneous, post-traumatic, or associated with bleeding disorders and a variety of ocular disorders.

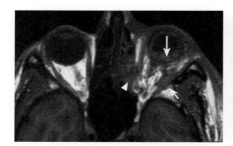

Fig. 4.10 Bulbar and retrobulbar hemorrhage. A poorly defined hemorrhage of intermediate signal intensity is seen in the posterior aspect of the vitreous (arrow) and the retrobulbar fat (small arrow) and left ethmoidal sinus (arrowhead) (T1WI).

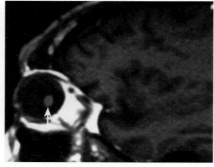

a

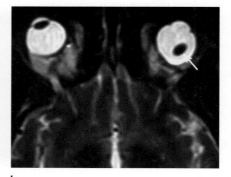

b

Fig. 4.11 Traumatic dislocation of the lens. The lens (arrow) is dislocated in the posterior vitreous without signal abnormalities in the latter (**a**: T1WI, sagittal; **b**: T2WI, axial).

Table 4.2 Optic nerve sheath lesions

Disease	MRI Findings	Comments
Increased intracranial pressure	Bilateral tortuous and thickened optic nerve sheath complex. The swollen subarachnoid space surrounding the normal optic nerve is best appreciated on T2WI.	Elevation of the intracranial cerebrospinal fluid (CSF) pressure transmitted to the perioptic subarachnoid space results in distension of the optic sheath.
Optic neuritis	Focal or diffuse thickening of the optic nerve is seen with increased signal intensity on T2WI. Plaques of multiple sclerosis may be best seen with fat-suppression techniques. After intravenous Gd-DTPA administration localized or diffuse enhancement occurs, best seen on fat-suppressed T1WI.	Sporadic or an early manifestation of multiple sclerosis (MS). Patients present with decreased visual acuity or visual field defects occurring over hours to days. Approximately half of the patients with idiopathic optic neuritis eventually develop MS.
Optic perineuritis (Fig. 4.12)	Ragged edematous enlargement of the optic nerve sheath complex with marked perineural enhancement after intravenous Gd-DTPA administration producing a "tram-track" sign.	Localized form of *orbital pseudotumor*. May simulate optic neuritis. In contrast to the latter, pain is exacerbated with retrodisplacement of the globe. Primary or secondary involvement of the optic nerve sheath complex is rarely also found with *viral*, *tuberculous*, and *syphilitic infections*, *radiation therapy*, and *sarcoidosis*.
Optic nerve glioma (Figs. 4.13, 4.14)	Marked, well-defined, fusiform enlargement of the typically kinked optic nerve that appears isointense to white matter on T1WI and hyperintense to both white matter and orbital fat on T2WI. Moderate to marked contrast enhancement occurs after intravenous Gd-DTPA administration. Tumor heterogeneity is occasionally caused by mucinous or cystic changes. Intracranial extension along the optic pathway through the eroded optic foramen is common. Bilateral involvement is characteristic of neurofibromatosis.	Presents with decreased vision and minimal axial proptosis. Seventy-five percent occur in children under 10 years of age. One-third of patients have neurofibromatosis type 1. Fifteen percent of patients with neurofibromatosis have optic nerve or optic chiasm glioma. Histologically, optic nerve gliomas in children are usually *pilocytic astrocytomas*, whereas in adults they are usually *glioblastomas* with much more aggressive behavior.

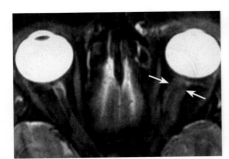

Fig. 4.**12**   **Optic perineuritis.** Ragged edematous enlargement of the optic nerve sheath complex (arrows) in the left orbit is seen (T2WI).

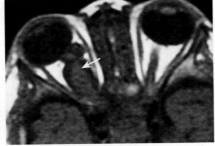

Fig. 4.**13**   **Optic glioma.** A well-defined fusiform enlargement of the right optic nerve (arrow) with low signal intensity is seen (T1WI).

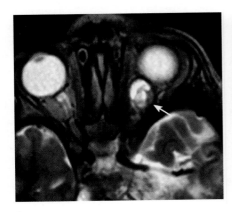

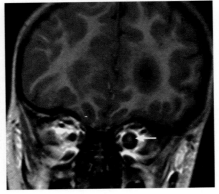

a

b

Fig. 4.**14**   **Optic glioma.** A heterogeneous focal enlargement of the left optic nerve (arrow) is seen (**a**: T2WI, axial; **b**: STIR, coronal).

Table 4.2 Optic nerve sheath lesions

Disease	MRI Findings	Comments
Optic nerve sheath meningioma (perioptic meningioma) (Fig. 4.15)	Tubular thickening of the optic nerve sheath complex, or, less commonly, eccentric localized mass that is hypointense to gray matter on T1WI and isointense to the periorbital fat on T2WI. Intense contrast enhancement occurs after intravenous Gd-DTPA administration best seen on fat suppressed T1WI. The enhanced perioptic meningioma may appear tram-track-like on axial and ring-like on coronal images. Contiguous intracranial extension may occur, but, when present, is limited to a short distance along the prechiasmatic optic nerve sheath.	On CT tumor calcifications and hyperostosis around the enlarged optic canal are characteristic. Occurs most often in middle-aged females and occasionally in children with neurofibromatosis type 2. Presents with progressive loss of vision over months.
Optic nerve sheath metastases	Local spread of retinoblastomas occurs in 25% of patients. Direct extension from uveal melanoma is less common. Lymphoma and leukemia may infiltrate the perioptic nerve sheath as part of systemic disease and present similarly to meningiomas in this location. Hematogenous metastases to the optic nerve sheath complex are rare.	*Hemangiomas* and *hemangiopericytomas* may rarely originate in the perioptic nerve sheath. The optic nerve has no Schwann cells. Therefore tumors deriving from these cells (schwannoma and neurofibroma) do not arise from the optic nerve, but may engulf it secondarily.

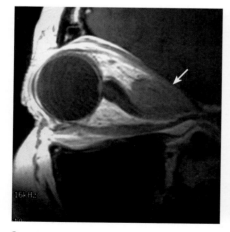

a

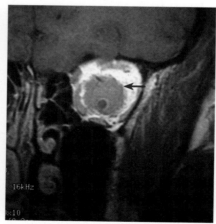

b

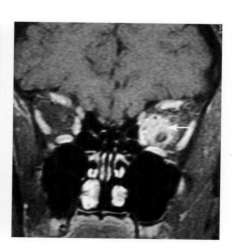

c

Fig. 4.15 **Optic nerve sheath meningioma.** An eccentric mass (arrow) is seen surrounding the hypointense optic nerve. The lesion is hypointense to the retrobulbar fat in (**a**) (sagittal T1WI) and in (**b**) (coronal T1WI), and after contrast enhancement hyperintense in (**c**) (T1WI, FS, +C).

Table 4.3 Extraocular (intraconal and extraconal) lesions

Disease	MRI Findings	Comments
Optic nerve sheath lesions	See Table 4.2	
Orbital pseudotumor (Fig. 4.16)	Unilateral inhomogeneous retrobulbar infiltrate or mass (tumefactive type, common) or involvement of one or more extraocular muscles including their tendinous insertions (myositic type, less common) with variable signal intensity, but more or less isointense to brain on both T1WI and T2WI. Absence of both bony erosion and distortion of orbital contents differentiates this lesion from true neoplasm. Marked contrast enhancement after intravenous Gd-DTPA administration is characteristic. Associated findings include infiltration of the retrobulbar fat (76%), proptosis (71%), extraocular muscle enlargement (57%), optic nerve sheath thickening (38%), thickening of the sclera near Tenon's capsule (33%), and enlargement of the lacrimal gland (5%).	Most common intraorbital mass lesion in adults caused by nongranulomatous inflammatory process. May be associated with Wegener granulomatosis, sarcoidosis, fibrosing mediastinitis, retroperitoneal fibrosis, sclerosing cholangitis, vasculitis, and lymphoma. Presents with unilateral painful ophthalmoplegia, proptosis, and chemosis. Rapid and lasting response to steroid therapy is characteristic. Pseudotumors are an acute or subacute inflammation involving the anterior orbit, the retrobulbar or apical orbit, the extraocular muscles, the lacrimal gland or diffusely the entire orbit. *Tolosa-Hunt syndrome* is considered to be a regional variant of the orbital pseudotumor involving the cavernous region with extension into the orbital apex.
Orbital cellulitis and abscess formation (Fig. 4.17)	Orbital involvement from sinusitis occurs in five stages: 1) inflammatory edema, 2) subperiosteal phlegmon and subsequent subperiosteal abscess formation, 3) orbital cellulitis, 4) orbital abscess formation, and 5) ophthalmic vein and cavernous sinus thrombosis. Edema and cellulitis present as a poorly defined infiltrate with low signal intensity on T1WI and high signal intensity on T2WI progressing from the preseptal space (anterior to the orbital septum) and/or the medial wall of the orbit to the periorbital and retroorbital fat. Abscesses present as space-occupying lesions with liquefied, necrotic centers and enhancing walls, sometimes containing gas evident as signal void. Ophthalmic vein thrombosis is evident as an engorged vein with abnormal (increased) signal intensity on spin-echo sequences.	Most often secondary to sinusitis, but may also develop from an infectious process of the skin or pharynx, or may be secondary to trauma, foreign body, or septicemia. Bacterial, viral, fungal, or parasitic organisms may be the causative agents. *Mycotic infections* in diabetic and immunocompromised hosts demonstrate a much more aggressive course with early bone destruction and invasion of arteries and veins (e.g., *mucormycosis* and *aspergillosis*). *Mucoceles* originating in the frontal or ethmoidal sinuses may erode through the adjacent orbital wall and present as a nonenhancing homogeneous mass of greatly variable signal intensity on both T1WI and T2WI, depending on the concentration and viscosity of its content.

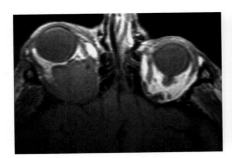
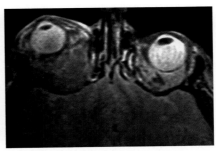

a **b**

Fig. 4.**16** **Orbital pseudotumor.** A retrobulbar lesion which is isointense to the brain in both (**a**) (PDWI) and (**b**) (T2WI) is evident on the right side. The lesion also causes a right exophthalmos.

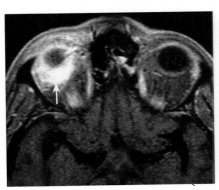
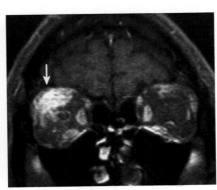

a **b**

Fig. 4.**17** **Orbital cellulitis.** After intravenous Gd-DTPA administration, marked enhancement of a poorly defined lesion (arrow) is seen (T1WI, FS, +C. Axial [**a**], coronal [**b**]).

Table 4.3 (Cont.) Extraocular (intraconal and extraconal) lesions

Disease	MRI Findings	Comments
Sarcoidosis	Unilateral or bilateral lacrimal gland or optic nerve sheath complex enlargement which may simulate a primary neoplasm of these structures.	Ocular manifestations include chorioretinitis, keratoconjunctivitis, and conjunctival inflammatory nodules.
Wegener granulomatosis	Diffuse retrobulbar infiltration similar to pseudotumor, but involvement is bilateral and bony destruction is common. Nasal and sinus manifestations are almost always also evident.	Orbital involvement is present in approximately 20% of patients. Ocular manifestations include scleritis, episcleritis, uveitis, and retinal vasculitis.
Lacrimal gland inflammation	Diffuse enlargement of the lacrimal gland with low signal intensity on T1WI, high signal intensity on T2WI, and marked contrast enhancement after intravenous Gd-DTPA administration. In the acute phase, scleritis and lateral rectus muscle myositis may be associated.	*Acute*: bacterial or viral dacryadenitis, usually unilateral. *Chronic*: Sjögren syndrome (lymphocytic infiltration of lacrimal and salivary glands). Secondary form is most commonly associated with rheumatoid arthritis, but also with other connective tissue diseases, lymphoma, AIDS, and graft-versus-host disease. *Mikulicz syndrome*: nonspecific enlargement of lacrimal and salivary glands that may be associated with sarcoidosis, lymphoma, and leukemia. *Pseudotumor* is a frequent inflammatory cause of unilateral lacrimal gland enlargement.
Thyroid ophthalmopathy (Graves disease or orbit) (Fig. 4.18)	Enlargement of the extraocular muscles with sparing of the tendinous attachments to the globe is characteristic. (DD: pseudotumor with tendon involvement). Disease may be limited to a single muscle belly (10%) or affect several muscles bilaterally (80%). The inferior rectus muscle is most frequently involved, followed by the medial and superior rectus, levator palpebrae, lateral rectus, and superior oblique muscles. On T2WI areas of high signal intensity may be present within the involved muscle. Proptosis and increase in retroglobular fat are common. Late findings include apical crowding causing dilatation of both ophthalmic veins and the perioptic subarachnoid space, stretching of the optic nerve with or without tenting of the posterior globe, engorgement of the lacrimal glands, uveal-scleral thickening, and eventually edema in the orbital fat.	Most common cause of unilateral or bilateral exophthalmos in adults. Usually in females (80%) with signs of hyperparathyroidism. However, 10% of patients have neither clinical nor laboratory evidence of hyperparathyroidism ("euthyroid ophthalmopathy"). *Acromegaly* may also be associated with extraocular muscle enlargement. *Myositis* and hematoma (spontaneous and posttraumatic) must be considered in the differential diagnosis of a single (rarely multiple) extraocular muscle enlargement.

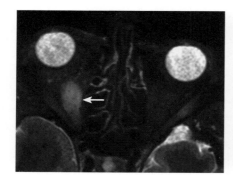

a

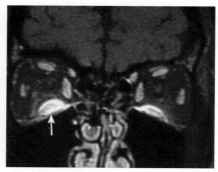

b

Fig. 4.18 **Thyroid ophthalmopathy (Graves disease of orbit).** Enlargement of the belly of the right inferior rectus muscle (arrow) with sparing of its tendinous attachment is seen causing proptosis of the right globe in (**a**) (T2WI, axial) and after contrast enhancement in (**b**) (T1WI, FS, +C, coronal).

Table 4.**3** (Cont.) Extraocular (intraconal and extraconal) lesions

Disease	MRI Findings	Comments
Cavernous hemangioma (Fig. 4.19)	Round to oval, usually intraconal mass that often spares the orbital apex. The lesion appears poorly marginated and uniformly hypointense on T1WI and well marginated, heterogeneous, and hyperintense on T2WI. Intense homogeneous or inhomogeneous (when partially thrombosed). Contrast enhancement occurs after intravenous Gd-DTPA administration. Intraorbital structures are displaced but not invaded by the lesion.	Most common orbital tumor occurring usually in adults aged 20–40 years, with female predilection. Presents as unilateral proptosis with diplopia and diminution of vision due to optic nerve compression. Radiographically small phleboliths are occasionally evident. The bony orbit may be expanded or remodeled but is never eroded by the lesion.
Capillary hemangioma	Poorly marginated heterogeneous lesion with low signal intensity on T1WI and high signal intensity on T2WI and marked contrast enhancement after intravenous Gd-DTPA administration. The lesion is most frequently located in the superomedial quadrant and may span intraconal and extraconal areas.	Presents usually in infants with proptosis and swelling of the eyelid and conjunctiva that increases with crying. The tumor frequently increases in the first 10 months of life and then begins to regress spontaneously.
Hemangio-endothelioma and hemangio-pericytoma	Signal characteristic and contrast enhancement pattern similar to capillary hemangioma. Lesion may invade adjacent tissue and erode underlying bone.	Benign or malignant vascular neoplasms occurring in adulthood.
Lymphangioma (Fig. 4.20)	Multilobulated, often infiltrative, heterogeneous lesion in extraconal or intraconal location with variable signal intensity ranging from low to high on T1WI and usually very high on T2WI. Contrast enhancement ranges from minimal to marked. Hemorrhage within the lesion is common and larger cystic areas with rim enhancement and occasionally fluid–fluid levels are sometimes seen (cystic lymphangioma).	Presents in infants and growing children with proptosis and periorbital swelling. Lesions on the lid, cheek, and oral mucosa may be associated. Gradual enlargement of the lesions occurs during the growing years and may lead to bony remodeling. Intratumoral hemorrhages may cause an abrupt increase in size. Spontaneous involution does not occur.

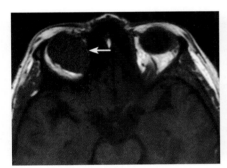

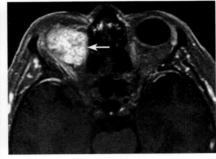

a   b

Fig. 4.**19** **Cavernous hemangioma.** **a** A uniformly hypointense lesion (arrow) is seen on the right side (T1WI). **b** After intravenous Gd-DTPA administration a marked inhomogeneous contrast enhancement occurs in the lesion (arrow) (T1WI, FS, +C).

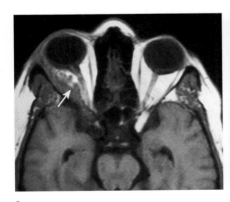

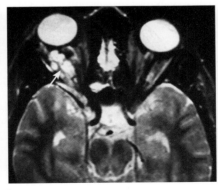

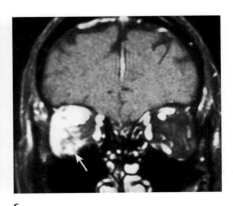

a   b   c

Fig. 4.**20** **Lymphangioma.** A heterogeneous lesion (arrow) is seen that is hypointense in (**a**) (T1WI) and hyperintense in (**b**) (T2WI). After intravenous Gd-DTPA administration marked contrast enhancement is seen in the lesion sparing only its cystic components (**c**: coronal T1WI, FS, +C).

Table 4.3 (Cont.) Extraocular (intraconal and extraconal) lesions

Disease	MRI Findings	Comments
Dermoid	Well-defined, cystic lesion with thick capsule containing fatty material located either superolaterally (60%) or superomedially (25%) between the globe and orbital periosteum. The lesion depicts high signal intensity on both T1WI and T2WI and does not enhance after intravenous Gd-DTPA administration. May contain calcifications (teeth) which may be evident as signal void. Expansion or pressure erosions of the bony orbit may be associated.	Most common benign orbital tumor in childhood. *Epidermoids* are less common and can be differentiated from dermoids by their low signal intensity on T1WI and the absence of calcifications. *Teratomas* are evident at birth as grossly visible cystic orbital masses.
Lacrimal gland tumor (Fig. 4.21)	Round or oblong, often bulky extraconal mass in the superolateral aspect of the orbit with low signal intensity on T1WI, high signal intensity on T2WI and moderate to marked enhancement after intravenous Gd-DTPA administration. Erosion or destruction of the contiguous bone may be associated. Tumors have a tendency for posterior extension. Benign and malignant tumors cannot be reliably differentiated, though the latter may display a serrated margin indicative of infiltration.	Epithelial tumors of the lacrimal gland consist equally of benign mixed pleomorphic adenomas and a variety of carcinomas of which the adenocystic is the most common. Malignant degeneration of pleomorphic adenomas occurs in a significant number of untreated or recurrent tumors. Radiographically calcifications are more frequently observed in malignant lacrimal gland tumors.
Schwannoma (neuroma) and neurofibroma	Sharply marginated, oval or fusiform, usually intraconal lesions with low to intermediate signal intensity on T1WI, moderately high signal intensity on T2WI and uniform contrast enhancement after intravenous administration of Gd-DTPA. The optic nerve is usually displaced or may be engulfed by the tumor.	Benign slow-growing nerve sheath tumors originating from the Schwann cells and accounting for 5% of all orbital tumors. They arise from cranial nerves other than the optic nerve, since the latter has no Schwann cells.
Meningioma	May involve the extraconal space from above or from either side. Relative to orbital fat they are hypointense on T1WI and isointense on T2WI. Intense and uniform contrast enhancement is typical. Calcifications within the tumor may be visualized as foci of signal void.	On CT sclerotic or lytic involvement of the adjacent orbital bone is invariably evident. Sphenoid wing meningioma is the most common meningioma in the extraconal space. Intraconal perioptic meningiomas are much more common (see Table 4.2).
Rhabdomyosarcoma (Fig. 4.22)	Large intraconal and/or extraconal mass with low signal intensity on T1WI and high signal intensity on T2WI extending commonly into the eyelid, adjacent sinus, and intracranial cavity. Bone destruction is frequently associated. Moderate to marked contrast enhancement occurs after intravenous Gd-DTPA administration.	Most common primary malignant orbital tumor in childhood presenting with rapidly developing unilateral proptosis arising from undifferentiated mesenchyma of orbital soft tissue or extraocular muscles. *Osteosarcomas* and *malignant fibrous histiocytomas* may be seen following radiation to the orbit for retinoblastoma.
Lymphoma (Fig. 4.23)	Well-defined extraconal mass, most common about the lacrimal gland, or diffuse infiltration of the intraconal space, or, occasionally more circumscribed involvement of the optic nerve sheath complex. Lymphomas typically have a uniform signal intensity that is low or intermediate on T1WI and intermediate to high (often isointense to fat) on T2WI. Contrast enhancement is only mild to moderate. Involvement may be unilateral or bilateral. Generally, lymphoma manifestations mold themselves to pre-existing structures without significant displacement and bony erosions, thus frequently mimicking orbital pseudotumors.	Usually non-Hodgkin lymphoma. Present frequently without evidence of systemic disease. Clinically painless swelling of the eyelids may be the first symptom. Exophthalmos and limitation of extraocular muscle movement occur later in the course. Seventy-five percent of patients either have or will eventually develop systemic lymphoma. *Leukemic infiltrates* of the orbits may present in a similar fashion on MRI. In acute myelogenous leukemia the infiltrate may form a mass lesion referred to as *chloroma*.
Metastases (Fig. 4.24)	Direct extension from malignant tumors originating in the globe, the adjacent paranasal sinuses, nose, bony orbit, and cranium is readily visualized and, depending on both origin and nature of the lesion, may have distinct features.	Hematogenous metastases to the extraocular portions of the orbit are much less common than intraocular metastases and account for only approximately 12% of all orbital metastases.

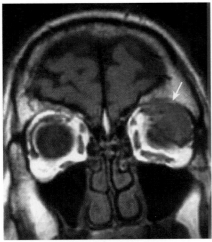

Fig. 4.**21** **Lacrimal gland carcinoma.** A poorly defined lesion (arrow) is seen originating in the superolateral aspect of the left orbit with low signal intensity (T1WI), coronal).

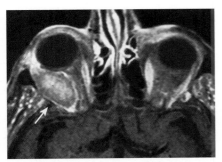

Fig. 4.**22** **Rhabdomyosarcoma.** After intravenous Gd-DTPA administration, inhomogeneous enhancement of a large intraconal and extraconal lesion (arrow) with destruction of the lateral orbital wall is seen on the right side (T1WI, FS, +C).

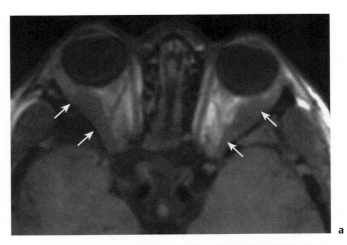

a

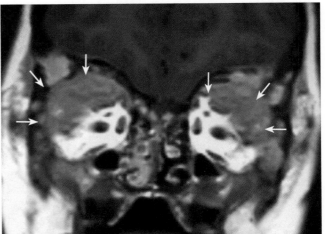

b

Fig. 4.**23** **Leukemic orbital infiltrates.** Bilateral symmetric infiltrates (arrows) of intermediate signal intensity are seen predominantly involving the superolateral aspects of both orbits (T1WI, axial [**a**], coronal [**b**]).

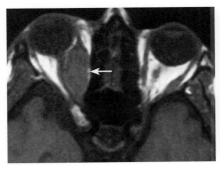

a

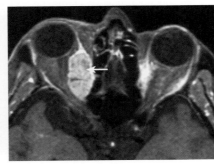

b

Fig. 4.**24** **Melanoma metastasis.** **a** An oblong lesion (arrow) of intermediate signal intensity is seen in the medial extraconal space (T1WI). **b** After intravenous Gd-DTPA administration the lesion (arrow) enhances considerably (T1WI, FS, +C).

Table 4.3 (Cont.) Extraocular (intraconal and extraconal) lesions

Disease	MRI Findings	Comments
Orbital varix	Well-defined round, tubular, or lobulated, intraconal structure with variable signal intensity. Flow void will be seen on SE sequences with rapid flow. With slow or turbulent flow increased signal intensity is evident on all pulse sequences. Homogeneous intense contrast enhancement is seen in noncomplicated varix after intravenous Gd-DTPA administration. Varix enlarges with Valsalva maneuver. Both thrombosis and spontaneous hemorrhage are frequent complications. The signal intensity of clots and hemorrhages varies with the age of these complications.	Congenital or acquired massive dilation of the superior and/or inferior orbital vein. Phleboliths may be seen with plain radiography or CT. *Congenital varices* are caused by a weakness in the venous wall or a venous malformation. *Acquired varices* are caused by an intraorbital or intracranial AVM.
Carotid-cavernous fistula **(Fig. 4.25)**	Dilatation of the cavernous sinus, superior ophthalmic vein, facial vein, and jugular vein with flow void is seen. Edematous enlargement of the extraocular muscles with increased signal intensity on T2WI may be associated. Phase contrast magnetic resonance angiography with directional emphasis demonstrates the reversal of flow in the enlarged superior ophthalmic vein. Associated findings may include partial venous thrombosis in the lumen of the superior ophthalmic vein or cavernous sinus.	Spontaneous or posttraumatic communication between the cavernous carotid artery and the cavernous sinus causes chemosis, suffusion of the globe and orbit, pulsating exophthalmos, and a bruit on auscultation. Restricted ocular movement and loss of vision due to increased intraocular pressure occur in a more advanced stage. Radiographically sellar erosion and enlargement of the superior orbital fissure may occasionally be seen.

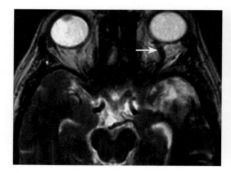
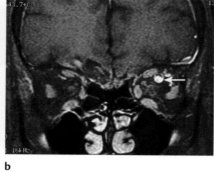
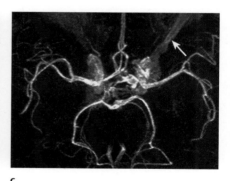

a   b   c

Fig. 4.**25** **Carotid-cavernous fistula.** An enlarged left superior orbital vein (arrow) is seen as flow void in (**a**) (T2WI, axial), contrast enhanced in (**b**) (T1WI, FS, +C, coronal), and on MRA in (**c**).

Table 4.**3** (Cont.) Extraocular (intraconal and extraconal) lesions

Disease	MRI Findings	Comments
Superior ophthalmic vein thrombosis	Enlarged superior ophthalmic vein without flow void and without contrast enhancement when completely thrombosed. Central clots present with absent central flow void and rim enhancement after intravenous Gd-DTPA administration. Ipsilateral cavernous sinus is usually enlarged.	Presents with ophthalmoplegia. May be associated with cavernous sinus thrombosis that is frequently a late complication of advanced paranasal sinus infection.
Subperiosteal hematoma (Fig. 4.26)	Sharply defined, mound-like extraconal lesion with its broad base abutting the bony orbit, displacing the peripheral fat toward the center of the orbit. Subacute hematomas containing methemoglobin appear hyperintense on both T1WI and T2WI and do not enhance after intravenous Gd-DTPA administration. An incompletely resorbed hematoma may eventually progress to a *hematic cyst*.	Present as painful unilateral proptosis, often after a recent history of trauma. Spontaneous hematomas occur in patients with bleeding diathesis. Almost exclusively found in children and young adults, presumably because the orbital periost is not firmly adherent to the bone.

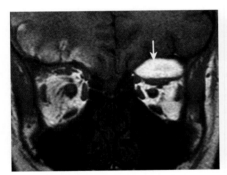

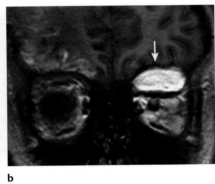

a   b

Fig. 4.**26** **Subperiosteal orbital hematoma.** A sharply defined, extraconal lesion (arrow) is seen in the roof of the left orbit displacing its content inferiorly. Because of methemoglobin formation the hematoma is hyperintense in both (**a**) (T1WI, coronal) and (**b**) (STIR, coronal). Increased signal intensity in the inferiorly displaced orbital content is caused by subacute hemorrhage.

5 Paranasal Sinuses and Nasal Cavity

The paranasal sinuses are present at birth and continue to grow until they attain their full size in the late teens. The sinuses vary considerably in size from hypoplastic and even absent to very large. They tend to be symmetric in an individual, but occasionally considerable size differences occur.

Hypoplastic or absent paranasal sinuses may be a congenital anomaly or associated with fibrous dysplasia, Paget disease, thalassemia, cretinism, Down syndrome, Kartagener (immotile cilia) syndrome, and a variety of dysplasias. A pneumocele is an expansion of a sinus into the orbit.

Computed tomography (CT) remains the imaging modality of choice for the evaluation of bone pathology including fractures, bone dysplasias, osteomyelitis, and primary bone neoplasms. Although CT is more specific in the diagnosis of bone infections and tumors, MRI is more sensitive in displaying their soft-tissue extent. MRI is superior to CT in differentiating inflammatory conditions from neoplastic processes. Most tumors of the sinonasal cavities are not as hyperintense as the retained secretions with surrounding inflammations. Furthermore, after intravenous administration of Gd-DTPA inflammatory processes with retained secretions tend to demonstrate intense peripheral or ring-like contrast enhancement, whereas the contrast enhancement in tumors and tumor-like conditions tends to be only moderate and homogeneous.

Air-fluid levels in the paranasal sinuses are most often associated with acute sinusitis and fractures (blood or cerebrospinal fluid [CSF]). Other causes include antral lavage, surgical procedure, barotrauma, and spontaneous hemorrhages associated with bleeding disorders or anticoagulation. A larger retention cyst may mimic an air-fluid level when its upper surface flattens out. However, the convex polypoid appearance of its upper and lower border differentiates it from a true air-fluid level. The differential diagnosis of lesions in the nasal cavity and paranasal sinuses is discussed in Table 5.1.

Table 5.1 Lesions in the nasal cavity and paranasal sinuses

Disease	MRI Findings	Comments
Choanal atresia or stenosis	Unilateral or bilateral, bony (85%) or membranous (15%) atresia or stenosis of the posterior nasal cavity. The obstructing choanal membranes may be either thin tissue layers or thick plugs with low signal intensity on all pulse sequences.	Approximately half are isolated congenital anomalies and the other half are associated with other congenital defects. A major component of all bony atresia is an abnormal widening of the vomer. Hypoplasia of the nasal cavity is frequently associated. CT is the imaging modality of choice.
Cephalocele	Extracranial herniation of meninges (meningocele) or brain parenchyma and meninges (encephalocele) through a defect in the anterior cranial fossa accounts for 25% of all congenital cephaloceles. MRI determines the composition of the cephalocele, visualizes the route of herniation, and diagnoses frequently associated brain anomalies such as dysgenesis of the corpus callosum, intracranial lipomas, and dermoids.	Congenital cephaloceles involving the anterior cranial fossa typically present as cystic midline lesions in the nasal or pharyngeal space. They may be visible (sincipital) or not visible (basal). Sincipital encephaloceles (15%) are frontoethmoidal cephaloceles originating at or near the foramen cecum and are subdivided into nasofrontal, nasoethmoidal, and naso-orbital lesions. Basal cephaloceles (10%) are divided into transethmoidal, sphenoethmoidal, spheno-orbital, and sphenomaxillary subtypes.
Nasal dermoid	Fusiform mass of fat density presenting with very high signal intensity on T1WI, intermediate to high signal intensity on T2WI and without contrast enhancement is seen in the nasal septum.	May present with a dimple or fistula containing a hair over the dorsum of the nose. An enlarged foramen cecum, bifid crista galli, or broadened nasal septum may be present when a dermal sinus tract exists between the lesion and the anterior cranial fossa.
Nasal glioma (Fig. 5.1)	Extranasal (60%), intranasal (30%), or mixed midline lesion appearing isointense or hyperintense to gray matter on both T1WI and T2WI. Fifteen percent have fibrous connection to the subarachnoid space, but no CSF connection exists (DD: cephalocele).	Benign extracranial rest of glial tissue and not a neoplastic lesion. Intranasal gliomas appear as large, polypoid submucal lesions. They may extend inferiorly toward or near the nostril and may expand the nasal fossa, widen the nasal bridge, and deviate the septum contralaterally.

Table 5.**1** (Cont.) Lesions in the nasal cavity and paranasal sinuses

Disease	MRI Findings	Comments
Sinusitis (Figs. 5.2 and 5.3)	*Acute*: Smooth or nodular, edematous mucosal thickening with marked contrast enhancement and/ or watery secretions presenting as an air–fluid level are characteristic. *Chronic*: Persistent mucosal thickening, which may be associated with inflammatory polyps and partial to complete obliteration of the sinus lumen with secretions of variable signal intensity. With increasing protein concentration and subsequent desiccation the signal intensity of the secretions changes on T1WI from low to high to low and eventually to signal void, and on T2WI from high to low and finally to signal void. Diffuse thickening and sclerosis of the contiguous sinus wall may be associated. Signs of chronic rhinitis including mucosal thickening, inflammatory polyps, and hyperplasia of the turbinates may also be evident. Destructive sinus wall changes with or without focal thickening and sclerosis suggests secondary osteomyelitis.	The most common cause of sinus disease. Acute sinusitis is usually viral, but secondary bacterial infections, especially by hemophilus and pneumococcus, may supervene. In one-third of all MRI examinations, mild mucosal thickening of one or more sinuses is found as an incidental finding in asymptomatic patients. *Allergic sinusitis* is found in 10% of the population and presents as bilateral, often symmetric mucosal thickening. Sinonasal polyps are frequently associated.

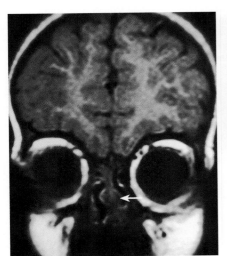

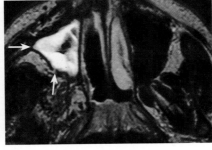

a

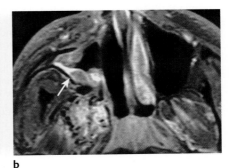

b

Fig. 5.**2** **Acute sinusitis. a** Hyperintense nodular mucosal thickening (arrows) is seen in the right maxillary sinus (T2WI).

b After intravenous Gd-DTPA administration considerable enhancement of the mucosal thickening (arrow) is seen (T1WI, FS, +C). Similar mucosal abnormalities are also evident in the left nasal cavity.

Fig. 5.**1** **Nasal glioma.** An intranasal midline lesion (arrow) of intermediate signal intensity is seen (T1WI, coronal).

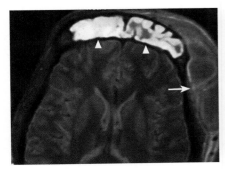

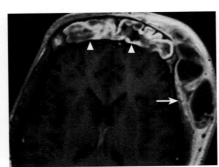

Fig. 5.**3** **Chronic sinusitis with secondary osteomyelitis. a** Hyperintense mucosal thickening (arrowheads) in the frontal sinus is associated with osteomyelitis (arrow) in the left frontal bone (T2WI). **b** After intravenous Gd-DTPA administration, enhancement of the mucosa (arrowheads) and the periphery of the left frontal osteomyelitis with intracranial soft-tissue extension (arrow) is seen (T1WI, FS, +C).

a   **b**

Table 5.1 (Cont.) Lesions in the nasal cavity and paranasal sinuses

Disease	MRI Findings	Comments
Fungal sinusitis (Fig. 5.4)	Nodular mucosal thickening with high signal intensity on T2WI affecting multiple sinuses is common. Findings are similar to chronic sinusitis, but bony destruction tends to be more frequent and more extensive and fungal concretions (desiccated secretions, often containing microcalcifications) of very low signal intensity on both T1WI and T2WI are commonly present.	Mucor and aspergillus are the most common offending organisms affecting primarily diabetic and immunocompromised patients. In the immunocompetent patient fungal sinus disease may present as a slow-growing, extramucosal fungus ball with heterogeneous low signal intensity on all pulse sequences.
Infectious granulomatous sinonasal disease	Nodular or tumor-like masses in the nasal cavity and/or paranasal sinuses, commonly associated with bony destruction. External nasal involvement may also be present.	Bacterial infections include actinomycosis nocardiosis, tuberculosis, syphilis, leprosy, and glanders. *Rhinoscleroma* is a tumor-like expansion of the nose and upper lip caused by klebsiella rhinoscleromatis.
Cocaine nose	Granuloma of the nasal septum, which eventually may be eroded. Nonspecific mucosal inflammation of the nasal cavity may be associated.	Secondary to necrotizing vasculitis with prolonged cocaine abuse.
Idiopathic midline granuloma	Destructive mass in the nasal septum leading to perforation. With progression the disease spreads to nose, face, hard and soft palates, adjacent sinuses and orbits with extensive bone destruction.	Lymphoreticular disorder (also referred to as malignant midline reticulosis) that can lead to non-Hodgkin lymphoma. *Sarcoidosis* may also present as granulomatous sinonasal disease with external nasal involvement.
Wegener granulomatosis	Presents with usually bilateral, irregular mucosal thickening and soft-tissue nodules with predilection for the maxillary sinuses and nose. Extensive bony destruction may occur without associated large soft-tissue masses.	Necrotizing granulomatous vasculitis that may also affect lungs and kidneys in addition to the sinonasal involvement. ANCA (antineutrophil cytoplasmotic autoantibodies) assay is usually positive.
Inflammatory sinonasal polyposis	Mucosal thickening with polypoid lesions measuring up to 1 cm in diameter, which blend at least partially with the mucosa. Solitary inflammatory polyps occur and can even be larger. Partial or complete replacement of the sinus lumen occurs with polyposis depicting low signal intensity on T1WI and very high signal intensity on T2WI. Nose and maxillary sinuses are most commonly affected, and bilateral involvement is common.	Most common complication of chronic sinusitis. Extensive bilateral sinonasal polyposis is far more common in allergic than infectious sinusitis, reflecting the water content in the redundant mucosa. Polyps in children may be associated with cystic fibrosis and Kartagener (immotile cilia) syndrome.
Retention cyst	Solitary or multiple homogeneous spherical lesions with low signal intensity on T1WI and very high signal intensity on T2WI. In larger cysts the upper surface may flatten out and thus simulate an air-fluid level. Retention cysts are frequently not associated with mucosal thickening and edema, otherwise they cannot be differentiated from inflammatory polyps.	Caused by obstruction of a submucosal seromucinous gland. Commonly found in asymptomatic patients as incidental finding. If large enough it may become symptomatic by obstructing the sinus drainage.
Antrochoanal polyp	Homogeneous cystic lesion originating in the maxillary sinus. May prolapse through the sinus ostium into the ipsilateral nasal cavity or through the choana into the nasopharynx.	Very large mucous retention cyst, occurring usually in teenagers or young adults. Usually unilateral, but bilateral maxillary sinusitis is sometimes associated.
Mucocele (Fig. 5.5)	Nonenhancing expansile sinus mass of varying signal intensity depending on its content. With time, watery secretions (hypointense on T1WI and hyperintense on T2WI) become more concentrated and viscous (hyperintense on both T1WI and T2WI). When the secretions become progressively more viscid first the signal intensity on T1WI and later on T2WI decreases to become eventually signal voids on both T1WI and T2WI with complete desiccation. Expansion of the sinus is frequently associated with erosion of its wall and extension into the orbit or skull base.	Caused by inflammatory (rarely post-traumatic or neoplastic) obstruction of the ostium of either a sinus or a compartment of a septated sinus. Occurs in frontal (60%), ethmoidal (30%), maxillary (10%), or sphenoidal sinus (rare). In chronically infected mucoceles (*mucopyoceles*) a surrounding zone of thick bone sclerosis is frequently evident radiographically.
Esthesioneuroblastoma (olfactory neuroblastoma) (Fig. 5.6)	Originates in the high nasal vault near the cribriform plate, which is frequently destroyed. Extension into the ethmoidal and sphenoidal sinuses, anterior cranial fossa, and/or orbits occur and is associated with destruction of the intervening bony walls. The lesion is of low signal intensity on T1WI and of mixed intermediate to high signal intensity on T2WI. After intravenous Gd-DTPA administration moderate contrast enhancement occurs.	Slow-growing malignant tumor that occurs at any age but has a predilection for the second and sixth decade of life. Presenting clinical symptoms include nasal obstruction, episodic epistaxis, hyposmia, headache, and/or visual disturbance.

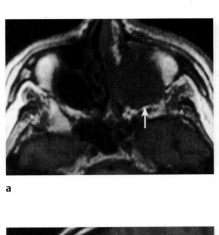

a

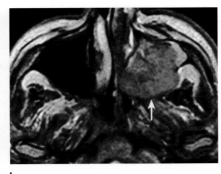

b

Fig. 5.**4** **Fungal sinusitis (aspergillus).** Soft-tissue mass (arrow) with mixed signal intensity, which is low in (**a**) (T1WI) and intermediate in (**b**) (T2WI), is seen in the left maxillary sinus.

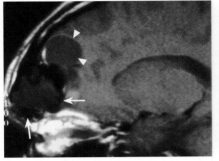

a

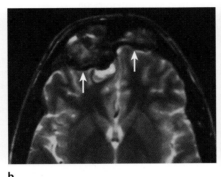

b

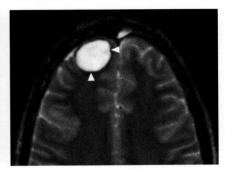

c

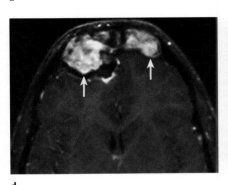

d

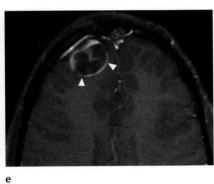

e

Fig. 5.**5** **Chronic frontal sinusitis with mucocele formation.** **a** Irregular low-density mucosal thickening (arrows) in the frontal sinus is associated with a homogeneous spherical low-density lesion (arrowheads) (T1WI, sagittal). **b, c** In T2WI the mucosal thickening (arrows) remains hypointense and inhomogeneous, whereas the mucocele (arrowheads) becomes uniformly hyperintense. **d, e** After intravenous Gd-DTPA administration considerable contrast enhancement is seen in the thickened mucosa (arrows), whereas in the mucocele (arrowheads) the contrast enhancement is largely limited to a thin peripheral line (T1WI, FS, +C).

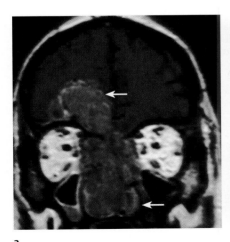

a

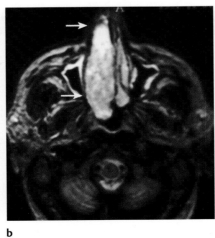

b

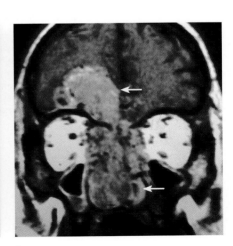

c

Fig. 5.**6** **Esthesioneuroblastoma.** A lesion (arrows) extending from the anterior cranial fossa through the cribriform plate into the nasal cavity depicts intermediate signal intensity in (**a**) (T1WI, coronal) and high signal intensity in (**b**) (T2WI, axial). After intravenous Gd-DTPA administration, moderate heterogeneous contrast enhancement is seen in the lesion (arrows) (T1WI, +C, coronal).

Table 5.1 (Cont.) Lesions in the nasal cavity and paranasal sinuses

Disease	MRI Findings	Comments
Juvenile nasopharyngeal angiofibroma (Fig. 5.7)	Invasive mass originating from the roof of the posterior nasal cavity or anterior nasopharynx with early extension through the sphenopalatine foramen into the pterygopalatine fossa (89%), resulting in widening of this fossa and anterior bowing of the posterior ipsilateral antral wall. Extension in the sphenoidal sinus (61%), maxillary sinus (43%), and ethmoidal sinus (35%) occurs. Intracranial extension (10%) occurs usually via orbit through the infraorbital fissure and from there through the superior orbital fissure into the middle cranial fossa. The tumor demonstrates intermediate signal intensity on T1WI and relatively high signal intensity on T2WI, interspersed with flow voids due to large tumor vessels. Intense contrast enhancement is seen after intravenous Gd-DTPA administration.	Benign, but locally aggressive highly vascular tumor that can grow to enormous size. It is exclusively found in male adolescents and young adults with a mean age of 15 years at time of diagnosis. Patients present with nasal obstruction and severe recurrent epistaxis.
Papilloma (Fig. 5.8)	Usually solitary (75%) nasal mass with uniform, relatively high signal intensity on T2WI and diffuse moderate contrast enhancement after intravenous Gd-DTPA administration. Presents as small nasal polypoid lesion or expansile mass causing bowing of the nasal septum to the contralateral side and remodeling of the lateral nasal wall without frank bone destruction. Fungiform papillomas arise from the nasal septum. Inverted papillomas arise from the lateral nasal wall and frequently extend into the ipsilateral maxillary and/or ethmoidal sinus.	Sinonasal (schneiderian) papillomas are classified as fungiform (50%), inverted (47%), and cylindric cell (3%) papillomas. They are preferentially found in adult males presenting with nasal obstruction, epistaxis, and anosmia. Inverted papillomas have a tendency for local recurrence and are associated in about 10% of cases with carcinomas that may be concurrent or develop subsequent to therapy. Cylindric cell papillomas are similar to inverted papillomas in both clinical and MRI presentation.
Squamous cell carcinoma (Fig. 5.9)	Poorly marginated soft-tissue mass with extensive destruction of adjacent bone. The majority of tumors originate in the maxillary sinus, followed by nasal cavity (30%), ethmoidal sinus (10%), and rarely in the frontal and sphenoidal sinuses. The tumors appear homogeneous with a signal intensity that is low to intermediate on T1WI and only slightly higher on T2WI. Focal areas of intermediate to high signal intensity on both T1WI and T2WI within the tumor represent subacute hemorrhages, whereas areas of low signal intensity on T1WI and high signal on T2WI are consistent with necrosis. After intravenous administration of Gd-DTPA contrast, enhancement is minimal to moderate and less than normal mucosa. Regional lymph nodes (retropharyngeal, submandibular, and/or jugular) are involved in 15% at the time of diagnosis. Invasion of the pterygopalatine fossa, orbit, middle cranial fossa, maxillary alveolar ridge, hard palate, buccal space, and/or nose occurs frequently.	By far the most common tumor of the sinuses and nose (80–90%). Often clinically silent until advanced. First symptoms are usually from secondary obstructive sinusitis. *Adenocarcinoma* (in woodworkers and cabinet makers), *adenoid cystic carcinoma*, and *mucoepidermoid carcinoma* cannot be differentiated on MRI from squamous cell carcinoma. *Staging* T1: tumor limited to antral mucosa; T2: bony destruction limited to hard palate or lateral wall of nose; T3: tumor invades posterior antral wall, orbital wall, anterior ethmoidal sinus, or skin; T4: tumor invades orbital contents, cribriform plate, posterior ethmoid, sphenoidal sinus, nasopharynx, soft palate, nasopharyngeal masticator space, or skull base.
Lymphoma (Fig. 5.10)	Often bilateral, homogeneous soft-tissue mass with low to intermediate signal intensity on T1WI and intermediate to high on T2WI. After intravenous Gd-DTPA administration contrast enhancement is uniform and usually moderate. Bone erosions occur occasionally. Nasal fossa and maxillary sinuses are the most common locations.	Sinonasal lymphoma occurs with or without associated cervical or systemic nodal disease and is usually of the non-Hodgkin variety.

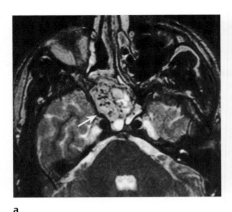

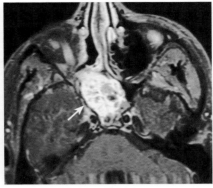

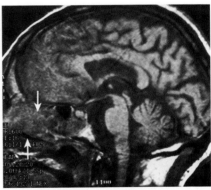

a

b

Fig. 5.7 Juvenile nasopharyngeal angiofibroma. A lesion (arrow) originating from the anterior nasopharynx demonstrates high signal intensity interspersed with flow voids due to large tumor vessels in (**a**) (T2WI). After intravenous Gd-DTPA administration, intense, inhomogeneous contrast enhancement is seen in the lesion in (**b**) (T1WI, FS, +C).

Fig. 5.8 Recurrent inverted papilloma. A lesion (arrow) with intermediate signal intensity is seen in the right maxillary sinus extending into the right nasal cavity (T1WI). A carcinoma is associated in 10% and cannot be excluded from this examination.

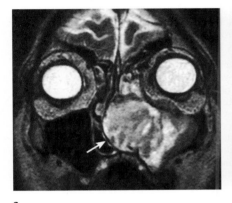

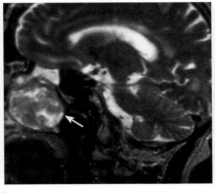

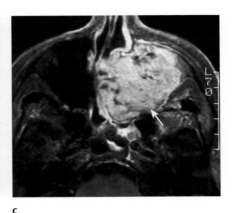

a

b

c

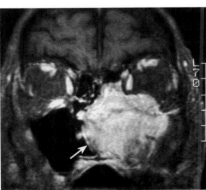

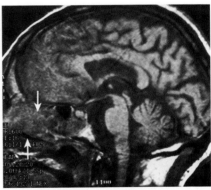

d

Fig. 5.9 Squamous cell carcinoma. An inhomogeneous lesion (arrow) with intermediate to high signal intensity is seen in the left maxillary sinus in (**a**) (T2WI, coronal) and (**b**) (T2WI, sagittal). After intravenous Gd-DTPA administration, marked inhomogeneous contrast enhancement of the lesion (arrow) is seen in (**c**) (T1WI, FS, +C, axial) and (**d**) (T1WI, FS, +C, coronal).

Fig. 5.10 Lymphoma. A relatively inhomogeneous lesion (arrows) of intermediate signal intensity is seen involving frontal and ethmoidal sinuses and skull base (spoiled GRE, sagittal).

Table 5.1 (Cont.) Lesions in the nasal cavity and paranasal sinuses

Disease	MRI Findings	Comments
Metastases (Fig. 5.11)	Osteolytic (hypointense on T1WI and hyperintense on T2WI) or osteoblastic (hypointense on both T1WI and T2WI) lesions with or without associated soft-tissue component.	Common primary sites include kidney, lung, breast, and prostate. *Multiple myeloma* manifestations cannot be differentiated from osteolytic metastases.
Fracture (Fig. 5.12)	Besides visualization of the actual fracture site with accompanying hematoma, indirect fracture signs include air-blood or air-fluid level (CSF) in a sinus, pneumocephalus (intracranial air or air-fluid level), and subcutaneous emphysema. In a blowout fracture herniation of orbital fat, inferior rectus muscle, and inferior oblique muscle can easily be diagnosed and differentiated from each other.	CT is the imaging modality of choice for evaluation of facial fractures. *Postoperative changes* may also present with bony defects, air-fluid levels in sinuses, soft-tissue emphysema, edema and hematoma, and eventual fibrosis and scarring. Obliteration of the sinus cavity is sometimes achieved by packing it with abdominal muscle or fatty tissue.
Hemorrhage (Fig. 5.13)	Diffuse or polypoid mucosal thickening, blood-fluid level, or complete air replacement by blood are manifestations of sinus bleeding. The signal intensity varies with the age of the blood.	Occurs with trauma, surgery, neoplasm, vascular malformations, bleeding disorders, anticoagulation, and barotrauma (e.g., in divers and pilots of unpressurized aircraft).
Rhinolith and sinolith	Foreign body in the sinonasal cavity acting as nidus may become encrusted with mineral salts and present with low signal intensity or even signal void on all pulse sequences.	Radiographically a calcified nasal or sinal mass is evident. On MRI a *mycetoma, desiccated secretions*, an *intrasinus tooth* in the maxillary sinus, or an *osteoma* in the frontal or ethmoidal sinus can all present similarly to a sinolith.
Bone lesions (Figs. 5.14–5.17)	Diffuse bone enlargement with variable signal intensity and marked contrast enhancement is seen with Paget disease, fibrous dysplasia, and neurofibromatosis. Nonenhancing, well-defined, homogeneous lesions appearing hypointense on T1WI and hyperintense on T2WI include simple bone cyst and a variety of dentigerous cysts such as keratocyst, dentigerous cyst (with focus of signal void caused by crown of molar tooth), radicular cyst, and fissural cyst. Well-defined lesions consisting largely or completely of opaque material or dense bone presenting as signal void on all pulse sequences include bone island, osteoma, osteoblastoma, odontoma, osteoblastic metastases, well-differentiated sclerotic osteosarcoma, and sclerosing osteomyelitis.	Enhancing, well-defined, often expansile lesions with or without cortical violation include giant cell tumor, giant cell granuloma, aneurysmal bone cyst, brown tumor of hyperparathyroidism, eosinophilic granuloma, ossifying granuloma, ameloblastoma, plasmocytoma, and Brodie's abscess. Poorly defined, destructive bone lesions with associated soft-tissue mass include osteomyelitis, eosinophilic granuloma, ameloblastoma, malignant fibrous histiocytoma, plasmocytoma, Ewing sarcoma, chondrosarcoma, and osteosarcoma.

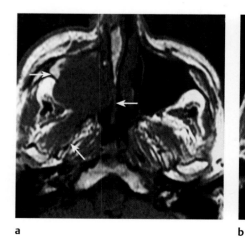
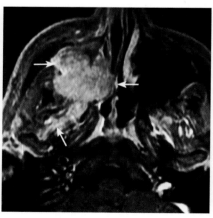

a   b

Fig. 5.**11** **Soft-tissue sarcoma metastasis.** A large lesion (arrows) is seen extending into the right maxillary sinus. The lesion appears homogeneous in (**a**) (T1WI) and demonstrates considerable contrast enhancement in (**b**) (T1WI, FS, +C).

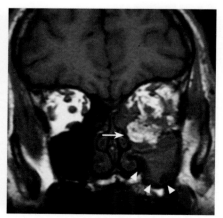

Fig. 5.**12** **Blowout fracture, left orbit.** Herniation (arrow) of both orbital fat and inferior rectus muscle into the left maxillary sinus is seen. Blood in the left maxillary sinus and small subperiosteal hematomas (arrowheads) are also evident (T1WI, coronal).

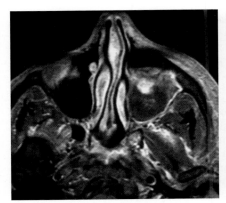

Fig. 5.**13**   **Subacute maxillary sinus hemorrhage.** Blood in the left maxillary sinus demonstrates heterogeneous signal intensity due to both clot and methemoglobin formation (T1WI).

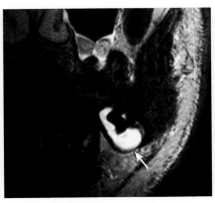

Fig. 5.**14**   **Dentigerous cyst.** A hyperintense cystic lesion (arrow) containing a crown of a tooth, evident as an area of signal void, is seen in the mandible (T2WI, coronal).

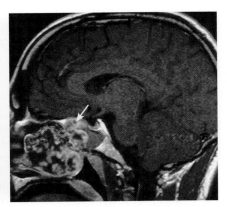

Fig. 5.**15**   **Chondrosarcoma of the nasal septum.** A heterogeneous lesion (arrow) with greatly variable signal intensity is seen (T1WI, sagittal).

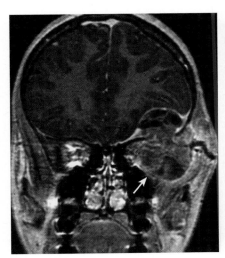

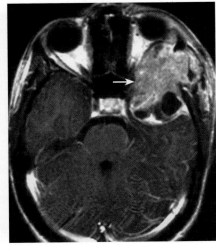

Fig. 5.**16**   **Ewing sarcoma.**   **a** A heterogeneous lesion (arrow) of intermediate signal intensity is seen originating from the skull base (GRE, coronal).   **b** Considerable contrast enhancement occurs in the lesion (arrow) after intravenous Gd-DTPA administration (T1WI, +C, axial).

a

b

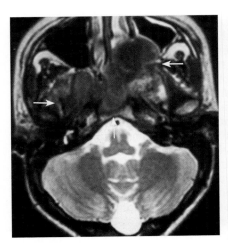

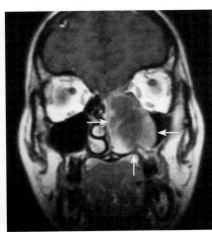

Fig. 5.**17**   **Osteosarcoma.**   **a** A poorly defined, heterogeneous lesion (arrows) with variable intermediate signal intensity is seen (T2WI, axial).   **b** After intravenous Gd-DTPA administration, contrast enhancement is preferentially located in the periphery of the lesion (arrows) (T1WI, +C, coronal).

a

b

6 Upper Neck

The upper neck includes the nasopharynx, oropharynx, oral cavity, and surrounding bone and soft-tissue structures. The deep cervical fascia consists of three layers, permitting subdivision of the soft tissues of the neck into different anatomic compartments (Fig. 6.1).

The *pharyngeal mucosal space* is comprised of the nasopharynx and oropharynx. The pharyngeal mucosa with its minor salivary glands, tonsils, and adenoids are the most important structure with regard to nosogenesis. The mucosal signal is either isointense or slightly hyperintense to muscle on T1WI and hyperintense on T2WI. Mucosal contrast enhancement occurs after intravenous Gd-DTPA administration and is often intense. Squamous cell carcinomas frequently originate in the pharyngeal mucosa. Other benign and malignant neoplasms occur in the minor salivary glands. Tonsils and adenoids may harbor abscesses and lymphoma. A Thornwaldt cyst is found midline in the posterior wall of the upper nasopharynx.

The *retropharyngeal space* is located posterior to the pharynx and contains the retropharyngeal lymph nodes embedded in fat. Common lesions in the retropharyngeal space include lymphoma and lymph node metastases. Primary tumor and abscess formation rarely occur in the retropharyngeal space, but extension of these conditions from a neighboring compartment into the retropharyngeal space is very frequent.

The *prevertebral space* is separated from the retropharyngeal space by the deep (prevertebral) layer of the deep cervical fascia. The prevertebral space is contiguous lateroposteriorly with the paraspinal space and contains the brachial plexus, phrenic nerve, and vertebral artery and vein. Common lesions in the prevertebral space originate from the cervical spine and include osteophytes, osteomyelitis, chordoma, and metastases. Schwannoma and neurofibroma may derive from the branchial plexus.

The *parapharyngeal space* has no mucosa, muscle, bone, lymph nodes, or salivary gland tissue within its boundaries. Consequently it is unusual for a disease process to originate in the parapharyngeal space. It is a fatty crescent-shaped tube extending from the skull base to the superior corner of the hyoid bone and serves as an "elevator shaft" through which infection and tumor originating from adjacent spaces may travel.

The *masticator space* is composed of the four muscles of mastication (masseter, temporalis, medial and lateral pterygoid). The cephalad extension of the masticator space is the temporal fossa (also referred to as the suprazygomatic masticator space), where the temporalis muscle originates. The nasopharyngeal portion of the masticator space is the infratemporal fossa (also referred to as the nasopharyngeal masticator space) confined by the pterygopalatine fossa medially and zygomatic arch laterally. Anteriorly the masticator space extends without boundary in the buccal space. The posteromedial masticator space borders the parapharyngeal space. Directly posterior to the masticator space is the parotid space. Besides the already mentioned mastication muscles and their nerves, part of both mandible and parotid duct (Stensen's duct) are in the masticator space and buccal space, respectively. Common lesions in the masticator space include odontogenic ab-

scesses, bone and soft-tissue sarcomas, and lymphoma. An accessory parotid gland and masseteric hypertrophy may both mimic these mass lesions.

The *parotid space* is the most lateral space in the upper neck extending from the external auditory canal to the mandibular angle. Anterior to the parotid space is the masticator space; medial, the parapharyngeal space; and posteromedial, the posterior belly of the digastric muscle and its fascia, which separates the parotid from the carotid space. Because of its fat content the normal parotid gland appears inhomogeneous with an overall intermediate to high signal intensity on T1WI and low to intermediate on T2WI. On fast T2WI its signal intensity is intermediate to high. Besides the parotid gland, the parotid space contains the intraparotid lymph nodes, facial nerve, and external carotid artery. Lesions in the parotid space are mostly related to inflammatory and neoplastic processes involving the parotid gland or the 20 to 30 intraparotid lymph nodes.

The *carotid space* extends from the skull base to the aortic arch. It is surrounded by the parotid space laterally, the parapharyngeal space anteriorly, and the retropharyngeal space medially. The carotid space is enveloped in the carotid sheath, which is formed by the condensed three layers of the deep cervical fascia, preventing disease outside the carotid space from getting in and vice versa. The carotid space contains the internal carotid artery and jugular vein, the cranial nerves IX, X, XI, XII, the sympathetic plexus, and lymph nodes. Frequent pathology in the carotid space includes paragangliomas (glomus tumors), schwannomas, lymph node metastases, and vascular lesions.

The *sublingual space* is located superomedial to the mylohyoid muscle, which forms the floor of the oral cavity. The sublingual space contains the sublingual glands and ducts, the deep portion of the submandibular gland, and the submandibular gland duct (Wharton's duct). Inflammatory and neoplastic mass lesions in the sublingual space commonly originate from the salivary glands and ducts. Squamous cell carcinomas from the tongue frequently invade the sublingual space. Ludwig angina is a severe form of cellulitis or abscess formation in the sublingual and submandibular space secondary to a periodontal abscess or tooth extraction from the lower alveolar ridge.

The *submandibular space* is located inferolateral to the mylohyoid muscle and superior to the hyoid bone. It communicates posteriorly with both the sublingual and inferior parapharyngeal spaces. The submandibular space contains the superficial portion of the submandibular gland and the submandibular and submental lymph nodes. Inflammatory and neoplastic mass lesions in the SMS originate commonly from the submandibular gland or may be caused by benign or malignant lymph node enlargement. Congenital cysts (second branchial cleft cyst at the mandibular angle and suprahyoid thyroglossal duct cyst in the midline) may be evident in characteristic locations.

The differential diagnosis of pharyngeal lesions is discussed in Table 6.1, lesions involving the carotid and masticator space in Table 6.2, parotid lesions in Table 6.3, and lesions involving the oral cavity including the sublingual and submandibular spaces in Table 6.4.

Table 6.**1** Pharyngeal and parapharyngeal lesions

Disease	MRI Findings	Comments
Asymmetric lateral pharyngeal recess (fossa of Rosenmüller)	Unilaterally collapsed recess and unilateral hypertrophic adenoid tissue, which is isointense to muscle on T1WI and hyperintense on T2WI, may both mimic a mass lesion. Maintenance of normal soft-tissue planes in the adjacent parapharyngeal and retropharyngeal spaces strongly argues against a true mass lesion.	The pharyngeal recess is located behind the opening of the eustachian tube. A collapsed lateral pharyngeal recess can frequently be opened with a modified Valsalva maneuver.
Asymmetric pterygoid venous plexus	After intravenous Gd-DTPA administration, a racemose, intensely enhancing area along the medial border of the lateral pterygoid muscle is best seen on fat suppressed T1WI.	Normal variant that should not be mistaken for a focal vascular tumor.
Thornwaldt's cyst	Midline cystic lesion measuring up to 3 cm in diameter in the posterior roof of the nasopharynx without bone erosion.	Usually an asymptomatic finding on head MRI. May become symptomatic when secondarily infected. DD: *Rhatke's pouch*, a small epithelial cyst in the sphenoid body anterocephalad of Thornwaldt's cyst.
Atypical (parapharyngeal) second branchial cleft cyst	Cystic mass with usually low and occasionally high (proteinaceous content) signal intensity on T1WI and high signal intensity on T2WI, projecting into the lateral wall of the pharynx from the palatine tissue toward the skull base.	Presents in a child or young adult with laterally displaced parotid gland and bulging posterolateral pharyngeal wall, often after a respiratory tract infection.
Mucous retention cyst (postinflammatory)	Well-circumscribed 1–2 cm cystic lesion in the pharyngeal mucosal space. In the lateral pharyngeal recess it is usually oblong and may obstruct the eustachian tube, leading to fluid accumulation in the middle ear.	Usually an incidental finding.
Pleomorphic adenoma	Round or oval well-circumscribed mass either pedunculating into the lumen of the nasopharynx or oropharynx or centered within the parapharyngeal space surrounded by fat. The lesion appears homogeneous, isointense to muscle on T1WI and hyperintense on T2WI, and demonstrates moderate uniform contrast enhancement.	These benign mixed tumors arise either from minor salivary glands of the pharyngeal mucosa or from ectopic salivary gland tissue in the parapharyngeal space.
Lipoma	Circumscribed fatty lesion with high signal intensity on T1WI and intermediate signal intensity on T2WI in the parapharyngeal or retropharyngeal space.	Rare. *Dermoid* (encapsulated fatty lesion, usually in the midline) must be differentiated.

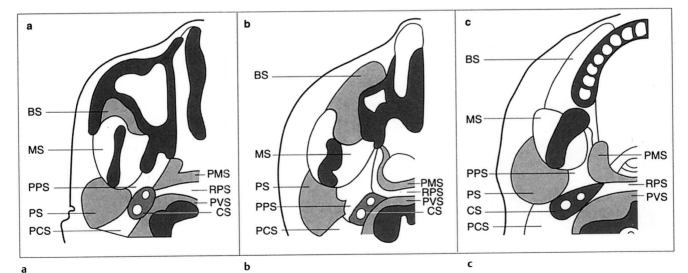

Fig. 6.1 Axial anatomy of the upper neck. a Mid nasopharynx. **b** Low nasopharynx (level of soft palate). **c** Mid oropharynx. BS: buccal space; CS: carotid space; MS: masticator space; PCS: posterior cervical space; PMS: pharyngeal mucosal space; PPS: parapharyngeal space; PS: parotid space; PVS: prevertebral space; RPS: retropharyngeal space.

Table 6.1 (Cont.) Pharyngeal and parapharyngeal lesions

Disease	MRI Findings	Comments
Hemangioma (Fig. 6.2)	Poorly marginated (T1WI) or well-marginated (T2WI) lesion, isointense to muscle on T1WI and hyperintense with areas of heterogeneity on T2WI. Phleboliths may cause signal voids. Thrombi containing methemoglobin or interspersed fatty tissue may produce foci of high signal intensity on T1WI. Contrast enhancement is usually intense.	Located anywhere in the nasopharynx and oropharynx and occasionally multicentric. Occurs commonly in children and young adults with female predominance.
Juvenile nasopharyngeal angiofibroma (Fig. 6.3)	Aggressive, large mass in the nasopharynx with intermediate signal intensity on T1WI, relatively high signal intensity on T2WI interspersed with flow voids due to large tumor vessels and intense contrast enhancement. Extension in neighboring structures such as nose, paranasal sinuses, and middle cranial fossa through existing foramina or bone erosion is frequent.	Benign, but locally aggressive, highly vascular tumor presenting exclusively in male adolescents and young adults with nasal obstruction and severe recurrent epistaxis.
Squamous cell carcinoma (Figs. 6.4 and 6.5)	Polypoid or infiltrating soft-tissue mass originating in the pharyngeal mucosal space of the nasopharynx or oropharynx with early invasion of the fat in the adjacent parapharyngeal or retropharyngeal space. The signal intensity of the lesion is homogeneous and similar to normal mucosa, appearing isointense to muscle on T1WI and hyperintense on T2WI. Contrast enhancement is usually uniform and moderate (similar to mucosa, but considerably more than muscle). Larger tumors may undergo central necrosis evident as increased signal intensity on T2WI and absent contrast enhancement. Nodal metastases, occasionally with central necrosis, are common in the retropharyngeal space (retropharyngeal and upper deep cervical lymph nodes). With superior extension, invasion and/or destruction of the skull base may be associated.	By far the most common malignant tumor, the majority being of the nonkeratizing epidermoid type, previously known as "lymphoepithelioma." Most patients present with known primary tumor for staging by MRI. Occasionally the patient presents with malignant lymphadenopathy and occult primary tumor. TNM staging: *Nasopharynx* T1 Tumor limited to one subsite* T2 Tumor invades more than one subsite T3 Tumor invades nasal cavity or oropharynx T4 Tumor invades skull or cranial nerves *Oropharynx* T1 Tumor <2 cm T2 Tumor 2–4 cm T3 Tumor >4 cm T4 Tumor invades spine, soft tissue of neck, deep muscle of tongue *Lymph nodes* N1 Single ipsilateral node <3 cm N2 Single ipsilateral node 3–6 cm or multiple nodes <6 cm N3 Node(s) >6 cm *Nasopharyngeal subsites include posterosuperior wall, lateral wall (fossa of Rosenmüller, and antero-inferior wall).
Minor salivary gland malignancy	Indistinguishable from squamous cell carcinoma when originating in the pharyngeal mucosal space. Tumor with its epicenter outside the pharyngeal mucosal space may originate from ectopic salivary gland tissue.	Histologically these tumors include adenocarcinoma, mucoepidermoid carcinoma, adenoid cystic carcinoma, and pleomorphic adenocarcinoma.

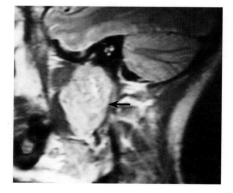

Fig. 6.2 **Hemangioma.** A well-marginated, slightly heterogeneous lesion (arrow) with high signal intensity extends into the parapharyngeal space (T2WI, sagittal).

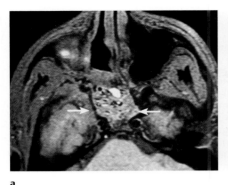

a

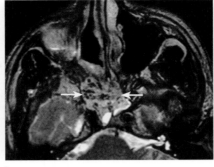

b

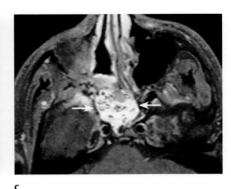

c

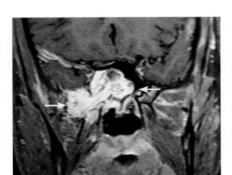

d

Fig. 6.**3 Juvenile nasopharyngeal angio-fibroma.** An irregularly shaped lesion (arrows) with numerous small foci devoid of signal representing flow voids originates in the nasopharynx and depicts intermediate signal intensity in (**a**) (T1WI, axial) and slightly higher signal intensity in (**b**) (T2WI, axial). After intravenous administration of Gd-DTPA, intense contrast enhancement is seen in the lesion (arrows) in (**c**) (T1WI, FS, +C, axial) and in (**d**) (T1WI, FS, +C, coronal).

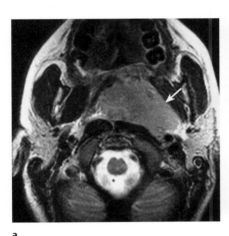

a

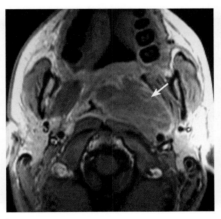

b

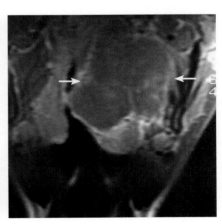

c

Fig. 6.**4 Squamous cell carcinoma. a** A large homogeneous mass (arrow) of intermediate signal intensity extends from the nasopharynx into the adjacent spaces (T2WI). **b, c** After intravenous Gd-DTPA administration only minimal enhancement of the lesion itself (arrows) is seen (axial and coronal, T1WI, +C).

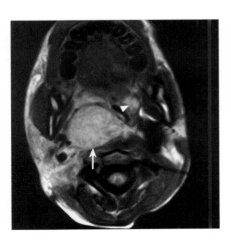

Fig. 6.**5 Squamous cell carcinoma.** A large, relatively homogeneous lesion (arrow) of intermediate signal intensity is seen in the right parapharyngeal and retropharyngeal space. Edematous changes extend from the lesion into the right subcutis. A lymph node metastasis (arrowhead) is also evident (PDWI).

Table 6.**1** (Cont.) Pharyngeal and parapharyngeal lesions

Disease	MRI Findings	Comments
Lymphoma (Fig. 6.6)	In the pharyngeal mucosal space, lymphoma may originate from lymphatic tissue of the Waldeyer's ring resulting in enlargement of the tonsils and adenoids. Nodal lymphoma may originate in the retropharyngeal space but not in the parapharyngeal space, since the latter does not contain lymph nodes. Lymphoma has signal characteristics (hypointense on T1WI and hyperintense on T2WI) and an enhancement pattern (uniform and moderate) similar to squamous cell carcinoma. Lymphomas of the nasopharynx and oropharynx appear well circumscribed but, unlike squamous cell carcinomas, tend to lack deep invasion despite their bulky size. Associated multiple large non-necrotic lymph nodes in unusual drainage locations may further support the diagnosis of lymphoma.	Usually non-Hodgkin lymphoma. Malaise, fever, distant adenopathy, and hepatosplenomegaly differentiate lymphoma clinically from squamous cell carcinoma. When the lymphoma is confined to the pharynx and cervical lymph nodes it may present indistinguishable from metastatic squamous cell carcinoma. Under these conditions the only clue suggesting lymphoma rather than squamous cell carcinoma may rest in the anatomic location of the affected lymph nodes that do not fit a lymphatic drainage pattern.
Lymph node metastases (See Fig. 6.5)	Usually multiple lymph nodes exceeding 1 cm in diameter in the retropharyngeal space, sometimes with necrotic center and rim enhancement. Besides pharyngeal carcinoma, which is by far the most common cause for retropharyngeal node involvement, melanoma and thyroid carcinoma have a propensity for this location.	*Reactive lymph node hyperplasia* is a benign enlargement of the retropharyngeal nodes commonly, but not always, associated with pharyngitis, tonsillitis, or upper respiratory tract infection. It is usually found in children and young adults. The lymph nodes rarely exceed 1 cm in diameter.
Pharyngeal hematoma	Bulging submucosal lesion with smooth outline and variable signal intensity depending on its age. Hyperintense areas due to methemoglobin formation are usually present on all pulse sequences.	Secondary to iatrogenic instrumentation, trauma, and foreign bodies or spontaneous in bleeding diathesis.
Parapharyngeal or retropharyngeal abscess (Fig. 6.7)	Abscess located in the parapharyngeal or retropharyngeal space originates from a different space (e.g., pharyngitis, tonsillitis, and spondylitis). Poorly defined mass with necrotic liquefied center and enhancing wall is characteristic. A retropharyngeal abscess spreading from side to side may assume a characteristic "bow tie" appearance.	Patients with parapharyngeal or retropharyngeal abscess are very sick, presenting with fever and elevated white blood cell count. In penetrating trauma the parapharyngeal and retropharyngeal spaces may be primarily involved. An infected hematoma can be difficult to differentiate from an abscess.
Tonsillitis and tonsillar abscess	Tonsillitis presents as tonsillar enlargement with increased signal intensity on T2WI due to inflammation and edema. Inflammatory changes may extend into the soft palate, parapharyngeal space, and medial pterygoid muscle. A tonsillar abscess (lesion with enhancing wall and liquefied center containing occasionally gas) frequently extends into the parapharyngeal or submandibular space.	Presents usually in younger patients with sore throat and fever, followed by painful swallowing with pharyngeal wall mass. *Adenoidal tonsillitis and abscess formation* is much less common and presents on MRI similar to palatine tonsillar involvement.

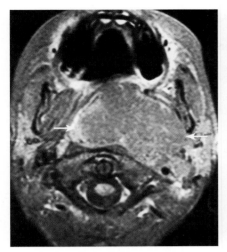
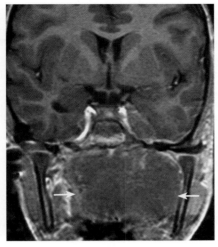

a

b

Fig. 6.**6** **Non-Hodgkin lymphoma.** A large homogeneous lesion (arrows) with only minimal contrast enhancement is seen. **a** Axial T1WI, FS, +C. **b** Coronal T1WI, FS, +C.

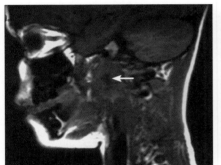
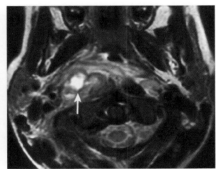

a

b

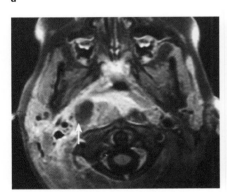
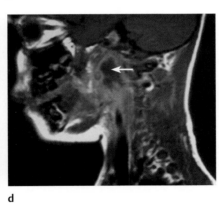

c

d

Fig. 6.**7** **Retropharyngeal abscess.** A poorly defined retropharyngeal abscess is seen spreading into the neighboring spaces. The liquefied abscess center containing pus (arrow) appears hypointense in (**a**) (T1WI, sagittal), hyperintense in (**b**) (T2WI, axial) and does not enhance in (**c**) and (**d**) (axial and sagittal T1WI, FS, +C). However, both abscess wall and extensive surrounding inflammatory changes enhance markedly.

Table 6.2 Masticator space and carotid space lesions

Disease	MRI Findings	Comments
Masseteric hypertrophy	Unilateral or bilateral homogeneous enlargement of the masseter muscle.	Acquired form is usually secondary to nocturnal teeth clenching.
Accessory parotid gland	Soft-tissue mass with identical signal characteristics as the adjacent parotid gland located on the lateral surface of the masseter muscle.	Occurs in 21% of population, but when asymmetric or unilateral may be mistaken for a lateral masticator space mass.
Hemangioma (Fig. 6.8)	Poorly marginated (T1WI) or well-marginated (T2WI) lesion, isointense to muscle on T1WI and heterogeneous hyperintense on T2WI. Phleboliths may cause signal voids. Thrombi containing methemoglobin or interspersed fatty tissue may produce foci of high signal intensity on T1WI. Hyperintense signal on T2WI reflects slow-flowing, relatively stagnant blood. Contrast enhancement is usually intense.	Occurs in children and young adults with female predilection and may progressively enlarge.
Schwannoma (neuroma) (Fig. 6.9 and 6.9*)	Well-defined fusiform mass with homogeneous low signal intensity on T1WI and high signal intensity on T2WI. After intravenous Gd-DTPA administration, moderate and uniform contrast enhancement is seen. Larger lesions may become heterogeneous due to areas of cystic degeneration. Common locations include the carotid space (cranial nerves IX-XII) and the prevertebral space (brachial plexus and cervical spine rootlets), whereas the masticator space (trigeminal nerve branches) and parotid space (fascial nerve) are less frequently involved. Splaying or displacing neighboring structures (e.g., carotid vessels) and smooth scalloping of adjacent bone (e.g., jugular foramen) is characteristic.	Slow-growing mass that may become painful with associated cranial neuropathy when the jugular foramen becomes involved. May be multiple in patients with neurofibromatosis type 2. *Meningioma* may descend from the jugular foramen into the carotid space. On MRI a dural tail may be visible, and the contrast enhancement is more intense than in schwannomas. CT may show intratumoral calcifications and hyperostosis in the adjacent skull base.
Neurofibroma (Fig. 6.10)	Usually indistinguishable from schwannomas, unless they undergo diffuse fatty degeneration increasing the signal intensity on T1WI and decreasing it on T2WI or it contains a central fibrous core presenting with low signal intensity on all pulse sequences.	Solitary neurofibromas occur in young adults. Multiple lesions are associated with neurofibromatosis type 1.

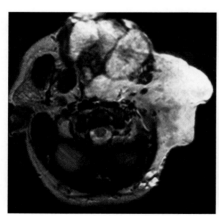

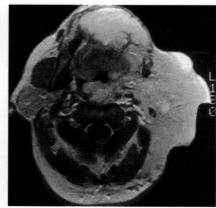

Fig. 6.8 **Hemangioma. a** A large left facial hemangioma presents as a well-defined, somewhat heterogeneous, hyperintense lesion consisting of several loosely connected components extending into the oral cavity (PDWI). **b** After intravenous Gd-DTPA administration, intense contrast enhancement of the lesion occurs (T1WI, +C).

a   b

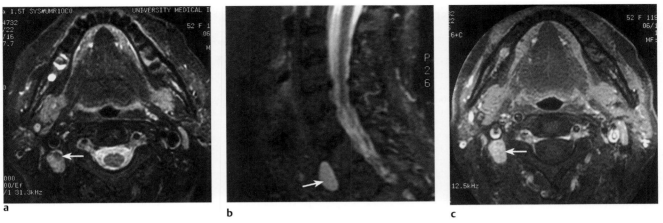

Fig. 6.**9**   **Schwannoma.** A hyperintense lesion (arrow) originating from the vagus nerve is seen in **a** (T2WI, axial) and **b** (T2WI, sagittal). After intravenous Gd-DTPA administration considerable contrast enhancement of the tumor (arrow) is evident in **c** (T1WI, FS, +C, axial).

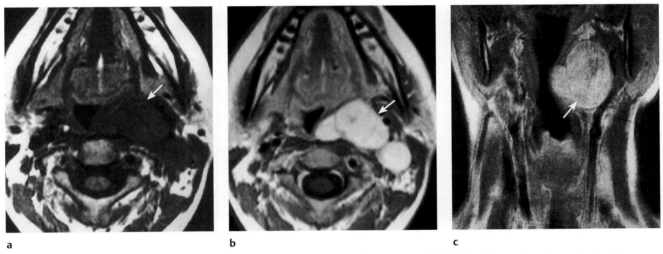

Fig. 6.**9***   **Schwannoma.** Well-defined mass (arrow) is seen with low signal intensity in (**a**) (T1WI) and considerable contrast enhancement in (**b**) and (**c**) (axial and coronal T1WI, +C).

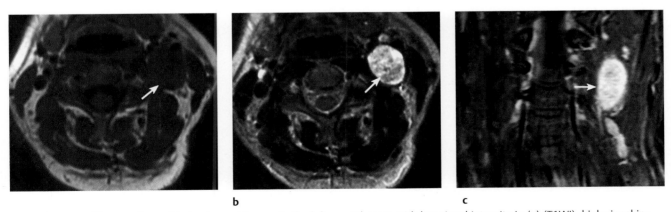

Fig. 6.**10**   **Neurofibroma.** An oval lesion (arrow) is seen in the left carotid space with low signal intensity in (**a**) (T1WI), high signal intensity in (**b**) (T2WI), and considerable contrast enhancement in (**c**) (T1WI, FS, +C, coronal).

Table 6.2 (Cont.) Masticator space and carotid space lesions

Disease	MRI Findings	Comments
Glomus tumor (paraganglioma) (Figs. 6.11–6.13)	Heterogeneous, often ovoid or tubular mass with low to intermediate signal intensity on T1WI and relatively high signal intensity on T2WI. Characteristic are serpiginous flow voids due to enlarged tumor vessels and "salt-and-pepper" appearance reflecting tumor hypervascularity. Intense contrast enhancement is seen after intravenous Gd-DTPA administration. Erosion of the skull base (e.g., jugular foramen) is irregular and permeative. Glomus tumors are found throughout the carotid space from skull base to carotid bifurcation and originate from the glomus jugulare (skull base at jugular foramen), the glomus vagale (near jugular foramen with propensity to grow caudad) or the carotid body (at carotid bifurcation).	Slow-growing tumors arising from nonchromaffin paraganglion cells of neuroectodermal origin. Can occur at any age but have a predilection for middle-aged women, eventually presenting with variable cranial neuropathy. Multiple tumors are seen in 3–5% of cases and in 20–30% of patients with family history. Occur anywhere in the paraganglionic tissue between the glomus jugulotympanicum and the base of the urinary bladder. Malignant transformation occurs in approximately 4% of cases.
Lymphoma	Single or, more commonly, multiple enlarged lymph nodes in the carotid space of typically homogeneous signal intensity that is low on T1WI (similar to muscle) and intermediate to moderately high on T2WI (similar to fat). May progress with extracapsular spread to an infiltrating mass that by itself cannot be differentiated from another malignancy.	The *jugulodigastric node*, located at the intersection between the posterior belly of the digastric muscle and internal jugular vein, is the largest deep cervical (internal jugular) lymph node measuring up to 1.2 cm in its longest diameter. All other cervical lymph nodes normally do not exceed 1 cm in diameter. In benign *reactive hyperplasia* the lymph node size rarely exceeds 1.5 cm in diameter. The initial presentation of both Hodgkin disease and non-Hodgkin lymphoma commonly involves the deep cervical lymph nodes.
Metastases (Figs. 6.14 and 6.15)	Nodal metastases in the carotid space present with single or multiple round to oval masses exceeding 1.5 cm in diameter. A central signal intensity that is decreased on T1WI and increased on T2WI is always abnormal, regardless of lymph node size. Metastatic involvement of the masticator space occurs by direct extension from a malignancy of the oral cavity or oropharynx. Mandibular destruction is frequently associated.	In most cases the patient has a known primary lesion in the upper aerodigestive tract, usually a squamous cell carcinoma. Occasionally lymph node metastases are found in the carotid space with clinically and radiologically occult primary lesions.

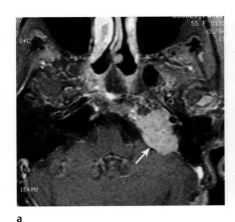

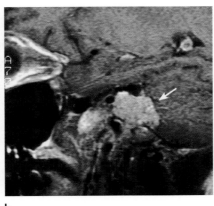

Fig. 6.**11** **Glomus jugulare tumor.** After intravenous Gd-DTPA administration a markedly enhanced lesion with "salt-and-pepper" appearance is in the jugular foramen with intracranial extension. **a** Axial T1WI, FS, +C. **b** Sagittal T1WI, FS, +C.

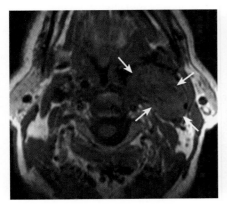

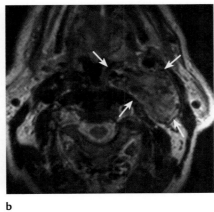

Fig. 6.**12** **Glomus vagale tumor.** A lesion (arrows) is seen with small foci of flow void caused by enlarged tumor vessels. The lesion depicts low signal intensity in (**a**) (T1WI) and intermediate signal intensity in (**b**) (T2WI).

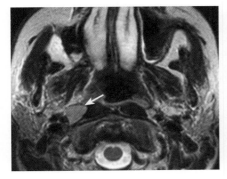

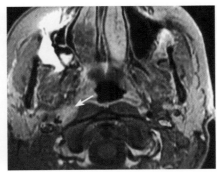

Fig. 6.**13** **Carotid body tumor.** A small bullet-shaped lesion (arrow) is seen at the carotid bifurcation with relatively high signal intensity in (**a**) (T2WI) and marked contrast enhancement in (**b**) (T1WI, +C).

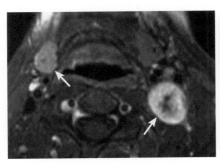

Fig. 6.**14** **Squamous cell carcinoma metastases with unknown primary.** Two enlarged lymph nodes (arrows) are seen, the larger right deep cervical node depicting a necrotic center (T1WI, FS, +C).

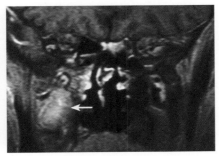

Fig. 6.**15** **Soft-tissue sarcoma metastasis.** An enhancing lesion (arrow) is seen in the masticator space (coronal T1WI, FS, +C).

Table 6.2 (Cont.) Masticator space and carotid space lesions

Disease	MRI Findings	Comments
Bone and soft-tissue sarcomas (Fig. 6.16)	Poorly defined infiltrating mass with low signal intensity on T1WI and heterogeneous high signal intensity on T2WI and usually inhomogeneous contrast enhancement. Mandibular infiltration or frank destruction is common. *Chondrosarcomas* arise from the region of the temporomandibular joint, *osteosarcomas* and *Ewing sarcomas* from any part of the mandible. A *rhabdomyosarcoma* originating in the muscles of mastication is the most common soft-tissue sarcoma.	On CT chondrosarcomas depict chondroid calcifications within the mass, whereas osteosarcomas demonstrate tumorous new bone formation. *Malignant schwannoma* originates from the mandibular branch of the trigeminal nerve and may present as a tubular mass with destruction of the mandibular foramen and canal.
Odontogenic cellulitis and abscess	Swollen masticator space due to inflammation and edema presents with increased signal intensity on T2WI or frank abscess formation with a nonenhancing liquefied center and an enhancing wall. Originates commonly from parodontal and periapical abscess in the mandible that may demonstrate signs of osteomyelitis. Infection may spread cephalad in the masticator space and may eventually cause osteomyelitis of the skull base.	In patients with bad dentition or a history of dental manipulation presenting with trismus. Masticator space cellulitis and abscess formation may also occur as a complication of zygomatic fractures, especially when treated with internal fixation.
Jugular vein thrombophlebitis and thrombosis	In thrombophlebitis the enlarged thrombus-filled vein depicts high signal intensity on both T1WI and T2WI due to methemoglobin formation within the clot. The soft-tissue planes surrounding the jugular vein are inflamed and edematous. After intravenous Gd-DTPA administration the vasa vasorum in the venous wall may enhance intensely. In chronic jugular vein thrombosis the clot may be of low signal intensity due to fibrosis and hemosiderin formation. This finding should not be mistaken for the flow void seen in a normal jugular vein. No enhancement occurs in the thrombosed area of the jugular vein.	Patients present with a tender red neck mass in acute thrombophlebitis or a hard, nontender mass in the chronic thrombotic phase. A history of central venous catheterization, intravenous drug abuse, or malignancy is often available. Normal variations in the jugular vein, ranging from unilateral absence to considerable dilatation with flow void, should not be mistaken for a pathologic process.
Carotid artery lesions (Fig. 6.16*	A mural thrombus or complete thrombosis presents as partial or complete loss of the normal carotid artery flow void. The clot often shows a complex mixture of signal intensities, especially on T1WI because of the different ages of the blood within the clot. Aneurysm and pseudoaneurysm are evident as fusiform or eccentric dilatation with or without mural thrombosis. The demonstration of an internal flap indicative of dissection requires gradient-echo sequences or intravenous administration of Gd-DTPA. MR angiography may display the carotid artery lesion to even greater detail.	Dissection and pseudoaneurysm formation are often sequelae of penetrating trauma or deceleration injury. An *ectatic common* or *internal carotid artery* may present clinically as a pulsatile mass and on MRI as a flow void in a dilated, tortuous, tubular structure that may fold on itself and should not be mistaken for an aneurysm or avascular tumor.

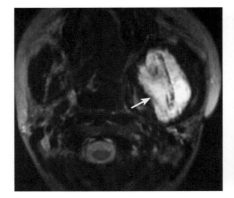

a

Fig. 6.16 Ewing sarcoma of the mandible. a A heterogeneous expansile lesion (arrow) of the left ramus mandibulae is seen with large soft-tissue component and overall increased signal intensity (T2WI, axial).

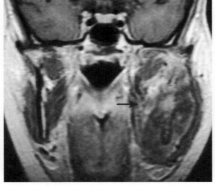

b

b After intravenous Gd-DTPA administration, inhomogeneous enhancement of the lesion (arrow) is seen (T1WI, FS, +C, coronal).

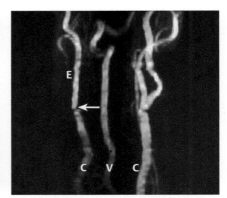

Fig. 6.**16*** **Internal carotid artery occlusion.** MRA: The right internal carotid artery is completely occluded at its take-off (arrow). C. common carotid artery. V: vertebral artery.

Table 6.3 Parotid lesions

Disease	MRI Findings	Comments
First branchial cleft cyst (Fig. 6.17 and 6.17*)	Cystic mass with varying wall thickness depending on the degree of inflammation located either within the parotid gland or around its periphery. The cyst content is usually hypointense on T1WI and hyperintense on T2WI. A proteinaceous cyst content increases the signal intensity on T1WI. After intravenous Gd-DTPA administration the cyst wall enhances.	Occurs most often in middle-aged women, presenting with history of "multiple parotid abscesses unresponsive to treatment." Otorrhea may be present when the cyst connects with the external auditory canal. An external sinus opening is occasionally seen at the angle of the mandible.
Capillary hemangioma	Poorly marginated lobulated mass with heterogeneous signal intensity that is usually low on T1WI and high on T2WI. Prior hemorrhages may increase the signal intensity on T1WI. After intravenous Gd-DTPA, contrast enhancement is pronounced.	The lesion is usually discovered shortly after birth as a soft and compressible tumor in the area of the parotid gland with bluish discoloration of the overlying skin. Rapid enlargement can occur in the first year of life; may then regress spontaneously.
Cystic lymphangioma (hygroma) (Fig. 6.18)	Thin-walled multiloculated cystic lesion with low signal intensity on T1WI and high signal intensity on T2WI involving the parotid gland. Fluid-fluid levels may be present and are best seen on T2WI. Intracystic hemorrhage and infections may complicate the lesion and alter the signal characteristics of the cystic content. Minimal contrast enhancement of the cyst walls unless they are thickened by infection.	Lymphangiomas are classified into simple (capillary), cavernous, and cystic subtypes. Cystic lymphangioma is by far the most common subtype in the neck. Ninety percent are diagnosed before the age of 3. Spontaneous involution does not occur. Sudden enlargement is associated with either hemorrhage or infection. Cystic lymphangiomas rarely occur in adulthood and may be post-traumatic.

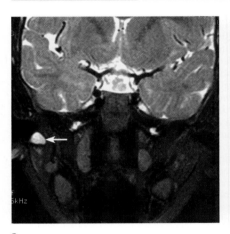

a

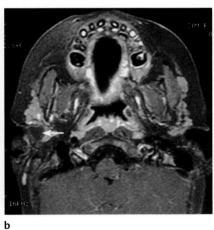

b

Fig. 6.**17** **First branchial cleft cyst.** A hyperintense cystic lesion (arrow) is seen in **a** projecting between the external auditory canal and parotid gland (T2WI, coronal).

After intravenous Gd-DTPA administration contrast enhancement is limited to the wall (arrow) of the cyst (**b**: T1WI, FS, +C, axial).

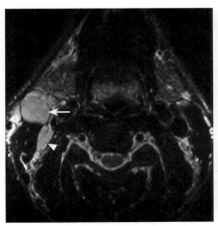

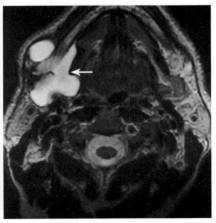

Fig. 6.**17*** **Infected first branchial cleft cyst.** An infected cyst (arrow) with fistula (arrowhead) is seen in the posterior aspect of the left parotid gland (T2WI).

Fig. 6.**18** **Cystic lymphangioma.** A multiloculated cystic lesion (arrow) with high signal intensity is seen in the right parotid

Table 6.3 (Cont.) Parotid lesions

Disease	MRI Findings	Comments
Pleomorphic adenoma (Fig. 6.19)	Sharply marginated round or lobulated mass with fairly homogeneous signal intensity that is low on T1WI and high on T2WI. A low signal intensity "capsule" is often seen on T2WI. The signal intensity of larger tumors becomes inhomogeneous, with areas of hemorrhage appearing hyperintense on both T1WI and T2WI and regions of necrosis or cystic degeneration usually hypointense on T1WI and hyperintense on T2WI. Contrast enhancement is variable but moderate at best.	Most common benign parotid tumor (80%) consisting of a mixture of epithelial and myoepithelial cells and usually presenting in patients over 50 years of age with a slow-growing mass in the cheek. Dystrophic calcifications are occasionally seen radiographically. Malignant degeneration of pleomorphic adenomas may reach 25% when left untreated.
Warthin's tumor (papillary cystadenoma lymphomatosum) (Fig. 6.20)	Small (less than 4 cm in diameter), ovoid, smoothly marginated, solid and/or cystic lesion frequently located in the tail (posterior superficial lobe) of the pancreas. Solid tumors have similar signal characteristics as small pleomorphic adenomas, but tend to be more heterogeneous. Compared with their solid counterparts, cystic lesions have decreased signal intensity on T1WI and increased signal intensity on T2WI. Contrast enhancement is minimal to moderate and limited to the noncystic components. Larger lesions may project outside of the normal gland contour. Multiple lesions in one parotid gland (30%) and bilateral involvement (10%) occur.	Second most common parotid tumor (10%). Arises from heterotopic salivary gland tissue within parotid lymph nodes. Presents in patients over 40 years of age, with male predominance, as a slow-growing mass in the parotid tail region. Other benign parotid gland tumors include *oncocytoma, clear cell adenoma, basal cell adenoma*, and *sebaceous lymphadenoma*. *Facial nerve schwannoma* (Fig. 6.21) or *neurofibroma* and *lipomas* occur also in the parotid gland.
Parotid carcinoma (Figs. 6.22–6.24)	Findings depend on the degree of malignancy. *Low-grade carcinomas* cannot be differentiated from pleomorphic adenomas presenting with well-delineated smooth borders, low signal intensity on T1WI and high signal intensity on T2WI. Hemorrhagic, necrotic, and cystic changes may be present and alter the signal characteristics accordingly. *High-grade carcinomas* have indistinct infiltrating margins and tend to be solid with intermediate signal intensity on both T1WI and T2WI. Besides metastasizing to subcutaneous tissues, lymph nodes, bone, and lung, perineural tumor spread along the facial nerve occurs.	Presents at any age including childhood (peak range 20–50 years) with hard parotid mass and pain or itching in the facial nerve distribution. Facial nerve paralysis is an ominous sign. *Mucoepidermoid carcinoma* is the most common malignant lesion of the parotid gland. *Adenoid cystic carcinoma* has the greatest propensity for perineural tumor spread. *Acinic cell carcinoma* may be multiple and/or bilateral. *Malignant mixed tumor* (carcinoma ex-pleomorphic adenoma) is associated with a (benign) pleomorphic adenoma. TNM staging of salivary glands: T1 Tumor <2 cm T2 Tumor 2–4 cm T3 Tumor 4–6 cm T4 Tumor >6 cm N1 Single ipsilateral node <3 cm N2 Single ipsilateral node 3–6 cm or multiple nodes <6 cm N3 Node(s) >6 cm

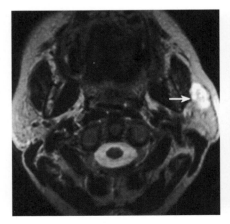

a

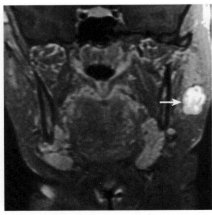

b

Fig. 6.19 Pleomorphic adenoma. A heterogeneous hyperintense lesion (arrow) is seen in the left parotid gland in (**a**) (T2WI). After intravenous Gd-DTPA administration, inhomogeneous enhancement of the lesion (arrow) is seen in (**b**) (coronal T1WI, FS, +C).

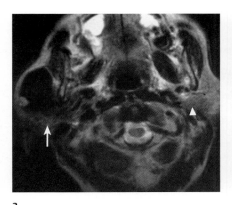

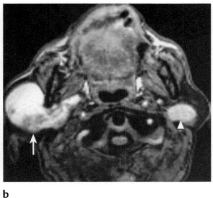

a

b

Fig. 6.**20** **Warthin's tumor.** A predominantly cystic lesions (arrow) is seen in the tail of the right parotid gland and appears hypointense in (**a**) (T1WI) and hyperintense in (**b**) (T2WI). A smaller lesion (arrowhead) is evident in the left parotid gland.

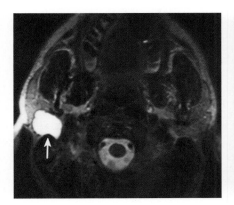

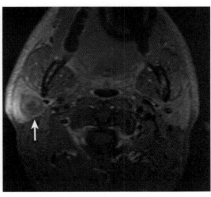

a

b

Fig. 6.**21** **Facial nerve schwannoma.** A lesion (arrow) is seen within the right parotid gland with uniformly low signal intensity on T1WI (not shown), high signal intensity on T2WI (**a**), and ring enhancement after intravenous Gd-DTPA administration in (**b**) (T1WI, FS, +C).

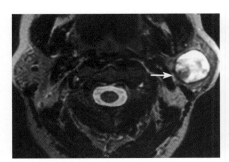

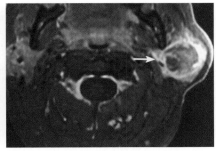

a

b

Fig. 6.**22** **Mucoepidermoid parotid carcinoma.** **a** A large left parotid lesion (arrow) with necrotic hyperintense center is seen on T2WI. **b** After intravenous Gd-DTPA administration, contrast enhancement in the periphery of the necrotic center is seen (T1WI, FS, +C).

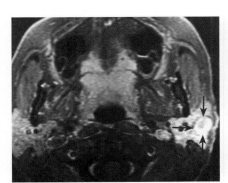

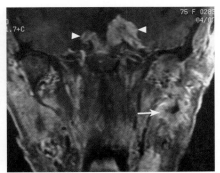

Fig. 6.**23** **Parotid carcinoma.** After intravenous Gd-DTPA administration a small nodule (arrows) with hypointense center is seen (T1WI, FS, +C). The lesion cannot be differentiated from a pleomorphic adenoma.

Fig. 6.**24** **Parotid carcinoma with perineural intracranial metastasis.** After intravenous Gd-DTPA administration a left parotid lesion (arrow) is seen with peripheral enhancement and central necrosis in the left parotid gland. Perineural tumor spread resulted in an intracranial metastasis (arrowheads) with the same signal characteristics as the primary lesion (coronal T1WI, FS, +C).

Table 6.3 (Cont.) Parotid lesions

Disease	MRI Findings	Comments
Parotid metastases and lymphoma	Single or multiple focal lesions or diffuse enlargement and infiltration of entire gland with usually homogeneous and intermediate signal intensity on both T1WI and T2WI. Inhomogeneous signal intensity due to central necrosis is frequently seen with squamous cell carcinoma metastases. Intraparotid lymphadenopathy caused by inflammation or infection tends to have a higher signal intensity on T2WI than neoplastic adenopathy.	Intraparotid and periparotid lymph nodes drain the external ear and part of the ipsilateral scalp and face. Melanomas and squamous cell carcinomas located in these areas frequently metastasize to the parotid gland. Carcinomas of the mouth, pharynx, and sinuses can also metastasize to the intraglandular parotid lymph nodes. Hematogenous metastases from carcinomas of lung, kidney, and breast rarely occur.
Acute suppurative parotitis and abscess formation (Fig. 6.25)	Unilateral enlargement of the parotid gland with increased signal intensity on T2WI and blurring of the normally seen internal architecture of the gland. Because of inflammatory and edematous changes in the surrounding tissue the parotid gland is poorly demarcated. Marked contrast enhancement occurs after intravenous Gd-DTPA administration. An intraglandular abscess is diagnosed by its enhancing wall and the nonenhancing liquefied center.	Patients present with acute, unilateral, painful swelling of the parotid gland. Purulent exudate may be evident in the buccal orifice of Stensen's duct. The most common offending agents include staphylococci, streptococci, pneumococci, haemophilus, and escherichia coli. Bacterial parotitis must be differentiated from endemic parotitis or mumps, which is bilateral and caused by an RNA virus of the paramyxovirus group.
Chronic recurrent parotitis	Unilaterally enlarged parotid gland with heterogeneous signal intensity that is low on T1WI and intermediate to high on T2WI. After intravenous Gd-DTPA administration, moderate, nonuniform contrast enhancement is seen.	Presents with recurrent painful swelling of the parotid gland. Focal stricture of Stensen's duct with or without calculus and prestenotic sialectasis is evident on sialograms.
Granulomatous parotitis	Multiple small nodules distributed throughout the gland or a solitary mass is seen in a diffusely enlarged parotid gland. Compared with the normal parotid tissue, the intraglandular nodules or mass are hypointense on T1WI and hyperintense on T2WI. The involvement is unilateral or, less commonly, bilateral.	Presents as progressive painless glandular enlargement. Associated with *tuberculosis, syphilis, cat-scratch fever*, or *actinomycosis*. In *sarcoidosis* it may be associated with uveitis and facial nerve paralysis (*Heerfordt syndrome*).
Sialosis and sialadenosis	Bilateral, slightly enlarged parotid glands due to fatty replacement and/or fibrosis of the interlobular septa. Depending on the dominant underlying process, signal intensity is increased with fatty replacement on T1WI or decreased with fibrosis on both T1WI and T2WI.	Non-neoplastic, noninflammatory, nontender, chronic or recurrent enlargement of the parotid glands. May be caused by cirrhosis, alcoholism, diabetes, malnutrition, hormonal imbalance, and a variety of drugs. In *postirradiation sialadenitis* a smaller than normal parotid gland with fibrosis is seen.
Sjögren syndrome (Fig. 6.26)	Unilateral or, more commonly, bilateral enlarged parotid glands. Dilatation of the most peripheral intraglandular ducts and acini with uniform distribution measuring one to a few millimeters and presenting with discrete collections of low signal intensity on T1WI and high signal intensity on T2WI. Sialogram reveals a normal central duct system and numerous punctate contrast material collections.	*Primary*: Sicca syndrome (Mikulicz disease) presents with xerostomia, xerorhinia, and keratoconjunctivitis sicca and is usually seen in middle-aged females or as recurrent parotitis in children. *Secondary*: Associated with rheumatoid arthritis or other connective-tissue disorders, AIDS, or graft-versus-host disease. Associated with increased risk of developing lymphoma in intraparotid or extraparotid sites.
Lymphoepithelial cysts (lesions) in AIDS (Fig. 6.27)	Usually bilateral parotid gland enlargement with intraglandular cysts, hypointense on T1WI and hyperintense on T2WI and varying in size from a few millimeters to several centimeters (rare). Intraparotid lymph nodes may also be enlarged. Cervical lymphadenopathy caused by reactive hyperplasia is almost invariably associated.	Lymphoepithelial cysts in the parotid gland may be secondary to incomplete ductal obstruction by periductal lymphocytic infiltration or arise within the intraparotid lymph nodes. Occurs in HIV positive patients and may be the first manifestation of the disease.

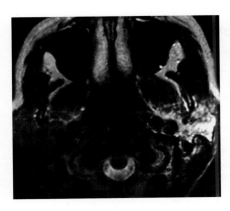

Fig. 6.**25** **Acute suppurative parotitis.** Inflammatory and edematous changes in the left parotid gland produce an increase in signal intensity and blurring of the normal structures (T2WI).

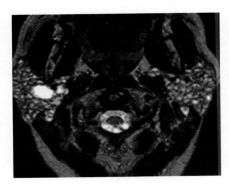

Fig. 6.**26** **Sjögren syndrome.** Bilateral enlarged parotid glands with uniformly distributed, tiny, hyperintense cystic lesions in both glands (T2WI). The larger solitary cystic lesion in the right parotid gland is not typical for Sjögren syndrome and probably unrelated.

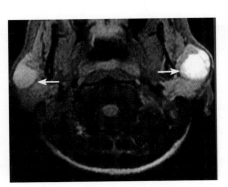

Fig. 6.**27** **Lymphoepithelial cysts (lesions) in AIDS.** Bilateral hyperintense lesions (arrows) are seen in the slightly enlarged parotid glands (PDWI, FS).

Table 6.4 Lesions in the oral cavity, sublingual space, and submandibular space

Disease	MRI Findings	Comments
Pedunculated parotid lesion	A pedunculated parotid mass or cyst may be located in the mandibular angle area and mimic a posterior submandibular space lesion.	Frequently pedunculated parotid lesions include Warthin's tumor (may be cystic), pleomorphic adenoma, and first branchial cleft cyst (may be associated with sinus tract opening in overlying skin).
Second branchial cleft cyst (Fig. 6.28)	Unilocular cystic mass with thin wall, low signal intensity on T1WI and high signal intensity on T2WI. After infection the cyst wall becomes thicker and often irregular and the signal intensity of the cyst content may increase on T1WI. Contrast enhancement is limited to the cyst wall. Most common location is near the angle of the mandible displacing the submandibular gland anteromedially, the sternocleidomastoid muscle posterolaterally, and the carotid artery and jugular vein posteromedially. A beak on the cyst pointing medially between internal and external carotid arteries is pathognomonic when present.	Second branchial cleft anomalies represent 95% of all branchial disorders, and cysts are far more common than sinuses and fistulas. Twenty percent are diagnosed in infants and young children and 75% in patients between 20 and 40 years old, usually after a respiratory infection clinically mimicking a suppurative jugulodigastric lymphadenitis. A second branchial cleft cyst may be associated with a fistula that opens into the tonsillar fossa. The fistula may descend along the anterior border of the sternocleidomastoid muscle and may open onto the skin anywhere along this path, frequently just above the clavicle.
Thyroglossal duct cyst (suprahyoid) (Fig. 6.29)	Cystic mass in the midline or paramedian location, extending from the hyoid bone region upward into the submandibular space.	Presents as a midline mass in the suprahyoid region with fullness in the floor of the mouth. Only 20% of thyroglossal duct cysts are suprahyoid, the rest are hyoid (15%) and infrahyoid (65%).
Lingual thyroid	Lobular midline mass extending from the tongue base (foramen cecum) into the sublingual space. Signal intensity of the thyroid tissue is intermediate on both T1WI and T2WI and similar to the tongue musculature. The lingual thyroid is best delineated after intravenous Gd-DTPA administration, since it enhances considerably more than the tongue.	Normal undescended thyroid tissue found more commonly in females and becoming mildly symptomatic during adolescence in 80% of cases. In addition to the base of the tongue, ectopic thyroid tissue of the neck can be found anywhere along the path of the thyroglossal duct.
Cystic lymphangioma (hygroma) (Fig. 6.30)	Cystic, often multilocular lesion with or without fluid levels, more commonly in the submandibular than sublingual space. May extend posteriorly from the submandibular into the sublingual space or anteriorly into the contralateral submandibular space. The cystic lesions appear hypointense on T1WI and hyperintense on T2WI with focal inhomogeneities corresponding to fibrous septae.	Submandibular and sublingual spaces are relatively common locations in adults, although 90% of all lymphangiomas are clinically apparent before the age of 3 years with predilection for the left posterior triangle of the neck bordered by sternocleidomastoid and trapezius muscles and clavicle. Simple (capillary) and cavernous lymphangiomas are less common at these sites.
Capillary hemangioma	Poorly marginated heterogeneous lesion in the sublingual or submandibular space with low signal intensity on T1WI and high signal intensity on T2WI; marked inhomogeneous contrast enhancement.	In infants, often increases in size during the first 10 months of life and then usually begins to involute spontaneously.
Cavernous hemangioma (Fig. 6.31)	Rounded or lobulated mass appearing as poorly marginated and uniformly hypointense on T1WI and well-marginated, heterogeneous and hyperintense on T2WI. Intense homogeneous or inhomogeneous (when partially thrombosed) contrast enhancement occurs after intravenous Gd-DTPA administration.	Usually diagnosed in the second to fourth decades of life with female predilection. Radiographically small phleboliths within the lesion are occasionally seen and are virtually diagnostic.
Lipoma	Homogeneous nonenhancing fatty lesion with high signal intensity on T1WI and intermediate signal intensity on T2WI occurring in the cheek, tongue (usually within the oral part), sublingual and submandibular space.	Often incidental findings. In the submandibular space they are occasionally mistaken on clinical examination for an enlarged lymph node (e.g., during staging of squamous cell carcinoma).

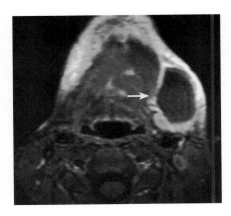

Fig. 6.**28** **Second branchial cleft cyst.**
After intravenous Gd-DTPA administration
a hypointense, unilocular, cystic lesion
(arrow) with contrast enhancement limited
to the cyst wall is seen near the mandibular angle (T1WI, FS, +C).

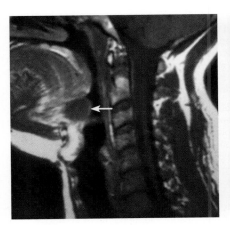

a

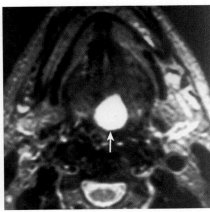

b

Fig. 6.**29** **Thyroglossal duct cyst.** A cystic
lesion (arrow) at the foramen cecum of the
tongue is seen presenting with uniformly
low signal intensity in (**a**) (T1WI, sagittal)
and high signal intensity in (**b**) (T2WI,
axial).

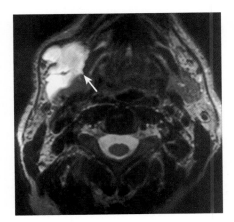

Fig. 6.**30** **Cystic lymphangioma.** A multilocular cystic lesion (arrow) is seen (T2WI).

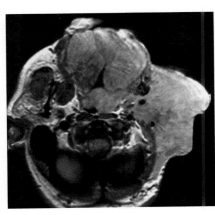

a

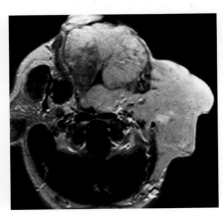

b

Fig. 6.**31** **Cavernous hemangioma.** **a** An extensive, well-defined and
slightly inhomogeneous lesion is seen involving the oral cavity and left side of the
face (PDWI). **b** After intravenous Gd-
DTPA administration the lesion enhances
markedly (T1WI, +C).

Table 6.4 (Cont.) Lesions in the oral cavity, sublingual space, and submandibular space

Disease	MRI Findings	Comments
Epidermoid and dermoid (Figs. 6.32 and 6.33)	Usually located in the floor of the mouth (sublingual or submandibular space), occasionally in lips, tongue, and buccal mucosa. Epidermoids are cystic lesions of low signal intensity on T1WI and high signal intensity on T2WI. Dermoids are at least partially hyperintense on T1WI due to a variable amount of fat and hemorrhage (methemoglobin). The cyst wall of both lesions frequently enhances after intravenous Gd-DTPA administration.	Present as a slow-growing mass most commonly located in the anterior aspect of the floor of the mouth. Usually diagnosed in the second or third decade of life. Epidermoids are cysts with a fibrous wall lined by simple squamous epithelium. Dermoids have, in addition, a variable number of skin appendages such as hair follicles and sebaceous glands.
Pleomorphic adenoma	Well-circumscribed mass originating in the submandibular or, less commonly, sublingual salivary gland. The signal intensity is fairly homogeneous, low on T1WI and high on T2WI. Hemorrhage and cystic necrosis may complicate larger lesions.	Presents as slow-growing mass in the submandibular or sublingual space.
Sublingual and submandibular gland carcinomas (Fig. 6.34)	Low-grade carcinomas cannot be differentiated from pleomorphic adenomas. High-grade carcinomas have indistinct infiltrating margins and tend to be solid with intermediate signal intensity on both T1WI and T2WI.	Adenoid cystic carcinomas are the most common malignancy in these locations, followed by mucoepidermoid carcinomas. Primary sublingual tumors are malignant in 70%, submandibular tumors in 60%, whereas parotid tumors are only malignant in 20% of cases.
Oral cavity carcinoma (Fig. 6.35)	Poorly marginated infiltrative mass with distortion of normal structures and surrounding fat planes. The tumor tends to be isointense to muscle on T1WI and hyperintense on T2WI. After intravenous Gd-DTPA administration the contrast enhancement is variable but more than the surrounding musculature. Mandibular involvement is frequent and may be demonstrated on T1WI by replacement of bone marrow, even in the absence of cortical destruction. Carcinomas of the oral tongue spread along the intrinsic muscle to the floor of the mouth. Carcinomas of the base of the tongue invade the floor of the mouth from posterior to anterior. Carcinomas originating in the floor of the mouth tend to spread in all directions. Regional lymph nodes include submental, submandibular, and internal jugular nodes.	Squamous cell carcinomas represent over 90% of malignant lesions in the oral cavity. They commonly present in middle-aged men with a long history of alcohol and tobacco abuse and tend to affect the dependent portions of the oral cavity. Regional lymph nodes are involved in almost half the patients at the time of initial presentation. Carcinomas of the oral cavity originate in the lower lip (38%), tongue (22%), floor of the mouth (17%), gingiva (6%), palate (5%), upper lip (4%), buccal mucosa (2%), and other areas (6%).

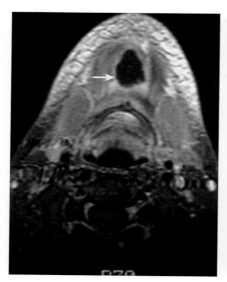

a

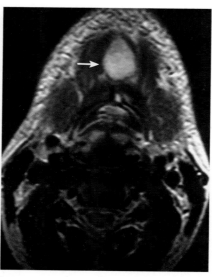

b

Fig. 6.32 Epidermoid. A small cystic midline lesion (arrow) is seen in the tongue presenting with low signal intensity and without contrast enhancement in (**a**) (T1WI, FS, +C) and high signal intensity in (**b**) (T2WI).

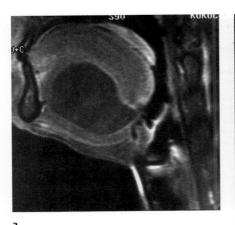
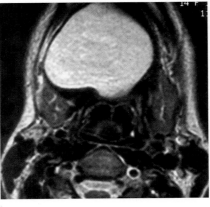

a

b

Fig. 6.**33**   **Dermoid.** A large cystic lesion is seen in the floor of the mouth presenting with a somewhat cloudy hypointense cystic content in (**a**) (sagittal T1WI, FS, +C) and isointense to subcutaneous fat in (**b**) (T2WI, axial).

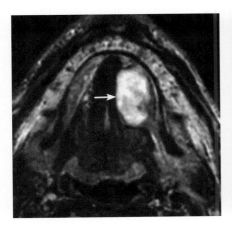
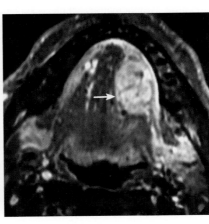

a

b

Fig. 6.**34**   **Sublingual carcinoma.   a** An inhomogeneous, hyperintense lesion (arrow) originates from a left sublingual gland (T2WI) and   **b** enhances considerably after intravenous GD-DTPA administration (T1WI, FS, +C).

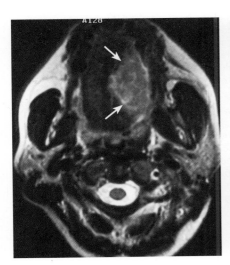
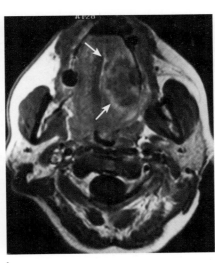

a

b

Fig. 6.**35**   **Carcinoma of the tongue.   a** A poorly defined, heterogeneous lesion (arrows) with increased signal intensity is seen in the left side of the tongue (T2WI).   **b** After intravenous Gd-DTPA administration moderate inhomogeneous enhancement of the lesion (arrows) is evident (T1WI, +C).

Table **6.4** (Cont.) Lesions in the oral cavity, sublingual space, and submandibular space

Disease	MRI Findings	Comments
Tonsillar carcinoma (Fig. 6.36)	Poorly marginated, infiltrating mass. Originates from the anterior tonsillar pillar or the tonsil itself, with invasion of the surrounding tissue planes and a tendency to spread inferiorly to the base of the tongue and floor of the mouth, posterolaterally into the parapharyngeal space, laterally to the pterygoid muscles, and superiorly into the nasopharynx. The tumor demonstrates low signal intensity on T1WI, high signal intensity on T2WI, and moderate contrast enhancement. Lymphatic spread occurs to submandibular, deep jugular, and retropharyngeal lymph nodes.	Tonsillar carcinoma is the most common malignancy of the oropharynx and usually of squamous cell origin. Presents most often in elderly men with mild sore throat and a history of cigarette and alcohol abuse. Seventy-five percent of patients have regional lymph node metastases at the time of presentation.
Lymph node metastases and lymphoma (Figs. 6.37 and 6.38)	Submental and/or submandibular lymph nodes exceeding 1.5 cm in size are considered malignant. Central necrosis, evident as low signal intensity on T1WI and high signal intensity on T2WI, is frequently seen in squamous cell carcinoma metastases originating from the oral cavity, anterior sinuses, face, and nose. Lymphomatous lymph nodes tend to be larger, usually homogeneous and commonly associated with more widespread cervical lymphadenopathy.	Besides squamous cell carcinoma metastases, central necrotic or cystic changes in lymph nodes may be found in undifferentiated AIDS-related lymphoma, Burkitt lymphoma, and following chemotherapy and/or radiotherapy. In Hodgkin disease a heterogeneous pattern may be seen caused by intranodal granuloma formations. Suppurative adenitis may also produce central nodal necrosis.
Ludwig angina (cellulitis and abscess formation) (Fig. 6.39)	Cellulitis of the sublingual and submandibular space presents as thickening of the overlying skin, inflammatory and edematous changes in the subcutaneous fat and adjacent muscles with obliteration of the corresponding fascial planes. The inflamed, edematous soft tissues demonstrate decreased signal intensity on T1WI, increased signal intensity on T2WI, and marked diffuse contrast enhancement. An abscess is formed when frank nonenhancing pus is surrounded by a markedly enhanced rim representing the abscess wall. Abscesses may be multiloculated and tend to conform to the sublingual or submandibular space. Mandibular osteomyelitis is commonly associated. Enlarged submental and/or submandibular lymph nodes due to inflammation or suppuration, the latter often depicting central necrosis, rarely exceed 1.5 cm in diameter.	Extensive infection of the floor of the mouth precipitated by a mandibular molar extraction or manipulation 2 to 4 days earlier. Cellulitis and abscess formation in the floor of the mouth may also be secondary to suppurative sublingual and particularly submandibular sialadenitis, which are often secondary to ductal stenosis or calculus formation. CT is superior to MRI for identifying possible inciting factors such as a calculus in the submandibular (Wharton's) duct or mandibular osteomyelitis secondary to molar infection.
Sublingual or submandibular sialadenitis (Fig. 6.40)	In acute suppurative sialadenitis inflammatory and edematous changes in an enlarged gland may be associated with intraglandular abscess formation. In both chronic recurrent and granulomatous sialadenitis a mottled signal intensity may be seen with all pulse sequences in an enlarged gland.	Patients with acute sialadenitis present with painful swelling of the involved gland. Chronic recurrent submandibular sialadenitis is typically associated with a calculus and/or focal stenosis in Wharton's duct. Granulomatous sialadenitis is found with tuberculosis, cat-scratch fever, actinomycosis, or sarcoidosis.
Ranula (simple or diving) (Figs. 6.41 and 6.42)	A simple ranula is a sharply marginated, thin-walled, cystic lesion without septation (DD: cystic lymphangioma) conforming to the sublingual space. The cyst content is homogeneous with low signal intensity on T1WI and high signal intensity on T2WI. A diving ranula herniates from the posterior sublingual space into the submandibular space, where the bulk of the cyst is seen, but a characteristic thin extension into the sublingual space ("tail-sign") remains.	A simple ranula is a postinflammatory retention cyst of a sublingual gland with epithelial lining. A diving ranula is an enlarged simple ranula that ruptured out the back of the sublingual space into the submandibular space. It is a pseudocyst since it has no epithelial lining. A retention cyst of the submandibular gland can be differentiated from a diving ranula by the submandibular gland involvement.

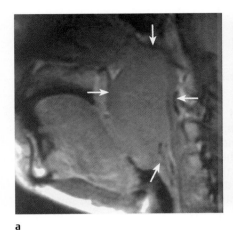

a

Fig. 6.36 Tonsillar carcinoma. a A large mass (arrows) originating from the tonsillar fossa and spreading posteriorly, superiorly, and inferiorly appears homogeneous and isointense to the tongue (T1WI, sagittal). After intravenous Gd-DTPA administration,

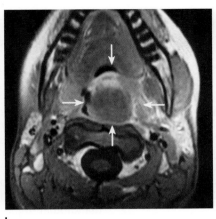

b

contrast enhancement is largely limited to the periphery of the lesion (arrows), whereas the tumor itself enhances only minimally in (**b**) (T1WI, +C, axial).

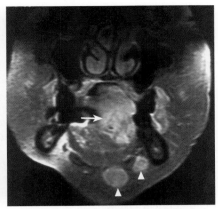

Fig. 6.37 Submandibular lymph node metastases from carcinoma of the tongue (arrow). Two enlarged submandibular lymph nodes (arrowheads) are seen (coronal T1WI, FS, +C).

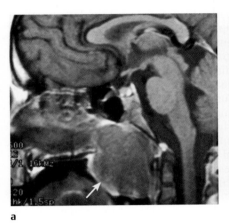

a

Fig. 6.38 Lymphoma. A large bulging mass (arrow) with only minimal contrast enhancement and two markedly enlarged

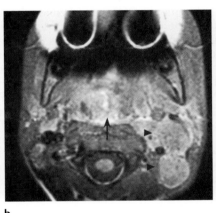

b

lymph nodes (arrowheads) are seen.
a Sagittal T1WI, +C.   **b** Axial T1WI, FS, +C).

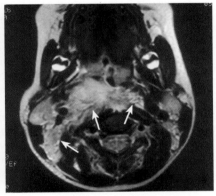

Fig. 6.39 Cellulitis and abscess formation. Inflammatory and edematous changes (arrows) present as poorly defined, inhomogeneous and hyperintense infiltrates (arrows) spreading within different cervical spaces (T2WI).

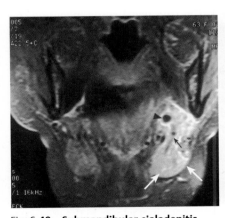

Fig. 6.40 Submandibular sialadenitis secondary to calculus formation in Wharton's duct. An enlarged and markedly enhanced left submandibular gland (long arrows) with obstructed submandibular (Wharton's) duct (short arrow) by a calculus (arrowhead) presenting as signal void is seen after intravenous Gd-DTPA administration (T1WI, FS, +C, coronal).

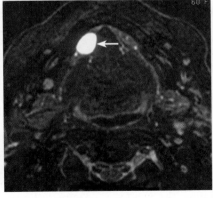

Fig. 6.41 Simple Ranula. A sharply marginated, cystic lesion (arrow) without septation is seen in the sublingual space (T2WI, FS).

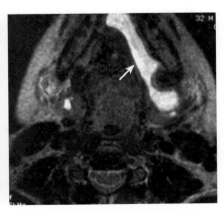

Fig. 6.42 Diving ranula. A cystic lesion (arrow) with homogeneous high signal intensity extends from the sublingual into the submandibular space (T2WI).

7 | Lower Neck, Larynx, and Hypopharynx

The cervical neck from the mandible to the clavicles is divided by the *sternocleidomastoid muscle* into two large triangles, the *anterior* and *posterior triangles*. The anterior triangle contains the *submandibular space*, the *visceral (anterior) space*, the *carotid (lateral) space*, and the *posterior cervical space* (Fig. 7.1). As in the upper neck, these spaces are by and large defined by the three layers of the deep cervical fascia.

The middle layer of the deep cervical fascia envelops the *visceral space* containing the larynx and trachea, the hypopharynx and esophagus, the thyroid and parathyroid glands, the recurrent laryngeal nerves, and the juxtavisceral lymph nodes. The visceral space extends from the hyoid bone to the mediastinum. The *carotid space* is completely encircled by the carotid sheath, which is made up of all three layers of the deep cervical fascia. The carotid space extends from the skull base (jugular foramen) to the aortic arch and in the lower neck contains the common carotid artery, internal jugular vein, vagus nerve, sympathetic chain, and deep cervical lymph nodes.

The *posterior cervical space* represents the lateroposterior compartment of the neck confined anteriorly by the carotid space, medially by the deep layer of the deep cervical fascia enveloping the perivertebral space, and laterally by the superficial layer of the deep cervical fascia. The posterior cervical space extends from a small superior tip at the skull base to the clavicles. When viewed from the side it has the shape of a posteriorly tilted triangle. It contains the spinal accessory nerve, spinal accessory lymph nodes chain, and preaxillary brachial plexus.

The *prevertebral space* is a misnomer, since it is made up of not only the anterior perivertebral space but also its lateral and posterior compartments. It is completely enclosed by the deep or prevertebral layer of the deep cervical fascia. It contains the cervical spine, vertebral arteries and veins, spinal nerves (including the phrenic nerve), and proximal brachial plexus, but no lymph nodes.

The *retropharyngeal space* is sandwiched between the visceral space anteriorly and the prevertebral space posteriorly and extends from the skull base to the third thoracic vertebral body. Retropharyngeal lymph nodes are only present in the suprahyoid portion of the retropharyngeal space, whereas the infrahyoid portion of the retropharyngeal space only contains fat.

The *deep cervical (internal jugular) lymph nodes* are the most important group of the lower neck. They are confined to the carotid space and divided into the upper, middle, and lower groups. The most prominent node is the *jugulodigastric node* located at the intersection between the posterior belly of the digastric muscle and the internal jugular vein. This level is also the boundary between the upper and middle deep cervical lymph nodes. The *juguloomohyoid node* is located at the crossing of the omohyoid muscle and the jugular vein, dividing the middle from the lower deep cervical group. The *superficial cervical lymph nodes* extend along the external jugular vein superficial to the sternocleidomastoid muscle. The *spinal accessory (posterior cervical) lymph node chain* runs along the spinal accessory nerve and lies in the posterior cervical space just behind the carotid space. *Prelaryngeal, paratracheal*, and *paraesophageal lymph nodes* are all located in the visceral space. Both *submental* and *submandibular lymph nodes* are contained within the submandibular space. The former are located between the anterior bellies of the digastric muscles, and the latter surround the submandibular glands and extend from the middle of the mandibular rami to the mandibular angles.

The *deep cervical lymph nodes* are located in the proximity of the internal jugular vein and carotid artery. Tributaries to these vessels demonstrate flow void on spin-echo (SE) sequences and can be differentiated from lymph nodes depicting intermediate signal intensity on all pulse sequences and only moderate contrast enhancement. Deep cervical lymph nodes normally measure 1 cm or less in their longest diameter, with the exception of the jugulodigastric node that can measure up to 1.2 cm. Inflammation of the cervical lymph nodes secondary to pharyngitis and tonsillitis is frequent, causing a benign nodal enlargement that is often referred to as reactive lymph node hyperplasia. In this condition the cervical lymph nodes may attain a maximum diameter of 1.5 cm and only in exceptional cases are longer. Furthermore, the lymph nodes maintain their oval shape and homogeneous internal architecture. When the cervical lymph nodes exceed 1.5 cm in diameter, metastatic or lymphomatous involvement is suspected. Generalized central necrosis in cervical lymph nodes presenting with decreased signal intensity on T1WI and increased signal intensity on T2WI is always abnormal, regardless of the lymph node size. In the neck it is most commonly caused by either metastases from a squamous cell carcinoma or by an aggressive infection (suppurative adenopathy).

The *larynx* can be divided into three compartments. The *supraglottis* extends from the tip of the epiglottis to the laryngeal ventricles and contains the epiglottis, aryepiglottic folds, arytenoid cartilages, and false vocal cords. The *glottis* is composed of the true vocal cords including the anterior and posterior commissures. The *subglottis* extends from the undersurface of the true vocal cords to the inferior surface of the cricoid cartilage. The thyroid, cricoid, and greater part of arythenoids consist of hyaline cartilage with high signal intensity on T2WI before they become progressively ossified with advancing age. The epiglottis, apices of arythenoids, corniculate and cuneiform cartilages consist of elastic fibrocartilage with little tendency to calcification.

Of malignant larynx tumors, 98% are squamous cell carcinomas. Approximately one-third originate in the supraglottis, two-thirds in the glottis, and a small fraction (5%) in the subglottis.

Supraglottic carcinomas have metastases in the deep cervical lymph nodes at the time of presentation in over half of all cases. Epiglottic carcinomas grow circumferentially and spread initially into the pre-epiglottic space and subsequently into the base of the tongue above and the periglottic space below. Carcinomas of the aryepiglottic folds (marginal supraglottic carcinomas) grow exophytically, invading the epiglottis medially and the periglottic space inferiorly. False vocal cord and laryngeal ventricle carcinomas initially spread submucosally into the periglottic space with subsequent destruction of the thyroid cartilage and invasion of the true vocal cords and the subglottis.

Glottic (vocal cord) carcinomas spread anteriorly into the anterior commissure; posteriorly into the posterior commissure, arytenoid cartilage, and cricoarytenoid joints; inferiorly into the subglottis; and superiorly into the periglottic space. The anterior commissure represents the midline anterior meeting point of the true vocal cords. On MRI less than 1 mm of tissue should be discernible at this location. A soft-tissue density in excess of 1 mm at the anterior commissure is indicative of malignant invasion. The posterior commissure is the mucosal surface on the anterior surface of the cricoid cartilage between the arytenoid cartilages. The soft tissues in the posterior commissure should not exceed 1 mm on quiet respiration.

The rare *subglottic carcinoma* is well visualized with MRI because of the absence of normal soft tissue between the cricoid cartilage and the airway below the true vocal cords. Any soft tissue visualized in this area is abnormal. Subglottic tumors frequently spread to the hypopharynx, trachea, and thyroid gland. It has to be emphasized that subglottic extension of a glottic or even supraglottic tumor is much more common than a primary lesion arising in the subglottis.

Laryngeal injuries iatrogenic or caused by blunt or penetrating trauma. Evaluation of injury to the larynx is the domain of computed tomography (CT) despite the improved ability of MRI to discern various soft tissues. The appearance of laryngeal cartilage varies considerably, depending on the degree of ossification and the amount of fatty marrow in its ossified medullary region. Subcutaneous emphysema indicative of a mucosal tear, soft-tissue hematoma, and airway obstruction are readily diagnosed by MRI.

Supraglottic injuries may involve hyoid bone, epiglottis, thyroid cartilage, and aryepiglottic folds. Fractures of the hyoid bone are better delineated by CT than MRI. Laceration or avulsion of the epiglottis, the latter associated with rupture of the thyroepiglottic ligament, may be associated with thyroid cartilage fractures. A longitudinal fracture of the thyroid cartilage is the most common type of injury, but transverse, oblique, and comminuted fractures occur also. A late sequela of a longitudinal thyroid cartilage fracture may present as overlap of the thyroid ala at the original fracture site associated with larynx located slightly off midline. An aryepiglottic fold hematoma suggests cricoarytenoid joint disruption.

In *glottic injuries* avulsion and deep laceration of the vocal cord, fixation of the arytenoid cartilage by hematoma, or dislocation of the arytenoid cartilage in an anterior or anterosuperior direction may be evident on MRI. The anterior arytenoid dislocation can mimic a paralyzed vocal cord on both physical examination and radiologic imaging studies.

The most common *subglottic injury* is a fracture of the cricoid cartilage that is often associated with immediate, severe airway obstruction. Since the cricoid cartilage is the only complete cartilaginous ring in the airway, fractures occur in two places. Dislocation of the cricothyroid joint, seen on MRI as widening of the cricothyroid space, is often associated with injury to the recurrent laryngeal nerve. Rarely the trachea may be severed from the larynx.

The *hypopharynx* consists of three major components. The *pyriform sinus* looks like two symmetric stalactites

hanging from the hypopharynx behind the larynx. The *postcricoid hypopharynx* (pharyngoesophageal junction) extends from the level of the arytenoid cartilages to the inferior border of the cricoid cartilage. The *posterior pharyngeal wall* extends from the level of the valleculae to the level of the cricoarytenoid joints.

Carcinomas of the hypopharynx are most common in the pyriform sinus (60%), followed by the postcricoid areas (25%) and the posterior pharyngeal wall (15%). Histologically the majority are squamous cell carcinomas. They usually occur in men with a history of tobacco and alcohol abuse. Hypopharyngeal carcinoma occasionally complicates *Plummer-Vinson syndrome* that occurs more frequently in women and is characterized by atrophic mucosa, achlorhydria, and sideropenic anemia.

The *pyriform sinus carcinoma* tends to spread posterolaterally into the soft tissues of the neck and frequently destroys the posterior aspect of the ipsilateral thyroid cartilage ala. At presentation 50% of patients already have nodal metastases. In the case of malignant cervical adenopathy with unknown primary, the piriform sinus is, besides the nasopharynx and the Waldeyer's lymphatic ring (lingual and palatine tonsil area), a common location where the primary tumor may hide.

The *postcricoid carcinoma* carries the worst prognosis of all hypopharyngeal carcinomas. The inherent signal intensity difference between tumor and adjacent prevertebral and inferior constrictor muscles with greatly variable thickness may at times be insufficient for accurate tumor delineation and require contrast enhancement with fat suppressed imaging sequences.

The *posterior pharyngeal wall carcinoma* invades the retropharyngeal space early and spreads in both cephalad and caudad directions. The retropharyngeal lymph nodes, which are only found above the hyoid bone, are frequently the sole cervical lymph nodes involved.

Thyroid lesions are primarily evaluated with radionuclide scanning and ultrasonography. On MRI the normal thyroid parenchyma has intermediate intensity on T1WI and T2WI. Regions of high signal intensity on T1WI usually are due to either hemorrhage or colloid cyst. Diffuse increase in signal intensity on both T1WI and T2WI is found in Graves disease and occasionally in de Quervain thyroiditis. A focal homogeneous or heterogeneous increase in signal intensity is seen on T2WI with nearly all lesions, including benign adenomas and carcinomas. Cystic areas in the thyroid are found with noncolloid and colloid cysts (especially in goiters), intranodular hemorrhage, liquefaction necrosis in neoplasm, and abscess formation. Nodular, cystic, or diffuse enlargement of the thyroid gland is referred to as goiter. Calcifications are evident as foci devoid of signal on MRI, but are better appreciated with CT. Dystrophic calcifications occur with similar frequency in benign (11%) and malignant (17%) lesions. Psammoma bodies (peripheral punctate or linear microcalcifications) are common in papillary carcinomas.

The differential diagnosis of lesions of the visceral space is discussed in Table 7.1, laryngeal lesions in Table 7.2, thyroid gland lesions in Table 7.3, and lesions of both the lower neck carotid space and posterior cervical space in Table 7.4.

Table 7.1 Lesions in the visceral space

Disease	MRI Findings	Comments
Laryngeal lesions	See Table 7.2	See Table 7.2
Thyroid gland lesions	See Table 7.3	See Table 7.3
Cervical thymic cyst	Usually unilateral, unilocular cyst. Located anywhere below the mandibular angle in the anterior mid and lower neck extending parallel to the sternocleidomastoid muscle with or without continuation into the anterior mediastinum.	Forms along the migratory tract of thymic tissue into the mediastinum. Presents usually in childhood as an asymptomatic, slow-growing mass. When in contact with the thyroid, it may be indistinguishable from a thyroidal cyst.
Thyroglossal duct cyst (Fig. 7.2)	Midline or paramedian, anterior 2–4 cm cystic lesion above (20%), at (15%), or just below (65%) the hyoid bone. The latter is nestled in the infrahyoid strap muscles that appear to "beak" over the edges of the cyst. It may bulge into the pre-epiglottis and displace the epiglottis posteriorly.	Develops anywhere within the thyroglossal duct along which the thyroid gland descends from the foramen cecum in the base of the tongue through the area anterior to the hyoid bone to its final lower neck location.
Parathyroid cyst	Thin-walled, 1–10-cm cystic lesion typically located posterior to the thyroid with compression and displacement of the ipsilateral thyroid lobe anteriorly.	Usually diagnosed in the fourth or fifth decade of life. Large cysts may compress the adjacent trachea, esophagus, and recurrent laryngeal nerve producing hoarseness. Rarely functional, producing hyperparathyroidism.
Parathyroid adenoma (Figs. 7.3–7.4)	Well-defined mass larger than 5 mm in diameter. Typically located between the longus colli muscle posteriorly and the posterior aspect of the thyroid gland lobe anteriorly, or may have an ectopic location. The homogeneous mass depicts low to intermediate signal intensity on T1WI (similar to muscle and thyroid) and high signal intensity on T2WI (isointense or hyperintense to fat). Hyperintensity on T1WI may be seen after intratumoral hemorrhage. Parathyroid carcinoma cannot be differentiated from an adenoma. Ectopic parathyroid adenomas may be difficult to differentiate from normal lymph nodes, since both signal characteristics and enhancement patterns are very similar.	Normal parathyroid glands (5 x 3 x 1 mm) are often not seen on MRI. Most people have four parathyroid glands located behind the upper and lower poles of the thyroid gland. Ectopic glands may be located within the thyroid gland or at any distance below the lower poles of the thyroid gland in the cervicothoracic junction or upper mediastinum. Primary hyperparathyroidism is caused by a solitary adenoma in 85%, multiple adenomas in 4%, diffuse hyperplasia in 10%, and parathyroid carcinoma in 1%.
Hypopharyngeal carcinoma (Fig. 7.5)	Infiltrating mass with signal intensity similar to normal mucosa appearing isointense to muscle on T1WI and hyperintense on T2WI. Contrast enhancement after intravenous administration of Gd-DTPA is usually moderate (similar to mucosa, but considerably more than muscle). Larger tumors may undergo central necrosis evident as increased signal intensity on T2WI and absent contrast enhancement. Pyriform sinus carcinomas (60%) tend to invade the posterior aspect of the thyroid ala, cricothyroid space, and soft tissues of the neck. Postcricoid carcinomas (25%) invade the larynx at an early stage. Posterior wall carcinomas (15%) extend into the retropharyngeal space, cephalad into the oropharynx and frequently into retropharyngeal lymph nodes.	Over 90% are squamous cell carcinomas occurring usually in men with a history of tobacco and alcohol abuse. In women it may be associated with *Plummer–Vison syndrome* (atrophic mucosa, achlorhydria, and sideropenic anemia). Early symptoms are vague and include sore throat and intolerance to hot and cold liquids. More advanced disease presents with dysphagia and cervical adenopathy (50% incidence at time of diagnosis). TNM staging of hypopharyngeal carcinoma: T1 Tumor limited to one subsite* T2 Tumor invades more than one subsite* or an adjacent site, *without* fixation of the hemilarynx T3 As T2, but *with* fixation of the hemilarynx T4 Tumor invades thyroid or cricoid cartilages or soft tissue of neck N1 Single ipsilateral node <3 cm N2 Single ipsilateral node 3–6 cm or multiple nodes <6 cm N3 Node(s) >6 cm *Hypopharyngeal subsites include pyriform sinus, postcricoid area, and posterior pharyngeal wall.
Esophageal carcinoma	Poorly marginated, infiltrating mass originating from the wall of the esophagus with or without intraluminal component. Tumor delineation in the invaded soft-tissue structures can be improved with contrast-enhanced fat suppressed imaging.	Diagnosis is established with barium swallow, endoscopy, and biopsy. MRI may be performed for staging (tumor extension and lymph node metastases).

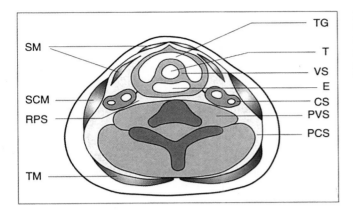

Fig. 7.**1** **Axial anatomy of the lower neck** at the first tracheal ring level. CS: carotid space; E: esophagus; PCS: posterior cervical space; PVS: prevertebral space; RPS: retropharyngeal space; SCM: sternocleidomastoid muscle; SM: strap muscles (sternohyoid and sternothyroid muscles); T: trachea; TG: thyroid gland; TM: trapezius muscle; VS: visceral space.

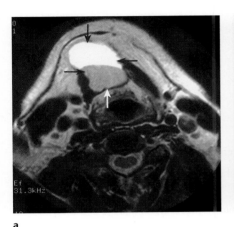

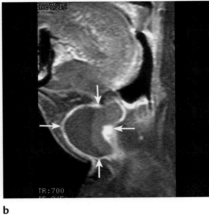

a

b

Fig. 7.**2** **Infected thyroglossal duct cyst**
a A cystic lesion (arrows) with hyperintense supernatant fluid and debri of intermediate signal intensity on the bottom is seen (T2WI, axial).   **b** After intravenous Gd-DTPA administration the contrast enhancement is limited to the cyst wall (T1WI, FS, +C, sagittal).

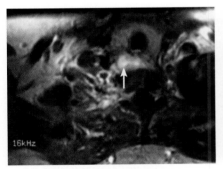

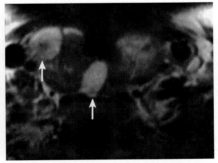

Fig. 7.**3** **Parathyroid adenoma.** After intravenous Gd-DTPA administration a markedly enhanced adenoma (arrow) is seen (T1WI, FS, +C).

Fig. 7.**4** **Multiple parathyroid adenomas.** After Gd-DTPA administration two adenomas (arrows) are identified as markedly enhanced lesions (T1WI, FS, +C).

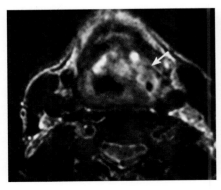

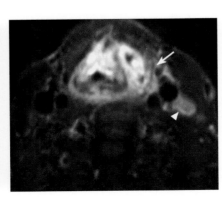

a

b

Fig. 7.**5** **Pyriform sinus carcinoma.**
a A poorly defined heterogeneous lesion (arrow) with increased signal intensity originates from the left pyriform sinus and infiltrates the larynx (T2WI). After intravenous Gd-DTPA administration, inhomogeneous enhancement of the tumor is seen including a deep cervical lymph node metastasis (arrowhead) (T1WI, FS, +C).

Table **7.1** (Cont.) Lesions in the visceral space

Disease	MRI Findings	Comments
Lymph node metastases and lymphoma	Usually multiple nodular lesions exceeding 1.5 cm in diameter, with low to intermediate signal intensity on T1WI and intermediate to high signal intensity on T2WI along the trachea and esophagus. Central necrosis is frequently associated with squamous cell carcinomas from the larynx, hypopharynx, or cervical esophagus and with thyroid carcinomas ("cystic" metastases).	Juxtavisceral lymph nodes include prelaryngeal, paratracheal, and paraesophageal lymph nodes. Exclusive involvement of these nodes frequently occurs with thyroid carcinoma at an early stage. Lymphoma is virtually always associated with other cervical adenopathy.
Abscess	Poorly marginated mass with nonenhancing center surrounded by an enhancing rim. Compared with the abscess wall, the center representing pus tends to be hypointense on T1WI and hyperintense on T2WI.	Rare. In the visceral space it is usually secondary to penetrating trauma. A *hematoma* depicts variable signal intensity, but in the subacute stage it is at least partially hyperintense on T1WI due to methemoglobin formation.
Zenker's diverticulum	Cystic lesion with an air-fluid level in the posterior visceral space below the pharyngoesophageal junction where it originates.	Outpouching of the posterior wall of the upper esophagus presenting sometimes with dysphagia or chronic aspiration.

Table **7.2** Laryngeal lesions

Disease	MRI Findings	Comments
Mucosal cyst	Thin-walled, homogeneous cystic lesion measuring up to several centimeters in diameter with low signal intensity on T1WI and high signal intensity on T2WI. May arise in any part of the larynx that contains submucosal glands and protrude into the airway. A vallecular cyst bulges between the base of the tongue and the free anterior margin of the epiglottis.	Mucosal (mucous retention) cysts occur at any age of life and have a predilection for the supraglottic area. *Congenital laryngeal cysts* originate in the aryepiglottic fold and may bulge into the laryngeal vestibule, pre-epiglottic space, or lateral neck.
Laryngocele (Fig. 7.6)	Cystic mass secondary to obstruction and enlargement of the normal ventricular appendix (saccule), which is a 5–15-mm-long blind pouch originating from the anterior part of the ventricle and ascending bilaterally between epiglottis and thyroid cartilage. Three types are differentiated: *Internal* laryngoceles are confined to the soft tissue of the larynx. May extend either anterosuperiorly into the pre-epiglottic space or posterosuperiorly into the aryepiglottic fold. *External* laryngoceles extend laterally through the thyrohyoid membrane, presenting as an anterolateral neck cyst just below the mandibular angle. *Mixed* laryngoceles have cystic components both medial and lateral to the thyrohyoid membrane. Laryngoceles are bilateral in 20% of cases.	The normal ventricular appendix (saccule) is usually not visible with MRI. A dilated ventricular appendix may be filled with air (laryngeal aerocele), fluid (laryngocele), or pus (pyolaryngocele). Laryngoceles result from functional or, less commonly, mechanical obstruction of the ventricular appendix, either at its opening into the ventricle or more peripherally. Chronic increase in intraglottic pressure (chronic cough, trumpet player, glass blower) or chronic granulomatous and neoplastic diseases may be the underlying cause. Over 90% of laryngoceles occur in adults, presenting either with hoarseness or stridor (internal laryngocele) or anterior neck mass that may expand with valsalva maneuver. A dilated ventricle (e.g., in ipsilateral vocal cord paralysis) should not be mistaken for a laryngeal aerocele.

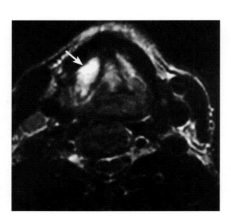

Fig. 7.**6** **Laryngocele.** A cystic lesion (arrow) is seen within the larynx consistent with an internal laryngocele (T2WI).

Table 7.2 (Cont.) Laryngeal lesions

Disease	MRI Findings	Comments
Subglottic stenosis	Eccentric or circumferential subglottic narrowing.	Congenital or acquired (e.g. prolonged intubation or sequela of cricoid cartilage fracture).
Croup	Edematous swelling of both vocal cords and sub-glottic mucosa.	Parainfluenza or respiratory syncytial virus infection in young children, and, rarely, adults.
Epiglottitis	Symmetric edematous swelling of epiglottis and aryepiglottic folds	Caused by haemophilus, pneumococcus, or streptococcus. *Angioneurotic edema* presents identically on MRI.
Rheumatoid disease	Cricoarytenoid subluxation, thickening of the true vocal cords, sometimes with polypoid rheumatoid nodules.	Laryngeal abnormalities are seen in up to 50% of patients with advanced rheumatoid arthritis.
Amyloidosis	Submucosal thickening and nodules more or less isointense to muscle on all pulse sequences are seen in the epiglottis and vocal cords.	Localized form of amyloidosis, which, besides the larynx, may also involve the trachea and bronchi. Less commonly, laryngeal amyloidosis may be part of systemic disease.
Granulomatous disease	Diffuse or, less commonly, focal thickening of epiglottis, aryepiglottic folds and glottis with signal characteristics and enhancement pattern similar to squamous cell carcinoma.	In sarcoidosis, tuberculosis, mycotic infections, and Wegener granulomatosis laryngeal involvement is usually part of more widespread disease.
Hematoma	Variable signal abnormalities with or without mass effect in the pre-epiglottic space, aryepiglottic folds, true and false vocal cords, and around the cricoid cartilage.	Laryngeal hemorrhages are usually associated with trauma, with or without cartilage fracture. Spontaneous hemorrhage occurs with bleeding disorders and anticoagulation.
Fibrous and fibro-angiomatous polyp	Nodular lesion on the free margin of the true vocal cord commonly located at the junction of the anterior and middle thirds. Frequently bilateral and occasionally multiple lesions.	Non-neoplastic stromal reaction in patients with history of vocal abuse (e.g., singers, professional speakers).
Papilloma and papillomatosis	Solitary or multiple small nodular lesions, frequently located in the anterior half of the larynx at the level of the vocal cords. Subglottic extension with spread to the trachea and bronchi may be associated.	Squamous cell papilloma caused by the papova virus is the most common benign laryngeal tumor. Usually multiple in children under 10 years of age and solitary in adults.
Chondroma and low-grade chondro-sarcomas	Hyperintense mass on T2WI with scattered foci devoid of signal due to intratumoral calcifications. The lesion arises from laryngeal cartilages, most commonly from the inner surface of the posterolateral portion of the cricoid cartilage. The involved cartilage may be expanded.	Chondromas are more common than chondrosarcomas, which are usually low-grade malignant lesions. They cannot be differentiated by MRI from each other. *High-grade chondrosarcomas* tend to destroy the laryngeal cartilage similar to squamous cell carcinomas.
Hemangioma	Hypointense on T1WI, hyperintense on T2WI and marked contrast enhancement. *Cavernous hemangiomas* occur in adults and tend to be glottic (especially true vocal cords) or supraglottic. *Capillary hemangiomas* occur in infants with predilection for the subglottic area.	Capillary hemangiomas may cause airway obstruction in the first year of life before they begin to regress spontaneously. Radiographically small phleboliths are occasionally seen in cavernous hemangiomas. *Paragangliomas* (very rare) may mimic a hemangioma in the supraglottis.
Schwannoma and neurofibroma	Single or multiple (neurofibromatosis) submucosal tumors with homogeneous low signal intensity on T1WI and high signal intensity on T2WI, unless complicated by hemorrhage or necrosis.	Other rare benign mesenchymal tumors include lipoma (hyperintense on T1WI), leiomyoma, rhabdomyoma, and *granular cell tumor* (may mimic squamous cell carcinoma in true vocal cord).

Table 7.2 (Cont.) Laryngeal lesions

Disease	MRI Findings	Comments
Squamous cell carcinoma (Figs. 7.7–7.9)	Poorly marginated mass with low to intermediate signal intensity on T1WI, intermediate to high on T2WI, and moderate contrast enhancement. Compared with muscle the tumor is isointense on T1WI and hyperintense on both T2WI and after enhancement. Compared with fat or marrow fat in the ossified laryngeal cartilage, the tumor is hypointense on T1WI and isointense on both T2WI and after contrast enhancement on T1WI unless fat suppression techniques are used. Compared with the nonossified thyroid and cricoid cartilage, the tumor is isointense on T1WI, mildly hyperintense on T2WI, and hyperintense after enhancement. *Supraglottic carcinomas* (30%) arise in the epiglottis (circumferential growth with early spread into the pre-epiglottic space), aryepiglottic fold (exophytic growth with spread to epiglottis and periglottic space), or false vocal cord and laryngeal ventricle (spread to periglottic space, or inferiorly into the glottis and subglottis). Deep cervical lymph node metastases occur early. *Glottic carcinomas* (60%) originate in the vocal cord and spread anteriorly into the anterior commissure, which should not exceed 1 mm in thickness, posteriorly into the arytenoid and cricoid cartilages and posterior commissure, inferiorly into the subglottis, and superiorly into the periglottic space. Nodal lymph node metastases are late. *Subglottic carcinomas* (5%) are diagnosed by demonstrating any soft tissue inside the cricoid cartilage, since there is no normal tissue between this cartilage and the mucosa.	Ninety-eight percent of malignant laryngeal tumors are squamous cell carcinomas. Chondrosarcomas (2%) represent the largest group of the remaining laryngeal malignancies. History of tobacco abuse is often present. Both supraglottic and subglottic carcinomas are symptomatic only late in the course of the disease and thus present usually in an advanced stage at the time of diagnosis. Glottic carcinomas are diagnosed early due to hoarseness. TNM staging: *Supraglottis* T1 Tumor limited to one subsite* T2 Tumor invades more than one subsite* or glottis with normal cord mobility T3 Tumor limited to larynx with fixation of vocal cord and/or extension into the postcricoid area, medial wall of pyriform sinus, or pre-epiglottic space T4 Tumor extends beyond larynx to oropharynx or invades thyroid cartilage *Subsites include epiglottis, aryepiglottic folds, and false vocal cords including the laryngeal ventricles. *Glottis* T1 Tumor limited to one or both vocal cords including anterior or posterior commissures with normal cord mobility T2 Tumor extends to supraglottis and/or subglottis or associated with impaired vocal cord mobility, or both T3 Tumor limited to larynx with vocal cord fixation T4 Tumor invades thyroid cartilage and/or soft tissue of the neck *Subglottis* T1 Tumor confined to subglottis T2 Tumor invades vocal cord(s) with normal or impaired mobility T3 Tumor limited to larynx with vocal cord fixation T4 Tumor invades thyroid or cricoid cartilage and/or soft tissue of neck *Lymph nodes* N1 Single ipsilateral node <3 cm N2 Single ipsilateral node 3–6 cm or multiple nodes <6 cm N3 Node(s) >6 cm
Metastases and lymphoma	Metastatic and lymphomatous involvement of the larynx is usually by direct extension from neighboring structures. Primary laryngeal lymphoma and hematogenous metastases are exceedingly rare.	Hematogenous metastases may originate from melanomas, renal cell carcinomas, breast and lung primaries. Leukemic infiltrates may rarely occur too.

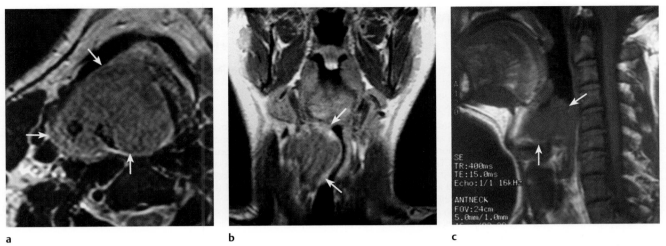

a   b   c

Fig. 7.**7** **Supraglottic carcinoma.** A large mass (arrows) extending from the supraglottic area into the right oropharynx is seen (T1WI: axial, coronal, and sagittal).

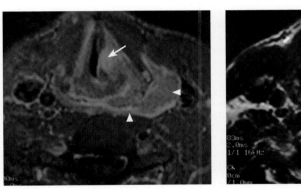

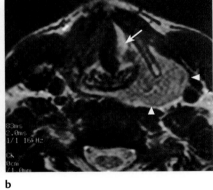

a   b

Fig. 7.**8** **Glottic carcinoma.** A hyperintense vocal cord lesion (arrow) is seen with extension into the left pyriform sinus (arrowheads) (**a**: T1WI, FS, +C. **b**: T2WI).

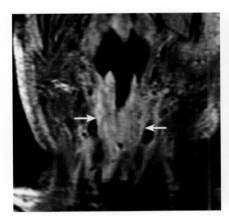

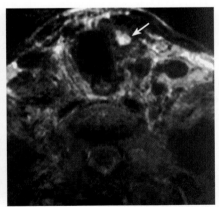

Fig. 7.**9** **Larynx carcinoma.** After intravenous Gd-DTPA administration an enhanced lesion (arrows) is seen extending from the supraglottic to the subglottic space (T1WI, FS, +C, coronal).

Fig. 7.**10** **Thyroid cyst.** A hyperintense focus (arrow) is seen in an enlarged left thyroid lobe (T2WI).

Table 7.3 Thyroid gland lesions

Disease	MRI Findings	Comments
Pyramidal lobe	Midline or, less commonly, paramedian anterosuperior extension of normal thyroid tissue with intermediate signal intensity on both T1WI and T2WI into the distal remnant of the thyroglossal duct.	Normal variant present in 10–40% of population
Thyroid cyst (Fig. 7.10)	*Noncolloid cyst* is hypointense on T1WI and hyperintense on T2WI. *Colloid cyst* is homogeneous and hyperintense on both T1WI and T2WI. *Hemorrhagic cyst* is relatively hyperintense on both T1WI and T2WI and may depict a hypointense rim best seen on T2WI ("rim sign" secondary to hemosiderin-laden macrophages). *Cystic degenerated adenoma* or *carcinoma* may be either hyperintense or hypointense (hyaline degeneration) on T2WI.	Most thyroid cysts represent cystic degeneration of adenomas. Hyperproteinaceous colloid accumulation occurs in a macrofollicle (primary colloid cyst) or with colloid cystic degeneration of a solid lesion. A *cervical thymic cyst* in contiguity with the lower pole of the thyroid may mimic a thyroidal cyst.
Thyroid granuloma	Single or multiple well-circumscribed nodules with low signal intensity on T1WI and high signal intensity on T2WI. May be calcified.	Rare.
Suppurative thyroiditis	Focal or diffuse swelling of the inflamed thyroid gland with decreased signal intensity on T1WI and increased signal intensity on T2WI. Progress to abscess formation is frequent, occasionally with subsequent capsular rupture and spread to the soft tissues of the neck.	Most commonly a streptococcal or pneumococcal infection presenting with acute onset of pain and swelling of the thyroid gland. Associated with fever and dysphagia.
De Quervain thyroiditis	Diffuse, heterogeneous enlargement of the entire thyroid gland with increased signal intensity on both T1WI and T2WI.	Subacute, probably viral thyroiditis presenting with pain, fever, and fatigue after an upper respiratory tract infection. Toxic hyperthyroidism is initially present in 50%, followed by euthyroidism at 1–2 months, hypothyroidism at 2–4 months, and return to the euthyroid state at 6 months. Most commonly affects middle-aged females.
Riedel thyroiditis	Unilateral or bilateral, often asymmetric and irregular enlargement of the thyroid gland with obliteration of the adjacent soft-tissue planes simulating an infiltrative mass. Characteristic is the decreased signal intensity on both T1WI and T2WI due to extensive fibrosis.	Patients present with an enlarging mass causing compression of the trachea, hoarseness, and difficulty in swallowing. Predilection for women. Hypothyroidism, retroperitoneal and mediastinal fibrosis, sclerosing cholangitis, and orbital pseudotumor may be associated.
Hashimoto thyroiditis (Fig. 7.11)	Symmetrically and diffusely enlarged thyroid gland with heterogeneous, sometimes nodular appearance demonstrating usually increased signal intensity on T2WI with low-density fibrous bands. Rarely, signal intensity may be decreased on T2WI.	Most common chronic thyroiditis (autoimmune disease) occurring at any age (peak incidence between 40 and 60 years) with strong female predilection. Hyperthyroidism develops in 50%. Predisposition for non-Hodgkin lymphoma.
Graves disease (Fig. 7.12)	Diffusely enlarged thyroid gland with heterogeneous signal intensity that is increased on both T1WI and T2WI. Usually no focal mass is evident (diffuse toxic goiter).	Most common cause of hyperthyroidism. Women are affected 10 times more often than men; mean age at diagnosis 45 years. Autoimmune disease with thyroid stimulating antibodies (LATS) producing hyperplasia of thyroid gland.
Multinodular goiter	Nodular enlargement of the thyroid gland with very heterogeneous signal intensity that is overall decreased on T1WI and increased on T2WI. Besides cyst-like lesions appearing hypointense on T1WI and hyperintense on T2WI, hemorrhagic adenomas and hemorrhagic or colloid cysts demonstrate high signal intensity on T1WI, and foci of calcifications or hyaline degeneration depict low signal intensity on T2WI. With intrathoracic extension, the mass is usually located in the anterior mediastinum in front of the great vessels. The intrathoracic goiter is usually continuous with the cervical thyroid, but rarely may originate from ectopic thyroid tissue in the chest.	Multinodular (adenomatous) goiters may or may not be associated with functional thyroid abnormalities. Iodine-deficiency goiters occur in endemic areas. In *toxic nodular goiter (Plummer disease)* hyperthyroidism is caused by the autonomous function of one or more adenomas. The disease is three times more common in females and occurs usually in the fourth and fifth decade of life.

Table 7.**3** (Cont.) Thyroid gland lesions

Disease	MRI Findings	Comments
Thyroid adenoma	Well-defined, homogeneous or inhomogeneous 1–4-cm lesion, usually hypointense to nearly isointense to normal thyroid tissue on T1WI and hyperintense on T2WI. Liquefaction of the lesion may decrease the signal intensity on T1WI and increase it on T2WI. Intratumoral hemorrhage or colloid degeneration may produce hyperintensity on T1WI. Calcifications and hyaline degeneration may produce low signal intensity on T2WI. Adenomas cannot reliably be differentiated from carcinomas. Multiple adenomas may produce an asymmetrically enlarged thyroid gland and are often referred to as adenomatous hyperplasia.	Nonfunctioning thyroid adenomas are the most common cause of "cold nodules" in scintigraphy. The majority of "cold nodules" are caused by degenerated adenomas, nodular hemorrhage, cysts, inflammatory conditions, or amyloid deposition. Functioning thyroid adenomas are "hot nodules" on scintigraphy and are 90% benign. A toxic adenoma is an autonomous functioning adenoma that usually exceeds 3 cm in diameter before it produces clinically apparent hyperparathyroidism.
Thyroid carcinoma (Fig. 7.13)	Unilateral thyroidal mass with infiltrating margins obliterating adjacent soft-tissue planes, or intrathyroidal mass with well-defined margins simulating a benign lesion. On T1WI the signal intensity of the lesion is intermediate and similar to normal thyroid tissue; on T2WI the tumor appears heterogeneous and hyperintense. Cystic components are evident in 38% of tumors. Calcifications including psammomatous bodies (punctate or linear in the tumor periphery) occur in approximately one-third of all cases, but are difficult to appreciate as foci of signal void. Lymphangitic spread to the paratracheal nodes, which may have a cystic appearance, occurs early. Hematogenous spread to lung and bone is frequent.	Occurs usually in the fifth to seventh decade with female predilection. Five types: papillary (60%), follicular (25%), anaplastic (10%), medullary (4%), Hürthle cell (1%). Medullary carcinomas occur in adolescence when associated with multiple endocrine neoplasia (MEN) syndrome. MEN 1: pituitary and parathyroid adenoma, pancreatic island cell tumor. MEN 2: parathyroid adenoma, medullary thyroid carcinoma, pheochromocytoma. MEN 3: medullary thyroid carcinoma, pheochromocytoma, ganglioneuromatosis.
Thyroid lymphoma	Solitary mass (80%) or multiple nodules (20%) with homogeneous signal intensity that is low to intermediate on T1WI and high on T2WI.	In primary non-Hodgkin lymphoma of the thyroid, a history of Hashimoto thyroiditis is almost always present. The two conditions may be difficult to differentiate with MRI because of considerable overlap in signal characteristics.
Thyroid metastases	Usually multiple nodular lesions demonstrating low signal intensity on T1WI and high signal intensity on T2WI. Carcinomas of kidney and lung are the most common sources.	Thyroid metastases usually are clinically occult. At autopsy 2–4% of cancer patients have thyroidal metastases.

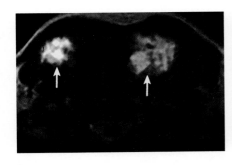

a

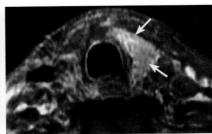

b

Fig. 7.**11 Hashimoto thyroiditis. a** Diffuse enlargement of the thyroid is seen with bilateral regions of inhomogeneous increased signal intensity (arrows) (T2WI).

b After intravenous Gd-DTPA administration, marked enhancement (arrows) of the regions depicting increased signal intensity on the precontrast T2WI is seen (T1WI, FS, +C).

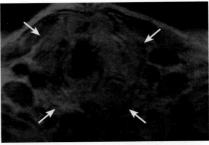

Fig. 7.**12 Graves disease.** A diffusely enlarged thyroid gland (arrows) is seen with heterogeneous and slightly increased signal intensity (PDWI).

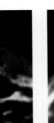

a   b

Fig. 7.**13 Thyroid carcinoma (medullary type).** A lesion (arrows) is seen in the left thyroid lobe that is isointense to the normal thyroid tissue in (**a**) (T1WI) and hyperintense in (**b**) (T2WI).

Table 7.**4** Lesions of the lower carotid space and posterior cervical space

Disease	MRI Findings	Comments
Atypical second branchial cleft cyst	Unilocular cystic mass along the anterior border of the common carotid artery or protruding posteriorly into the posterior cervical space from its normal location at the angle of the mandible.	Second branchial cleft cysts account for 95% of all branchial cleft anomalies. They may be diagnosed in infancy or become apparent in young adulthood after viral upper respiratory tract infection or trauma.
Third branchial cleft cyst	Unilocular cystic mass centered in the posterior cervical space.	Presents as painless fluctuant mass in the posterior triangle of the neck.
Cystic lymphangioma (hygroma) (Fig. 7.**14**)	Multilocular cystic mass in the posterior cervical space.	Posterior cervical space and mediastinum are primary locations in infants.
Capillary hemangioma	Poorly marginated heterogeneous lesion in the posterior cervical space with low signal intensity on T1WI and high signal intensity on T2WI with intense inhomogeneous contrast enhancement.	In infants, often increases in the first 10 months of life and then usually begins to involute spontaneously. *Cavernous hemangiomas* (Fig. 7.**15**) in this location occur in adolescents and adults.
Carotid body tumor (paraganglioma) (Figs. 7.**16** and 7.**17**)	Heterogeneous ovoid mass located in the carotid bifurcation with splaying of the external and internal carotid arteries. Signal intensity is low to intermediate on T1WI and relatively high on T2WI. Characteristic serpiginous flow voids and "salt-and-pepper" appearance reflect tumor hypervascularity. Intense contrast enhancement occurs after intravenous Gd-DTPA administration.	Presents as slow-growing painless neck mass below the angle of the mandible. The lesion is firm and pulsatile, laterally mobile, but vertically fixed. Bilateral involvement occurs in 5% and malignant transformation in 6%.
Schwannoma (neuroma) (Fig. 7.**18**)	Well-defined, sometimes eccentric mass protruding from the trunk of a nerve, with homogeneous signal intensity that is low on T1WI and high on T2WI. Moderate, uniform contrast enhancement occurs after intravenous Gd-DTPA administration. Larger lesions may become heterogeneous due to areas of cystic degeneration.	Occurs in both the carotid and posterior cervical space as a slow-growing mass with or without symptoms related to the involved nerve. May be multiple in neurofibromatosis.

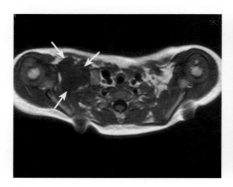
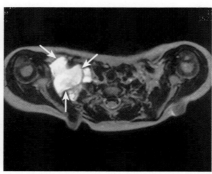
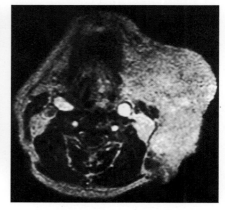

a   b

Fig. 7.**14**   **Cystic lymphangioma (hygroma).** A multiloculated cystic lesion with low signal intensity in **a** (T1WI) and high signal intensity in **b** (T2WI) is seen.

Fig. 7.**15**   **Cavernous hemangioma.** After intravenous Gd-DTPA administration a considerably enhancing mass is seen extending from the face into the posterior neck (T1WI, FS, +C).

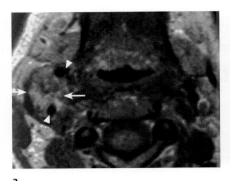

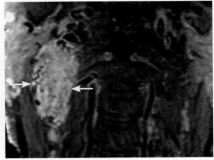

a

b

Fig. 7.**16** **Carotid body tumor.** **a** A heterogeneous ovoid lesion (arrows) with low signal intensity is located in the carotid bifurcation and causes splaying of the external and internal carotid arteries (arrowheads) presenting with signal void (T1WI, axial).

b After intravenous Gd-DTPA administration, intense contrast enhancement of the lesion (arrows) is seen (T1WI, FS, +C, coronal).

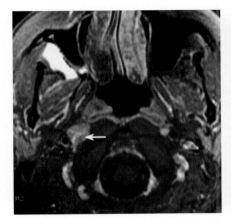

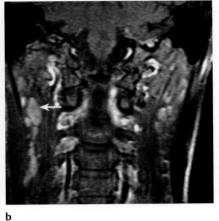

a

b

Fig. 7.**17** **Carotid body tumor.** After intravenous Gd-DTPA administration an intensely enhanced small lesion (arrow) is seen (axial and coronal T1WI, FS, +C).

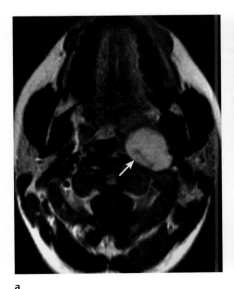

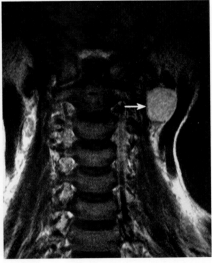

a

b

Fig. 7.**18** **Schwannoma.** After intravenous Gd-DTPA administration a markedly enhanced lesion (arrow) is seen (axial and coronal T1WI, +C).

Table 7.**4** (Cont.) Lesions of the lower carotid space and posterior cervical space

Disease	MRI Findings	Comments
Neurofibroma (Figs. 7.19 and 7.20)	Well-defined fusiform mass with signal characteristics and contrast enhancement similar to schwannomas, unless it undergoes diffuse fatty degeneration (increased signal intensity on T1WI and decreased on T2WI) or contains a central core of fibrous tissue producing a "target" appearance on T2WI with central hypointense focus.	Presentation and symptomatology similar to schwannomas. Only 10% of patients with neurofibromas have neurofibromatosis. Solitary neurofibromas most frequently occur in the third decade of life.
Lipoma	Most common location of lipomas in the head and neck is the posterior cervical space. The lesion has signal characteristics identical to subcutaneous fat on all pulse sequences without discernable contrast enhancement after intravenous Gd-DTPA administration.	*Liposarcoma* should be considered when the fatty mass depicts significant internal stranding or signal inhomogeneity, or demonstrates partial contrast enhancement. Liposarcomas are, however, very rare in this area.
Lymphoma (Fig. 7.21)	Unilateral or bilateral enlargement of the middle and lower deep cervical lymph nodes is the most common manifestation. Lymphoma may involve the upper deep cervical lymph nodes (above the jugulodigastric node), either alone or, more often, together with the middle and lower deep cervical lymph nodes. Upper deep and/or superficial cervical lymph node involvement tends to indicate lymphoma rather than metastases from an unknown primary. *Non-Hodgkin lymphoma* typically demonstrates a homogeneous low signal intensity (similar to muscle) on T1WI and a homogeneous, relatively high signal intensity (similar to fat) on T2WI. In *Hodgkin disease* low signal intensity on T1WI is often associated with a pattern of mixed low and high signal intensity on T2WI. *Response to treatment* is evident by a decrease in lymph node size, often associated with heterogeneous signal intensity that decreases overall on T1WI and increases overall on T2WI due to inflammation and necrosis. Successful treatment eventually results in *lymph node fibrosis,* producing low signal intensity on both T1WI and T2WI.	Both non-Hodgkin lymphoma (75%) and Hodgkin disease (25%) occur in the head and neck region. Patients present with painless neck masses (nodes). Extranodal involvement is uncommon and usually limited to non-Hodgkin lymphoma. Besides involvement of the deep cervical lymph nodes in the carotid space, lymphoma may also involve all the other superficial and deep cervical lymph node groups, including the spinal accessory chain in the posterior cervical space. Non-Hodgkin lymphomas that may present as necrotic cystic areas prior to therapy include undifferentiated AIDS-related lymphoma and Burkitt lymphoma.
Metastases (Fig. 7.22)	Deep cervical lymph nodes measuring more than 1 cm in diameter are abnormal, except for the jugulodigastric node that normally measures up to 1.2 cm. Enlarged lymph nodes may be inflamed or neoplastic. Lymph nodes exceeding 1.5 cm in diameter are considered malignant for practical purposes. A lymph node with a necrotic or cystic center is abnormal, regardless of size. Central necrosis is common with squamous cell carcinoma metastases. This is in contrast to fatty lymph node replacement, frequently commencing in the hilum of the node and referred to as fibrolipomatosis. It is found after chronic inflammation and irradiation or as an involutional process in the elderly. When the metastases extend beyond the lymph node, its margin becomes ill defined.	Squamous cell carcinoma metastases found in the middle or lower deep cervical lymph nodes with unknown primary tumor suggest that the primary lesion may hide in the nasopharynx, palatine tonsil, base of the tongue, or pyriform sinus. With metastatic involvement of the lower deep lymph nodes alone, the primary tumor is commonly located in the thyroid, thorax, or abdomen. Metastases in the spinal accessory (posterior cervical) lymph nodes, located in the posterior cervical space behind the deep cervical lymph nodes of the carotid space, originate most often from nasopharyngeal malignancies.

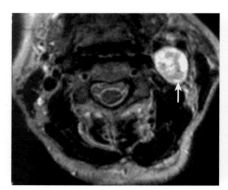

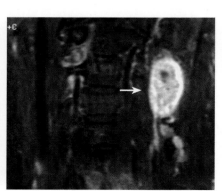

Fig. 7.**19** **Neurofibroma.** After intravenous Gd-DTPA administration an inhomogeneously enhanced lesion (arrow) is seen (axial and coronal T1WI, FS, +C).

a   b

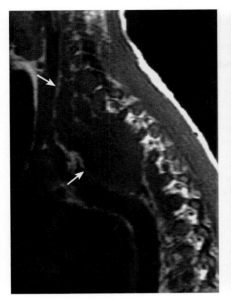
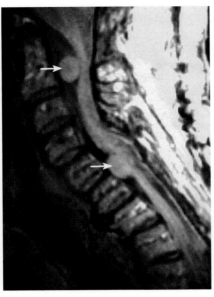

Fig. 7.**20** **Neurofibromatosis.** **a** A large paravertebral mass (arrows) with low signal intensity is seen (T1WI, sagittal). **b** Two neurofibromas (arrows) are visible in the spinal canal (T2WI, sagittal).

a

b

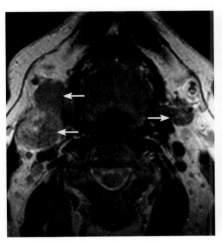
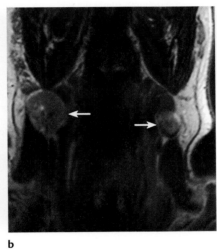

Fig. 7.**21** **Non-Hodgkin lymphoma.** Markedly enlarged, well-delineated, homogeneous lymph nodes (arrows) are seen presenting with intermediate signal intensity in (**a**) (T2WI, axial) and without significant contrast enhancement in (**b**) (T1WI, FS, +C, coronal).

a

b

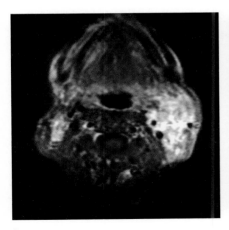
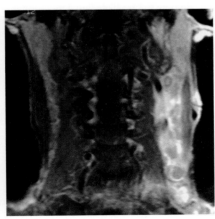

Fig. 7.**22** **Squamous cell carcinoma metastases.** After intravenous Gd-DTPA administration, bilateral, largely confluent, necrotic deep cervical lymph node metastases are seen, which are much more advanced on the left side (axial and coronal T1WI, FS, +C).

a

b

Table 7.**4** (Cont.) Lesions of the lower carotid space and posterior cervical space

Disease	MRI Findings	Comments
Inflammatory or infectious lymphadenopathy (Fig. 7.23)	In *reactive hyperplasia* the deep cervical lymph nodes may by definition enlarge to a maximum diameter of 1.5 cm, but maintain their normal oval shape and their homogeneous internal architecture. In *suppurative adenopathy* the normal intermediate signal intensity of lymph nodes on all pulse sequences is decreased on T1WI and increased on T2WI. Intranodal abscesses are evident as cystic areas appearing hypointense on T2WI. In *tuberculous adenopathy* a heterogeneous pattern with overall decreased signal intensity on T1WI and increased signal intensity on T2WI is seen, or a tuberculous nodal abscess appearing hypointense on T1WI and hyperintense on T2WI with an enhancing rim. Calcified lymph nodes demonstrate low signal intensity on all pulse sequences. Involved nodes may coalesce to form a single necrotic mass ("cold abscess").	Reactive hyperplasia is a nonspecific lymph node reaction to any inflammation or infection in its draining area. Differentiation between suppurative adenopathy and squamous cell carcinoma metastases, both of which frequently present with enlarged lymph nodes with central necrosis, should easily be possible, when the clinical picture is taken into consideration. Atypical mycobacterial infections (e.g., in AIDS) and a variety of granulomatous infections produce lymph node changes on MRI similar to tuberculosis.
Abscess (Fig. 7.24)	Carotid space abscesses are relatively small since they are usually contained within the tenacious carotid sheath. A central area of nonenhancing pus is surrounded by the poorly defined, markedly enhancing abscess wall.	Carotid space abscess is a surgical emergency. It arises from extracapsular spread of suppurative lymphadenitis or is due to penetrating trauma, vascular surgery, or intravenous drug abuse.
Trauma (Fig. 7.25)	Fresh blood appears similar to other fluids. Subsequent intrasellar deoxyhemoglobin formation causes progressive decrease in signal intensity on T2WI. With intracellular methemoglobin formation the hematoma becomes progressively hyperintense on T1WI, progressing from the periphery towards the center. Extracellular methemoglobin secondary to red blood cell lysis is associated with increased signal intensity, particularly on T1WI but also on T2WI. *Carotid artery injuries* include subintimal hematoma, partial wall tear seen as an intraluminal flap, dissection with subsequent aneurysm formation, and partial or complete thrombosis. *Traumatic brachiocephalic plexopathy* may or may not be associated with cervical fracture. A hematoma may be the only visible abnormality. In acute nerve root avulsion fluid may be seen in the adjacent soft tissues with T2WI.	Arteriosclerotic changes in the carotid artery, such as thrombotic plaques, localized stenosis, and localized ectasia or an asymmetrically enlarged carotid bulb, have to be differentiated from acute carotid injury. The brachiocephalic plexus is a transpatial neural structure that originates from the spinal cord (C5–T1 roots) and crosses the perivertebral and posterior cervical space in its course to the axillary apex. Lesions involving the brachiocephalic plexus are discussed in Chapter 13.
Jugular vein thrombophlebitis (Figs. 7.26 and 7.27)	Enlargement of the internal jugular vein by intraluminal thrombus, demonstrating high signal intensity on both T1WI and T2WI due to methemoglobin within the clot. The soft-tissue planes surrounding the jugular vein are inflamed and edematous. After intravenous Gd-DTPA administration the vasa vasorum in the venous wall may enhance intensely.	The patient presents with a tender neck mass mimicking an abscess. A history of central venous catheter placement or intravenous drug abuse is often available.

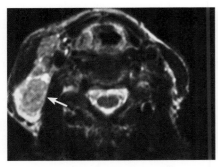

Fig. 7.**23** **Tuberculous adenopathy.** An enlarged deep cervical lymph node (arrow) with central necrosis is seen post intravenous Gd-DTPA administration (T1WI, FS, +C).

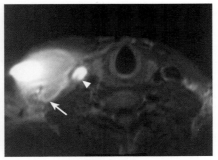

Fig. 7.**24** **Tuberculous abscess.** The abscess (arrow) presents as an area of increased signal intensity adjacent to the thrombosed internal jugular vein (arrowhead), evident as a round hyperintense focus (T2WI, FS).

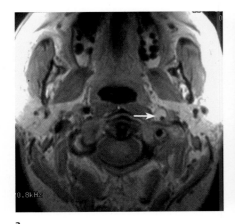

a

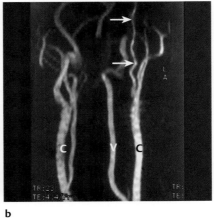

b

Fig. 7.**25** **Subintimal hematoma of the internal carotid artery.** A hyperintense crescent shaped hematoma (arrow) is seen in **a** surrounding the markedly narrowed and eccentrically located lumen of the left internal carotid artery evident as flow void (PDW1, axial). The markedly narrowed lumen of the left internal carotid artery (arrows) is well appreciated with MRI in **b** (C: Common carotid artery. V: Vertebral artery).

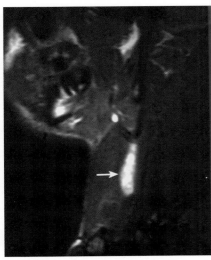

Fig. 7.**26** **Jugular vein thrombosis.** A fresh thrombus in the right internal jugular vein (arrow) presents with high signal intensity (sagittal T1WI, FS).

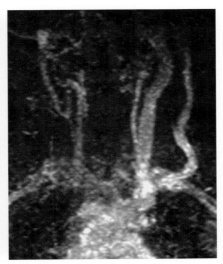

Fig. 7.**27** **Jugular vein occlusion.** Chronic thrombosis with complete occlusion of the right internal jugular vein and development of collaterals is seen on MRA.

Section III

Spine

8 Spine and Spinal Cord

MRI is a powerful imaging modality for evaluating normal spinal anatomy and pathologic conditions involving the spine and sacrum. Because of the high soft-tissue contrast resolution of MRI and multiplanar imaging capabilities, pathologic disorders of bone marrow (e.g., neoplasm, inflammatory diseases), epidural soft tissues, discs, thecal sac, spinal cord, intradural and extradural nerves, ligaments, facet joints, and paravertebral structures are readily discerned to a much greater degree than on CT.

The normal spine is comprised of seven cervical, 12 thoracic, and five lumbar vertebrae. The upper two cervical vertebrae have different configurations than the other vertebrae. The atlas (C1) has a horizontal ring-like configuration with lateral masses that articulate with the occipital condyles superiorly and superior facets of C2 inferiorly. The dorsal margin of the upper dens is secured in position in relation to the anterior arch of C1 by the transverse ligament. Various anomalies occur in this region such as atlanto-occipital assimilation, altered segmentation (e.g., block vertebrae), basiocciput hypoplasia, condylis tertius, and os odontoideum. The lower five cervical vertebral bodies have more rectangular shapes with progressive enlargement inferiorly. Superior projections from the cervical vertebral bodies laterally form the uncovertebral joints. The transverse processes are located anterolateral to vertebral bodies and contain the transverse foramina within which vertebral arteries are located. The posterior elements consist of paired pedicles, articular pillars, laminae, and spinous processes. The cervical spine has a normal lordosis.

The twelve thoracic vertebral bodies and five lumbar vertebral bodies progressively increase in size caudally. The posterior elements include the pedicles, transverse processes, laminae, and spinous processes. The transverse processes of the thoracic vertebrae also have articulation sites for ribs. The thoracic spine has a normal kyphosis and the lumbar spine a normal lordosis. Anterior and posterior longitudinal ligaments connect the cervical vertebrae, and interspinous ligaments and ligamentum flavum provide stability for the posterior elements.

The cortical margins of the vertebral bodies have dense compact bone structure that result in low signal on T1WI and T2WI (Fig 8.1). The medullary compartments of the vertebrae consists of bone marrow and trabecular bone (Fig 8.1). The signal intensity of the medullary compartment is primarily due to the proportion of red to yellow marrow. The proportion of yellow to red marrow progressively increases with age, resulting in increased marrow signal on T1WI. Similar changes are pronounced in patients who have received spinal irradiation. Pathologic processes (such as tumor, inflammation, infection) cause increased T1 and T2 relaxation coefficients, resulting in decreased signal on T1WI and increased signal on T2WI. MRI with fat-suppression (FS) techniques (short tau inversion recovery [STIR] sequence and fat-frequency saturated T1W and T2W sequences) provide optimal contrast between normal and pathologic marrow. Corresponding abnormal Gd-contrast enhancement is also usually seen at the pathologic sites, which can also be optimized using fat-frequency saturated T1W sequences. Because of direct visualization of these pathologic processes in the marrow, MRI can often detect these abnormalities sooner than CT, which relies on later indirect signs of trabecular destruction for confirmation of disease.

The intervertebral disks enable flexibility of the spine. The two major components (nucleus pulposis and annulus fibrosis) of normal disks are usually well seen with MRI. The outer annulus fibrosis is made of dense fibrocartilage and has low signal on T1WI and T2WI (Fig 8.2). The central nucleus pulposis is made of gelatinous material and usually has high signal on T2WI (Fig 8.2). The combination of various factors such as decreased turgor of the nucleus pulposis and loss of elasticity of the annulus with or without tears results in degenerative changes in the disks. MRI features of disk degeneration include decreased disk heights, decreased signal of nucleus pulposis on T2WI, disk bulging and associated posterior vertebral body osteophytes. Tears of the annulus fibrosis often have high signal on T2WI at the site of injury. Annular tears can be transverse, oriented parallel to the outer annular fibers, and are sometimes referred to as annular fissures. Annular tears can also be radial, extending from the central portion of the disk to the periphery. Radial tears are often clinically significant and are associated with disk herniations. The term "disk herniation" usually refers to extension of nucleus pulposis through an annular tear beyond the margins of the adjacent vertebral body endplates. Disk herniations can be further subdivided as protusions (when the head of the herniation equals the neck in size), extrusions (when the head of the herniation is larger than the neck), or extruded fragments (when there is separation of the herniated disk fragment from the disk of origin). Disk herniations can occur in any portion of the disk. Posterior and posterolateral herniations can cause compression of the thecal sac and contents, as well as compression of extradural nerve roots in the lateral recesses or within the intervertebral foramina. Lateral and anterior disk herniations are less common but can cause hematomas in adjacent structures. Disk herniations occurring superiorly or inferiorly result in focal depressions of the endplates, i.e, Schmorl's nodes. Recurrent disk herniations can be delineated from scar or granulation tissue because, unlike scar tissue, herniated disks do not typically enhance after Gd-DTPA contrast administration.

The thecal sac is a meningeal covered compartment containing cerebrospinal fluid (CSF) that is contiguous with the basal subarachnoid cisterns and extends from the upper cervical level to the level of the sacrum. The thecal sac contains the spinal cord and exiting nerve roots (Figs. 8.1, 8.2). The distal end of the conus medullaris is normally located at the T12-L1 level in adults. Lesions within the thecal sac are categorized as intradural, intramedullary, or extramedullary. Intramedullary lesions directly involve the spinal cord, whereas extramedullary lesions do not primarily involve the spinal cord. Extradual or epidural lesions refer to spinal lesions outside of the thecal sac.

The high soft-tissue contrast resolution of MRI enables evaluation of the normal spinal cord and various in-

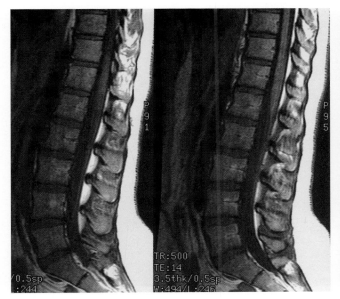

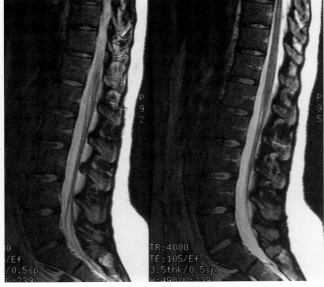

a   **b**

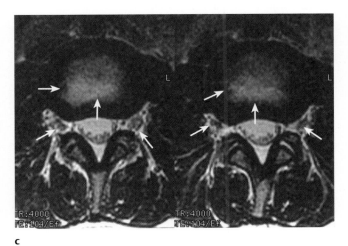

c

Fig. 8.**1** Sagittal T1WI (**a**) and T2WI (**b**) of the lumbar spine show normal configuration and MR signal of the vertebral marrow and disks. **c** Axial T2WI shows the normal appearance of lumbar disks with high signal in the nucleus pulposis centrally (arrows) surrounded by a low signal annulus. The subarachnoid fluid has high signal and contains multiple nerve roots. Nerve roots can also be seen in the foramina (arrows).

tramedullary pathologic conditions–such as congenital malformations, neoplasms, benign mass lesions (e.g., dermoid, arachnoid cyst), inflammatory/infectious processes, traumatic injuries (contusions, hematomas) and ischemia/infarction–as well as the adjacent CSF and nerve roots. MRI after intravenous administration of Gd-contrast is useful for evaluating lesions within the spinal cord as well as neoplastic or inflammatory diseases within the thecal sac.

The normal blood supply to the spinal cord consists of seven or eight radicular arteries that enter the spinal canal through the intervertebral foramina to supply the three main vascular territories of the spinal cord (cervicothoracic: cervical and upper three thoracic levels; mid thoracic: T3 level to T7 level; and thoracolumbar: T8 level to lumbosacral plexus). Cervicothoracic vascular distribution is supplied by radicular branches arising from the vertebral arteries and costocervical trunk. The midthoracic territory is often supplied by a radicular branch arising from the 3rd, 4th or 5th intercostal artery. The thoracolumbar territory is supplied by a single artery arising from the ninth, 10th, 11th, or 12th intercostal arteries (75%); the fifth, sixth, seventh, or eighth intercostal arteries (15%); or the first or second lumbar arteries (10%). The radicular arteries supply the longitudinally oriented anterior spinal artery; located in the midline anteriorly adjacent to the spinal cord, it supplies the gray matter and central white matter of the spinal cord. The radicular arteries also supply the two major longitudinally oriented posterior spinal arteries, which course along the posterolateral sulci of the spinal cord and supply one-third to one-half of the outer rim of the spinal cord via a peripheral anastomotic plexus. Ischemia or infarcts involving the spinal cord represent rare disorders associated with atherosclerosis, diabetes, hypertension, abdominal aortic aneurysms, and abdominal aortic surgery. Vascular malformations can be seen within the thecal sac, with or without involvement of the spinal cord.

Epidural structures of clinical importance include: 1) the lateral recesses (anterolateral portions of the spinal canal located between the thecal sac and pedicles that contains nerve roots, vessels, and fat); 2) dorsal epidural fat pad; 3) posterior elements and facet joints; 4) posterior longitudinal ligament and ligamentum flavum. The intervertebral foramina represent the bony channels between the pedicles through which the nerves traverse.

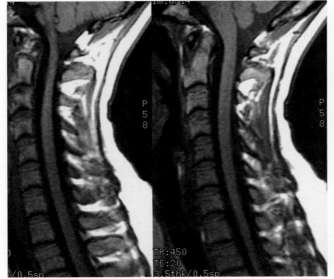

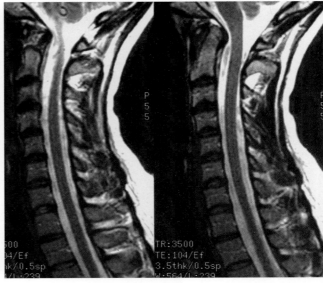

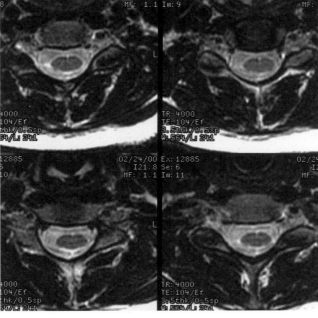

Fig. 8.**2**   Sagittal T1WI (**a**) and T2WI (**b**) of the cervical spine show normal configuration and MR signal of the vertebral marrow and disks, subarachnoid space, and spinal cord.   **c** Axial T2WI show the normal appearance of cervical disks, foramina, subarachnoid fluid, and spinal cord.

Narrowing of the thecal sac, lateral recesses, and intervertebral foramina can result in clinical signs and symptoms. Narrowing can result from disk herniations, posterior vertebral body osteophytes, hypertrophy of ligamentum flavum and facet joints, synovial cysts, excessive epidural fat, epidural neoplasms, abscesses, hematomas, spinal fractures, spondylolisthesis, or spondylolysis. MRI is useful for evaluating for these disorders and for categorizing the degree of narrowing of the thecal sac as well as compression of nerve roots in the lateral recesses and intervertebral foramina.

Table 8.1 Intramedullary lesions

Disease	MRI Findings	Comments
Congenital		
Chiari I malformation (Fig. 8.3)	Cerebellar tonsils extend more than 5 mm below the foramen magnum in adults, 6 mm in children below 10 years. Syringohydromyelia in 20–40%. Hydrocephalus in 25%. Basilar impression in 25%. Less common association: Klippel-Feil, atlanto-occipital assimilation.	Cerebellar tonsilar ectopia. Most common anomaly of CNS. Not associated with myelomeningocele.
Chiari II malformation (Arnold-Chiari) (Fig. 8.4)	Small posterior cranial fossa with gaping foramen magnum through which there is an inferiorly positioned vermis associated with a cervicomedullary kink. Beaked dorsal margin of the tectal plate. Myeloceles or myelomeningoceles in nearly all patients. Hydrocephalus and syringohydromyelia are common. Dilated lateral ventricles posteriorly (colpocephaly).	Complex anomaly involving the cerebrum, cerebellum, brainstem, spinal cord, ventricles, skull, and dura. Failure of fetal neural folds to develop properly results in altered development affecting multiple sites of the central nervous system (CNS).

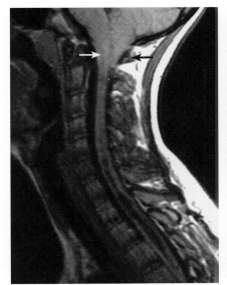
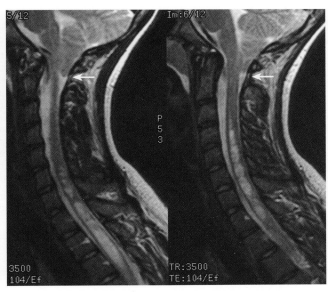

a

b

Fig. 8.3 Chiari I malformation. Sagittal T1WI (**a**) and T2WI (**b**) show the cerebellar tonsils extending through the foramen magnum with the inferior margins below the posterior arch of C1 (arrows). A syrinx is seen in the spinal cord associated with the Chiari I malformation.

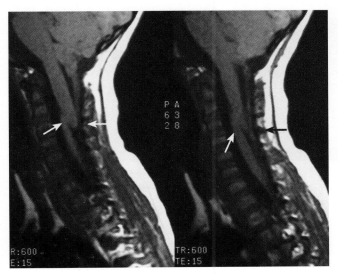

Fig. 8.4 Chiari II malformation (Arnold-Chiari). Sagittal T1WI shows a small posterior cranial fossa with gaping foramen magnum, through which there is an inferiorly positioned vermis associated with a cervicomedullary kink (arrows).

Table 8.1 (Cont.) **Intramedullary lesions**

Disease	MRI Findings	Comments
Chiari III malformation	Features of Chiari II plus lower occipital or high cervical encephalocele.	Rare anomaly associated with high mortality.
Myelomenigocele/ myelocele (Fig. 8.5)	MRI usually performed after surgical repair of myeloceles or myelomeningoceles. Posterior protrusion of spinal contents and unfolded neural tube (neural placode) through defects in the bony dorsal elements of the involved vertebrae or sacral elements. The neural placode is usually located at the lower lumbosacral region with resultant tethering of the spinal cord. If the neural placode is flush with the adjacent skin surface, the anomaly is labeled a myelocele. If the neural placode extends above the adjacent skin surface, the anomaly is labeled a myelomeningocele. Syringohydromyelia may be associated.	Failure of developmental closure of the caudal neural tube results in an unfolded neural tube (neural placode) exposed to the dorsal surface in the midline without overlying skin. Other features associated with myelomeningoceles and myeloceles include: dorsal bony dysraphism, deficient dura posteriorly at the site of the neural placode, and Chiari II malformations. By definition the spinal cords are tethered. Usually repaired surgically soon after birth.
Terminal myelocystocele (Fig. 8.6)	Posterior lower spina bifida through which the distal portion of a tethered spinal cord (containing a localized cystic dilatation), CSF and meninges extends beneath the dorsal subcutaneous fat.	Represent 1–5% of skin-covered masses at dorsal lumbosacral region. Anomalous development of the lower spinal cord, vertebral column, sacrum, and meninges. With or without associated anomalies of genitourinary tract (epispadias, caudal regression syndrome, anomalies of the genitourinary system and hindgut).
Lipomyelocele/lipomyelomeningocele (Fig. 8.7)	Unfolded caudal neural tube (neural placode) covered by a lipoma that is contiguous with the dorsal subcutaneous fat through defects (spina bifida) involving the bony dorsal vertebral elements. The neural placode is usually located at the lower lumbosacral region with resultant tethering of the spinal cord, with or without syringohydromyelia. With lipomyelomeningocele, the dorsal lipoma that extends into the spinal canal is asymmetric resulting in rotation of the placode and meningocele.	Failure of developmental closure of the caudal neural tube results in an unfolded neural tube (neural placode) covered by a lipoma which is continuous with the subcutaneous fat. The overlying skin is intact, although the lipoma usually protrudes dorsally. The nerve roots arise from the placode. Features associated with lipomyelomeningoceles and lipomyeloceles include: tethered spinal cords, dorsal bony dysraphism, deficient dura posteriorly at the site of the neural placode. Not associated with Chiari II malformations. Diagnosis often in children, occasionally in adults.
Intradural lipoma (Fig. 8.8)	Focal dorsal dysraphic spinal cord attached to a lipoma, which has high signal on T1WI. Lipoma often extends from the central canal of the spinal cord to the pial surface, intact dorsal dural margins and posterior vertebral elements.	Intradural lipomas are usually in the cervical or thoracic region.

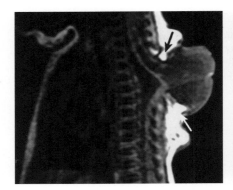

a

Fig. 8.5   **Thoracic myelomeningocele.**
Sagittal T1WI (**a**) and axial T2WI (**b**) show a thoracic myelomeningocele with posterior protrusion of spinal contents consisting of

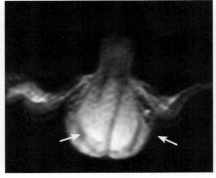

b

an unfolded neural tube (neural placode), meninges and CSF through defects in the bony dorsal elements.

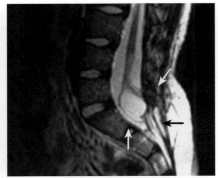

Fig. 8.6   **Repaired terminal myelocystocele.** Sagittal T2WI shows the distal portion of a tethered spinal cord containing a localized cystic dilatation (arrows).

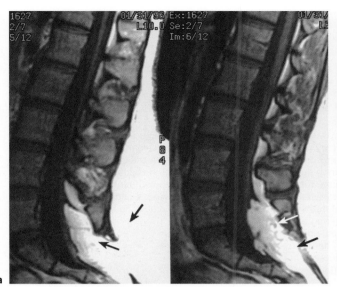

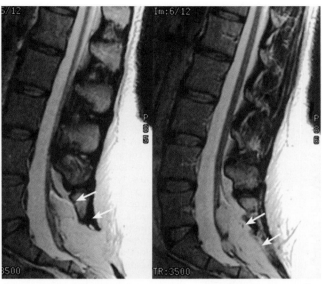

Fig. 8.**7** **Lipomyelocele/lipomyelomeningocele.** Sagittal T1WI (**a**) and T2WI (**b**) show an unfolded caudal neural tube (neural placode) covered by a lipoma which is contiguous with the dorsal subcutaneous fat through defects (spina bifida) involving the bony dorsal vertebral elements (arrows). The neural placode is located at the L5 and sacral region with resultant tethering of the spinal cord.

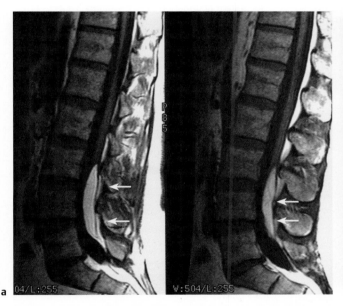

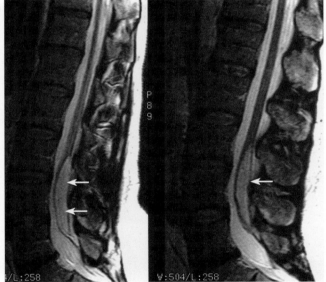

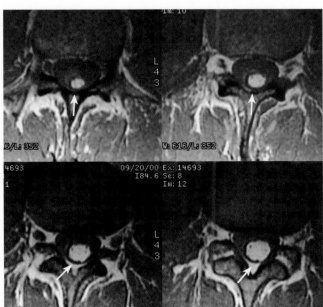

Fig. 8.**8** **Intradural lipoma.** Sagittal T1WI (**a**) and T2WI (**b**) show a focal dorsal dysraphic spinal cord attached to a lipoma which has high signal (arrows). **c** Axial proton density weighted image shows the high signal lipoma extending from the central canal of the spinal cord to the pial surface. Intact dorsal dural margins and posterior vertebral elements are present.

Table 8.1 (Cont.) Intramedullary lesions

Disease	MRI Findings	Comments
Fibrolipoma of the filum terminale (Fig. 8.9)	Thin linear zone of high signal on T1WI along the filum terminale, usually less than 3 mm in diameter. Normal position of conus medullaris (typically not associated with tethering of spinal cord).	Asymptomatic incidental finding with incidence of approximately 5 %.
Diastematomyelia (Fig. 8.10)	Division of spinal cord into two hemicords usually from T9 to S1; fibrous or bony septum may partially or completely separate the two hemicords. Hemicords located either within a common dural tube (50 %, type II) or within separate dural tubes (50 %, type I). With or without associated syringo-hydromyelia at, above, or below zone of diastematomyelia. Often associated with tethering of the conus medullaris, osseous anomalies (spina bifida with laminar fusion, butterfly vertebrae, hemivertebrae, block vertebrae). Diastematomyelia seen in 15 % of patients with Chiari II malformations.	Developmental anomalies related to abnormal splitting of the embryonic notochord with abnormal adhesions between the ectoderm and endoderm. Can present in children with clubfeet, or in adults and children with neurogenic bladder, lower extremity weakness, and chronic pain. With or without associated nevi, lipomas.
Ventriculus terminalis of the conus medullaris (Fig. 8.11)	Discrete intramedullary zone with low signal on T1WI and high signal on T2WI (equivalent to CSF) located in conus medullaris. Intramedullary cystic zone usually measures 25–40 mm craniocaudad x 17–25 mm axial plane surrounded by a thin rim of spinal cord up to 2 mm thick. No Gd-contrast enhancement. No syrinx above level of intramedullary cystic zone in conus medullaris.	Ventriculus terminalis is a congenital anomaly which consists of a persistent ependymal-lined dilated lumen containing CSF located in the conus medullaris. This lumen forms during embyonic development of the spinal cord during the stage of secondary neurulation (approximately 5 weeks of gestation).

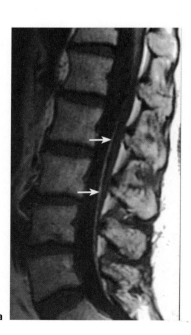

Fig. 8.9 **Fibrolipoma of the filum terminale.** Sagittal T1WI (**a**) and axial proton density weighted image (**b**) show a thin linear zone of high signal along the filum terminale measuring less than 3 mm in diameter (arrows). A normal position of conus medullaris is present.

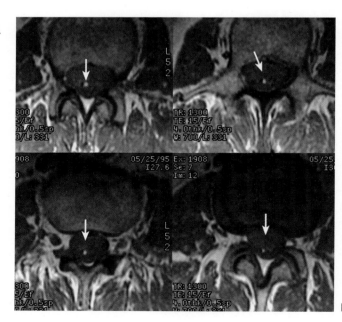

a

b

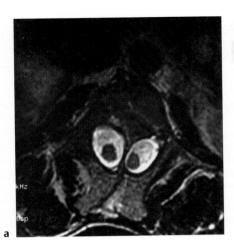

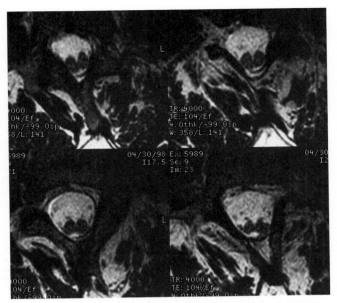

Fig. 8.10 Diastematomyelia.
a Axial T2WI shows division of spinal cord into two hemicords with a bony septum completely separating the two hemicords (type I).
b Axial T2WI in another patient shows hemicords located within a common dural tube (type II). Sagittal (**c**) and coronal (**d**) T2WI of patient in (**b**) above shows tethering of the conus medullaris.

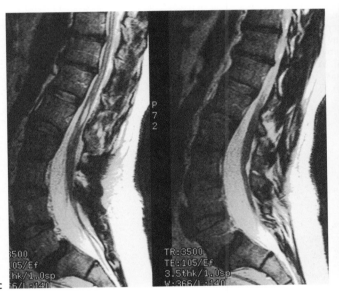

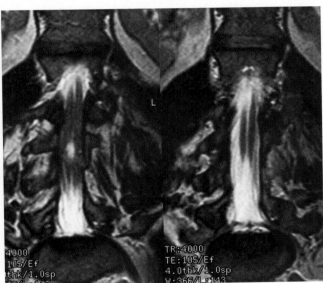

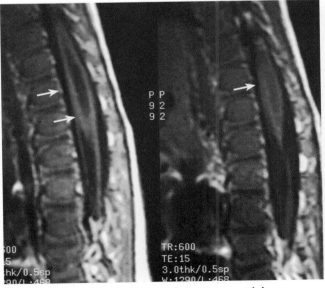

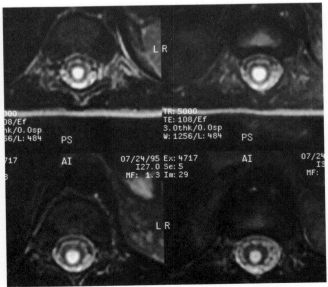

Fig. 8.11 Ventriculus terminalis of the conus medullaris. **a** Sagittal T1WI show a discrete intramedullary cystic zone with low signal associated with slight expansion of the conus medullaris (arrows). **b** Axial T2WI shows a well-circumscribed zone of high signal within the conus.

Table 8.1 (Cont.) Intramedullary lesions

Disease	MRI Findings	Comments
Inflammatory:		
Demyelinating disease		
Multiple sclerosis (MS) (Fig. 8.12)	Intramedullary lesion or multiple lesions in spinal cord, usually have low to intermediate signal on T1WI and high signal on T2WI. With or without Gd-contrast enhancement. Usually located in peripheral portions of spinal cord, occupy less than 50 % of cross-sectional area of cord, typically two vertebral segments or less. Gd-contrast enhancement usually in acute/early subacute phase of demyelination. Acute/subacute demyelinating lesions may mildly expand the spinal cord.	MS is the most common acquired demyelinating disease usually affecting women (peak age 20–40 years). Plaques in spinal cord associated with atrophy often associated with relapsing/remitting type of MS. Devic disease is a variant of MS that consists of optic neuritis and progressive demyelination of spinal cord without evidence of demyelination in the brain. Other demyelinating diseases include: acute disseminated encephalomyelitis (ADEM)–immune mediated demyelination after viral infection; toxins (exogenous from environmental exposure or ingestion–alcohol, solvents etc.–or endogenous from metabolic disorder–leukodystrophies, mitochondrial encephalopathies, etc.), radiation injury, trauma, vascular disease.
ADEM (Fig. 8.13)	Intramedullary lesion or multiple lesions in spinal cord with low to intermediate signal on T1WI and high signal on T2WI. Lesions located in peripheral white matter of spinal cord; may or may not involve central portions of spinal cord (gray matter); mild cord expansion may be associated. With or without Gd-contrast enhancement usually in acute/early subacute phases of demyelination.	ADEM is a noninfectious monophasic inflammatory/demyelination process involving the spinal cord and/or brain, occurring several weeks after viral infection or vaccination. More common in children than adults. Associated with various bilateral motor and sensory deficits.

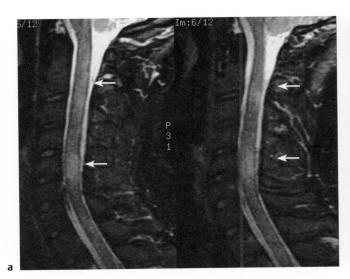

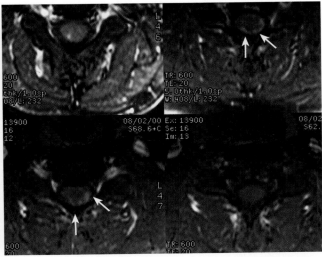

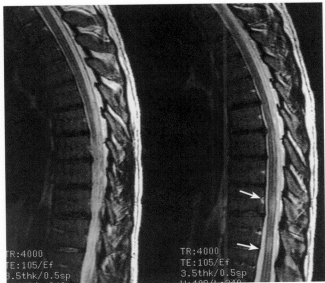

Fig. 8.**12** **MS.** **a** Sagittal inversion recovery (STIR) image shows two intramedullary lesions with high signal in the cervical spinal cord (arrows). Minimal expansion of the spinal cord is seen associated with the lesions. **b** Postcontrast FS axial T1WI shows enhancement in the peripheral portions of the spinal cord, indicating sites of recent active demyelination (arrows). **c** Sagittal T2WI also shows two lesions with high signal in the lower thoracic spinal cord (arrows).

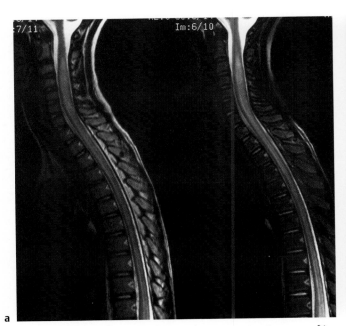

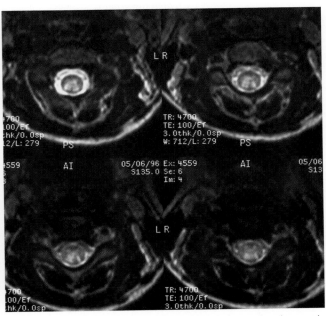

Fig. 8.**13** **ADEM.** **a** Sagittal T2WI shows an extensive zone of intramedullary high signal involving most of the spinal cord associated with mild expansion. **b** Axial T2WI shows the abnormal high signal involves both white and gray matter of the spinal cord.

Table 8.1 (Cont.) Intramedullary lesions

Disease	MRI Findings	Comments
Transverse myelitis (Fig. 8.14)	Intramedullary lesion or multiple lesions in spinal cord with low to intermediate signal on T1WI and high signal on T2WI. Involves thoracic spinal cord more commonly than cervical spinal cord. Usually located in central portion of spinal cord. Lesions typically occupy more than two-thirds of cross-sectional area of cord (88%) on T2WI; commonly extend three to four vertebral segments (53%); with or without mild cord expansion (47%). Gd-contrast enhancement (focal or peripheral) seen in 53%, usually in acute/early subacute phase of demyelination.	Transverse myelitis is a noninfectious inflammatory process involving both halves of the spinal cord as well as gray and white matter. Multiple causes include: demyelination after viral infection or vaccination (possibly a variant of ADEM), autoimmune diseases/collagen vascular diseases (SLE), paraneoplastic syndromes, atypical MS, idiopathic. Can be diagnosis of exclusion. More common in males than females, mean age 45 years. Associated with various bilateral motor and sensory deficits. Pathologic changes considered to be a combination of demyelination and arterial or venous ischemia.
Other noninfectious inflammatory disease involving the spinal cord		
Sarcoidosis (Fig. 8.15)	Poorly marginated intramedullary zone of high signal on T2WI and low to intermediate signal on T1WI; usually with Gd-contrast enhancement (patchy, multifocal, more commonly peripheral than central). With or without mild expansion of spinal cord and associated leptomeningeal enhancement along pial surface. Cervical/upper thoracic spinal cord more common than mid and lower thoracic spinal cord.	Sarcoidosis is a multisystem noncaseating granulomatous disease of uncertain cause that which involves the CNS in approximately 5–15%. Rarely involves the spinal cord. Association with severe neurologic deficits if untreated. May mimick intramedullary neoplasm.
Infectious diseases of spinal cord		
Viral	Intramedullary lesion or multiple lesions in spinal cord with low to intermediate signal on T1WI and high signal on T2WI. With or without minimal cord expansion. With or without mild Gd-contrast enhancement and leptomeningeal enhancement (cytomegalovirus [CMV], herpes).	Direct infection of spinal cord, common viruses include: polio virus, coxsackievirus, herpes zoster, CMV, human immunodeficiency viruses, JC virus.
Abscess/nonviral infectious myelitis	Early findings of myelitis and spinal cord abscess include: intramedullary zone of high signal on T2WI with a poorly defined peripheral zone of contrast enhancement on T1WI. The zone of peripheral enhancement can become better defined over time. Both high signal abnormalities on T2WI and enhancement can resolve with antibiotic therapy. Residual myelomalacia may be associated. With or without leptomeningeal enhancement (*Mycobacterium tuberculosis*, syphilis).	Infection can result from hematogenous dissemination or spread within CSF. Organisms reported to result in spinal cord abscess or nonviral myelitis include *Streptococcus milleria, S. pyogenes, Mycobacterium tuberculosis*, atypical mycobacteria, syphilis, *Schistosoma mansoni*, and *Fungi* (*Crytococcus, Candida*, and *Aspergillus*). In immunocompromised patients.

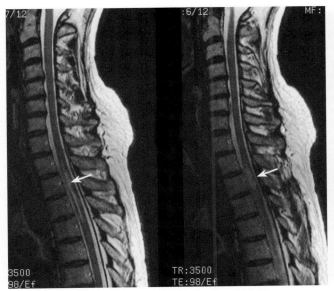

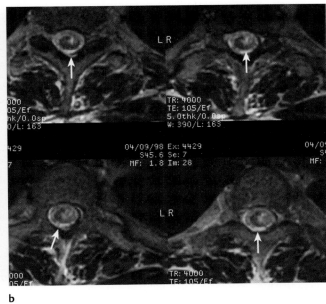

a   **b**

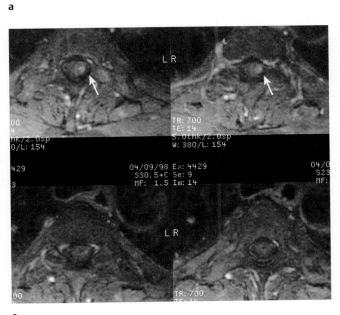

c

Fig. 8.**14** **Transverse myelitis.** Sagittal (**a**) and axial (**b**) T2WI shows an intramedullary zone of abnormal high signal involving the thoracic spinal cord. The signal abnormality involves up to two-thirds of the cross-sectional area of spinal cord. **c** Postcontrast FS axial T1WI shows mild peripheral enhancement associated with the lesion (arrows).

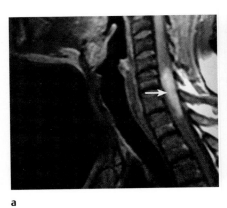

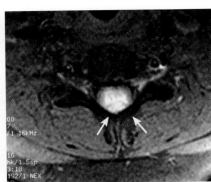

a   **b**

Fig. 8.**15** **Sarcoidosis.** Postcontrast FS sagittal (**a**) and axial (**b**) T1WI shows an irregularly marginated enhancing intramedullary lesion involving the cervical spinal cord (arrows). Expansion of the spinal cord is seen associated with this lesion.

Table 8.1 (Cont.) Intramedullary lesions

Disease	MRI Findings	Comments
Parasitic (Fig. 8.16)	Poorly marginated intramedullary zone of high signal on T2WI and low to intermediate signal on T1WI, usually with Gd-contrast enhancement. Lesions often located in thoracic spinal cord. With or without leptomeningeal enhancement. Concurrent lesions in brain are usually present.	Parasitic infection of the spinal cord is rare. The most common type of parasite to involve the spinal cord is *Toxoplasma gondii* in immunocompromised patients. Toxoplasmosis rarely involves the spinal cord, unlike cerebral infection. *Schistosoma mansoni* can involve the spinal cord in immunocompetent patients in Asia/Africa. Associated with rapid decline in neurologic function related to site of lesion in spinal cord.
Radiation injury	Focal lesion in spinal cord with poorly defined zone of low to intermediate signal on T1WI and intermediate to high signal on T2WI; with or without Gd-contrast enhancement. With or without expansion of spinal cord. Late phase: gliosis/atrophy.	Usually occurs from 3 months to 10 years after radiation treatment, may be difficult to distinguish from neoplasm. Marrow in field of radiation treatment typically has high signal on T1WI because of loss of red marrow (increased proportion of yellow marrow to red marrow).
Vascular		
Intramedullary hemorrhage (Fig. 8.17)	The signal of the hematoma depends on its age, size, location, hematocrit, hemoglobin oxidation state, clot retraction, and extent of edema. *Hyperacute phase (4–6 hours):* Hemoglobin primarily as diamagnetic oxyhemoglobin (iron Fe +2 state), intermediate signal on T1WI, slightly high signal on T2WI. *Acute phase (12–48 hours):* Hemoglobin primarily as paramagnetic deoxyhemoglobin (iron, Fe +2 state), intermediate signal on T1WI and low signal on T2WI, surrounded by a peripheral zone of high T2 signal (edema). *Subacute phase (>2 days):* Hemoglobin becomes oxidized to the iron Fe+3 state, methemoglobin, which is strongly paramagnetic. When methemoglobin is initially intracellular the hematoma has high signal on T1WI, progressing from peripheral to central, and low signal on T2WI, surrounded by a zone of high T2 signal (edema). When methemoglobin eventually becomes primarily extracellular the hematoma has high signal on T1WI and on T2WI. *Chronic phase:* Hemoglobin as extracellular methemoglobin is progressively degraded to hemosiderin.	Can result from trauma, vascular malformations, coagulopathy, amyloid angiopathy, infarction, metastases, abscesses, viral infections (herpes simplex, CMV).
Posthemorrhagic lesions	Intramedullary zone with high signal on T2WI secondary to gliosis and myelomalacia. With or without localized thinning of spinal cord, with or without sites of low signal on T2WI where there is methemoglobin (also high signal on T1WI) and/or hemosiderin deposition. Typically no enhancement.	Sites of prior hemorrhage can have variable appearance depending on the relative ratios of gliosis, encephalomalacia, and blood breakdown products (methemoglobin, hemosiderin, etc).
Arteriovenous malformation (AVM) (Fig. 8.18)	Lesions with irregular margins that can be located in the spinal cord (white and/or gray matter), dura, or both locations. AVMs contain multiple tortuous tubular flow voids on T1WI and T2WI secondary to patent arteries with high blood flow; as well as thrombosed vessels with variable signal, areas of hemorrhage in various phases, calcifications, gliosis, and myelomalacia. The venous portions often show Gd-contrast enhancement. With or without associated ischemia (high signal on T2WI in spinal cord) related to venous congestion. Swelling of spinal cord may be associated. Usually not associated with mass effect except in cases of recent hemorrhage or venous occlusion.	Intracranial AVMs are much more common than spinal AVMs. Annual risk of hemorrhage. AVMs can be sporadic, congenital, or associated with a history of trauma. Multiple AVMs can be seen in syndromes: Rendu-Osler-Weber, AVMs in brain and lungs, and mucosal capillary telangiectasias; Wyburn-Mason, AVMs in brain and retina, and cutaneous nevi.

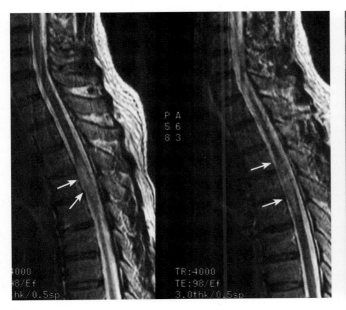

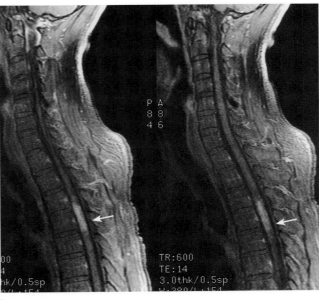

a

b

Fig. 8.**16**   **Intramedullary toxoplasmosis infection in an immunocompromised patient.**   **a** Sagittal T2WI shows an intramedullary lesion with high signal in the thoracic spinal cord associated with mild cord expansion (arrows).   **b** Postcontrast FS sagittal T1WI shows prominent enhancement of the lesion (arrows).

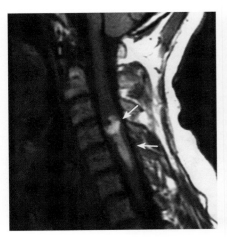

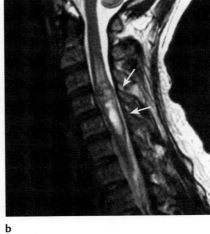

a

b

Fig. 8.**17**   **Subacute intramedullary hemorrhage.** Sagittal T1WI (**a**) and T2WI (**b**) show a subacute intramedullary hematoma with high signal and cord expansion (arrows) secondary to a vascular malformation confirmed later at surgery.

Fig. 8.**18**   **AVM.** Sagittal T2WI shows a large AVM involving the spinal cord and dura with multiple large and small tortuous tubular flow voids (arrows).

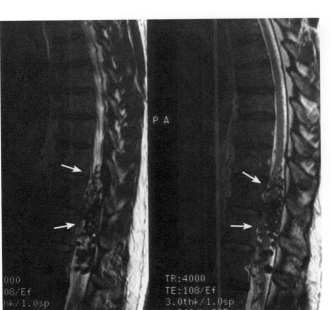

Table **8.1** (Cont.) Intramedullary lesions

Disease	MRI Findings	Comments
Cavernous hemangioma (Fig. 8.19)	Single or multiple multilobulated intramedullary lesions that have a peripheral rim or irregular zone of low signal on T2WI secondary to hemosiderin, surrounding a central zone of variable signal (low, intermediate, high, or mixed) on T1WI and T2WI depending on ages of hemorrhagic portions. Gradient echo (GRE) techniques useful for detecting multiple lesions.	Can occur as multiple lesions in brain, brainstem, and/or spinal cord. Association with increased risk of hemorrhage.
Venous angioma	On postcontrast T1WI, venous angiomas are seen as a Gd-contrast-enhancing vein draining a collection of small medullary veins (caput Medusa). The draining vein can be seen as a signal on T2WI.	Considered an anomalous venous formation typically not associated with hemorrhage. Usually an incidental finding except when associated with cavernous hemangioma.
Infarct/ischemia of spinal cord–Arterial etiology (Fig. 8.20)	Four MRI patterns of abnormalities associated with spinal cord ischemia related to vascular distribution of the anterior spinal artery (artery of Adamkiewicz): 1. Foci of high signal on T2WI involving the anterior horns of the gray matter of spinal cord. 2. Foci of high signal on T2WI involving both the anterior and posterior horns of the gray matter of spinal cord. 3. Diffuse zone of high signal on T2WI involving all of the gray matter of spinal cord and adjacent central white matter. 4. Diffuse zone of high signal on T2WI involving the entire cross-section of the spinal cord. With or without Gd-contrast enhancement. Expansion of spinal cord may be associated. Location: lower thoracic spinal cord and conus medullaris. May or may not be associated with bone infarcts in adjacent vertebral body/bodies.	Arterial infarcts, often in vascular territory of the anterior spinal artery that supplies the anterior two-thirds of the spinal cord, including white and gray matter. Ischemia or infarcts involving the spinal cord represent rare disorders associated with atherosclerosis, diabetes, hypertension, abdominal aortic aneurysms, and abdominal aortic surgery. Associated with clinical findings of rapid onset of bladder and bowel dysfunction. Ischemia/infarction of the spinal cord is most often seen in thoracolumbar vascular distribution (artery of Adamkiewicz).
Ischemia–Venous infarction/congestion (Fig. 8.21)	Poorly defined intramedullary zone of low to intermediate signal on T1WI and high signal on T2WI involves gray and white matter. With or without cord expansion and Gd-contrast enhancement. Dilated veins on pial surface of spinal cord.	Venous infarction of the spinal cord is associated with dural arteriovenous fistula or malformation, and thrombophlebitis. Results in coagulative necrosis of gray and white matter of spinal cord (subacute necrotizing myelopathy). MRI features may overlap those of arterial-related ischemia/infarction involving the spinal cord.

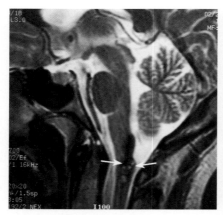

Fig. 8.**19** **Cavernous hemangioma. a** Sagittal T2WI shows a multilobulated intramedullary lesion with a peripheral irregular zone of low signal secondary to hemosiderin surrounding a central zone of mixed low and high signal in at the cervicomedullary junction (arrows).

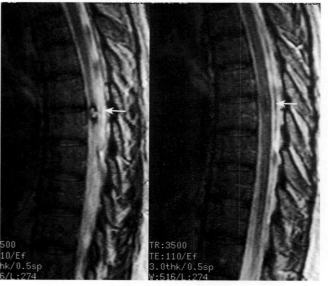

Fig. 8.**19 b** Sagittal T2WI in another patient shows an intramedullary lesion with signal characteristics similar to (**a**) (arrows).

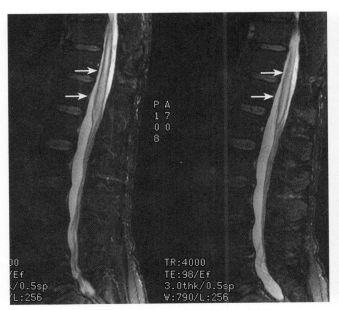

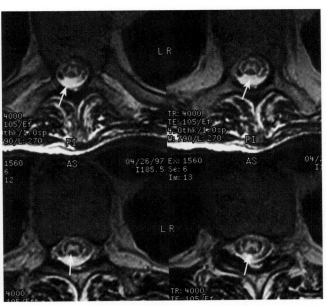

Fig. 8.**20** **Infarct/ischemia of spinal cord--arterial etiology.** **a** Sagittal FS T2WI shows abnormal high signal in the central portion of the lower spinal cord (arrows).

Fig. 8.**20 b** Axial T2WI shows abnormal high signal involving both the anterior and posterior horns of the gray matter of spinal cord (arrows).

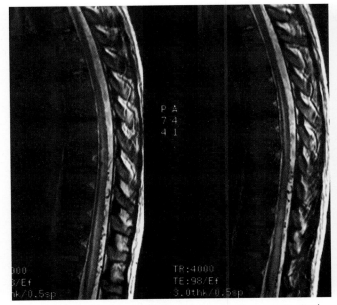

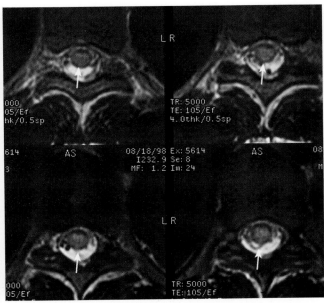

Fig. 8.**21** **Ischemia–venous infarction/congestion.** **a** Sagittal T2WI shows poorly defined intramedullary high signal in the lower spinal cord representing venous congestion secondary to a dural AVM. Note the multiple small flow voids along the dorsal margin of the spinal cord representing dilated hyalinized veins of the AVM.

Fig. 8.**21 b** Axial T2WI show abnormal high signal involving both the gray and white matter of the spinal cord (arrows).

Table **8.1** (Cont.) Intramedullary lesions

Disease	MRI Findings	Comments
Traumatic		
Spinal cord contusion (Fig. 8.22)	Poorly defined intramedullary zone of low to intermediate signal on T1WI and high signal on T2WI, involving gray and/or white matter. With or without cord expansion, with or without zones of high signal on T1WI (methemoglobin) or low signal on T2WI (intracellular methemoglobin). Usually no Gd-contrast enhancement. With or without avulsed nerve roots (Erbs palsy), vertebral fracture, and disruption of posterior longitudinal ligament.	Traumatic injury of spinal cord often secondary to large disk herniation, vertebral fracture, vertebral subluxation/dislocation, impression by foreign body, hyperflexion/extension injury, birth trauma.
Trauma shear injury	Foci and/or diffuse zones of high signal on T2WI involving gray and/or white matter of spinal cord, usually no enhancement.	Traumatic injury from acceleration/deceleration or shaking resulting in transection of axons. Often associated with other injuries such as vertebral fractures, traumatic subarachnoid or intramedullary hemorrhage.
Chronic injury (Fig. 8.23)	Poorly defined intramedullary zone of low to intermediate signal on T1WI and high signal on T2WI, involving gray and white matter. With or without cord atrophy, intramedullary zones of cavitation (discrete zones of low signal on T1WI and high signal on T2WI) or macrocystic change. No Gd-contrast enhancement. Syringohydromyelia may be associated.	Myelomalacic changes that can result from prior traumatic injuries, severe spinal stenosis, severe kyphosis, spondylolisthesis, radiation injury.
Syringohydromyelia (Fig. 8.24)	Enlarged spinal cord with intramedullary fluid-filled zone that is central or slightly eccentric. Usually there is a distinct interface between the intramedullary fluid and solid portions of the spinal cord. Septations along syrinx may be present. With or without zone of high signal surrounding syrinx (edema, gliosis). No enhancement if benign syringohydromyelia, with or without enhancement if syrinx associated with intramedullary neoplasm.	Hydromyelia refers to distention of the central canal of the spinal cord (lined by ependymal cells). Syringomyelia refers to dissection of CSF into the spinal cord (not lined by ependymal cells). Syringohydromyelia refers to combination of both. May be secondary to congenital/developmental anomalies (Chiari I, Chiari II malformations, basilar invagination), and also secondary to neoplasms of the spinal cord (astrocytoma, ependymoma, hemangioblastoma).

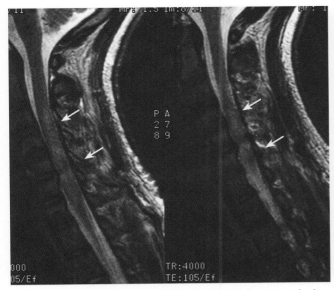

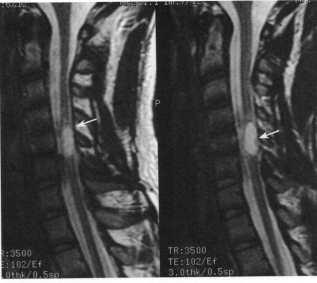

Fig. 8.**22** **Spinal cord contusion.** Sagittal T2WI shows poorly defined intramedullary high signal in a swollen contused cervical spinal cord secondary to trauma (arrows).

Fig. 8.**23** **Chronic injury.** Sagittal T2WI shows a post-traumatic syrinx in the cervical spinal cord (arrows).

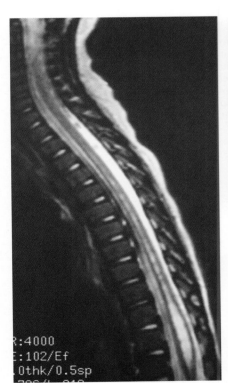

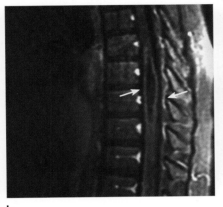

b

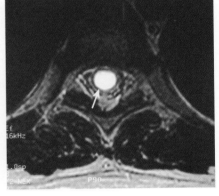

c

Fig. 8.**24** **Syringohydromyelia.** **a** Sagittal T2WI shows a long syrinx with high signal involving the mid and lower thoracic spinal cord. **b** Postcontrast FS sagittal T1WI in another patient shows a localized syrinx with cord expansion (arrows). No enhancement is seen at the syrinx. **c** Axial T2WI shows the syrinx to have uniform high signal (arrow).

a

Table 8.1 (Cont.) Intramedullary lesions

Disease	MRI Findings	Comments
Neoplastic		
Astrocytoma (Fig. 8.25)	Intramedullary expansile ill-defined eccentric lesions with low to intermediate signal on T1WI and intermediate to high signal on T2WI. Tumoral cysts (high signal on T2WI) may be present. Syringohydromyelia may be associated, usually with irregular enhancement. With or without peripheral high T2 signal (edema). Lesions often extends approximately seven vertebral segments. Locations in order of decreasing frequency: cervical spinal cord, upper thoracic spinal cord, conus medullaris.	Most common intramedullary tumor in children, second most common in adults. More common in children than adults. Astrocytomas involving the spinal cord usually are low grade (90% in children, 75% in adults) and slow growing. Anaplastic tumors account for the majority of the other astrocytomas, with glioblastoma accounting for only 1%. More common in males than females. Clinical presentation with pain and sensory deficits, motor dysfunction.
Ependymoma (Fig. 8.26)	Intramedullary circumscribed expansile lesions with low to intermediate signal on T1WI, intermediate to high signal on T2WI, and with or without peripheral rim of low signal (hemosiderin) on T2WI. Tumoral cysts may be present (high signal on T2WI). Syringohydromyelia may be associated. With enhancement (84%), with or without peripheral high T2 signal (edema). Often midline/central location in spinal cord, intramedullary locations: cervical spinal cord 44%, both cervical and upper thoracic spinal cord 23%, thoracic spinal cord 26%. Lesions often extends approximately 3.6 vertebral segments. Scoliosis and chronic bone erosion may be associated.	Most common intramedullary tumor in adults (60% of glial neoplasms). More common in adults than children. Intramedullary ependymomas involving the upper spinal cord often are cellular or mixed histologic types, whereas ependymomas at the conus medullaris or cauda equina usually are myxopapillary. Slight male predominance. Usually slow-growing neoplasms associated with long-duration neck or back pain, sensory deficits, motor weakness, bladder and bowel dysfunction.
Ganglioglioma (Fig. 8.27)	Circumscribed intramedullary tumor, variable mixed low to intermediate signal on T1WI and intermediate to high T2 signal on T2WI. Cysts may be present. Gd-contrast enhancement (85%), usually minimal or no surrounding edema (high signal on T2WI). Association with scoliosis (44%) and bone erosion (93%).	Rare tumors involving the spinal cord (1% of spinal neoplasms). May extend inferiorly from lesion in cerebellum, ganglioglioma (contains glial and neuronal elements), ganglioneuroma (contains only ganglion cells). Uncommon tumors, below 30 years, slow-growing neoplasms. gangliocytoma (contains only neuronal elements).

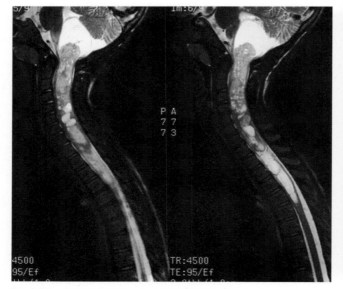

Fig. 8.**25** **Astrocytoma.** **a** Sagittal T2WI shows a large expansile intramedullary lesion with heterogeneous intermediate and high signal.

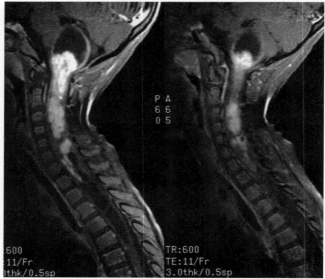

Fig. 8.**25 b** Postcontrast FS T1WI shows heterogeneous prominent enhancement of the lesion. Note the presence of a tumoral cyst superiorly (with a thin rim of enhancement) and a syrinx caudad to the enhancing lesion.

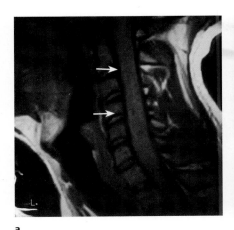
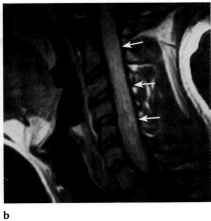

a

b

Fig. 8.**26** **Ependymoma.** **a** Sagittal T1WI shows an intramedullary circumscribed expansile lesion in the cervical spinal cord with intermediate signal (arrows). **b** Postcontrast sagittal T1WI shows enhancement of the lesion (arrows).

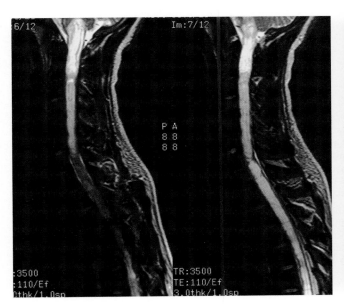

a

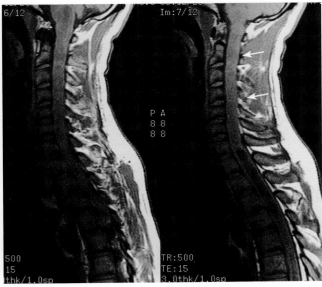

b

c

Fig. 8.**27** **Ganglioglioma.** **a** Sagittal T2WI shows a large expansile intramedullary lesion with high signal. **b** Sagittal T1WI shows an intramedullary circumscribed expansile lesion in the cervical spinal cord with intermediate signal (arrows). **c** Postcontrast T1WI shows heterogeneous prominent enhancement of the lesion (arrows). Note the presence of a syrinx caudad to the enhancing lesion.

Table 8.1 (Cont.) Intramedullary lesions

Disease	MRI Findings	Comments
Hemangioblastoma (Fig. 8.28)	Circumscribed tumors usually located in the superifical portion of the spinal cord. Small Gd-contrast-enhancing nodule, with or without cyst, or larger lesion with prominent heterogeneous enhancement with or without flow voids within lesion or at the periphery. Intermediate signal on T1WI, intermediate to high signal on T2WI. Occasionally lesions have evidence of recent or remote hemorrhage, usually associated with syrinx. Locations: thoracic spinal cord (50–60%), cervical spinal cord (40–50%).	Represent approximately 5% of spinal cord neoplasms. Usually intramedullary lesions, but occasionally extend into the intradural space or extradural location. Sporadic lesions usually occur in patients below 40. Multiple lesions occur in adolescents with von Hippel-Lindau disease.
Metastasis (Fig. 8.29)	Intramedullary lesion or superficial lesions with low to intermediate signal on T1WI and intermediate to high signal on T2WI; enhancement with surrounding edema (high signal on T2WI) in spinal cord or along the pial surface. Cysts rare. Often extend two to three vertebral segments.	Rare intramedullary lesions that can present with pain, bladder or bowel dysfunction, and paresthesias. Location: cervical spinal cord (45%), thoracic spinal cord (35%), lumbar region (8%). Usually solitary lesions, occasionally multiple; spread hematogenously via arteries, or direct extension into leptomeninges.with invasion of pial surface or central canal of the spinal cord. Primary CNS tumors include primary neuroectodermal tumors/medulloblastoma, glioblastoma. Primary tumors outside of CNS include: lung carcinoma (70%), breast carcinoma (11%), melanoma (5%), renal cell carcinoma (4%), colorectal carcinoma (3%), lymphoma (3%), others (4%).
Other		
Vitamin B12 deficiency (Fig. 8.30)	Symmetric, longitudinally oriented zones of high signal on T2WI involving the dorsal columns of the spinal cord, with or without mild expansion of the spinal cord, usually no Gd-contrast enhancement. Intramedullary signal abnormalities can resolve after correction of vitamin B12 deficiency.	The abnormalities involving the spinal cord caused by vitamin B12 deficiency are referred to as subacute combined degeneration. Histopathologic studies show lesions in the posterior and lateral columns of the spinal cord, as well as the cerebrospinal and corticospinal tracts.
Amyotrophic lateral sclerosis	Bilateral symmetric zones of abnormal high signal on T2WI in craniospinal motor tracts (anterior and lateral corticospinal tracts) extending from internal capsules and cerebral peduncles. Typically no enhancement. Atrophy of spinal cord may be associated.	Disorder affecting adults below 55 years with progressive muscle weakness and atrophy leading to death.

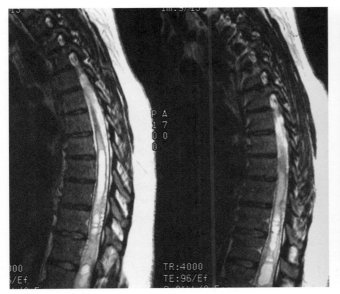

a

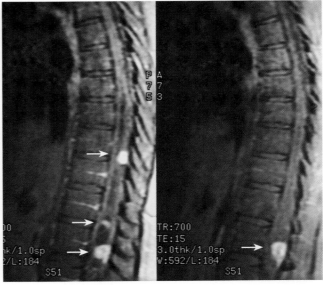

b

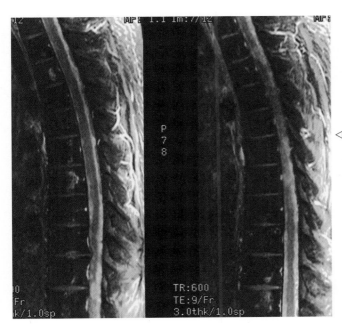

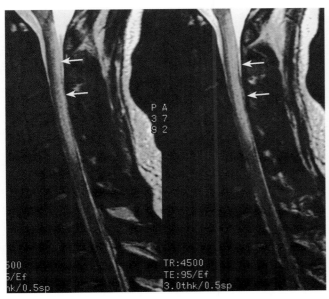

a

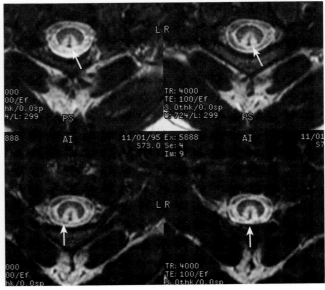

b

△
Fig. 8.**28**   **Hemangioblastomas/von Hippel-Lindau disease.   a** Sagittal T2WI show abnormal heterogeneous high signal of an expanded spinal cord.   **b** Postcontrast FS T1WI shows three nodular intramedullary zones of enhancement representing hemangioblastomas (arrows).

◁ Fig. 8.**29**   **Metastasis from disseminated medulloblastoma.** Postcontrast FS T1WI shows extensive abnormal enhancement in the spinal subarachnoid space with nodularity along the pial surface of the spinal cord. Note the multiple enhancing metastatic foci in the bone marrow, which otherwise has predominantly low signal secondary to extensive sclerotic metastatic lesions.

Fig. 8.**30**   **Vitamin B12 deficiency.** Sagittal (**a**) and axial (**b**) T2WI show symmetric, longitudinally oriented zones of high signal involving the dorsal columns of the spinal cord (arrows).
▽

Table 8.1 (Cont.) Intramedullary lesions

Disease	MRI Findings	Comments
Wallerian degeneration	Bilateral zones of abnormal high signal on T2WI in lateral corticospinal tracts below the site of spinal cord injury, and in the dorsal columns above the site of cord injury, usually seen 7 weeks or more after injury. Typically no enhancement.	Wallerian degeneration represents antegrade degeneration of axons and their myelin sheaths from injury to the cell bodies or proximal portions of axons. With spinal cord damage, wallerian degeneration is seen in the dorsal columns above the site of injury and in the corticospinal tracts below the site of injury. The size of intramedullary lesions/abnormalities is dependent on the number of axons affected. Neurodegenerative disorder involving one side of the brainstem and spinal cord related to neuronal/axonal loss in brain from cerebral infarction or cerebral hemorrhage.
Poliomyelitis (Fig. 8.31)	Acute infection appears as localized enlargement and high signal on T2WI involving the ventral horns of spinal cord. Chronic manifestations appear as foci of high signal on T2WI in one or both of the ventral horns of spinal cord.	Poliomyelitis virus targets the anterior horn cells in spinal cord (ventral horns) resulting in asymmetric flaccid paralysis. The native virus is virtually eradicated, although vaccine-associated paralytic poliomyelitis does rarely occur.
Superficial siderosis (Fig. 8.32)	Thin rims of low signal on T2WI and GRE images along the pial surface of the spinal cord and/or brain.	The low signal on T2WI and GRE images results from hemosiderin deposition from prior episodes of subarachnoid hemorrhage (ruptured aneurysm, trauma, coagulopathy, vascular malformation, etc.)

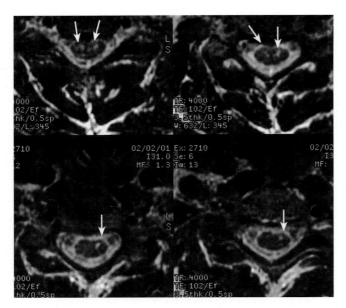

Fig. 8.**31**   **Poliomyelitis, chronic.** Axial T2WI shows small foci of high signal involving the ventral horns of the spinal cord (arrows).

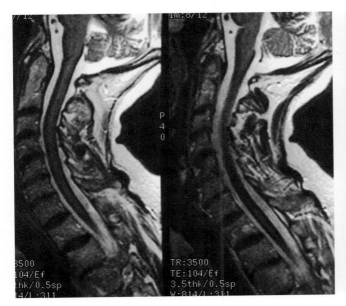

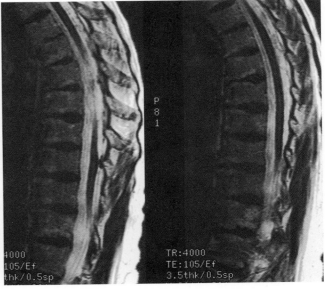

a

b

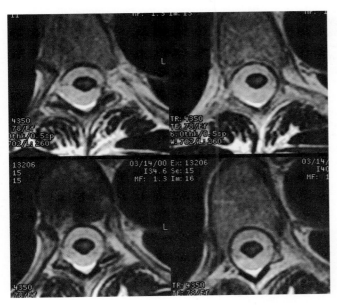

c

Fig. 8. **32   Superficial siderosis.** Sagittal (**a, b**) and axial (**c**) T2WI show thin rims of low signal along the pial surface of the spinal cord.

Table 8.2 Intradural extramedullary lesions

Disease	MRI Findings	Comments
Congenital		
Meningoceles (Fig. 8.33)	Protrusion of CSF and meninges through a dorsal vertebral defect, either from surgical laminectomies or congenital anomaly. Sacral meningoceles can alternatively extend anteriorly through a defect in the sacrum.	Acquired meningoceles are more common than meningoceles resulting from congenital dorsal bony dysraphism. Anterior sacral meningoceles can result from trauma or be associated with mesenchymal dysplasias (neurofibromatosis type 1, Marfan syndrome, syndrome of caudal regression).
Lipomyelomeningocele (Fig. 8.7)	Unfolded caudal neural tube (neural placode) covered by a lipoma which is contiguous with the dorsal subcutaneous fat through defects (spina bifida) involving the bony dorsal vertebral elements. The neural placode is usually located at the lower lumbosacral region with resultant tethering of the spinal cord. Syringohydromyelia may be associated.	Failure of developmental closure of the caudal neural tube results in an unfolded neural tube (neural placode) covered by a lipoma which is continuous with the subcutaneous fat. The overlying skin is intact, although the lipoma usually protrudes dorsally. The nerve roots arise from the placode. Features associated with lipomyelomeningoceles and lipomyeloceles include: tethered spinal cords, dorsal bony dysraphism, deficient dura posteriorly at the site of the neural placode. Not associated with Chiari II malformations. Diagnosis often in children, occasionally in adults.
Dural ectasia	Scalloping of the dorsal aspects of vertebral bodies, dilatation of optic nerve sheaths, dilatation of intervertebral and sacral foraminal nerve sheaths, lateral meningoceles.	Dural dysplasia associated with neurofibromatosis type 1
Tarlov cysts (perineural cysts) (Fig. 8.34)	Well-circumscribed cysts with MRI signal comparable to CSF involving nerve root sleeves associated with chronic erosive changes involving adjacent bony structures. Sacral (with or without widening of sacral foramina) more common than lumbar nerve root sleeves. Usually range from 15 to 20 mm in diameter, but can be larger.	Typically represent incidental asymptomatic anatomic variants.
Dorsal dermal sinus (Fig. 8.35)	Epithelial-lined tube with low signal on T1WI, extending internally from the dorsal skin of lower back, with or without extension into spinal canal through the median raphe or spina bifida. With or without associated dermoid or epidermoid in spinal canal (approximately 50 %).	Abnormality resulting from lack of normal developmental separation of superficial and neural ectoderm. Lumbar region more common than occipital region. Potential source of infection involving spine and spinal canal.

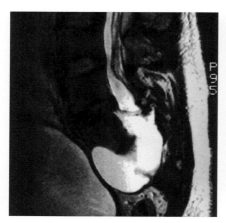

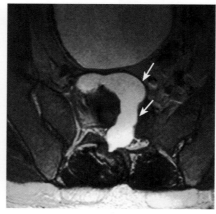

a   b

Fig. 8.**33** **Anterior sacral meningocele, post-traumatic.** Sagittal (**a**) and axial (**b**) T2WI show a well-circumscribed collection of high signal (CSF and meninges) extending anteriorly through a defect in the sacrum (arrows).

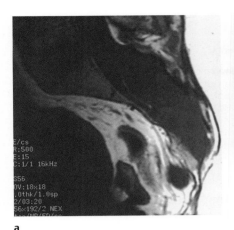

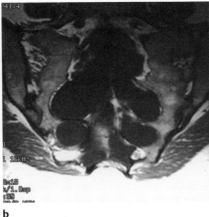

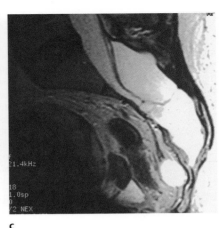

a

b

c

Fig. 8.**34**   **Tarlov cysts (perineural cysts).** Sagittal (**a**) and coronal (**b**) T1WI show large well-circumscribed cysts with low sig- | nal. Involve nerve root sleeves associated with chronic erosive changes involving the sacrum and sacral foramina.   **c** Sagittal | T2WI shows the cysts to have high signal similar to CSF.

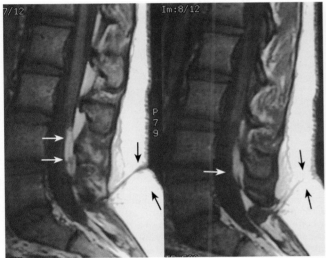

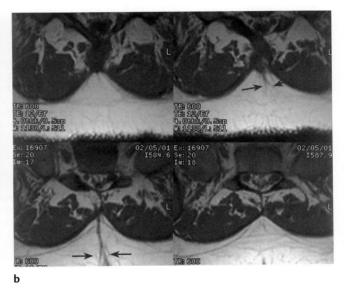

a

b

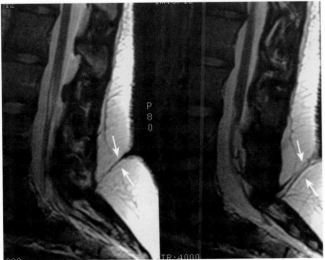

c

Fig. 8.**35**   **Dorsal dermal sinus.** Sagittal (**a**) and axial (**b**) T1WI show an epithelial-lined tube with low signal extending into the spinal canal from the dorsal skin of lower back (arrows). There is focal dilatation of the tract within the dorsal portion of the spinal canal. Note that there is a low-lying conus medullaris and a lipoma at the filum terminale (curved arrows).   **c** Sagittal T2WI shows the dorsal sinus tract to have low signal (arrows).

Table 8.2 (Cont.)   Intradural extramedullary lesions

Disease	MRI Findings	Comments
Dermoid (Fig. 8.36)	Well-circumscribed spheroid or multilobulated intradural extramedullary or intramedullary lesions, usually with intermediate to high signal on T1WI and and variable low, intermediate, and/or high signal on T2WI. No Gd-contrast enhancement. Fluid-fluid or fluid-debris levels may be present. Lumbar region most common location in spine. Can cause chemical meningitis if dermoid cyst ruptures into the subarachnoid space. Commonly located at or near midline.	Non-neoplastic congenital or acquired ectodermal-inclusion cystic lesions filled with lipid material, cholesterol, desquamated cells, and keratinaceous debris. Usually mild mass effect on adjacent spinal cord or nerve roots. In adults, slightly more common in males than females. With or without related clinical symptoms.
Epidermoid	Well-circumscribed spheroid or multilobulated intradural extramedullary lesion with low to intermediate signal on T1WI and high signal on T2WI similar to CSF. Mixed low, intermediate, or high signal on fluid attenuated inversion recovery (FLAIR) images. No Gd-contrast enhancement.	Non-neoplastic extramedullary epithelial-inclusion lesions filled with desquamated cells and keratinaceous debris. Usually mild mass effect on adjacent spinal cord and/or nerve roots. May be congenital (may be associated with dorsal dermal sinus, spina bifida, hemivertebrae) or acquired (late complication of lumbar puncture).
Fibrolipoma of the filum terminale (Fig. 8.9)	Thin linear zone of high signal on T1WI along the filum terminale, usually less than 3 mm in diameter. Normal position of conus medullaris (typically not associated with tethering of spinal cord).	Asymptomatic incidental finding with incidence of approximately 5%.
Neurenteric cyst	Circumscribed intradural extramedullary structures with low to intermediate signal on T1WI and high signal on T2WI. Usually no Gd-contrast enhancement. Location in order of decreasing frequency: thoracic, cervical, posterior cranial fossa, cranioverteberal junction, lumbar; usually midline in position and often ventral to the spinal cord.	Result from developmental failure of separation of the notochord and foregut, observed in patients below 40 years.
Neoplasm and other masses		
Ependymoma (Fig. 8.37)	Intradural circumscribed lobulated lesions at conus medullaris and/or cauda equina/filum terminale, rarely in sacrococcygeal soft tissues. Lesions usually have low to intermediate signal on T1WI and intermediate to high signal on T2WI; with or without foci of high signal on T1WI from mucin or hemorrhage, with or without peripheral rim of low signal (hemosiderin) on T2WI. Tumoral cysts (high signal on T2WI) may be present.	Ependymomas at conus medullaris or cauda equina/filum terminale usually are myxopapillary type, thought to arise from ependymal glia of filum terminale. Slight male predominance. Usually are slow-growing neoplasms associated with long duration of back pain, sensory deficits, motor weakness, bladder and bowel dysfunction. May be associated with chronic erosion of bone with scalloping of vertebral bodies and enlargement of intervertebral foramina.
Schwannoma (neurinoma) (Fig. 8.38)	Circumscribed or lobulated extramedullary lesions with low to intermediate signal on T1WI and high signal on T2WI; prominent Gd-contrast enhancement. High signal on T2WI and Gd-contrast enhancement can be heterogeneous in large lesions due to cystic degeneration and/or hemorrhage.	Encapsulated neoplasms arising asymmetrically from nerve sheath. Most common type of intradural extramedullary neoplasms, usual presentation in adults with pain and radiculopathy, paresthesias and lower extremity weakness. Multiple schwannomas seen with neurofibromatosis type 2.

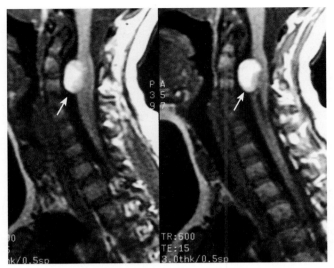

Fig. 8.**36   Dermoid.** Sagittal T1WI shows a well-circumscribed spheroid intradural extramedullary lesion with high signal located ventral to the spinal cord (arrows).

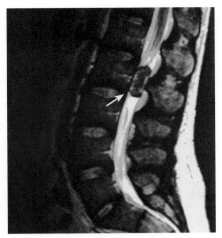

Fig. 8.**37   Ependymoma.   a** Sagittal T2WI shows an intradural circumscribed lesion with low to intermediate signal at the cauda equina (arrow).

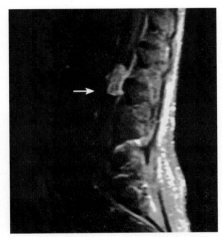

Fig. 8.**37 b**   Postcontrast FS sagittal T1WI shows prominent enhancement of the lesion (arrow).

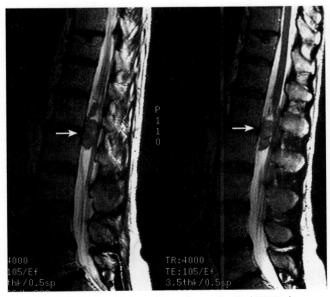

Fig. 8.**38   Schwannoma (neurinoma).   a** Sagittal T2WI show an intradural lobulated lesion with intermediate signal at the cauda equina (arrows).

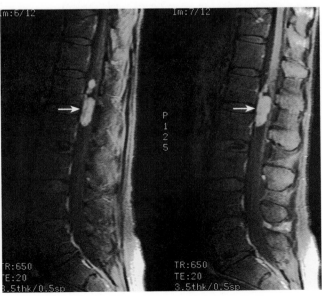

Fig. 8.**38 b**   Postcontrast FS sagittal T1WI show prominent enhancement of the lesion (arrows).

Table 8.2 (Cont.) Intradural extramedullary lesions

Disease	MRI Findings	Comments
Meningioma (Fig. 8.39)	Extradural or intradural extramedullary lesions with intermediate signal on T1WI and intermediate to slightly high signal on T2WI; usually prominent Gd-contrast enhancement. Calcifications may be present.	Usually benign neoplasms, typically occurs in adults (below 40 years), more common in females than males. Multiple meningiomas seen with neurofibromatosis type 2, can result in compression of adjacent spinal cord and nerve roots, rarely invasive/malignant types.
Neurofibroma (Fig. 8.40)	Lobulated extramedullary lesions with or without irregular margins, with or without extradural extension of lesion with dumbbell shape, low to intermediate signal on T1WI and high signal on T2WI, with prominent Gd-contrast enhancement. High signal on T2WI and Gd-contrast enhancement can be heterogeneous in large lesions. May be associated with erosion of foramina and scalloping of dorsal margin of vertebral body (chronic erosion or dural ectasia/neurofibromatosis type 1).	Unencapsulated neoplasms involving nerve and nerve sheath. Common type of intradural extramedullary neoplasms often with extradural extension. Usual presentation in adults with pain and radiculopathy, paresthesias and lower extremity weakness. Multiple neurofibromas seen with neurofibromatosis type 1.
Paraganglioma (Fig. 8.41)	Spheroid or lobulated intradural extramedullary lesion with intermediate signal on T1WI and intermediate to high signal on T2WI. With or without tubular zones of flow voids. Prominent Gd-contrast enhancement. With or without foci of high signal on T1WI from mucin or hemorrhage and peripheral rim of low signal (hemosiderin) on T2WI, usually located in region of cauda equina and filum terminale.	Paragangliomas are neoplasms that arise from paraganglion cells of neural crest origin. Usually occur at carotid body, jugular foramen, middle ear, and along vagus nerve. Rarely occur in spine.

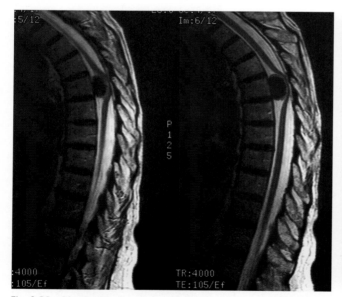

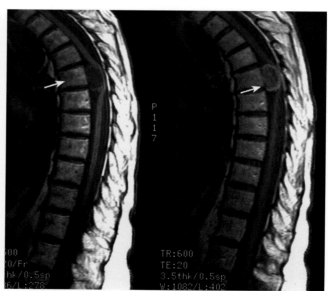

Fig. 8.39 **Meningioma.** **a** Sagittal T2WI shows an intradural circumscribed lesion with low signal (secondary to calcification) causing compression of the ventral margin of the thoracic spinal cord (arrows).

Fig. 8.39 b Precontrast and postcontrast sagittal T1WI show heterogeneous enhancement of the lesion (arrows).

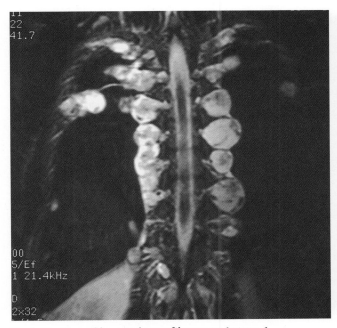

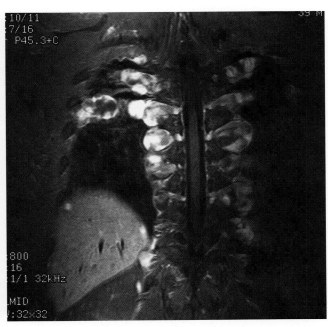

Fig. 8.**40** **Neurofibromas/neurofibromatosis type 1.**
a Coronal FS T2WI shows multiple spinal/paraspinal and intercostal neurofibromas with heterogeneous high signal.

Fig. 8.**40 b** Postcontrast FS coronal T1WI shows heterogeneous enhancement of the lesions.

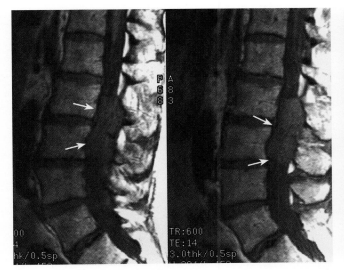

a

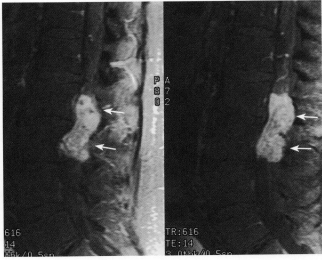

b

Fig. 8.**41** **Paraganglioma.** **a** Sagittal T1WI shows an intradural lesion with intermediate signal at the cauda equina (arrows). **b** Postcontrast FS sagittal T1WI shows prominent enhancement of the lesion (arrows). **c** Sagittal T2WI shows the lesion to have heterogeneous intermediate to high signal (arrows).

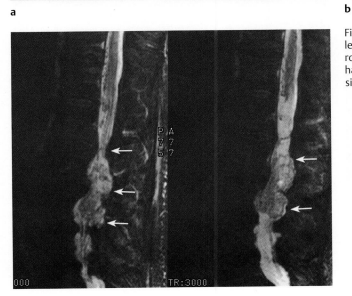

c

Table 8.2 (Cont.) Intradural extramedullary lesions

Disease	MRI Findings	Comments
Leptomeningeal metastases (Figs. 8.42, 8.43)	Single or multiple nodular enhancing lesions and/or focal or diffuse abnormal subarachnoid enhancement along pial surface of spinal cord. Low to intermediate signal on T1WI and intermediate to high signal on T2WI. Leptomeningeal tumor is best seen on postcontrast images.	Gd-contrast enhancement in the subarachnoid space (leptomeninges) usually is associated with significant pathology (neoplasm versus inflammation and/or infection). Primary neoplasms commonly associated with disseminated subarachnoid tumor include: primitive neuroectodermal tumors (e.g., medulloblastoma), glioblastoma, ependymoma, choroid plexus papilloma/carcinoma. Metastases within the CSF can result from direct extension through the dura or by hematogenous dissemination or via the choroid plexus. The most frequent primary neoplasms outside of the CNS within subarachnoid metastases include: lung carcinoma, breast carcinoma, melanoma, lymphoma, and leukemia.
Hemangiopericytoma	Extradural or intradural extramedullary lesions, can involve vertebral marrow, often well-circumscribed. Intermediate signal on T1WI, intermediate to slightly high signal on T2WI; prominent Gd-contrast enhancement (may resemble meningiomas). With or without associated erosive bone changes.	Rare neoplasms in young adults (more common in males than females), sometimes referred to as angioblastic meningioma or meningeal hemangiopericytoma. Arise from vascular cells, pericytes. Frequency of metastases > meningiomas.
Arachnoid cyst (Fig. 8.44)	Well-circumscribed intradural extramedullary lesions with low signal on T1WI and high signal on T2WI similar to CSF. No Gd-contrast enhancement.	Non-neoplastic congenital, developmental or acquired extra-axial lesions filled with CSF. Usually mild mass effect on adjacent spinal cord or nerve roots.

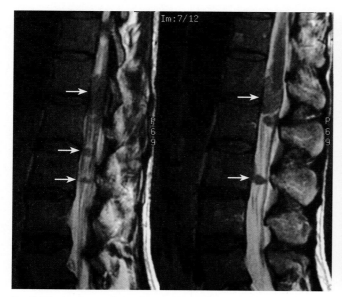

Fig. 8.42 **Leptomeningeal metastases from melanoma. a** Sagittal T2WI shows intradural lesions with intermediate signal in the lower thecal sac (arrows).

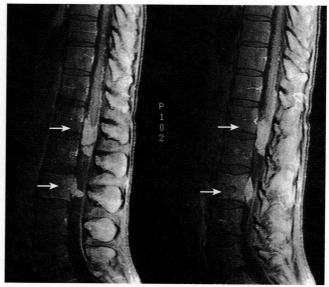

Fig. 8.42 b Postcontrast sagittal FS T1WI shows prominent enhancement of the intradural lesions (arrows). Abnormal enhancement is also seen in the L3 vertebral body extending into the adjacent epidural space consistent with metastatic skeletal disease.

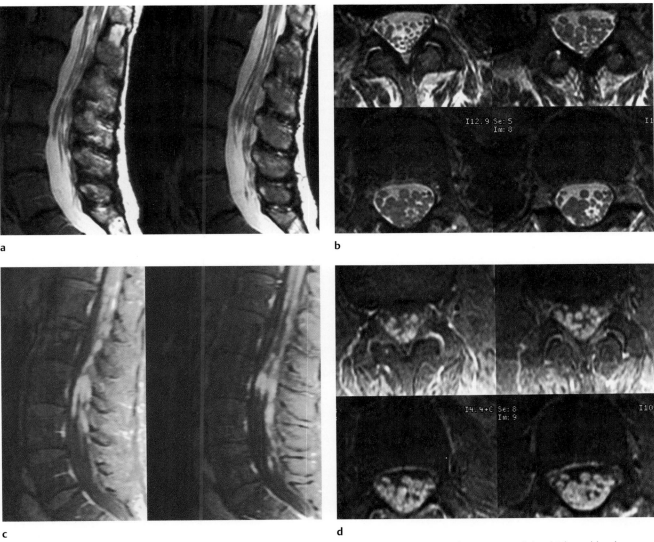

a

b

c

d

Fig. 8.**43** **Leptomeningeal lymphoma.** Sagittal (**a**) and axial (**b**) T2WI show abnormal thickening of multiple lumbar nerve roots within the thecal sac. Postcontrast FS sagittal (**c**) and axial (**d**) T1WI show prominent enhancement of the thickened lumbar nerve roots secondary to lymphoma.

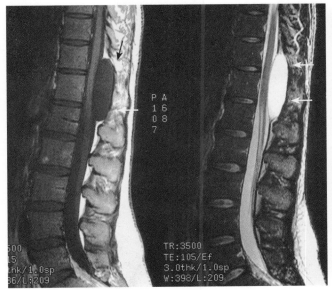

Fig. 8.**44** **Arachnoid cyst.** **a** Sagittal T1WI and T2WI show a well-circumscribed extramedullary lesion with low signal on the T1WI and high signal on the T2WI similar to CSF (arrows).

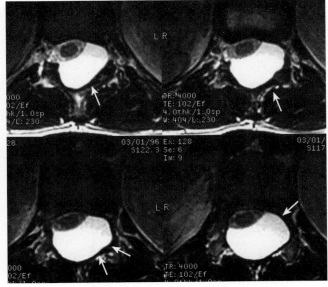

Fig. 8.**44 b** Axial T2WI shows the arachnoid cyst displacing the thecal sac anterolaterally to the right (arrows).

Table 8.2 (Cont.) Intradural extramedullary lesions

Disease	MRI Findings	Comments
Teratoma (Fig. 8.45)	Circumscribed lesions with variable low, intermediate, and/or high signal on T1WI and T2WI; with or without Gd-contrast enhancement. May contain calcifications, cysts, as well as fatty components that can cause a chemical meningitis if ruptured.	Second most common type of germ cell tumors, occurs in children, more common in males than females. Benign or malignant types, composed of derivatives of ectoderm, mesoderm, and/or endoderm.
Leptomeningeal infection/inflammation (Fig. 8.46)	Single or multiple nodular enhancing subarachnoid lesions or enhancement along the pial margin of the spinal cord. Low to intermediate signal on T1WI and intermediate to high signal on T2WI. Leptomeningeal inflammation often best seen on post-contrast images.	Gd-contrast enhancement in the subarachnoid space (leptomeninges) usually is associated with significant pathology (inflammation and/or infection versus neoplasm). Inflammation and/or infection of the leptomeninges can result from pyogenic, fungal, or parasitic diseases as well as tuberculosis. Neurosarcoidosis results in granulomatous disease in the leptomeninges producing similar patterns of subarachnoid enhancement.
Adhesive arachnoiditis (Fig. 8.47)	Clumping of nerve roots within the thecal sac and/or peripheral positioning of nerve roots within the thecal sac, "empty sac" sign. Usually no Gd-contrast enhancement.	Adhesive arachnoiditis is a chronic disorder that results in aggregation of nerve roots within the thecal sac or adhesion of nerve roots to the inner margin of the thecal sac. Can result from prior surgery, hemorrhage, radiation treatment, meningitis, myelography (Pantopaque).
Pyogenic arachnoiditis	Gd-contrast enhancement of one or more nerve roots within the thecal sac. With or without nerve root enlargement. With or without clumping of nerve roots within the thecal sac and/or peripheral positioning of nerve roots within the thecal sac, "empty sac" sign.	Pyogenic arachnoiditis can result from surgical complication, extension of intracranial meningitis, epidural abscess, vertebral osteomyelitis, immunocompromised status.

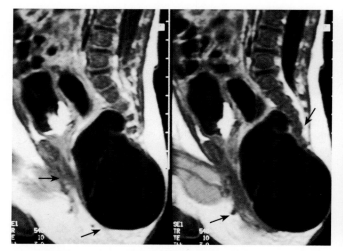 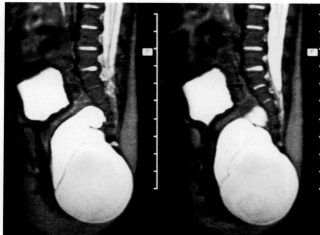

Fig. 8.**45** **Sacrococcygeal teratoma.** **a** Sagittal T1WI shows a large circumscribed septated cystic lesion with low signal (arrows).

Fig. 8.**45 b**   Sagittal T2WI shows the lesion to have high signal.

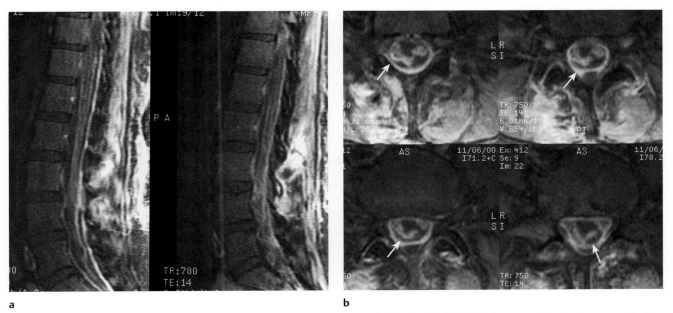

Fig. 8.**46**   **Leptomeningeal infection/streptococcus.** Postcontrast FS sagittal (**a**) and axial (**b**) T1WI show prominent enhancement of the abnormally thickened lumbar nerve roots secondary to streptococcal meningitis (arrows).

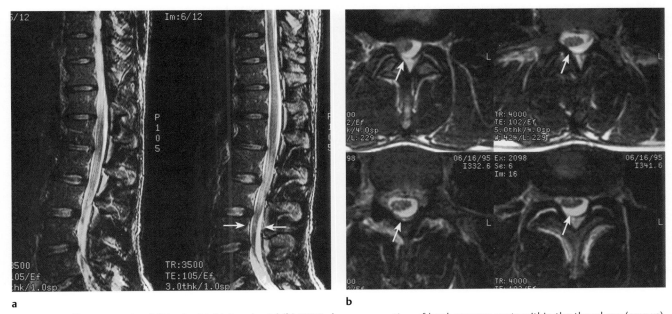

Fig. 8.**47**   **Adhesive arachnoiditis.** Sagittal (**a**) and axial (**b**) T2WI show aggregation of lumbar nerve roots within the thecal sac (arrows).

Table 8.2 (Cont.) Intradural extramedullary lesions

Disease	MRI Findings	Comments
Radiculitis	Gd-contrast enhancement of one or more intradural nerve roots. May be associated with nerve root enlargement and aggregation of one or more intradural nerve roots.	Gd-contrast enhancement of intradural nerves can be seen in two-thirds of asymptomatic volunteers–possibly secondary to enhancement of vessels adjacent to the nerves, but can also result from compression of nerve roots by disk herniations, inflammatory/infectious processes (e.g., CMV infection/AIDS patients, Guillain-Barre syndrome, sarcoidois).
AVM (Figs. 8.18, 8.21)	Lesions with irregular margins that can be located in the spinal cord (white and/or gray matter), dura, or both locations. AVMs contain multiple tortuous tubular flow voids on T1WI and T2WI secondary to patent arteries with high blood flow, as well as thrombosed vessels with variable signal, areas of hemorrhage in various phases, calcifications, gliosis, and myelomalacia. The venous portions often show Gd-contrast enhancement. Ischemia (high signal on T2WI in spinal cord) may be associated, related to venous congestion. With or without swelling of spinal cord. Usually not associated with mass effect except in cases of recent hemorrhage or venous occlusion.	Intracranial AVMs much more common than spinal AVMs. Annual risk of hemorrhage. AVMs can be sporadic, congenital, or associated with a history of trauma.
Hemorrhage within CSF (Fig. 8.48)	Hemorrhage into the CSF can result in prominent transient amorphous enhancement in the spinal leptomeninges/subarachnoid space. Low to intermediate signal on T1WI, high signal on T2WI similar to CSF. May be occult on T1WI and T2WI.	Hemorrhage into CSF from cranial or spinal surgery, trauma, vascular malformation, or neoplasm can result in leptomeningeal enhancement from chemical irritation within 2 weeks of surgery. Usually resolves after 2 weeks.
Other		
Intradural herniated disk	Amorphous structure with intermediate signal on T1WI, variable and/or mixed signal (intermediate, high) on T2WI. Occasionally with Gd-contrast enhancement if become vascularized (ingrowth of fibrovascular material).	Disk herniations rarely extend through dura into the thecal sac.

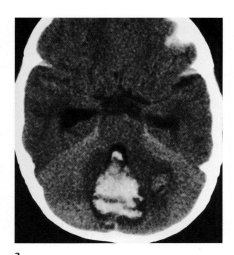

a

Fig. 8.**48** **Leptomeningeal enhancement from occult subarachnoid hemorrhage.** **a** Axial CT image show hemorrhage in the cerebellar vermis extending into the fourth ventricle secondary to a cerebellar AVM.

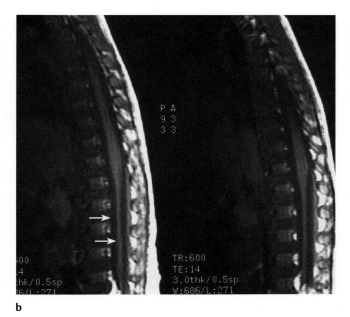

b

b Sagittal T1WI shows aggregation of lumbar nerve roots centrally (arrows). Postcontrast FS sagittal (**c**) and axial (**d**) T1WI show prominent diffuse abnormal leptomeningeal enhancement (arrows) resulting from reaction to the subarachnoid blood. This enhancement resolved 2 weeks later.

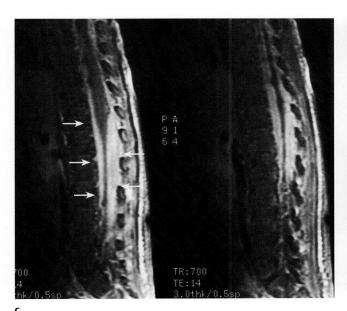

c

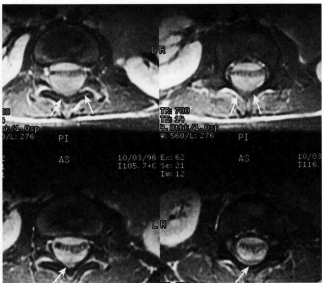

d

Table 8.3 Extradural lesions/abnormalities

Disease	MRI Findings	Comments
Congenital		
Os odontoideum	Separate corticated bony structure positioned superior to the C2 body at site of normally expected dens, often associated with enlargement of the anterior arch of C1 (may sometimes be larger than os odontoideum).	Normal variant representing an independent bony structure positioned superior to the C2 body at site of normally expected dens, often associated with hypertrophy of the anterior arch of C1; cruciate ligament incompetence/instability may be associated (with or without zone of high signal on T2WI in spinal cord). Os odontoideum associated with Klippel-Feil anomaly, spondyloepiphyseal dysplasia, Down syndrome, Morquio syndrome.
Short pedicles–Congenital/developmental spinal stenosis (Fig. 8.49)	Narrowing of the anteroposterior dimension of the thecal sac to less than 10 mm, resulting predominantly from developmentally short pedicles. May occur at one or multiple levels.	Developmental variation with potential predisposition to spinal cord injury from traumatic injuries or disk herniations, as well as early symptomatic spinal stenosis from degenerative changes.
Achondroplasia	*Anomalies of vertebrae* include: shortening and flattening of vertebral bodies, with or without anterior wedging of one or multiple vertebral bodies, shortened pedicles with spinal stenosis. *Anomalies at the craniovertebral junction* include: small foramen magnum, basioccipital hypoplasia, odontoid hypoplasia, basilar invagination, hypertrophy of posterior arch of C1, platybasia, atlanto-occipital dislocation.	Achondroplasia represents a congential type of osteochondrodysplasia that results in short-limbed dwarfism (decreased rate of endochondral bone formation). Usually autosomal dominant/sporadic mutations.
Klippel-Feil anomaly (Fig. 8.50)	Fusion of vertebral bodies that have either a narrow tall or wide flattened configuration, absent or small intervening disks, with or without fusion of posterior elements. Occipitalization of atlas, congenital scoliosis, kyphosis may be associated.	Represents congenital fusion of two or more adjacent vertebrae resulting from failure of segmentation of somites (third to eighth weeks of gestation). Can be associated with Chiari I malformations, syringohydromyelia, diastematomyelia, anterior meningocele, neurenteric cyst.
Hemivertebrae (Fig. 8.51)	Wedge-shaped vertebral body, with or without molding of adjacent vertebral bodies toward shortened side of hemivertebra.	Disordered embryogenesis in which the paramedian centers of chondrification fail to merge, resulting in failure of formation of the ossification center on one side of the vertebral body. Scoliosis.
Butterfly vertebra (Fig. 8.51)	Paired hemivertebrae with constriction of height in midsagittal portion of vertebral body. With or without molding of adjacent vertebral bodies toward midsagittal constriction.	Disordered embryogenesis in which there is persistence of separate ossification centers in each side of the vertebral body (failure of fusion).
Tripediculate vertebra	Wedge-shaped vertebral body containing two pedicles on enlarged side and one pedicle on the shortened side. May be multiple levels of involvement. With or without adjacent hemivertebrae and molding of adjacent vertebral bodies toward shortened side of involved segments. Scoliosis.	Disordered embryogenesis at more than one level with asymmetric malsegmentation. Scoliosis.
Spina bifida occulta	Minimal defect near midline where lamina do not fuse, no extension of spinal contents through defect. Most commonly seen at the S1 level, other sites include: C1, C7, T1, L5.	Mild anomaly with failure of fusion of dorsal vertebral arches (lamina) in midline; usually benign normal variation.

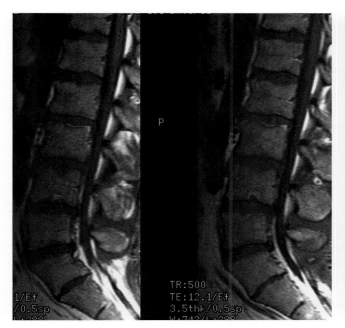

a

b

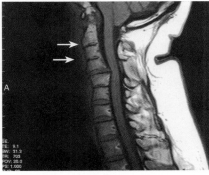

c

◁ Fig. 8.**49** **Short pedicles–congenital/developmental spinal stenosis.** Sagittal T1WI (**a**) and FS T2WI (**b**) as well as axial proton density weighted images (**c**) show narrowing of the anteroposterior dimension of the thecal sac to less than 10 mm at the four lower lumbar levels, resulting predominantly from developmentally short pedicles. Small posterior disk bulges are also evident at the lower four lumbar levels.

Fig. 8.**51** **Scoliosis secondary to multiple hemivertebrae and butterfly vertebrae.** Coronal T2WI shows two butterfly vertebrae (paired hemivertebrae) with constriction of height in midsagittal portion of vertebral body, with molding of adjacent vertebral bodies toward midsagittal constriction (arrows) and a hemivertebra (wedge-shaped vertebral body) (arrow). Other segmentation vertebral anomalies are also present.
▽

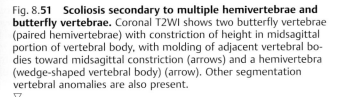

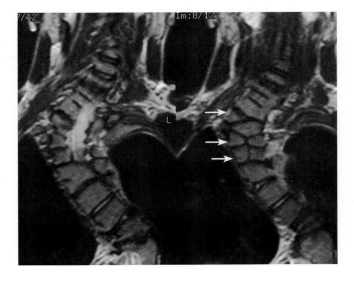

Fig. 8.**50** **Klipple Feil anomaly.** Sagittal T1WI shows partial fusion of the C2, C3, and C4 vertebral bodies that are shortened anteroposteriorly (arrows). Note small intervening disks. Degenerative disk disease is seen at the C4-C5 level below the fusion anomaly.

Table 8.3 (Cont.) Extradural lesions/abnormalities

Disease	MRI Findings	Comments
Spina bifida aperta (spina bifida cystica) (Fig. 8.52)	Wide defect where lamina are unfused and through which spinal contents extend dorsally (myelocele, myelomeningocele, meningocele, lipomyelocele, lipomyelomeningocele, myelocytocele).	Usually associated with significant clinical findings related to the severity and type of neural tube defect.
Myelomeningocele/ myelocele (Fig. 8.5)	MRI is usually performed after surgical repair of myeloceles or myelomeningoceles. Posterior protrusion of spinal contents and unfolded neural tube (neural placode) through defects in the bony dorsal elements of the involved vertebrae or sacral elements. The neural placode is usually located at the lower lumbosacral region with resultant tethering of the spinal cord. If the neural placode is flush with the adjacent skin surface, the anomaly is labeled a myelocele. If the neural placode extends above the adjacent skin surface, the anomaly is labeled a myelomeningocele. Syringohydromyelia may be associated.	Failure of developmental closure of the caudal neural tube results in an unfolded neural tube (neural placode) exposed to the dorsal surface in the midline without overlying skin. Other features associated with myelomeningoceles and myeloceles include: dorsal bony dysraphism, deficient dura posteriorly at the site of the neural placode, and Chiari II malformations. By definition the spinal cords are tethered. Usually repaired surgically soon after birth.
Meningoceles (Fig. 8.33)	Protrusion of CSF and meninges through a dorsal vertebral defect, either from surgical laminectomies or congenital anomaly. Sacral meningoceles can alternatively extend anteriorly through a defect in the sacrum.	Acquired meningoceles are more common than meningoceles resulting from congenital dorsal bony dysraphism. Anterior sacral meningoceles can result from trauma or be associated with mesenchymal dysplasias (neurofibromatosis type 1, Marfan syndrome, syndrome of caudal regression).
Lipomyelomeningocele (Fig. 8.7)	Unfolded caudal neural tube (neural placode) covered by a lipoma that is contiguous with the dorsal subcutaneous fat through defects (spina bifida) involving the bony dorsal vertebral elements. The neural placode is usually located at the lower lumbosacral region with resultant tethering of the spinal cord. Syringohydromyelia may be associated.	Failure of developmental closure of the caudal neural tube results in an unfolded neural tube (neural placode) covered by a lipoma which is continuous with the subcutaneous fat. The overlying skin is intact, although the lipoma usually protrudes dorsally. The nerve roots arise from the placode. Features associated with lipomyelomeningoceles and lipomyeloceles include: tethered spinal cords, dorsal bony dysraphism, deficient dura posteriorly at the site of the neural placode. Not associated with Chiari II malformations. Diagnosis often in children, occasionally in adults.
Diastematomyelia (Fig. 8.10)	Division of spinal cord into two hemicords usually from T9 to S1. Fibrous or bony septum may partially or completely separate the two hemicords. Hemicords located either within a common dural tube (50%) or within separate dural tubes (50%). May be associated with syringohydromyelia at, above, or below zone of diastematomyelia. Often associated with tethering of the conus medullaris, osseous anomalies (spina bifida with laminar fusion, butterfly vertebrae, hemivertebrae, block vertebrae). Diastematomyelia seen in 15% of patients with Chiari II malformations.	Developmental anomalies related to abnormal splitting of the embryonic notochord with abnormal adhesions between the ectoderm and endoderm. Can present in children with clubfeet or adults and children with neurogenic bladder, lower extremity weakness, and chronic pain. May be associated with nevi, lipomas.
Syndrome of caudal regression (Fig. 8.53)	Partial or complete agenesis of sacrum/coccyx, with or without involvement of lower thoracolumbar spine. Occurs as, in order of decreasing frequency: symmetric sacral agenesis, lumbar agenesis, lumbar agenesis with fused ilia, unilateral sacral agenesis. Prominent narrowing of thecal sac and spinal canal below lowermost normal vertebral level. May be associated with myelomeningocele, diastematomyelia, tethered spinal cord, thickened filum, lipoma.	Congenital anomalies related to failure of canalization and retrogressive differentiation resulting in partial sacral agenesis and/or distal thoracolumbar agenesis. Possible association with other anomalies such as imperforate anus, anorectal atresia/stenosis, malformed genitalia, renal dysplasia. May not have clinical correlates in mild forms. May be associated with distal muscle weakness, paralysis, hypoplasia of lower extremities, sensory deficits, lax sphincters, neurogenic bladders in others.

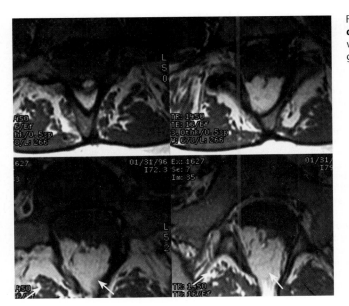

Fig. 8.**52** **Spina bifida aperta (spina bifida cystica)/lipomyelo-cele.** Axial proton density weighted images show a wide defect where lamina are unfused and through which a lipomyelomeningocele is contiguous with the dorsal subcutaneous fat (arrows).

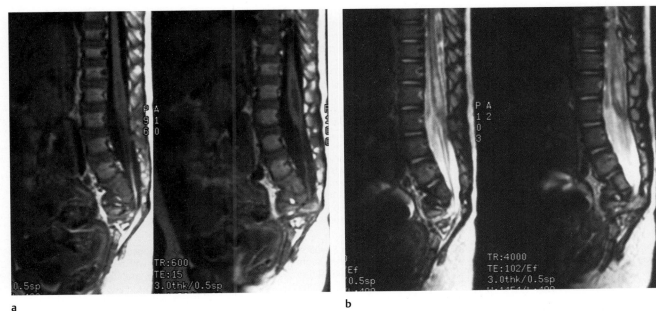

a

b

Fig. 8.**53** **Syndrome of caudal regression.** Sagittal T1WI (**a**) and T2WI (**b**) shows partial agenesis of the sacrum, associated with a tethered spinal cord and thickened filum. A syrinx is present in the conus medullaris.

Table **8.3** (Cont.) Extradural lesions/abnormalities

Disease	MRI Findings	Comments
Disk herniation		
Preoperative (Fig. 8.54)	*Disk herniation/protrusion:* Disk herniation in which the head of the protruding disk is equal in size to the neck on sagittal images. With or without zone of high signal on T2WI at site of annular/radial tear. Signal of disk herniation usually similar to disk of origin; occasionally disk herniations have high signal on T2WI. Can be midline in position, off-midline in lateral recess, posterolateral within intervertebral foramen, lateral or anterior. With or without compression or displacement of thecal sac and/or nerve roots in lateral recess and/or foramen.	*Disk herniation/protrusion:* Represents a disk herniation (focal more common than broad-based) that results from inner annular disruption or subtotal annular disruption with extension of nucleus pulposis toward annular weakening/disruption with expansive deformation.
	Disk herniation/extrusion: Disk herniation in which the head of the disk herniation is larger than the neck on sagittal images. With or without zone of high signal on T2WI at site of annular/radial tear. Signal of disk herniation usually similar to disk of origin; occasionally disk herniations have high signal on T2WI. Can be midline, off-midline in lateral recess, posterolateral within intervertebral foramen, lateral or anterior. Can extend superiorly, inferiorly, or both directions. With or without associated epidural hematoma. With or without compression or displacement of thecal sac and/or nerve roots in lateral recess and/or foramen.	*Disk herniation/extrusion:* Represents a disk herniation (focal more common than broad-based) with extension of nucleus pulposis through zone of annular disruption with expansive deformation. *Disk herniation/extruded disk fragment:* Herniation/extrusion: herniated fragment of nucleus pulposis without connection to disk of origin.
	Disk herniation/extruded disk fragment: Disk herniation that is not in continuity with disk or origin. With or without zone of high signal on T2WI at site of annular/radial tear. Signal of disk herniation usually similar to disk of origin; occasionally disk herniations have high signal on T2WI. Can be midline, off-midline in lateral recess, posterolateral within intervertebral foramen, lateral or anterior. Can extend superiorly, inferiorly, or both directions. Rarely extend into dorsal portion of spinal canal or into thecal sac. With or without associated epidural hematoma. With or without compression or displacement of thecal sac and/or nerve roots in lateral recess and/or foramen.	
Postoperative edema, scar/granulation tissue versus recurrent disk herniation (Fig. 8.55)	*Early postdiscectomy changes (less than 8 weeks after surgery):* Soft-tissue material located in anterior epidural space with intermediate signal on T1WI and intermediate to high signal on T2WI; with or without mass effect on thecal sac resulting from edema and tissue injury from surgery; Gd-contrast enhancement. Changes progressively involute after 2 months.	Initial postoperative changes discectomy consist of localized edema with or without mass effect on the thecal sac. Subsequently, granulation tissue and scar (peridural fibrosis) occurs at the surgical site which is associated with: enhancement without mass effect, with or without retraction of the adjacent structures. Recurrent disk herniations typically show no central enhancement except at sites of fibrovascular ingrowth.
	Scar (peridural fibrosis)/granulation tissue (more than 6–8 weeks after surgery): Often has higher signal on T2WI than annulus fibrosis or degenerated disk. Prominent Gd-contrast enhancement at surgical sites. Enhancement can be seen at site of discectomy.	
	Recurrent disk herniation: Signal of disk herniation usually similar to disk of origin; typically no enhancement of disk herniation centrally, enhancement at periphery of disk herniation. Rarely enhancement seen involving the central portion of disk.	

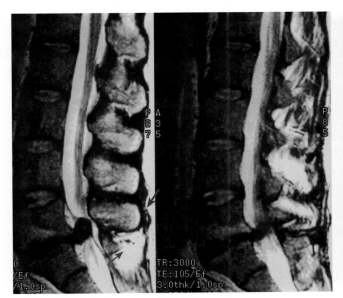

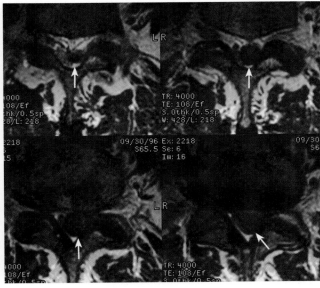

a

b

◁ Fig. 8.**54 Disk herniation/extrusion.** Sagittal (**a**) and axial (**b**) T2WI show a large posterior lumbar disk herniation/extrusion that severely compresses the thecal sac (arrows). **c** Sagittal T2WI in another patient shows a large posterior cervical disk herniation/extrusion that compresses the spinal cord (arrows).

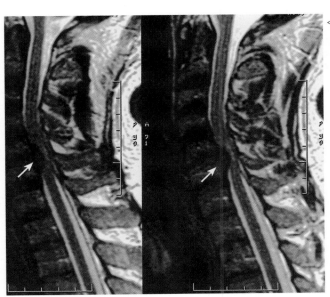

c

Fig. 8.**55 Recurrent disk herniation/extrusion. a** Sagittal T2WI shows a large recurrent disk herniation at the L3-L4 level (arrows). The signal of disk herniation is usually similar to disk of origin. **b** Postcontrast FS T1WI shows no enhancement of the disk herniation centrally, but thin enhancement at the periphery of the disk herniation (arrows).
▽

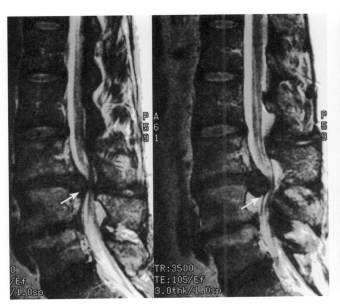

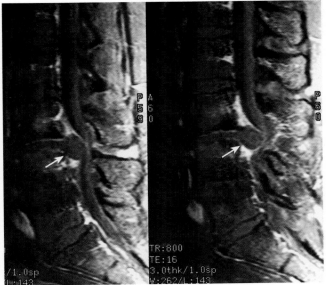

a

b

Table **8.3** (Cont.) Extradural lesions/abnormalities

Disease	MRI Findings	Comments
Degenerative changes		
Posterior disk bulge (Fig. 8.49)	Diffuse broad-based bulge of disk, usually with accompanying osteophytes from the adjacent vertebral bodies. Disks usually have decreased heights, intermediate signal on T1WI and low signal on T2WI related to disk degeneration and desiccation of the nucleus pulposus. May be associated with vacuum disk phenomenon (very low signal on T2WI). With or without linear zones of high signal on T2WI at annulus representing transverse tears or fissures.	With aging, altered disk metabolism, trauma, or biomechanical overload; the proteoglycan content in a disk can decrease resulting in disk desiccation, loss of turgor pressure in the disk, decreased disk height, bulging of the annulus fibrosis. May be associated with spinal canal stenosis, narrowing of the intervertebral foramina, and thickening of spinal ligaments.
Marrow changes related to degenerative disk disease (Fig. 8.56)	*Type 1:* Poorly defined zones with low to intermediate signal on T1WI (decreased relative to normal marrow), and slightly high signal on T2WI (increased relative to normal marrow) in marrow next to intact endplates. Often with Gd-contrast enhancement. Intervening disk usually with degenerative changes. *Type 2:* Poorly defined zones with intermediate to slightly high signal on T1WI (increased relative to normal marrow), and intermediate to slightly high signal on T2WI (isointense or increased relative to normal marrow) in marrow next to intact endplates. With or without Gd-contrast enhancement. Intervening disk usually with degenerative changes. *Type 1 and 2 marrow changes* can also be focal in association with degenerative disk disease and Schmorl's nodes.	Reactive changes in marrow from degenerative disk disease can result from fissuring of endplates with edematous changes and/or replacement with fibrovascular tissue in the subjacent marrow. The endplate margins typically appear intact as thin linear zones of low signal on T1WI and T2WI adjacent to a degenerated disk with low signal on T2WI. These latter two findings differ from the MRI features of vertebral osteomyelitis where there is often destruction of the endplates and annulus as well as high signal on T2WI within the disk.
Acquired spinal stenosis (Fig. 8.57)	Narrowing of the spinal canal or lateral recesses secondary to one or more of the following degenerative findings: posterior vertebral body osteophytes, posterior disk bulge (usually with low signal on T2WI and decreased height), hypertrophic degenerative changes involving the facet joints, and/or redundant ligamentum flavum, synovial cysts, spondylolisthesis, epidural lipomatosis.	Results from degenerative changes at the disks and facet joints, and occasionally from Paget disease, calcification of the posterior longitudinal ligament, synovial cysts. Usually occurs in middle-aged and elderly patients. Cervical and lumbar regions much more commonly involved than thoracic levels.

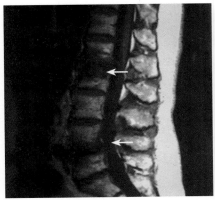

a

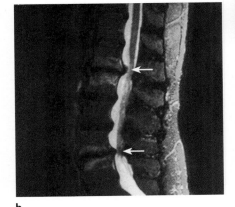

b

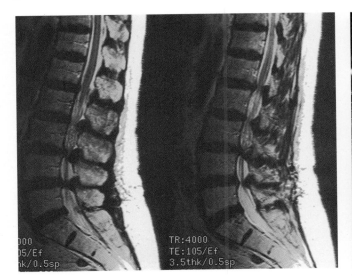

c

Fig. 8.**56** **Marrow changes related to degenerative disk disease.** Sagittal T1WI (**a**) and T2WI (**b**) show poorly defined zones of low signal on T1WI (decreased relative to normal marrow), and slightly high signal on T2WI (increased relative to normal marrow) in marrow next to intact endplates at the L1-L2 and L4-L5 levels (arrows): type 1 changes.   **c** Sagittal T1WI and T2WI show small, poorly defined zones with intermediate to slightly high signal on T1WI (increased relative to normal marrow) and intermediate to slightly high signal on T2WI (isointense or increased relative to normal marrow) in marrow next to intact endplates at the L5-S1 level (arrows): type 2 changes.

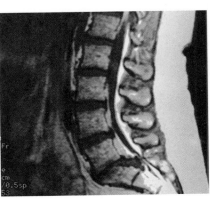

a

b

c

Fig. 8.**57** **Acquired spinal stenosis.** Sagittal (**a**) and axial (**b**) T2WI show severe narrowing of the spinal canal at multiple levels secondary to a combination of posterior vertebral body osteophytes, posterior disk bulge (usually with low signal on T2WI and decreased height), hypertrophic degenerative changes involving the facet joints, and redundant ligamentum flavum.   **c** Sagittal T1WI in another patient shows narrowing of the thecal sac from prominent epidural fat (epidural lipomatosis). A posterior disk herniation/ extrusion is also present at the L5-S1 level.

Table 8.3 (Cont.)   Extradural lesions/abnormalities

Disease	MRI Findings	Comments
Synovial cyst (Fig. 8.58)	Circumscribed structure located adjacent to the medial aspect of a degenerated facet joint. Thin low signal rim on T2WI surrounding a central zone that can have low or intermediate signal on T1WI and low, intermediate, or high signal on T2WI; typically no enhancement centrally.	Represents protrusion of synovium with fluid (ganglion cyst) from degenerated facet joint into spinal canal. Variable MRI signal related to contents that may include mucinous or serous fluid, blood, hemosiderin, or air.
Spondylolisthesis/lysis (Fig. 8.59)	Subluxation of one vertebral body anterior or posterior to the next level, usually associated with degenerative disk disease and facet arthropathy. May be associated with lysis at pars interarticularis regions (spondylolysis). With or without edema (high signal on T2WI in bone marrow adjacent to endplates (with or without enhancement) and/or in pars regions).	May result in acquired spinal stenosis or narrowing of the intervertebral foramina and lateral recesses.

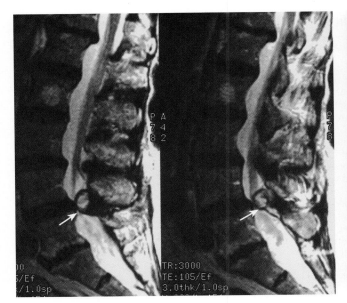

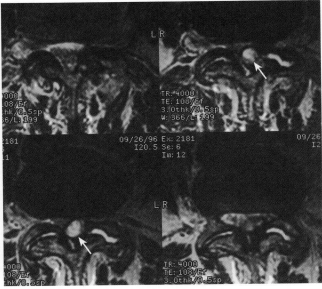

a

b

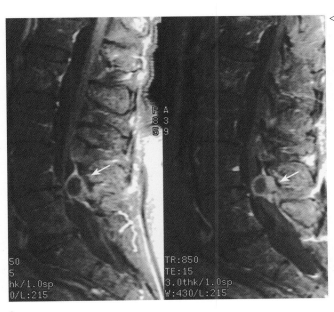

◁ Fig. 8.**58** **Synovial cyst.** Sagittal (**a**) and axial (**b**) T2WI show a circumscribed structure with a thin low signal rim surrounding a central zone with high signal located adjacent to the medial aspect of the degenerated left facet joint at the L4-L5 level (arrows). **c** Postcontrast sagittal FS T1WI shows a thin rim of peripheral enhancement at the lesion but no central enhancement (arrows).

Fig. 8.**59** **Spondylolisthesis/lysis.** Sagittal T2WI (**a, b**) shows prominent anterior subluxation of the L5 vertebral body relative to the sacrum associated with degenerative disk disease, and bilateral spondylolysis at the pars interarticularis regions of the L5 vertebra.
▽

c

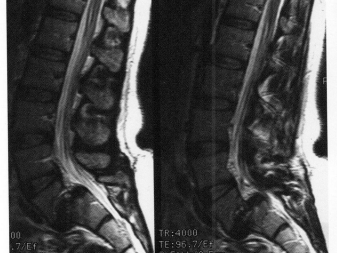

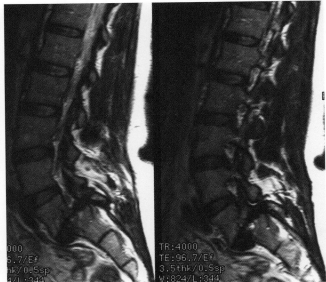

a

b

Table 8.3 (Cont.) Extradural lesions/abnormalities

Disease	MRI Findings	Comments
Fracture	*Traumatic vertebral fracture* (Fig. 8.**60**): Acute/sub-acute fractures have sharply angulated cortical margins, near-complete or complete abnormal signal (usually low signal on T1WI, high signal on T2WI [optimized with FS techniques] in marrow of affected vertebral body). Usually with Gd-contrast enhancement in early postfracture period. No destructive changes at cortical margins of fractured endplates. May be associated with: convex outward angulated configuration of compressed vertebral bodies; spinal cord and/or spinal canal compression related to fracture deformity; retropulsed bone fragments into spinal canal; subluxation; kyphosis; epidural hematoma. With or without high signal on T2WI involving marrow of posterior elements or between the interspinous ligaments. Chronic healed fractures usually have normal or near normal signal in compressed vertebral body. Occasionally, persistence of signal abnormalities in vertebral marrow results from instability and abnormal axial loading. *Osteopenic vertebral fracture* (Fig. 8.**61**): Acute/sub-acute fractures usually have sharply angulated cortical margins, near-complete or complete abnormal signal (usually low signal on T1WI, high signal on T2WI [optimized with FS techniques] in marrow of vertebral body). Usually with Gd-contrast enhancement in early postfracture period. No destructive changes at cortical margins of fractured vertebral bodies. May be associated with: compression deformities involving other vertebral bodies that have normal marrow signal (chronic/healed osteopenic fractures); convex outward angulated configuration of compressed vertebral bodies; spinal cord and/or spinal canal compression related to fracture deformity; retropulsed bone fragments into spinal canal; subluxation; kyphosis; epidural hematoma. Chronic healed fractures usually have normal or near normal signal in compressed vertebral body. Occasionally persistence of signal abnormalities in vertebral marrow results from instability and abnormal axial loading.	Vertebral fractures can result from trauma, primary bone tumors/lesions, metastatic disease, bone infarcts (steroids, chemotherapy, radiation treatment), osteoporosis, osteomalacia, metabolic (calcium/phosphate) disorders, vitamin deficiencies, Paget disease, and genetic disorders (e.g., osteogenesis imperfecta).

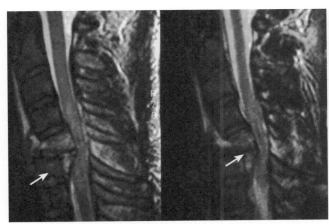
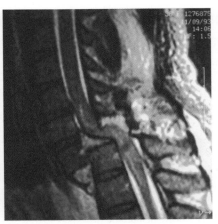

Fig. 8.60   Traumatic vertebral fractures.   a Sagittal T2WI shows acute fractures of the C5 and C6 vertebral bodies that have sharply angulated cortical margins, abnormal high signal in the marrow, and spinal cord compression (arrows). Abnormal high signal is seen in the cervical spinal cord representing contusion/edema.

Fig. 8.60 b   Sagittal T2WI in another patient shows fracture and dislocation at the C7-T1 level with severe contusion of the spinal cord.

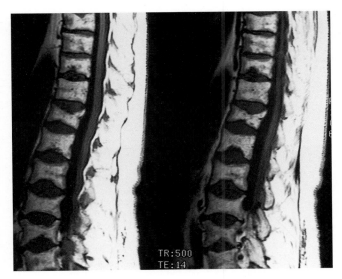

Fig. 8.61   Osteopenic vertebral fracture. Sagittal T1WI shows multiple healed fractures with sharply angulated cortical margins and normal marrow signal.

Table 8.3 (Cont.)   Extradural lesions/abnormalities

Disease	MRI Findings	Comments
Fracture	*Malignancy related vertebral fracture* (Fig. 8.**62**): Near-complete or complete abnormal marrow signal (usually low signal on T1WI, high signal on T2WI [optimized with FS techniques], occasionally low signal on T2WI for metastases with sclerotic reaction) in involved vertebra(e). Typically with Gd-contrast enhancement. May be associated with: destructive changes at cortical margins of vertebrae; convex outward-bowed configuration of compressed vertebral bodies; paravertebral mass lesions; spheroid or diffuse signal abnormalities/lesions in other noncompressed vertebral bodies.	
Epidural hematoma (Fig. 8.63)	*Acute hematoma (less than 48 hours):* Epidural collection with low to intermediate signal on T1WI, heterogeneous high signal on T2WI. With or without spinal cord compression and minimal central peripheral pattern of enhancement at hematoma. *Subacute hematoma (more than 48 hours):* Epidural collection with intermediate slightly high signal on T1WI, heterogeneous high signal on T2WI. With or without spinal cord compression and mixed central and/or peripheral patterns of enhancement of hematoma as well as adjacent dura. *Older hematoma:* Epidural collection with variable/heterogeneous signal on T1WI and T2WI. With or without spinal cord compression.	The MR signal of acute epidural hematoma typically is secondary to deoxyhemoglobin, and with subacute hematomas secondary to methemoglobin. Older epidural hematomas have mixed MR signal related to the various states of hemoglobin and breakdown products. Can be spontaneous or result from trauma or complication from coagulopathy, lumbar puncture, myelography, surgery.

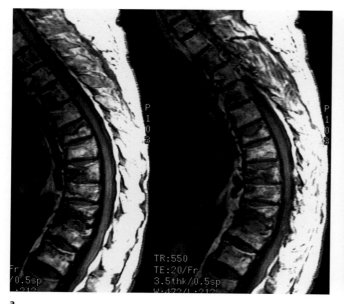

a

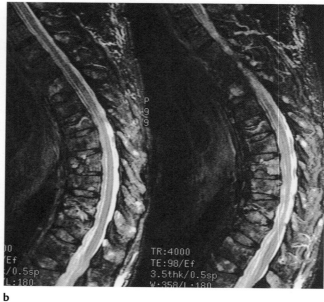

b

Fig. 8.62   Malignancy-related vertebral fractures. Sagittal T1WI (**a**), FS T2WI (**b**), and postcontrast FS T1WI (**c**) show multiple foci of abnormal signal and abnormal enhancement at multiple vertebrae associated with multiple fractures involving the vertebral body endplates in a patient with metastatic breast carcinoma.   **d** FS sagittal T2WI shows a malignant compression fracture deformity involving a thoracic vertebral body associated with compression of the spinal cord (arrows). Foci of abnormal high signal are also present in other vertebrae in this patient with multiple myeloma.

Fig. 8.**62 c, d** ▷

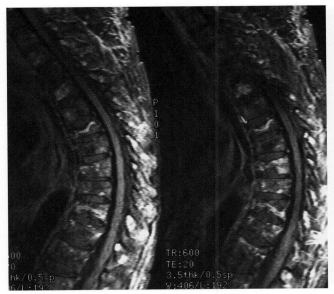

Fig. 8.**62 c**

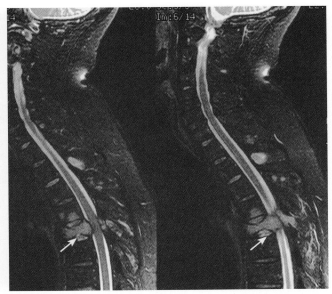

Fig. 8.**62 d**

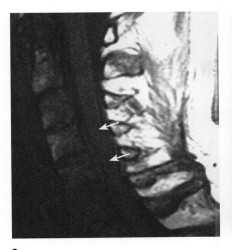

a

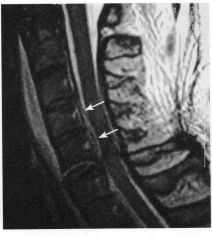

b

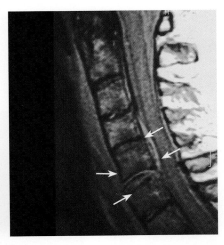

c

Fig. 8.**63   Post-traumatic acute epidural hematoma (less than 48 hours).** Sagittal T1WI shows an epidural hematoma with intermediate signal (arrows) (**a**) and hetero-geneous high signal on T2WI (arrows) (**b**) in this patient with ankylosing spondylitis.   **c** Sagittal proton density weighted image shows the hematoma to have high signal (arrows). Note disruption of thickened anterior longitudinal ligament (curved arrows).

Table 8.3 (Cont.) Extradural lesions/abnormalities

Disease	MRI Findings	Comments
Inflammation/infection		
Pyogenic vertebral osteomyelitis/diskitis (Fig. 8.64)	Poorly defined zones of low to intermediate signal on T1WI and high signal on T2WI and FS T2WI in marrow of two or more adjacent vertebral bodies and intervening disk(s). May involve paravertebral soft tissues. Irregular deficiencies of endplates may be associated (loss of linear low signal on T1WI and T2WI). Prominent Gd-contrast enhancement in marrow and paravertebral soft tissues; variable enhancement of disk (patchy zones within disk and/or thin or thick peripheral enhancement). Epidural/paravertebral abscess may be present (high signal collections on T2WI surrounded by a perpheral rim of Gd-contrast enhancement on T1WI). May be associated with vertebral compression deformity and spinal cord or spinal canal compression.	Vertebral osteomyelitis represents 3 % of osseous infections. Results from hematogenous source (most common) from distant infection or intravenous drug abuse, complication of surgery, trauma, diabetes, spread from contiguous soft-tissue infection. Initially involves end arterioles in marrow adjacent to endplates with eventual destruction and spread to the adjacent vertebra through the disk. Children and adults above 50 years. Gram-positive organisms (e.g., *Staphylococcus aureus, Staphylococcus epidermidis, Streptococcus*) account for 70 % of pyogenic osteomyelitis and Gram-negative organisms (e.g., *Pseudomonas aeruginosa, Escherichia coli, Proteus*) represent 30 %. Fungal osteomyelitis can appear similar to pyogenic infection of spine.
Vertebral osteomyelitis–Tuberculosis (Fig. 8.65)	Poorly defined zones of low to intermediate signal on T1WI and high signal on T2WI and FS T2WI in marrow of two or more adjacent vertebral bodies. Limited disk involvement early in disease process tends to spare disk until later in disease process. May involve paravertebral soft tissues. Irregular deficiencies of endplates may be associated (loss of linear low signal on T1WI and T2WI). Prominent Gd-contrast enhancement in marrow and paravertebral soft tissues. Epidural abscess may be present, often paravertebral abscesses (high signal collections on T2WI surrounded by perpheral rim(s) of Gd-contrast enhancement on T1WI). May be associated with vertebral compression deformity and spinal cord or spinal canal compression.	Tuberculous osteomyelitis initially involves marrow in the anterior portion of the vertebral body with spread to the adjacent vertebrae along the anterior longitudinal ligament, often sparing the disk until later in disease process. Usually associated with paravertebral abscesses that may be more prominent than the vertebral abnormalities.

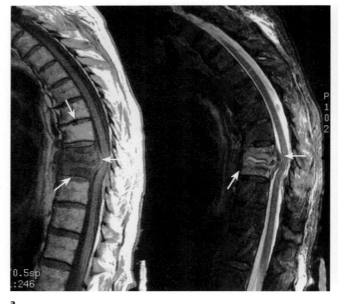

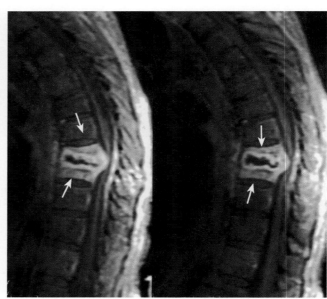

a

b

Fig. 8.**64 Pyogenic vertebral osteomyelitis/diskitis. a** Sagittal T1WI and FS T2WI shows poorly defined zones of low to intermediate signal on the T1WI and high signal on the FS T2WI in the marrow of two adjacent thoracic vertebral bodies and intervening disk (arrows), as well as irregular deficiencies of endplates. **b** Postcontrast FS T1WI shows prominent Gd-DTPA enhancement in the marrow with irregular peripheral enhancement at the intervening disk (arrows). A small dorsal epidural abscess is also present. Sagittal T1WI (**c**), T2WI (**d**), and postcontrast FS T1WI (**e**) show similar findings of pyogenic lumbar osteomyelitis/diskitis (arrows).

Fig. 8.**64 c–e** ▷

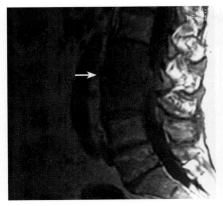

Fig. 8.**64 c**

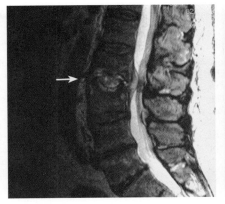

Fig. 8.**64 d**

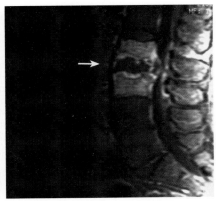

Fig. 8.**64 e**

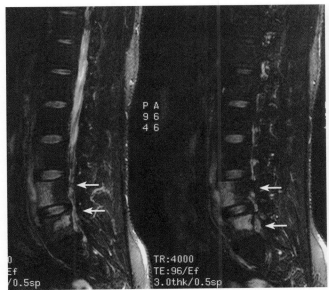

a

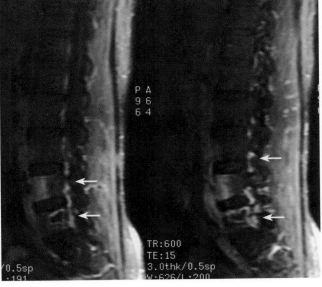

b

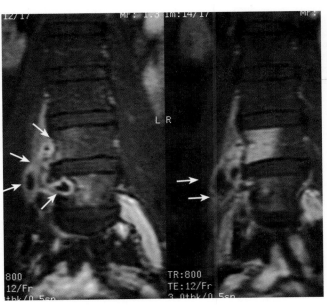

c

Fig. 8.**65**   **Vertebral osteomyelitis–tuberculosis.   a** FS T2WI shows poorly defined zones of high signal in two adjacent vertebral bodies (L4 and L5), without abnormal signal of the intervening disk (arrows). Postcontrast FS sagittal T1WI (**b**) and coronal T1WI (**c**) show abnormal enhancement in the L4 and L5 vertebral bodies, as well as in the right paravertebral soft tissues where there are loculated fluid collections/abscesses (arrows).

Table 8.3 (Cont.) Extradural lesions/abnormalities

Disease	MRI Findings	Comments
Epidural abscess (Fig. 8.66)	Epidural collection with low signal on T1WI and high signal on T2WI surrounded by a peripheral rim (thin or thick) of Gd-contrast enhancement. With or without associated vertebral osteomyelitis/diskitis. Air collections may be present (signal void on T1WI and T2WI). Often extend over two to four vertebral segments, can result in compression of spinal cord and spinal canal contents.	Epidural abscess can evolve from an inflammatory phlegmonous epidural mass, extension from paravertebral inflammatory process or vertebral osteomyelitis/diskitis. May be associated with complications from surgery, epidural anesthesia, diabetes, distant source of infection, immunocompromised status. Organisms commonly involved include *Staphylococcus aureus*, Gram-negative bacteria, tuberculosis, coccidiomycosis, candidiasis, Aspergillosis, blastomycosis. Clinical findings include back and radicular pain and possibly paresthesias and paralysis of lower extremities.
Rheumatoid arthritis (Fig. 8.67)	Erosions of vertebral endplates, spinous processes, and uncovertebral and apophyseal joints. Irregular enlarged enhancing synovium (pannus: low to intermediate signal on T1WI and intermediate to high signal on T2WI) at atlanto-dens articulation results in erosions of dens and transverse ligament. With or without destruction of transverse ligament with C1 on C2 subluxation and neural compromise. With or without basilar impression.	Most common type of inflammatory arthropathy that results in synovitis causing destructive/erosive changes of cartilage, ligaments, and bone. Cervical spine involvement in two-thirds of patients. Juvenile and adult types.
Ankylosing spondylitis (Fig. 8.63)	Squaring of vertebral bodies, thickening of anterior longitudinal ligament. With or without small zones of low signal on T1WI and high signal on T2WI at the anterosuperior and anteroinferior corners of vertebrae in early phases of disorder. Bony fusion may present at facet joints. May be associated with fracture at level of vertebral body or disks (increased incidence with AS) and destructive changes at disks and vertebral endplates (pseudoarthroses) mimicking vertebral osteomyelitis/diskitis.	Seronegative spondyloarthropathy with strong association with histocompatibilty antigen HLA-B27. More common in males than females (10 : 1), spinal involvement usually progresses superiorly from lumbosacral or thoracolumbar junctions. Inflammation initially located at insertion of outer fibers of the annulus fibrosis (enthesitis) with progressive erosive changes at the anterior vertebral corners with reactive sclerosis. Fibrosis/ossification eventually occurs along anterior longitudinal ligament and annular fibers resulting in ankylosis/rigid spine, increased susceptibility to fracture, pseudoarthrosis, subaxial subluxation, and kyphosis.
Eosinophilic granuloma (Fig. 8.68)	Single or multiple circumscibed soft-tissue lesions in the vertebral body marrow associated with focal bony destruction/erosion with extension into the adjacent soft tissues. Lesions usually involve the vertebral body and not the posterior elements, with low to intermediate signal on T1WI and mixed intermediate to slightly high signal on T2WI; Gd-contrast enhancement, with or without enhancement of the adjacent dura. Progression of lesion can lead to vertebra plana (collapsed flattened vertebral body), with minimal or no kyphosis and relatively normal-sized adjacent disks.	*Single lesion:* Commonly seen in males more than females, below 20 years of age. Proliferation of histiocytes in medullary cavity with localized destruction of bone with extension into adjacent soft tissues. *Multiple lesions:* Associated with syndromes such as: Letterer-Siwe disease (lymphadenopathy hepatosplenomegaly), children below 2 years; Hand-Schüller-Christian disease (lymphadenopathy, exophthalmos, diabetes insipidus), children 5–10 years.

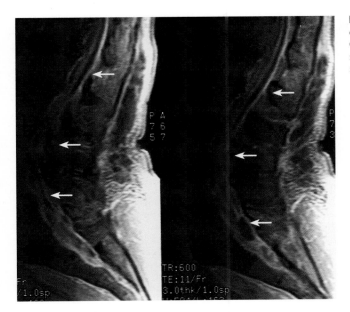

Fig. 8.**66** **Epidural abscess.** FS sagittal T1WI show an abnormal epidural fluid surrounded by a thick irregular peripheral rim of Gd-contrast enhancement involving the lower thoracic and lumbar spinal canal (arrows). There is prominent narrowing of the thecal sac.

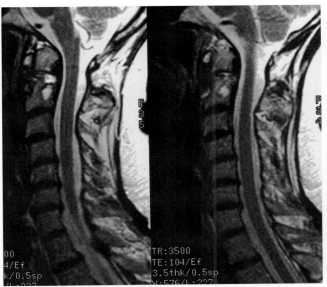

Fig. 8.**67** **Rheumatoid arthritis.** **a** Sagittal T2WI shows erosions of the dens.

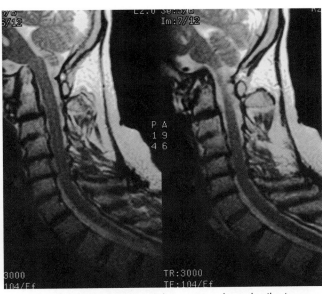

Fig. 8.**67 b** Sagittal T2WI in another patient shows basilar impression (secondary basilar invagination) secondary to destruction of the transverse ligament.

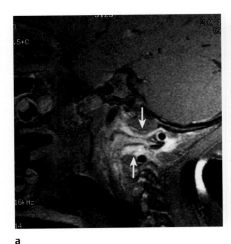

a

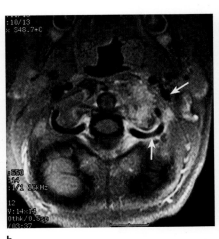

b

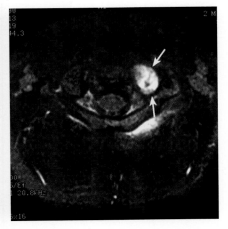

c

Fig. 8.**68** **Eosinophilic granuloma.** Post-contrast FS sagittal (**a**) and axial (**b**) T1WI show abnormal enhancement in the mar-row of left lateral mass of C1 associated with bone erosion and adjacent soft-tissue enhancement (arrows). **c** Axial FS T2WI shows abnormal high signal at the left lateral mass of C1 (arrows).

Table 8.3 (Cont.) Extradural lesions/abnormalities

Disease	MRI Findings	Comments
Neoplasms		
Metastatic tumor (Fig. 8.69)	Single or multiple well-circumscribed or poorly defined infiltrative lesions involving the vertebral marrow, dura, and/or leptomeninges. Low to intermediate signal on T1WI; low, intermediate, and/or high signal on T2WI; usually with Gd-contrast enhancement. May be associated with bone destruction, pathologic vertebral fracture, and compression of neural tissue or vessels. Leptomeningeal tumor often best seen on postcontrast images.	Metastatic tumor may have variable destructive or infiltrative changes involving single or multiple sites of involvement.
Lymphoma (Fig. 8.70)	Single or multiple well-circumscribed or poorly defined infiltrative lesions involving the vertebrae, dura, and/or leptomeninges. Low to intermediate signal on T1WI; intermediate to high signal on T2WI; usually with Gd-contrast enhancement. Bone destruction may be associated. Diffuse involvement of vertebra with Hodgkin lymphoma can produce an "ivory vertebra" that has low signal on T1WI and T2WI. Leptomeningeal tumor is often best seen on postcontrast images.	Lymphoma may have variable destructive or infiltrative marrow/bony changes involving single or multiple sites of vertebral involvement. Lymphoma may extend from bone into adjacent soft tissues within or outside of the spinal canal, or may initially involve only the epidural soft tissues or only the subarachnoid compartment. Can occur at any age (peak incidence third to fifth decades).

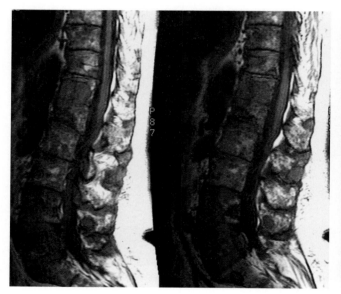

a

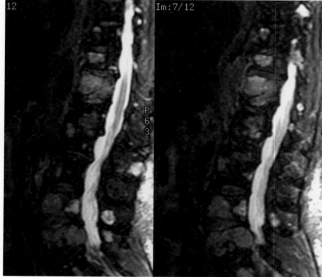

b

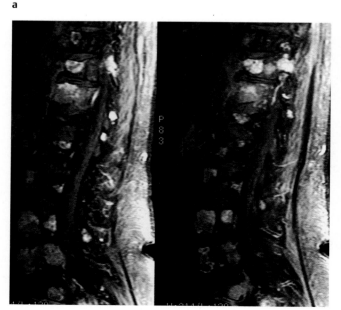

c

Fig. 8.**69 Metastatic tumor/breast carcinoma. a** Sagittal T1WI shows multiple foci of abnormal low signal throughout the visualized vertebrae. **b** Sagittal FS T2WI shows the lesions to have heterogeneous high signal. **c** Postcontrast FS sagittal T1WI show the lesions to have prominent enhancement.

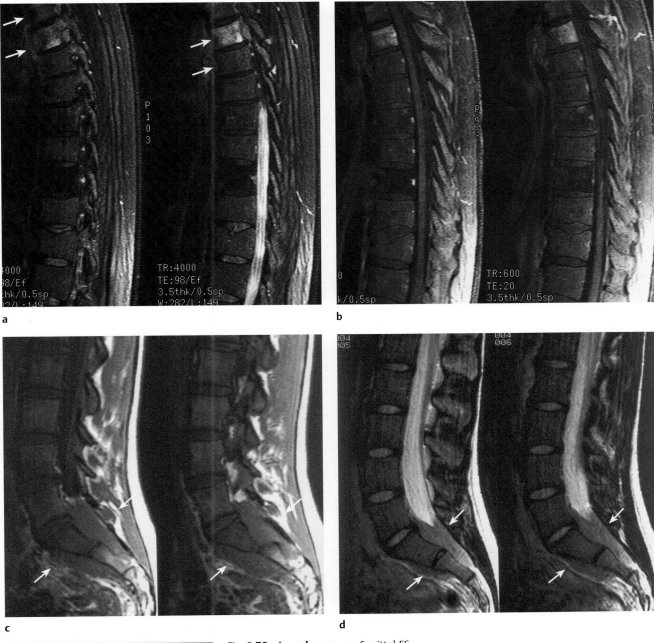

Fig. 8.**70 Lymphoma. a** Sagittal FS T2WI shows poorly defined zones of abnormal high signal in two upper thoracic vertebrae. **b** Postcontrast FS sagittal T1WI shows the lesions to have prominent enhancement. Sagittal T1WI (**c**), T2WI (**d**), and postcontrast FS T1WI (**e**) in another patient shows epidural lymphoma that has intermediate signal on the T1WI and T2WI and shows prominent enhancement (arrows). The epidural lymphoma extends through a widened sacral foramen into the presacral soft tissues.

a

b

c

d

e

Table 8.3 (Cont.) Extradural lesions/abnormalities

Disease	MRI Findings	Comments
Myeloma/plasma-cytoma (Fig. 8.62d)	Multiple (myeloma) or single (plasmacytoma) well-circumscribed or poorly defined diffuse infiltrative lesions involving the vertebra(e) and dura. Involvement of vertebral body typical, rarely involves posterior elements until late stages. Low to intermediate signal on T1WI and intermediate to high signal on T2WI; usually with Gd-contrast enhancement. Bone destruction may be associated.	Myeloma may have variable destructive or infiltrative changes involving the axial and/or appendicular skeleton.
Primary bone tumors		
Chordoma (Fig. 8.71)	Well-circumscribed lobulated lesions with low to intermediate signal on T1WI and high signal on T2WI; Gd-contrast enhancement (usually heterogeneous). Locally invasive associated with bone erosion/destruction, usually involves the dorsal portion of the vertebral body with extension toward the spinal canal. Also occurs in sacrum.	Rare, slow-growing tumors (approximately 3% of bone tumors). Usually occur in adults 30–70 years; more common in males than females 2 : 1). Occurs in sacrum (50%), skull base (35%), vertebrae (15%).
Enchondroma	Lobulated lesions with low to intermediate signal on T1WI and high signal on T2WI; with or without matrix mineralization–low signal on T2WI. Gd-contrast enhancement (usually heterogeneous). Locally invasive associated with bone erosion/destruction, usually involves posterior elements.	Rare, slow-growing tumors (approximately 12% of bone tumors), usually occur in children and young adults (10–30 years). Affects males and females equally.
Chondrosarcoma (Fig. 8.72)	Lobulated lesions with low to intermediate signal on T1WI and high signal on T2WI; with or without matrix mineralization–low signal on T2WI. Gd-contrast enhancement (usually heterogeneous). Locally invasive associated with bone erosion/destruction, encasement of vessels and nerves. Can involve any portion of the vertebra.	Rare, slow-growing tumors (approximately 16% of bone tumors), usually occurring in adults (peak in fifth to sixth decades), more common in males than females. Sporadic (75%). Malignant degeneration/transformation of other cartilaginous lesion, e.g., enchondroma, osteochondroma, (25%).
Osteochondroma	Circumscribed sessile lesion typically arising from posterior elements of vertebrae. Central zone with intermediate signal on T1WI and T2WI similar to marrow surrounded by a peripheral zone of low signal on T1WI and T2WI, with cartilaginous cap. Increased malignant potential when cartilaginous cap is more than 2 cm thick.	Benign cartilaginous tumors arising from defect at periphery of growth plate during bone formation with resultant bone outgrowth covered by a cartilaginous cap. Usually benign lesions unless associated with pain and increasing size of cartilaginous cap.
Osteogenic sarcoma	Destructive malignant lesions with low to intermediate signal on T1WI and mixed low, intermediate, high signal on T2WI; usually with matrix mineralization/ossification–low signal on T2WI. Gd-contrast enhancement (usually heterogeneous).	Malignant bone lesions rarely occur as primary tumor involving the vertebral column; locally invasive; high metastatic potential. Occur in children as primary tumors and in adults (associated with Paget disease, irradiated bone, chronic osteomyelitis, osteoblastoma, giant cell tumor, fibrous dysplasia).
Ewing sarcoma	Destructive malignant lesions involving the vertebral column. Low to intermediate signal on T1WI and mixed low, intermediate, high signal on T2WI; with or without matrix mineralization–low signal on T2WI. Gd-contrast enhancement (usually heterogeneous).	Usually occurs between the ages of 5 and 30; more common in males than females. Rarely occurs as primary tumor involving the spinal column. Locally invasive, high metastatic potential.
Osteoid osteoma	Intraosseous circumscribed vertebral lesion often less than 1.5 cm in diameter located in posterior elements. Central zone with low to intermediate signal on T1WI and high signal on T2WI (with prominent enhancement) surrounded by a peripheral rim of low signal on T1WI and T2WI (sclerosis); with or without high signal on T2WI in bone (edema) beyond zone of sclerosis or in adjacent soft tissues.	Benign osseous lesion containing a nidus of vascularized osteoid trabeculae surrounded by osteoblastic sclerosis. 14% of osteoid osteomas are located in the spine. Usually occurs between the ages of 5 and 25; more common in males than females. Focal pain and tenderness associated with lesion that is often worse at night, relieved with aspirin.
Osteoblastoma	Expansile vertebral lesion often greater than 1.5 cm in diameter located in posterior elements (90%), with or without extension into vertebral body (30%), with or without epidural extension (40%). Low to intermediate signal on T1WI and intermediate to high signal on T2WI, usually with enhancement. Spinal cord/spinal canal compression may be associated.	Rare benign bone neoplasm (2% of bone tumors) usually occur at age 6 to 30 years. One-third of osteoblastomas involve the spine.

Table 8.**3** (Cont.) Extradural lesions/abnormalities

Disease	MRI Findings	Comments
Giant cell tumor (Fig. 8.73)	Circumscribed extradural vertebral lesion with low to intermediate signal on T1WI and high signal on T2WI, with or without surrounding thin zone of low signal on T2WI, with Gd-contrast enhancement. Location in order of decreasing frequency: vertebral body, vertebral body and vertebral arch, vertebral arch alone. Spinal cord/spinal canal compression may be associated.	Giant cell tumors represent 5 % of primary bone tumors. Locally aggressive, rarely metastasize. Usually involve lone bones, only 4 % involve vertebrae. Usually occur in adolescents and adults (20–40 years).

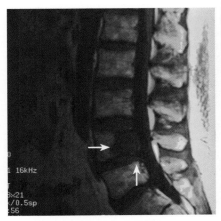

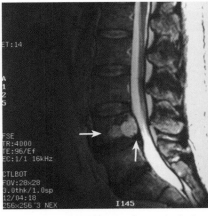

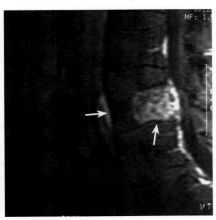

Fig. 8.**71** **Chordoma.** **a** Sagittal T1WI shows a well-circumscribed lesion with low to intermediate signal located in the posterior portion of the L4 vertebral body with dorsal extension toward the spinal canal (arrows).

Fig. 8.**71 b** Sagittal T2WI shows the lesion to have high signal (arrows).

Fig. 8.**71 c** Postcontrast FS T1WI shows the lesion to have heterogeneous prominent enhancement (arrows).

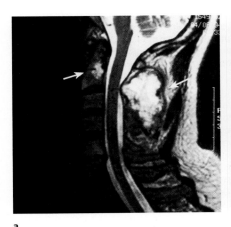

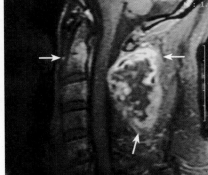

Fig. 8.**72** **Chondrosarcoma.** **a** Sagittal T2WI shows a well-circumscribed lobulated lesion with high signal involving the posterior portion of the C2 vertebra and dens (arrows). **b** Postcontrast FS T1WI shows the lesion to have heterogeneous, predominantly peripheral enhancement (arrows).

a

b

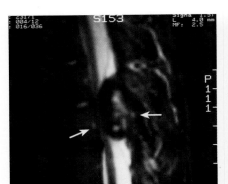

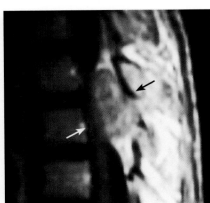

Fig. 8.**73** **Giant cell tumor.** **a** Sagittal T2WI shows a circumscribed extradural vertebral lesion with high signal on T2WI surrounded by an irregular zone of low signal (arrows). **b** Postcontrast T1WI shows enhancement of the lesion to have heterogeneous, predominantly peripheral enhancement (arrows).

a

b

Table 8.3 (Cont.) Extradural lesions/abnormalities

Disease	MRI Findings	Comments
Aneurysmal bone cyst	Circumscribed extradural vertebral lesion usually involving the posterior elements, with or without involvement of the vertebral body. Variable low, intermediate, high, and/or mixed signal on T1WI and T2WI, with or without surrounding thin zone of low signal on T2WI. Lobulations and one or multiple fluid-fluid levels may be present.	Expansile blood/debris filled lesions often occur in association with other bone lesions such as giant cell tumor, fibrous dysplasia, chondroblastoma, others. Most occur in patients below 30 years. Locations in order of decreasing frequency: lumbar, cervical, thoracic. Clinical findings can include neurologic deficits and pain.
Vascular		
Hemangioma (Fig. 8.74)	Circumscribed or diffuse vertebral lesion usually located in the vertebral body, with or without extension into pedicle or isolated within pedicle. Typically have intermediate to high signal on T1WI and high signal on T2WI and FS T2WI. Associated with thickened vertical trabeculae. Gd-contrast enhancement. Multiple (30%), thoracic (60%), lumbar (30%), cervical (10%).	Most common benign lesions involving vertebral column; more common in women than men. Composed of endothelial-lined capillary and cavernous spaces within marrow associated with thickened vertical trabeculae and decreased secondary trabeculae, seen in 11% of autopsies. Usually asymptomatic. Rarely cause bone expansion and epidural extension resulting in neural compression (usually in thoracic region). Increased potential for fracture with epidural hematoma.
Bone infarcts (Fig. 8.75)	Focal ring-like lesion or poorly defined zone with low to intermediate signal on T1WI and intermediate to high signal on T2WI centrally. With or without Gd-contrast enhancement involving the marrow depending on age/stage of infarction/healing. With or without associated fracture.	Bone infarcts can occur after radiation treatment, surgery, chemotherapy, or trauma.
Miscellaneous		
Paget disease (Fig. 8.76)	Expansile sclerotic/lytic process involving vertebrae with mixed low to intermediate or high signal on T1WI and variable mixed low, intermediate, high signal on T2WI; variable heterogenous enhancement. Irregular/indistinct borders between marrow and cortex.	Usually seen in older adults (osteitis deformans). Results from disordered osteoclastic and osteoblastic activity. Can result in narrowing of intervertebral foramina and spinal canal, and basilar impression with involvement of skull base.
Fibrous dysplasia	Zone of heterogeneous low to intermediate signal on T1WI and heterogeneous low, intermediate, high, or mixed signal on T2WI; usually with heterogeneous Gd-contrast enhancement located in marrow. With or without involvement of cortex.	Benign disorder with replacement of normal bone with abnormal fibrous tissue containing a malformed trabecular pattern. May be monostotic or polyostotic. Most common sites in order of decreasing frequency: long bones, ribs, facial/temporal bones, spine.
Morquio syndrome (Fig. 8.77)	Flattening and elongation of vertebral bodies with or without anterior fracture deformities, kyphosis, secondary expansion of intervertebral disks, dysplasia of odontoid process with or without atlantoaxial subluxation, dural thickening from deposition of abnormal metabolic byproducts, spinal stenosis.	Morquio syndrome is one of 13 types of mucopolysaccharidoses, which are lysosomal storage disorders resulting from enzymatic defects causing failure to properly metabolize and degrade glycoaminoglycans (mucopolysaccharides). Deposition of abnormal metabolic byproducts (e.g., dermatan sulfate, heparan sulfate, keratan sulfate) occurs in tissues with toxic effects. Types of mucopolysaccharidoses vary depending upon type of enzymatic defect. Craniocervical and vertebral abnormalities are also seen with Hurler and Maroteaux-Lamy syndromes and other types of mucopolysaccharidoses.

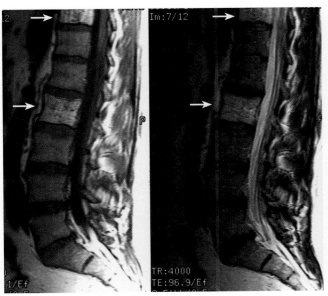

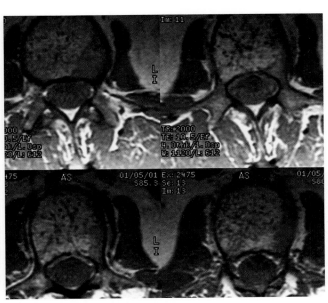

Fig. 8.**74** **Hemangioma.** **a** Sagittal T1WI and T2WI show diffuse high signal within the T11 and L2 vertebral bodies (arrows).

Fig. 8.**74**b Axial proton density weighted images show thickened vertical trabeculae within the hemangioma.

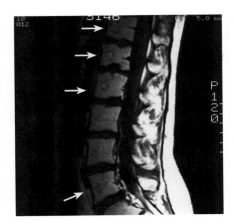

Fig. 8.**75** **Bone infarcts.** Sagittal T1WI shows focal ring-like lesion within the T12, L1, L2, and L5 vertebral bodies (arrows), representing infarcts secondary to radiation therapy.

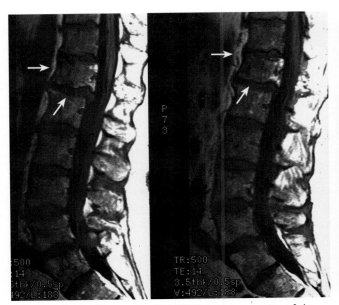

Fig. 8.**76** **Paget disease.** Sagittal T1WI shows expansion of the T12 vertebral body (arrows) with mixed low to intermediate and high signal in the marrow.

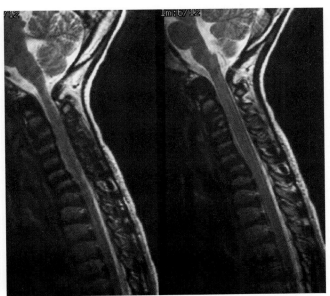

Fig. 8.**77** **Morquio syndrome.** Sagittal T2WI shows flattening and elongation of multiple vertebral bodies with anterior fracture deformities. Dysplasia of the odontoid process is present.

Section IV

Musculoskeletal System

9 Soft-Tissue Disease

MRI is far superior to CT for the visualization of soft-tissue pathology because of greater soft-tissue contrast, direct multiplanar imaging capability, and improved tissue characterization based on signal behavior on different pulse sequences and relaxation parameters. Skeletal muscle has low to intermediate signal intensity on conventional spin-echo (SE) and inversion-recovery (IR) sequences. Fat has high signal intensity on T1WI and an intermediate to relatively high signal intensity on T2WI. The signal intensities of normal tissue, edema, and blood are summarized for different pulse sequences in Table 9.1.

The response of skeletal muscle to physiologic conditions (e.g., exercise, immobilization) and pathologic conditions (e.g., neuromuscular disorders) is nonspecific and restricted to alteration in size (atrophy and hypertrophy) and tissue composition (muscle edema, fatty replacement, and fibrosis).

Muscle edema produces increased T1 and T2 relaxation times and accordingly presents with decreased and increased signal intensity, respectively, on T1 and T2-weighted SE images. Mild edema can at times be difficult to differentiate from early fatty infiltration. Under these circumstances fat suppression techniques (e.g., chemical shift methods or short tau inversion recovery [STIR] sequence) unequivocally permits the correct diagnosis. Muscle edema cannot be differentiated from a fresh muscle hemorrhage on any pulse sequence.

Muscle edema, evident by high signal intensity on T2WI and STIR images, is associated with a variety of neuromuscular disorders including denervation (acute stage), neuromuscular diseases (early stage), myonecrosis secondary to injury, myositis (infectious or idiopathic), and dermatomyositis (acute stage). Muscle strain, rupture, and overuse may also be associated with intramuscular edema and hemorrhage. The latter conditions may progress to compartment syndrome when contained within intact fascial boundaries. A physiologic transient increase of intramuscular water content is also observed after exercise. In glycogen storage diseases affecting primarily the muscles (e.g., type II or Pompe disease), this exercise-induced muscular enhancement on T2WI is largely absent and may reflect the impairment of muscle glycogenolysis.

In a later stage of many muscle diseases the degenerate and necrotic muscle fibers are often replaced by fat and fibrosis. On MRI, *fatty infiltration* can be differentiated from methemoglobin-containing subacute hemorrhages with fat suppression techniques. Fatty replacement of muscle may be complete and homogeneous or incomplete and inhomogeneous, but is not characteristic for a specific disease. It is observed as an idiopathic process, as well as being seen with muscular dystrophies, neuropathies, ischemias, and metabolic and systemic myopathies. Fatty replacement is rare in traumatized muscle, but fibrosis and ossification (traumatic myositis ossificans) are not uncommon.

A variety of inflammatory and infectious diseases present with diffuse edematous and leucocytic inflammatory changes. *Pyogenic bacterial myositis (pyomyositis)* is a localized muscle phlegmon that may progress to abscess formation. It is most often caused by staphylococcus aureus and less commonly by streptococcal species and other pathogens. Buttocks, thighs, and calves are the most common location. Bilateral symmetric muscle involvement is more characteristic of *polymyositis*, or if the skin is also affected, of *dermatomyositis*. In *thrombophlebitis* the edematous changes are predominantly found in the intermuscular fascia with relative sparing of the muscles. Demonstration of deep venous thrombosis may further support this diagnosis. *Necrotizing fasciitis,* a rare and rapidly progressing infection associated with severe systemic toxicity, presents also with thickening and edematous changes of the deep fascial sheaths. Edema in the adjacent muscles and subcutaneous tissue is usually associated. In *cellulitis* the inflammatory changes are most pronounced in the skin and subcutaneous tissue, both of which may be considerably thickened. Advanced cases of cellulitis and pyomyositis, however, cannot be reliably differentiated by MRI, when a disproportionate involvement of the skin and subcutaneous fat versus muscle is no longer evident. In both *vasogenic* and *lymphogenic edema* the edematous changes circumferentially involve skin, subcutaneous fat, and intermuscular fascia of the swollen extremity with relative sparing of the musculature itself. In the *compartment syndrome* the edematous and hemorrhagic changes are limited to the inside of intact fascial boundaries.

Normal tendons are uniformly low signal intensity structures with smooth contours and uniform thickness. Patients with tendinitis (tendinopathy) present with focal pain caused by chronic overuse, trauma, degeneration, or ischemia. An increased intratendinous signal intensity on T1WI generally indicates subacute hemorrhage or myxoid degeneration. If, however, normal tendons lie at an angle of approximately 55° from the direction of the static magnetic field, they may have intermediate signal intensity on short echo time (TE) images. This increased signal intensity observed on short TE images is termed the *"magic angle"* phenomenon and characteristically decreases with an increasing TE. Increased signal intensity within a tendon on T2WI is always abnormal and indicative of rupture or inflammation. Focal or diffuse tendon thickening is usually caused by edema and hemorrhage in acute inflammation and partial tears, or may result from fibrosis due to chronic tendinitis. Narrowing of a tendon is associated with partial tears and degeneration. Complete tendon discontinuity is diagnostic of a full-thickness tear and is usually associated with retraction of the torn ends and fluid or hematoma in the gap.

Differentiating acute or chronic tendinitis, degeneration, and partial tear is difficult. Both acute tendinitis and partial tears cause increased signal intensity mainly on T2WI and less so on T1WI in normal to slightly enlarged tendons. Contour irregularities of the tendon favor a partial tear over acute tendinitis. At a later stage a partial rupture may present as a stretched and focally attenuated tendon. In chronic tendinitis and degeneration the increased signal intensity is predominantly observed in T1WI, a finding that is also present in the "magic angle" effect discussed previously in this chapter.

Table 9.1 Signal intensities of normal and pathologic tissues

Tissue	SE T1-weighted	SE T2-weighted	GRE T2*-weighted	STIR
Muscle	Low	Low to intermediate	Intermediate	Low to intermediate
Ligaments and tendons	Low	Low	Low	Low
Fat	High	Intermediate to high	Intermediate	Low
Vessels	Low	Low	Intermediate to high	Low
Nerves	Low	Low to intermediate	Intermediate	Low
Bone marrow	High	Intermediate to high	Low to intermediate	Low
Cortical bone	Low	Low	Low	Low
Articular cartilage	Low to intermediate	Intermediate to high	High	Low to intermediate
Fibrocartilage	Low	Low	Low	Low
Edema and fluid	Low	High	High	High
Hematoma with oxyhemoglobin	Low	High	High	High
[1]Hematoma with deoxyhemoglobin	Low	Low to intermediate	Low to intermediate	Low to intermediate
[2]Hematoma with intracellular methemoglobin	High	Intermediate	Intermediate	High
[3]Hematoma with extracellular methemoglobin	High	High	High	High
[4]Hematoma with hemosiderin	Low	Low	Low	Low
Fibrosis/scar formation	Low	Low	Low	Low

[1] Intracellular deoxyhemoglobin formation begins after 1 hour and progressively decreases the signal intensity on T2WI.
[2] Intracellular methemoglobin formation begins after 1 day and progressively increases the signal intensity on T1WI.
[3] Extracellular methemoglobin accumulation secondary to red blood cell lysis begins after 1 week or even earlier and progressively increases the signal intensity on both T1WI and T2WI.
[4] Hemosiderin-laden macrophages begin to accumulate in the periphery of the hematoma after 1 month.

Tendon sheaths occur where tendons pass under ligamentous bands, retinacula, through fascial slings or osseofibrous tunnels. They consist of two concentric layers that are separated by a capillary film of synovial fluid and are continuous at the ends, thus resembling a closed, double-wall cylinder. Tenosynovitis is readily diagnosed with MRI by the increased amount of synovial fluid within the tendon sheath. With inflammation of a tendon without a tendon sheath (e.g., Achilles tendon) edematous changes may be observed in the loose connective tissue surrounding the tendon, which is termed the paratenon.

Similar to tendinitis chronic overuse is the most common cause for tenosynovitis. Both conditions are often present simultaneously. Because of its synovial lining, however, tenosynovitis is a common manifestation of rheumatoid arthritis and seronegative spondyloarthropathies. Septic and tuberculous infections occur, but are less common. Giant cell tumor of the tendon sheath is fairly frequent in the fingers and may produce low signal intensity within the lesion on both T1WI and T2WI because of its dense acellular fibrous stroma and hemosiderin deposition.

Tendinous and peritendinous calcifications are seen in calcific tendinitis, most often caused by calcium hydroxyapatite crystal deposition disease (HADD). Calcifications are devoid of signal on MRI. They may be missed on SE sequences within the low signal intensity tendon. Due to susceptibility artifacts the signal void caused by the calcifications is better appreciated on gradient echo (GRE) sequences where these low-signal foci will "bloom". Comparison with radiographs, however, is essential to arrive at the correct diagnosis in this condition.

The majority of bursae are located around joints and tendons. Bursae are subject to the same disease processes as the tendon sheath, since both possess identical synovial lining. The clinical symptoms of bursitis are often indistinguishable from tenosynovitis and tendinitis. An inflamed and fluid-distended bursa presents with high signal intensity on T2WI and low signal intensity on T1WI and, because of its precise anatomic location, can be differentiated from an adjacent tendinopathy.

MRI is the imaging modality of choice for diagnosing soft-tissue lesions. Because of its relative inability to detect soft-tissue calcifications it is essential to interpret MRI in conjunction with appropriate corresponding radiographs.

Differentiation between a benign and malignant soft-tissue lesion is not always feasible. Any rapidly growing solid tumor should be considered malignant regardless of its MRI features. Similarly, a large tumor size also favors malignancy. Benign neoplasms typically are sharply demarcated from adjacent structures. Malignant tumors commonly are less well demarcated and have a tendency to both infiltrate and displace adjacent tissues. The poor definition of malignant lesions frequently is more conspicuous on T2WI rather than T1WI. Inflammatory processes, on the other hand, typically obliterate adjacent fascial planes without mass effect. A sharp, smooth, well-defined border of low signal intensity between the lesion and adjacent tissue suggests the presence of a capsule indicating a benign rather than a malignant mass. Benign and malignant tumors usually have a uniform signal intensity on T1WI, but they tend to differ on T2WI with malignant tumors having inhomogeneous, and benign tumors homogeneous signal intensity. Exceptions to this rule are benign large nerve sheath tumors (schwannomas and neurofibromas) and hemangiomas, both of which present with inhomogeneous signal on T2WI. Thus, uniformity of signal on

T2-weighting suggests benignancy. Malignancies are generally larger and more likely to outgrow their vascular supply resulting in infarction and necrosis with an inhomogeneous signal intensity on T2WI.

Intravenous administration of Gd-DTPA may also contribute to further tissue characterization. Gd-DTPA enhances the signal intensity of many tumors on T1WI, thus enhancing tumor demarcation from surrounding tissues especially on fat suppressed images. Compared with benign neoplasms, the rate of enhancement is greater for malignant lesions, but because of considerable overlap this criterion is of limited use in an individual case. Differentiation between perineoplastic edema and tumor remains problematic, since both display similar low signal intensity on T1WI and high signal intensity on T2WI as well as marked contrast enhancement. In general, the contrast enhancement after bolus injection tends to be faster in the viable tumor than the peritumoral edema. Contrast enhancement is unequivocally useful in differentiating nonenhancing cystic from enhancing solid lesions, both of which may present as homogeneous high signal intensity masses on precontrast T2WI. Similarly contrast-enhanced MRI can separate cystic and necrotic areas from viable cellular regions within a tumor.

Since most lesions demonstrate prolonged T1 and T2 relaxation times, MRI remains limited in its ability to precisely characterize soft-tissue masses. There are instances, however, in which a more specific diagnosis can be made. Fatty lesions demonstrate a high signal intensity on T1WI and an intermediate to high signal intensity on T2WI. A subacute hematoma containing methemoglobin may present with similar signal intensities on SE images, but remains hyperintense with fat suppression techniques. Areas within a lesion containing fibrous tissue, calcifications,

sclerotic bones, or hemosiderin are characterized by low signal intensity on all sequences. Vascular lesions can be identified by their multiple serpiginous flow voids on SE images. The differential diagnosis of soft-tissue masses is discussed in Table 9.2.

MRI is valuable in monitoring tumor response to chemotherapy or radiotherapy and assessing tumor recurrence. A tumor responding to treatment demonstrates necrosis, granulation tissue formation, and eventual fibrous scarring. Similarly, postoperative changes may also include hematoma, granulation, and scar formation. Unfortunately most soft-tissue malignancies and granulation tissue have similar MRI features including low signal intensity on T1WI and high signal intensity on T2WI as well as considerable contrast enhancement. Stated differently, tumor recurrence and granulation tissue formation cannot be reliably differentiated based on MRI characteristics alone. On the other hand, tumor necrosis (cystic changes without contrast enhancement) and fibrosis (low signal intensity on all SE sequences with no or only minimal contrast enhancement) are readily diagnosed by MRI. Morphologic signs of good response of tumor to chemotherapy include reduction in overall tumor size, improved delineation (pseudocapsule formation) between tumor and neighboring muscle and fat planes, cystic changes (tumor necrosis), and fibrosis (scar formation). Tumor recurrence is suspected when the treated tumor mass is increasing in size, a growing spherical nodule with low signal intensity on T1WI and high signal intensity on T2WI is observed, or the surrounding soft-tissue planes are progressively more infiltrated with high signals on T2WI and/or depict increasing contrast enhancement with time. The cross-sectional musculoskeletal anatomy of the upper extremity, pelvis, and lower extremity is depicted in Figures 9.1-9.3.

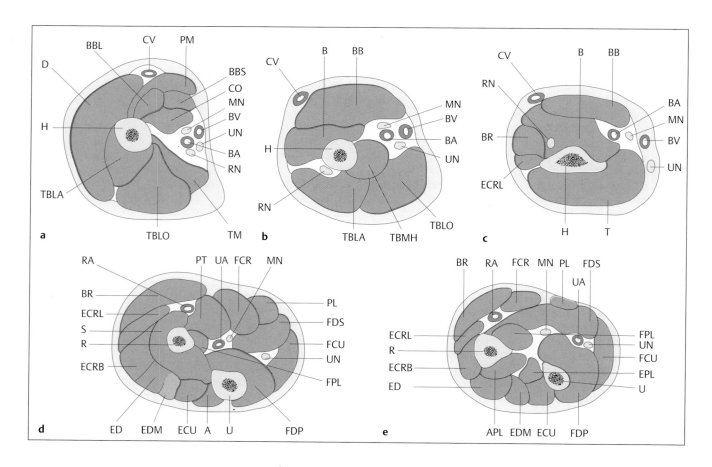

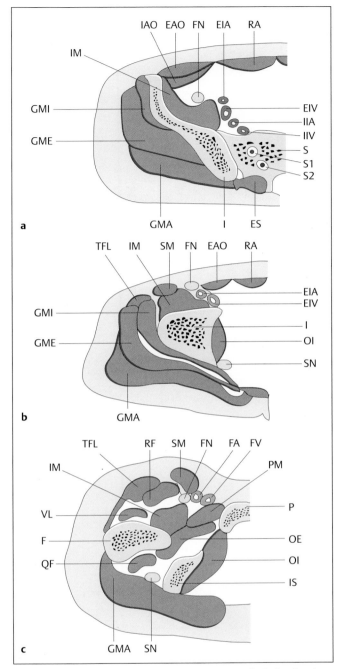

Fig. 9.1   Cross-sectional anatomy of the upper extremity.   a At junction of first and second quarters of humerus.   **b** At mid humerus.   **c** At junction of third and fourth quarters of humerus.   **d** At junction of first and second quarters of ulna.   **e** At mid ulna.

A: anconeus. APL: abductor pollicis longus. B: brachialis. BA: brachial artery. BB: biceps brachii. BBL: biceps brachii, long head. BBS: biceps brachii, short head. BR: brachioradialis. BV: basilic vein. CO: coracobrachialis. CV: cephalic vein. D: deltoid. ECRB: extensor carpi radialis brevis. ECRL: extensor carpi radialis longus. ECU: extensor carpi ulnaris. ED: extensor digitorum. EDM: extensor digiti minimi. EPL: extensor pollicis longus. FCU: flexor carpi ulnaris. FCR: flexor carpi radialis. FDP: flexor digitorum profundus. FDS: flexor digitorum superficialis. FPL: flexor pollicis longus. H: humerus. MN: median nerve. PL: palmaris longus. PM: pectoralis major. PT: pronator teres. R: radius. RA: radial artery. RN: radial nerve. S: supinator. T: triceps brachii. TBLA: triceps brachii, lateral head. TBLO: triceps brachii, long head. TBMH: triceps brachii, medial head. TM: teres major. U: ulna. UA: ulnar artery. UN: ulnar nerve.

Fig. 9.2   Cross-sectional anatomy of the musculoskeletal pelvis.   a At S1-S2 level.   **b** At acetabular roof level.   **c** At obturator foramen level.

EAO: external abdominal oblique. EIA: external iliac artery. EIV: external iliac vein. ES: erector spinae. F: femur. FA: femoral artery. FN: femoral nerve. FV: femoral vein. GMA: gluteus maximus. GME: gluteus medius. GMI: gluteus minimus. I: ilium. IAO: internal abdominal oblique. IIA: internal iliac artery. IIV: internal iliac vein. IM: iliopsoas. IS: ischium. OE: obturator externus. OI: obturator internus. P: pubis. PM: pectineus. QF: quadratus femoris. RA: rectus abdominis. RF: rectus femoris. S1: S1 nerve root. S2: S2 nerve root. S: sacrum. SM: sartorius. SN: sciatic nerve. TFL: tensor fasciae latae. VL: vastus lateralis.

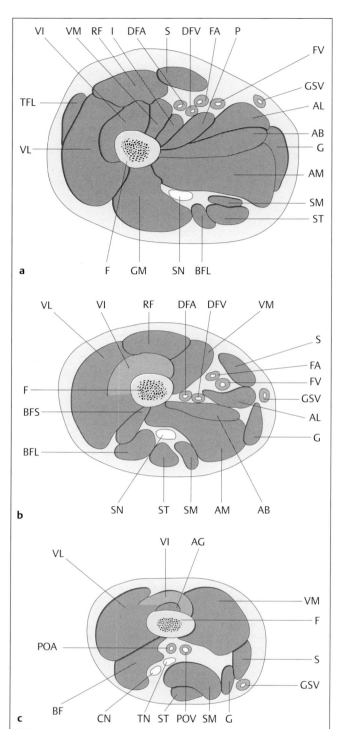

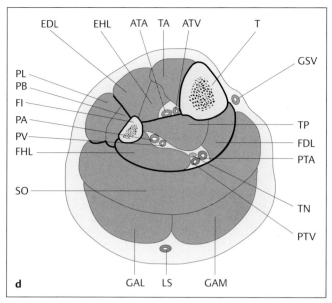

Fig. 9.**3** **Cross-sectional anatomy of the lower extremity.** **a** At junction of first and second quarters of femur. **b** At mid femur. **c** At junction of third and fourth quarter of femur. **d** At mid tibia.

AB: adductor brevis. AG: articularis genu. AL: adductor longus. AM: adductor magnus. ATA: anterior tibial artery. ATV: anterior tibial vein. BF: biceps femoris. BFL: biceps femoris, long head. BFS: biceps femoris, short head. CN: common peroneal nerve. DFA: deep femoral artery. DFV: deep femoral vein. EDL: extensor digitorum longus. EHL: extensor hallucis longus. F: femur. FA: femoral artery. FDL: flexor digitorum longus. FHL: flexor hallucis longus. FI: fibula. FV: femoral vein. G: gracilis. GAL: gastrocnemius, lateral head. GAM: gastrocnemius, medial head. GM: gluteus maximus. GSV: greater saphenous vein. I: iliopsoas. LS: lesser saphenous vein. P: pectineus. PA: peroneal artery. PB: peroneus brevis. PL: peroneus longus. POA: popliteal artery. POV: popliteal vein. PTA: posterior tibial artery. PTV: posterior tibial vein. RF: rectus femoris. S: sartorius. SM: semimembranosus. SN: sciatic nerve. SO: soleus. ST: semitendinosus. T: tibia. TA: tibialis anterior. TFL: tensor fasciae latae. TN: tibial nerve. TP: tibialis posterior. VI: vastus intermedius. VL: vastus lateralis. VM: vastus medialis.

Four fascial compartments of leg are demarcated in **d** and include the anterior compartment containing EDL, EHL, TA, ATA, and ATV, the lateral compartment containing PL and PB, the superficial posterior compartment containing SO, GAL, and GAM, and the deep posterior compartment containing TP, FDL, FHL, PA, PV, PTA, PTV, TN.

Table 9.2 Soft-tissue lesions

Disease	MRI Findings	Comments
Cyst **(Figs. 9.4 and 9.5)**	Sharply marginated, homogeneous lesion of low signal intensity on T1WI and high signal intensity on T2WI. Increased signal intensity on T1WI may be found with a high protein concentration of the cystic fluid content or after intracystic hemorrhage. No contrast enhancement occurs in uncomplicated cysts. Inflamed or infected cyst with wall enhancement may simulate an abscess. A popliteal (Baker) cyst represents a distended gastrocnemiosemimembranosus bursa communicating with the knee joint. It may dissect into the calf or rupture with the cyst content dissecting between the muscles of the leg.	Cystic lesions in the vicinity of a joint usually represent *synovial cysts* (herniation of synovial membrane through the joint capsule) or *distended bursae* (with or without communication with the adjacent articulation). These conditions result from chronic overuse or are of traumatic, degenerative, or inflammatory origin. Rheumatoid arthritis is the most common cause of a large synovial cyst. *Meniscal cysts* (Fig. 9.6) are small cystic lesions often associated with meniscal tears, most commonly occurring in the para-articular soft tissue adjacent to the lateral meniscus of the knee.

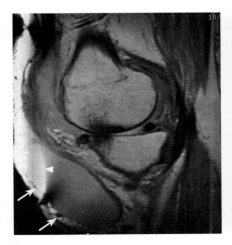

a

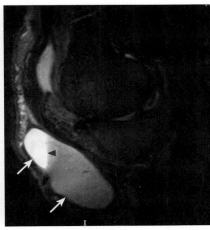

b

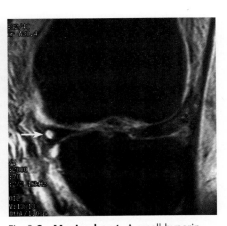

Fig. 9.**4** **Distended subcutaneous infrapatellar bursa.** A large oblong cystic lesion (arrows) with fluid-fluid level (arrowhead) is seen (**a**: PDWI; **b**: T2WI, FS). Arthritic changes secondary to CPPD (pseudogout) and sequela of patellectomy are also evident.

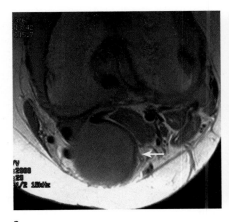

a

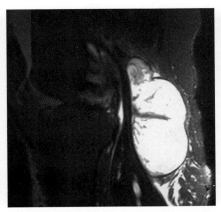

b

Fig. 9.**6** **Meniscal cyst.** A small hyperintense cystic lesion (arrow) is seen in the capsular attachment of the medial meniscus (T2WI). The patient also had a bucket handle tear of the lateral meniscus.

Fig. 9.**5** **Popliteal (Baker) cyst.** **a** A round homogeneous cystic lesion (arrow) of intermediate signal intensity is seen (PDWI, axial).

b The hyperintense lesion with incomplete septation projects behind the knee joint (T2WI, sagittal).

Table 9.2 (Cont.) Soft-tissue lesions

Disease	MRI Findings	Comments
Ganglion (Fig. 9.7)	Small unilocular or multilocular cyst, less than 3 cm in diameter, with round or lobular shape. Located adjacent to tendon sheaths or joint capsule, demonstrating low to intermediate signal intensity on T1WI and high signal intensity on T2WI. Sharply defined, delicate internal septation and small out-pouchings (pseudopodia) may be observed. Usually no contrast enhancement is present, but occasionally a peripheral rim enhancement occurs.	Asymptomatic or slightly tender cystic lesion containing viscous (myxomatous) material. Occurring most often in the dorsum of the wrist or adjacent to the interphalangeal joint of the hand and foot. Lesions may resolve spontaneously. A ganglion in the vicinity of the spinoglenoid notch of the scapula frequently causes entrapment of the suprascapular nerve. *Parosteal ganglion* causes scalloping of the adjacent bone due to extrinsic pressure defect. The majority of these lesions are found in the region of the pes anserinus.
Abscess (Fig. 9.8)	Poorly defined mass with low signal intensity on T1WI and high signal intensity on T2WI (early stage) or, more commonly, a well-defined cystic lesion with relatively thick wall, occasionally with septation, and necrotic center. The abscess wall is of low signal intensity on T1WI, of intermediate to high signal intensity on T2WI, and characteristically enhances considerably after intravenous Gd-DTPA administration. The necrotic center does not enhance and, depending on its content (frank pus versus necrotic debris), varies from homogeneous to inhomogeneous and high to intermediate signal intensity on T2WI. On T1WI abscesses are generally of similar to slightly lower signal intensity than muscle.	Common causes of soft-tissue abscesses include penetrating trauma, iatrogenic interventions, spread from a contiguous infection, and septic embolism. Calcification and gas formation within an abscess are difficult to appreciate with MRI, unless a gas-fluid level is formed. Presence of gas in the absence of iatrogenic interventions and penetrating trauma is rare, but virtually diagnostic. Nontuberculous abscesses rarely calcify. A *localized deep-seated cellulitis* or *phlegmon* composed of still viable tissue may be impossible to differentiate by MRI from an early abscess with liquefactive necrosis.
Hematoma (Figs. 9.9–9.11)	In the acute stage, a homogeneous mass or enlargement of the involved muscle is found with low signal intensity on T1WI and high signal intensity on T2WI. Subsequently a progressive decrease in signal intensity is observed on T2WI in the first few days due to intracellular deoxyhemoglobin formation. Deoxyhemoglobin is metabolized within the red blood cell to methemoglobin, producing an increase in signal intensity on T1WI. After 1 week the hematoma becomes inhomogeneous and hyperintense on both T1WI and T2WI due to extracellular methemoglobin accumulation secondary to red blood cell lysis. At a later stage a rim of low signal intensity may develop around the hematoma, caused by peripheral accumulation of hemosiderin-laden macrophages, fibrosis, and/or calcification. At that stage on GRE images the hematoma may depict a frayed, sometimes cauliflower-like appearance due to inhomogeneous magnetic susceptibility with resultant artifacts. Old hematomas are of low signal intensity on both T1WI and T2WI. Liquefaction of a hematoma occasionally occurs, producing a cystic lesion surrounded by a pseudocapsule. A subacute liquefied hematoma may demonstrate a fluid level (hematocrit effect) caused by settling of the cellular elements. A liquefied hematoma with enhancing rim mimics an abscess.	Soft-tissue hemorrhage occurs spontaneously, following trauma or surgery, with a variety of bleeding disorders, and during anticoagulation therapy. Bleeding into a tumor or abscess is a frequent complication. These conditions may at times be difficult to differentiate from a simple hematoma. A hemorrhagic tumor may be distinguished from a hematoma by the demonstration of a tumor nodule or an irregular rim of tumor tissue. An *infected hematoma* may depict similar signal characteristics and enhancement pattern to an abscess and cannot be reliably differentiated by MRI from the latter.

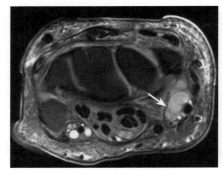

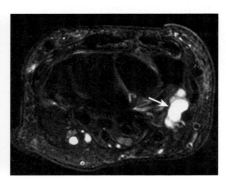

Fig. 9.7 **Ganglion.** A small lobulated multilocular cyst (arrow) is seen. The lesion depicts internmediate signal intensity in **a** (PDWI) and high signal intensity in **b** (T2WI, FS).

a

b

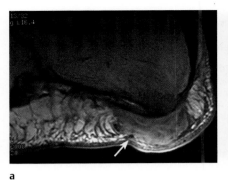
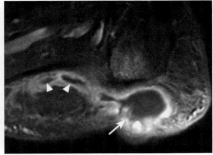

a

b

Fig. 9.**8** **Abscess.** **a** An inhomogeneous area (arrow) is seen in the heel pad that is hypointense to the adjacent fat (PDWI, sagittal). **b** After intravenous injection of Gd-DTPA marked enhancement of the abscess wall (arrow) is seen. Two smaller abscess cavities (arrowheads) are evident further distally (T1WI, FS, +C, sagittal).

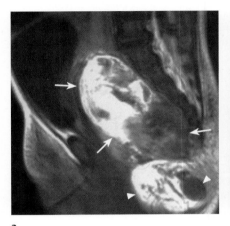
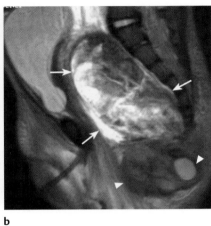

a

b

Fig. 9.**9** **Hematoma.** Spontaneous rupture of a coccygeal teratoma (arrowheads) produced a large subacute hematoma (arrows) with mixed low and high signal intensity located cephalad to the teratoma. (**a**: sagittal, T1WI; **b**: sagittal, T2WI).

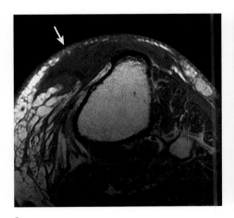
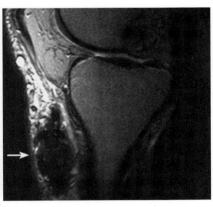

a

b

Fig. 9.**10** **Hematoma.** A poorly defined lesion of low to intermediate signal intensity within the subcutaneous fat anteromedially to the proximal tibia is seen (**a**: axial, T1WI; **b**: sagittal, T2WI).

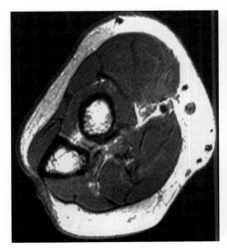
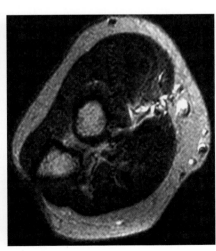

a

b

Fig. 9.**11** **Subacute muscle tear.** Inhomogeneous increased signal intensities isointense to fat are seen in several muscles of the forearm due to methemoglobin formation (**a**: T1WI; **b**: T2WI).

Table 9.2 (Cont.)   Soft-tissue lesions

Disease	MRI Findings	Comments
Myositis ossificans (pseudomalignant osseous tumor of soft tissue, heterotopic ossification)	MRI appearance varies with stage of lesion. Developing lesions *prior to radiographically visible mineralization* are inhomogeneous and poorly defined with intermediate to high signal intensity on T2WI and isointensity to muscle on T1WI. Curvilinear areas of decreased signal intensity develop in the periphery due to calcification and subsequent ossification. Irregular areas of decreased signal intensity coursing through the lesion correspond to areas of trabeculation. Adjacent cortex and bone marrow are usually not involved, differentiating myositis ossificans from a parosteal sarcoma. Rarely, however, mild adjacent bone marrow edema may be associated with myositis ossificans. Mature lesions have MRI signal characteristics of bone and bone marrow. Dense sclerotic lesions on radiographs demonstrate low signal intensity on all SE sequences. More often, signal intensity approximating fat is seen on both T1WI and T2WI, surrounded by a rim of low signal intensity. Areas of decreased signal intensity within the lesion correspond to ossification, fibrosis, and hemosiderin deposition.	History of trauma is apparent in a majority of cases. Remaining patients suffer from systemic problems associated with soft-tissue ossification such as neurologic disorders, burns, and tetanus, although spontaneous development does occur. Traumatic myositis ossificans occurs most often in the buttock, thigh, or calf of young adults, or around the shoulder and elbow. Radiographically, the earliest calcifications in the periphery of the soft-tissue mass may be apparent after 1 week and flocculent dense lesions within the mass after 2 weeks following trauma. Progression of peripheral and central calcifications with transformation to osseous structures occurs until maturity is reached at 6 months, when the lesion begins to shrink.
Amyloidosis (Fig. 9.12)	Soft-tissue infiltration and nodules with signal intensity between muscle and fibrous tissue on all sequences. Soft-tissue involvement occurs around the shoulder and olecranon and in the hand and wrist.	Amyloid deposits in the carpal tunnel may result in carpal tunnel syndrome. Extensive infiltration about the shoulders produces rubbery, hard masses resembling shoulder pads worn by football players.
Tophaceous nodule	Para-articular soft-tissue nodule of low signal intensity on T1WI and of mixed, low to relatively high inhomogeneous signal intensity on T2WI.	Tophaceous nodules consist of multicentric deposition of urate crystals, intercrystalline matrix and inflammatory and foreign body granulomatous reaction. They occasionally may calcify and occur in feet, hands, ankles, elbows (over olecranon), and knees.
Lipoma (Fig. 9.13)	Well-defined, usually homogeneous mass, identical in appearance to subcutaneous fat on all pulse sequences (high signal intensity on T1WI, intermediate to high on T2WI) without discernable contrast enhancement, is virtually diagnostic. Thin fibrous septations are occasionally seen, evident as linear areas of decreased signal intensity, and localized areas of calcification or ossification within the lesion, evident as foci of decreased signal intensity on all SE sequences. Parosteal lipomas may incite a localized hyperostosis in the adjacent bone. Lipomas originating in nonadipose tissue include intramuscular and intermuscular lipomas arising within or between skeletal muscle, synovial lipomas of tendon sheath (hand and wrist, less commonly ankle and foot) and joint (*lipoma arborescens*, usually in knee), as well as neural fibrolipomas (hand, wrist, and forearm, less commonly lower extremity). Invasion into the surrounding soft tissue or areas of nonfatty tissue within the lesion suggest the possibility of liposarcoma, although these findings might also be found with rare varieties of lipomas or with necrosis and hemorrhage within a lipoma.	Most common benign soft-tissue tumor. Predilection for the subcutaneous fat in patients between 30 and 50 years of age, with female predominance. Multiple in 5% of all patients. *Fibrolipoma*: lipoma with significant amount of fibrous tissue, presenting as a slowly enlarging mass in the volar aspect of the hand, wrist, or forearm. *Mesenchymoma*: lipoma with fibrous, vascular, smooth muscle, chondroid and osseous elements. *Angiolipoma*: noninfiltrating or infiltrating fatty tumors with angiomatous elements present in young adults with a heterogeneous pattern of high and low signal intensity on T1WI and T2WI. *Hibernoma*: rare hypervascular tumor of brown fat usually in shoulder region, chest wall, or thigh. *Lipoblastoma (lipoblastomatosis):* superficial infiltrating lipomatous lesion in the extremities occurring usually in infancy and early childhood. *Symmetric lipomatosis*: diffuse symmetric distribution of lipomas, usually extending from the neck into the axilla and back, often associated with a history of alcoholism or liver disease. *Macrodystrophia lipomatosa*: diffuse infiltrative lipomatosis in a limb resulting in grotesque overgrowth of one or more adjacent digits or, less commonly, the entire extremity.
Myxoma (Fig. 9.14)	Sharply marginated intramuscular lesion with decreased signal intensity compared with muscle on T1WI and very high signal intensity on T2WI simulating a cyst. From the latter, myxomas can be differentiated by their inhomogeneous contrast enhancement after intravenous Gd-DTPA administration. Occasionally, cystic components and calcifications are found within the lesion.	Intramuscular myxomas occur most often in the thigh of elderly patients, but are also found in the buttock, shoulder, arm, and other sites. Histologically they demonstrate an invasive pattern of growth with a high recurrence rate after resection. Myxomas have been associated with fibrous dysplasia of the adjacent bone. *Myxosarcoma* is the rare malignant counterpart.

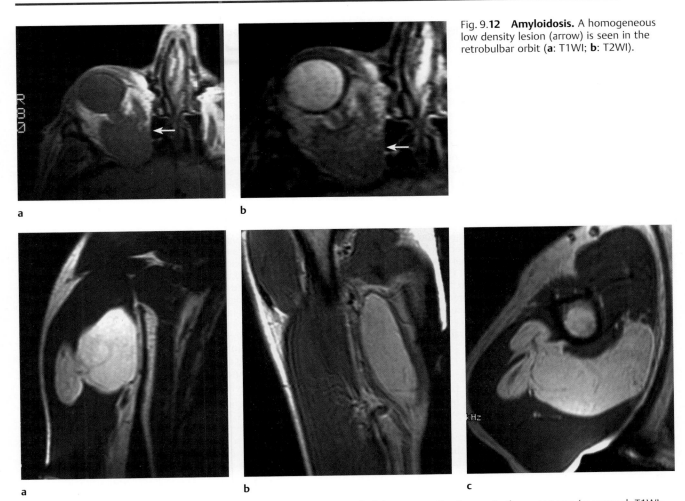

a   **b**

Fig. 9.**12** **Amyloidosis.** A homogeneous low density lesion (arrow) is seen in the retrobulbar orbit (**a**: T1WI; **b**: T2WI).

a   **b**   **c**

Fig. 9.**13** **Lipoma.** A well-circumscribed, homogeneous fatty lesion with delicate septation is seen in the upper arm (**a**: coronal, T1WI; **b**: sagittal, PDWI).   **c** After intravenous administration of Gd-DTPA the lesion does not enhance (axial, T1WI, +C).

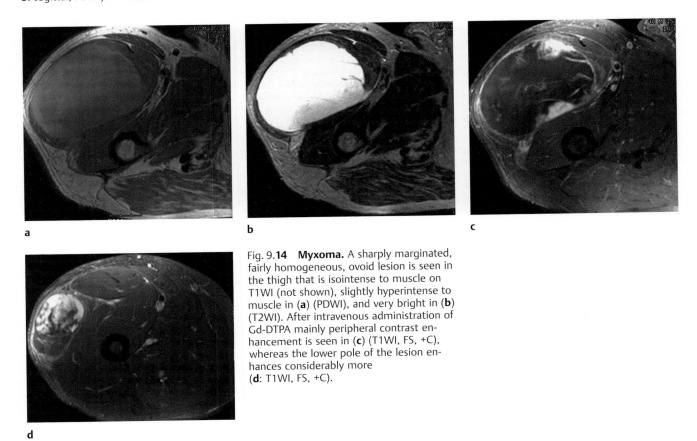

a   **b**   **c**

Fig. 9.**14** **Myxoma.** A sharply marginated, fairly homogeneous, ovoid lesion is seen in the thigh that is isointense to muscle on T1WI (not shown), slightly hyperintense to muscle in (**a**) (PDWI), and very bright in (**b**) (T2WI). After intravenous administration of Gd-DTPA mainly peripheral contrast enhancement is seen in (**c**) (T1WI, FS, +C), whereas the lower pole of the lesion enhances considerably more
(**d**: T1WI, FS, +C).

d

Table 9.**2** (Cont.) Soft-tissue lesions

Disease	MRI Findings	Comments
Benign fibrous histiocytoma (fibroxanthoma)	Well-defined homogeneous soft-tissue mass, hypointense on T1WI, hyperintense on T2WI, and with contrast enhancement.	Presents as painful soft-tissue mass in adults and children. *Xanthomatoses*: multiple xanthomas in soft tissues and tendons about fingers, elbow, knee, and neck, often associated with hypercholesterolemia and diabetes mellitus.
Desmoid tumor (localized fibromatosis) (Fig. 9.15)	Homogeneous or inhomogeneous lesion with irregular or smooth margins of usually low signal intensity on both T1WI and T2WI. Hypercellular lesions may produce a high signal intensity on T2WI interspersed with foci and bands of low signal intensity caused by collagen.	In young adults commonly located in abdominal wall (often after pregnancies), buttocks, thighs, and especially the shoulder region. Localized superficial fibromatosis includes *palmar fibromatosis (Dupuytren), plantar fibromatosis, penile fibromatosis (Peyronie),* and *knuckle pads.*
Fibromatosis	Variety of benign fibrous proliferations presenting as poorly defined, inhomogeneous soft-tissue lesions with signal intensity of muscle on T1WI and of fat on T2WI. Considerable variation in signal intensity is noted, however, depending on proportion and distribution of spindle cells, collagen, and mucopolysaccharide within the tumor. Moderate to marked enhancement is seen after intravenous Gd-DTPA administration.	*Aggressive fibromatosis* affects the musculature of adults and may be subdivided into extra-abdominal, abdominal, and intra-abdominal forms. The latter also involves the mesentery and may be associated with Gardner syndrome. *Congenital generalized fibromatosis* (Fig. 9.**16**) occurs in infants and may affect not only soft tissues but also viscera and bone. *Recurring digital fibromas* occur in fingers and toes of infants. *Juvenile aponeurotic fibromatosis* arises in the aponeurotic tissues of the hands and feet of children. May calcify.
Elastofibroma	Well-defined subscapular lesion of lenticular shape and heterogeneous signal intensity on T1WI and T2WI reflecting mature adipose tissue entrapped within the predominantly fibrous mass. Partial enhancement of the lesion occurs after intravenous Gd-DTPA administration.	Unilateral or bilateral reactive lesions (pseudotumors) in middle-aged and elderly persons, especially in manual laborers and weight lifters. Typical location is the area between inferior scapula and chest wall, presumably secondary to mechanical friction caused by the scapula tip.
Morton neuroma	Dumbbell-shaped mass between metatarsal heads most conspicuous on T1WI as an area of decreased signal intensity that is well demarcated from the adjacent fatty tissue. Lesions are isointense or slightly hypointense to fat on T2WI. Contrast enhancement is moderate. In two-thirds of cases intermetatarsal bursitis is associated.	Usually in females presenting with pain between the third and fourth or, less often, second and third metatarsal heads. Lesion is a pseudotumor caused by perineural fibrosis of the plantar digital nerve. True plantar neuromas can be differentiated by their high signal intensity on T2WI.
Schwannoma (neurilemoma) (Fig. 9.17)	Often inhomogeneous lesion with low to intermediate signal intensity on T1WI and high signal intensity on T2WI. A fibrous capsule is occasionally seen as a thin peripheral rim of low signal intensity (DD: neurofibromas have no capsule). Contrast enhancement is often irregular due to hemorrhagic, necrotic, or cystic areas found especially within larger lesions.	Occurs in adults between 20 and 50 years of age and typically arises from the spinal/nerve roots and the cervical, sympathetic, vagus, ulnar, or peroneal nerves. In contrast to intracranial schwannomas that are associated with neurofibromatosis type 2 in 5–20%, extracranial tumors are usually solitary.
Neurofibroma	Presents isointense to muscle on T1WI and with high signal intensity on T2WI. Target appearance on T2WI, consisting of a central zone of low signal intensity and a peripheral zone of high signal intensity, is characteristic but only present in a minority of cases. After intravenous GD-DTPA administration, contrast enhancement is usually moderate, but may sometimes be intense in the central area. A target pattern is occasionally also seen in schwannomas but not in the malignant counterparts (neurofibrosarcomas and malignant schwannomas).	Solitary neurofibromas usually occur in patients between 20 and 40 years of age and commonly arise in peripheral (cutaneous) nerves. Malignant transformation is very rare except in neurofibromatosis. Ten percent of patients with neurofibromas have neurofibromatosis type 1. *Plexiform neurofibromas* have heterogeneous signal intensity on both T1WI and T2WI and are always associated with neurofibromatosis.
Giant cell tumor of tendon sheath (Fig. 9.18)	Well-defined mass adjacent to a tendon. Isointense to muscle on T1WI. Inhomogeneous and hyperintense to muscle, but hypointense to fat on T2WI. Regions of low signal intensity correspond to fibrous tissue and hemosiderin deposition. Areas of higher signal intensity on T2WI reflect inflamed synovial tissue.	Second most frequent mass in the hand after ganglion. Occurs most commonly in the volar aspect of the first three fingers and first two toes of a young adult. *Pigmented villonodular synovitis* is histologically the identical counterpart involving large joints.

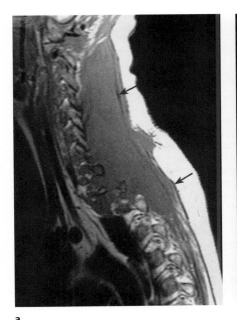

a

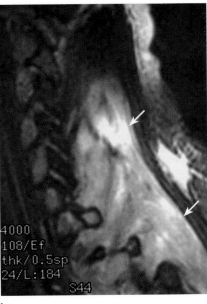

b

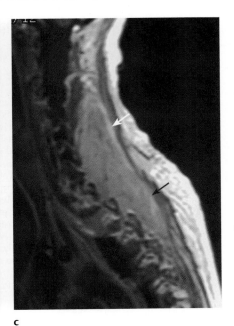

c

Fig. 9.**15**   **Desmoid tumor.** A relatively poorly marginated lesion (arrows) is seen in the posterior neck. The lesion appears

fairly homogeneous and of low signal intensity in (**a**) (T1WI, sagittal), and inhomogeneous and of high signal intensity in (**b**)

(T2WI, sagittal). After intravenous Gd-DTPA administration the lesion enhances moderately and unevenly (**c**: T1WI, FS, +C, sagittal).

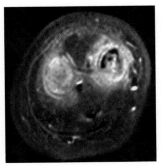

Fig. 9.**16**   **Congenital generalized fibromatosis.** A poorly defined, inhomogeneous, hyperintense soft-tissue infiltrate is seen surrounding and invading both tibia and fibula (T2WI).

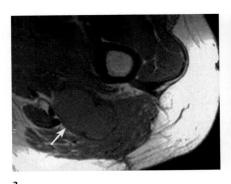

a

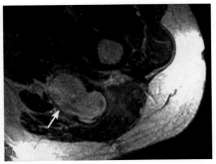

b

Fig. 9.**17**   **Schwannoma.** A well-defined, slightly inhomogeneous lesion with "figure 8" appearance (arrow) is seen in the poste-

rior thigh. The lesion is slightly hyperintense to muscle in (**a**) (PDWI) and isointense to fat in (**b**) (T2WI).

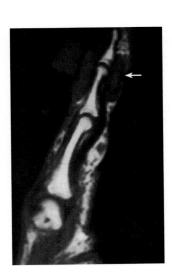

◁ Fig. 9.**18**   **Giant cell tumor of tendon sheath.** An inhomogeneous mass (arrow) isointense to muscle with pressure erosions in the volar aspect of the middle and distal phalanges of the index finger (T1WI).

Table 9.2 (Cont.) Soft-tissue lesions

Disease	MRI Findings	Comments
Hemangioma (cavernous) (Fig. 9.19)	Heterogeneous, poorly marginated lesion on T1WI with linear, lace-like, or coarse bands of high signal intensity representing fat interspersed between low intensity regions representing vascular spaces with slow-flowing or stagnant blood and other connective tissues. On T2WI the lesion is typically well marginated and markedly hyperintense compared with subcutaneous fat, reflecting the stagnant blood in the relatively uniform vascular spaces that are separated by fibrofatty septa of lower signal intensity. A fluid level (hematocrit effect) is occasionally seen in larger vascular spaces. Phleboliths may be evident as small rounded foci of signal void. Contrast enhancement is marked. Hemangiomas characteristically have little if any mass effect since involved muscle is replaced rather than displaced and becomes atrophic. Feeding and draining vessels with rapid flow (dark on SE and bright on GRE sequences) are only identified in a minority of cases.	Cavernous hemangiomas consist of large cavernous vascular channels. They also contain variable amounts of nonvascular tissues, the most common of which is fat, but also smooth muscle, fibrous tissue, and occasionally bone. On radiographs calcifications are relatively common and phleboliths are diagnostic when present. Superficial (subcutaneous) hemangiomas are usually diagnosed in infancy and early childhood, whereas deep (intramuscular) hematomas are manifest by 30 years of age with the highest prevalence in the limbs. *Capillary hemangiomas* (Fig. 9.**20**) are composed of capillary-sized vascular channels. They occur in infancy and grow rapidly in the first few months, beginning to spontaneously regress toward the end of the first year. They are poorly marginated on both T1WI and T2WI, mimicking a malignant vascular tumor. *Synovial hemangiomas* occur most frequently in the knees of an adolescent girl or young woman and may mimic hemophilia but invariably are monoarticular.
Hemangiopericytoma	Well or poorly marginated, relatively homogeneous lesion with low signal intensity on T1WI, high signal intensity on T2WI, and intense contrast enhancement after intravenous Gd-DTPA administration.	Slow-growing, deep-seated lesion arising in the musculature of the lower extremity, pelvis, or retroperitoneum of an adult. The majority of hemangiopericytomas are benign. *Glomus tumors* (paragangliomas) present as inhomogeneous oval masses with low signal intensity on T1WI, high signal intensity on T2WI, and intense contrast enhancement.
Arteriovenous malformation (AVM)	Serpentine, tangled tubular structures of signal void on all SE sequences and of high signal intensities on flow-sensitive GRE sequences secondary to rapidly circulating blood.	Congenital AVMs are composed of large tortuous arterial and venous vessels and thick capillaries. Acquired AVM usually are post-traumatic or iatrogenic, and rarely mycotic or neoplastic.
Aneurysm and pseudoaneurysm (Fig. 9.21)	Fusiform or saccular mass with signal voids in areas of flowing blood, often complicated by hemorrhage and thrombosis. Dark thrombi on both T1WI and T2WI are well organized and contain hemosiderin, bright lesions are unorganized and contain methemoglobin and inhomogeneous lesions are partially organized.	Popliteal artery aneurysm is the most common aneurysm of the extremities. The lesion is usually palpated on physical examination. Radiographically, curvilinear calcification may be noted in its wall.
Lymphangioma (Fig. 9.22)	Heterogeneous and isointense relative to muscle on T1WI and variably hyperintense on T2WI. Hyperintense foci on T1WI correspond to fat or methemoglobin. In larger cystic spaces fluid-fluid levels may be seen. Solid part of tumor, cyst walls, and internal septa enhance after Gd-DTPA administration.	Depending on the size of the lymphatic vessels the lesions are subdivided into capillary lymphangiomas, cavernous lymphangiomas, and cystic lymphangiomas, the latter presenting with unilocular or multilocular cystic spaces measuring up to several centimeters. The *cystic lymphangioma (hygroma)* is the most common type presenting usually in the neck of children. Occasionally it is associated with *Turner syndrome*.

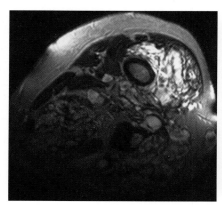
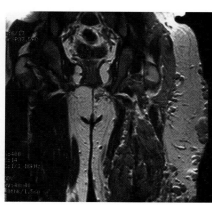

a   **b**

Fig. 9.**19** **Cavernous hemangioma (Kasabach-Merritt syndrome).** A heterogeneous poorly defined mass with variable signal intensity involving the subcutaneous fat and almost all muscles of the left thigh is seen (**a**: axial T1WI; **b**: coronal T2WI).

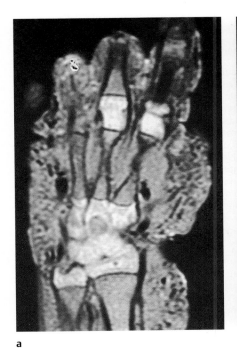
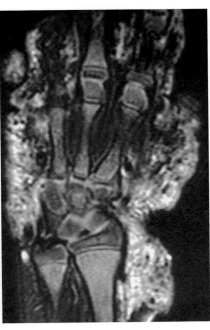

a   b

Fig. 9.**20** **Capillary hemangioma.** An extensive heterogeneous poorly marginated lesion involving the soft tissues of the hand is seen presenting with intermediate signal intensity in (**a**) (coronal T1WI) and high signal intensity in (**b**) (coronal T2WI).

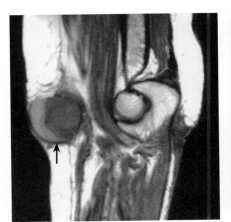
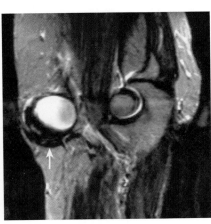

a   b

Fig. 9.**21** **Pseudoaneurysm (secondary to arteriovenous dialysis shunt).** A partially thrombosed pseudoaneurysm (arrow) with heterogeneous signal intensity is seen in the elbow (**a**: T1WI; **b**: T2WI).

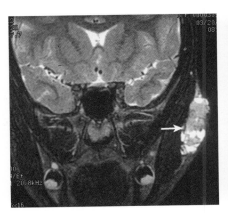
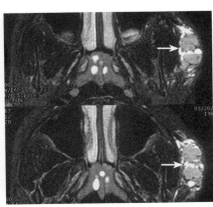

a   b

Fig. 9.**22** **Cystic lymphangioma (hygroma).** A heterogeneous lesion (arrows) is seen in the cheek consisting of both cystic (high signal intensity) and solid (intermediate signal intensity components) (T2WI, FS. **a**. coronal, b: axial).

Table 9.2 (Cont.) Soft-tissue lesions

Disease	MRI Findings	Comments
Liposarcoma (Figs. 9.23 and 9.24)	*Well-differentiated liposarcoma* presents as fatty mass with high signal intensity on T1WI and intermediate signal intensity on T2WI, containing irregularly thickened linear or nodular septa that appear hypointense on T1WI and may even be hyperintense on T2WI. In *myxoid, pleomorphic,* and *round cell liposarcomas* fatty tissue is only visible in about half of the cases. Myxoid liposarcomas present as well-defined homogeneous masses with decreased signal intensity on T1WI and increased signal intensity on T2WI. Pleomorphic and round cell liposarcomas are heterogeneous, poorly marginated tumors that are hypointense on T1WI, hyperintense on T2WI, and enhance considerably after Gd-DTPA administration.	Second most frequent soft-tissue sarcoma (after malignant fibrous histiocytoma), occurring commonly in the retroperitoneum, gluteal region, thigh, and leg of middle-aged and elderly patients. Four subtypes ranging from low-grade to high-grade malignancy include: 1) well-differentiated, 2) myxoid, 3) round cell, and 4) pleomorphic tumors. Myxoid liposarcoma is the most common subtype accounting for almost half of all liposarcomas. Calcifications occasionally occur in well-differentiated liposarcomas. A *dedifferentiated liposarcoma* (Fig. 9.25) is a bimorphic neoplasm consisting of a low-grade liposarcoma and a histologically different high-grade sarcoma.
Malignant fibrous histiocytoma (Fig. 9.26)	Poorly to relatively well defined inhomogeneous mass with intermediate signal intensity on T1WI (isointense to hyperintense to muscle) and high signal intensity on T2WI. Intratumoral hemorrhage and central necrosis are common. Contrast enhancement is considerable, but spares the necrotic areas. Erosion and infiltration of adjacent bone is fairly common. Rarely, low signal intensity on T2WI is observed when fibromatous tissue predominates histologically.	Most common soft-tissue tumor in adulthood (peak at 50 years of age) presenting as large painless mass located in the lower extremity (50%), upper extremity (25%), retroperitoneum (15%), and head and neck (5%). Male and Caucasian predominance. Histologically the following subtypes are differentiated: pleomorphic-storiform (50%), myxoid (25%), giant cell (10%), inflammatory (10%), and angiomatoid (5%). *Fibrosarcomas* have similar histologic and imaging features, but overall are slightly less malignant.

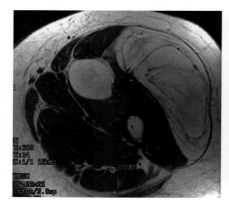

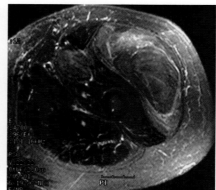

Fig. 9.**23** **Well-differentiated liposarcoma. a** A well-marginated fatty tumor consisting of a smaller nodular and a larger meniscus-shaped component with irregular septation is seen in the thigh (T1WI). **b** After intravenous Gd-DTPA administration inhomogeneous contrast enhancement occurs in the lesion (T1WI, FS, +C).

a

b

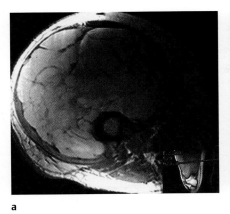

a

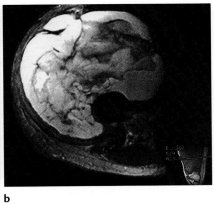

b

Fig. 9.**24** **Pleomorphic liposarcoma.** A large heterogeneous mass with intermediate to high signal intensity is seen in the thigh (**a**: PDWI; **b**: T2WI).

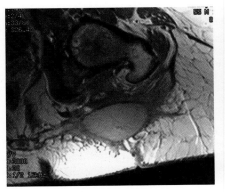

a

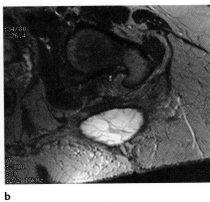

b

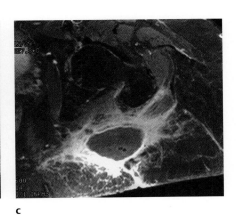

c

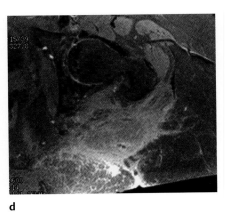

d

Fig. 9.**25** **Dedifferentiated liposarcoma.** A well-defined egg-shaped, septated and initially nonenhancing central core is surrounded by a poorly defined, infiltrating and markedly enhancing lesion located in the gluteus maximus (**a**: PDWI; **b**: T2WI; **c**: T1WI, FS, +C early; **d**: T1WI, FS, +C late).

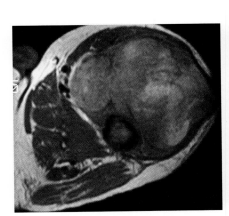

a

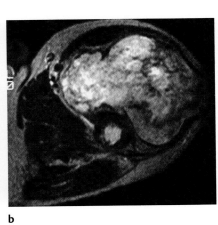

b

Fig. 9.**26** **Malignant fibrous histiocytoma.** A poorly defined, heterogeneous mass, slightly hyperintense to muscle in (**a**) (PDWI) and hyperintense in (**b**) (T2WI), is seen in the thigh.

Table 9.2 (Cont.) Soft-tissue lesions

Disease	MRI Findings	Comments
Synovial sarcoma (synovioma) (Fig. 9.27)	Well or poorly marginated, usually inhomogeneous mass isointense to muscle on T1WI and hyperintense to subcutaneous fat on T2WI. Occasionally, the lesion appears multiloculated with internal septation. Calcifications may be evident as area of decreased signal intensity on all pulse sequences. Osseous erosion or invasion is occasionally evident. Fluid-fluid levels secondary to previous hemorrhages occur rarely.	Slow-growing mass presenting in the extremities (two-thirds in lower limb) of young adults with female predominance. Extra-articular origin from tendon sheaths and bursae accounts for 95%, whereas intra-articular location is rare (5%). Tumor calcifications occur in approximately one-third of cases and are often located in the periphery of the lesion. Local recurrence and metastases occur in 80% but may be late (several years after initial diagnosis) and calcified.
Leiomyosarcoma, Rhabdomyosarcoma (Fig. 9.28)	Fairly well to poorly defined inhomogeneous soft-tissue mass isointense to muscle on T1WI and isointense or hyperintense to fat on T2WI. Central areas of necrosis, appearing hypointense on T1WI and hyperintense on T2WI, are common. Intratumoral hemorrhage is relatively frequent; erosion and invasion of adjacent bone rare.	Leiomyosarcomas arise in the retroperitoneum, major blood vessels, and peripheral soft tissue. They occur in middle-aged adults with a strong female predominance. Rhabdomyosarcomas occurring in adults under 50 years of age are located in the deep tissue of the extremities and torso. In children the tumor is predominant in the head, neck, and urogenital tract.
Malignant schwannoma and neurofibro-sarcoma (Figs. 9.29 and 9.30)	Poorly marginated inhomogeneous mass of low signal intensity on T1WI and high signal intensity on T2WI. Malignant and benign nerve sheath tumors cannot be reliably distinguished, although large (>5 cm) or increasing size, marked inhomogeneities, infiltrating margins, and irregular bone destruction favor malignancy.	Malignant counterpart of benign schwannoma and neurofibroma. Approximately half arise in patients with neurofibromatosis, and the other half occur as isolated phenomena, usually in the trunk and proximal portions of the extremities, in association with the sciatic nerve and brachial and sacral plexuses.
Angiosarcoma (malignant hemangioendothelioma)	Poorly defined, inhomogeneous lesion, isointense to muscle on T1WI and hyperintense on T2WI with marked contrast enhancement.	*Kaposi sarcoma*: Angiofibrosarcoma-like tumor, often associated with hemorrhage and hemosiderin deposition, found almost exclusively in homosexual male AIDS patients. Usually with obvious skin and/or mouth lesions.

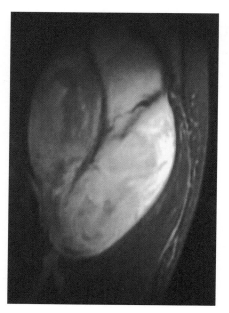

Fig. 9.**27** **Synovial sarcoma.** An ovoid, multiloculated mass with thick septation and heterogeneous high signal intensity is seen in the forearm (T2WI, FS).

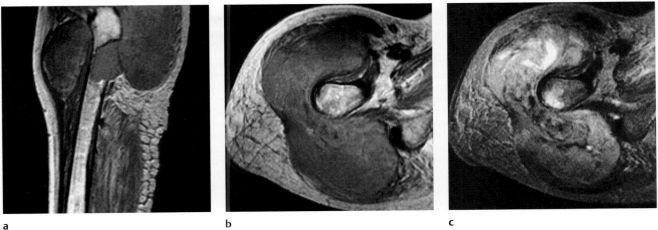

a b c

Fig. 9.**28** **Leiomyosarcoma. a** A large, fairly well-defined mass of low signal intensity wraps around the proximal femur and invades it (sagittal, PDWI). The lesion appears relatively homogeneous in (**b**) (axial, PDWI) and hyperintense and inhomogeneous in (**c**) (axial, T2WI).

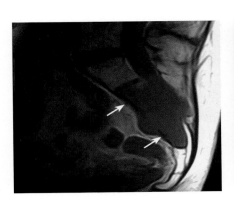

a b

Fig. 9.**29** **Malignant schwannoma.** A large, relatively homogeneous lesion (arrows) with destruction of the mid sacrum appears hypointense in (**a**) (sagittal, T1WI) and hyperintense in (**b**) (axial, T2WI).

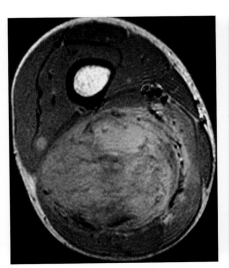

a b

Fig. 9.**30** **Neurofibrosarcoma. a** A poorly marginated, heterogeneous lesion of intermediate signal intensity is seen (PDWI). **b** After intravenous Gd-DTPA administration inhomogeneous and preferentially peripheral contrast enhancement is seen with necrotic/cystic foci presenting as hypointense regions (T1WI, FS, +C).

Table 9.2 (Cont.) Soft-tissue lesions

Disease	MRI Findings	Comments
Other soft-tissue malignancies (Figs. 9.31–9.35)	Fairly well to poorly defined, inhomogeneous lesions with decreased signal intensity on T1WI, increased signal intensity on T2WI, and considerable contrast enhancement. Low signal intensity on T2WI may be evident in heavily calcified or ossified lesions, and with extensive fibrosis or hemosiderin deposition. Melanoma can demonstrate increased signal intensity on T1WI resulting from the paramagnetic effect of melanin.	*Metastases, melanomas, lymphomas, extraosseous plasmacytomas, clear cell sarcomas* (arise in the vicinity of tendons and aponeuroses, most commonly in the foot and ankle), *alveolar soft-tissue sarcomas (malignant granular cell myoblastoma), epithelioid sarcomas* (arising primarily in fingers, hands, and forearms of young adults), *primitive neuroectodermal tumors* and *primary soft-tissue osteosarcomas, Ewing sarcomas*, and *chondrosarcomas. Primary benign* and *malignant bone tumors* extending into the soft tissues must be differentiated.

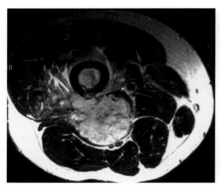

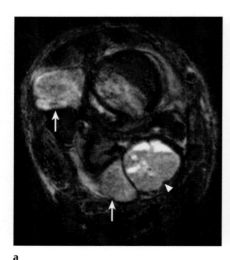

a

b

Fig. 9.**31** **Clear cell sarcoma. a** A poorly defined, heterogeneous lesion of high signal intensity is seen with extension into the medullary cavity of adjacent femur (T2WI). **b** After intravenous Gd-DTPA administration patchy heterogeneous contrast enhancement of the lesion is seen (T1WI, FS, +C).

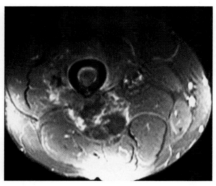
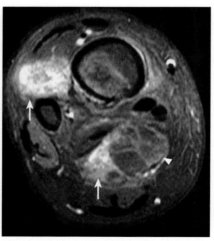

a

b

Fig. 9.**32** **Primitive neuroectodermal tumor complicated by aneurysmal bone cyst. a** Two poorly defined, heterogeneous hyperintense foci (arrows) represent primitive neuroectodermal tumors. The third well-defined nodule (arrowhead) with two small fluid-fluid levels may represent an aneurysmal bone cyst. Increased signal intensity in the tibial bone marrow is secondary to primitive neuroectodermal tumor infiltration (T2WI, FS). **b** After intravenous Gd-DTPA administration marked contrast enhancement in the two primitive neuroectodermal tumor lesions (arrows) is seen, whereas only peripheral and streaky contrast enhancement occurs in the aneurysmal bone cyst (arrowhead) (T1WI, FS, +C).

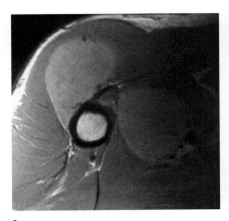
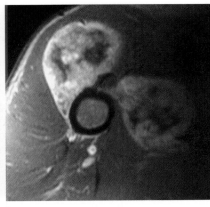

a

b

Fig. 9.**33 Ewing sarcoma. a** Two relatively well-defined, homogeneous nodules of intermediate signal intensity are seen in the soft tissue of the upper arm (PDWI). **b** After intravenous Gd-DTPA administration inhomogeneous contrast enhancement is seen (T1WI, FS, +C).

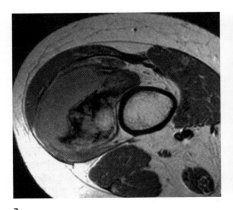
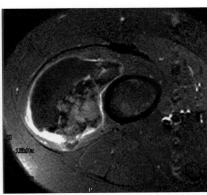

a

b

Fig. 9.**34 Chondrosarcoma. a** A well-defined lesion adjacent to the lateral aspect of the femur is seen, consisting of an inhomogeneous medial part and a homogeneous lateral part (proton density weighted image). **b** After intravenous Gd-DTPA administration, contrast enhancement occurs in the inhomogeneous medial part and the tumor periphery (T1WI, FS, with contrast enhancement).

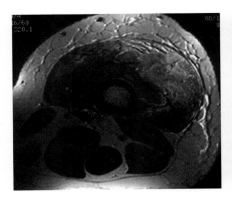
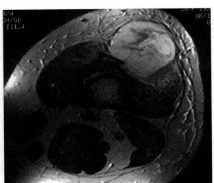

a

b

Fig. 9.**35 Non-Hodgkin lymphoma** (metastasis). A heterogeneous, poorly (9.35 **a**) to well defined (9.29 **b**) lesion is evident in the quadriceps muscle (T2WI).

10 Joint Disease

In articular disease both conventional radiography and CT can display osseous involvement better than any other imaging modality. These modalities, however, cannot provide the excellent soft-tissue contrast of MRI. Intra-articular and para-articular structures such as joint cartilage, tendons, ligaments, muscles, and bone marrow are depicted by MRI in unrivaled fashion. Similarly pathologic conditions such as edema, hemorrhage, and joint effusions can easily be visualized. Another benefit of MRI is its multiplanar image capability, allowing direct imaging of every joint in any desired plane. Nevertheless, MRI examinations should not be interpreted without plain radiographs, since calcifications, loose bodies, bony spurs, and fractures may be either missed or misdiagnosed.

Normal *articular (hyaline) cartilage* presents on spin-echo (SE) sequences as a line of intermediate signal intensity paralleling the subchondral cortical bone that has a low signal intensity. On gradient-echo (GRE) sequences the articular cartilage demonstrates a high signal intensity, resulting in the best contrast between the articular cartilage and bone. Meniscal fibrocartilage has a lower signal intensity on all pulse sequences when compared with the articular cartilage. Articular cartilage pathology can be diagnosed with MRI by demonstrating focal erosions, contour irregularities, and thinning of the joint cartilage. Decreased and inhomogeneous cartilage signal intensity on T1WI and especially GRE images indicates degeneration.

Normal *ligaments* demonstrate a homogeneous signal void on all MR sequences. Discontinuity of a ligament is direct evidence of a complete tear. Increased signal intensity within an intact ligament suggests a partial tear. Associated joint effusion, edema in the adjacent soft tissue, and hemorrhage at the site of ligamentous injury may be present and are well demonstrated on T2WI. Chronically torn ligaments may appear thickened or attenuated.

Normal *tendons* are devoid of signal on all pulse sequences. Increased intratendinous signal intensity on T1WI indicates either hemorrhage or myxoid degeneration, but may occasionally be normal (see "magic angle" phenomenon in Chapter 9, page 334). Increased signal intensity on T2WI, however, is always abnormal and indicative of rupture or inflammation. Morphologically, normal tendons exhibit smooth contours and uniform thickness. Tendon thickening can result from fibrosis due to chronic tendinitis or from edema and hemorrhage which accompany partial tears or acute inflammation. Focal narrowing of a tendon is usually caused by a partial tear. Complete discontinuity is diagnostic of a full-thickness tear and is usually associated with retraction of the torn ends, with fluid or hemorrhage in the gap.

Joint effusions demonstrate low signal intensity on T1WI and high signal intensity on T2WI. Fresh hemorrhage into a joint cannot be differentiated by MRI from a regular joint effusion, unless a fluid-fluid level is seen caused by the settling of the cellular elements ("hematocrit effect"). Such a phenomenon has to be differentiated from a fat/blood-fluid level seen with intra-articular fractures, where the lighter fat on top of the blood is recognized by its bright signal intensity on the T1WI. However, when the hemorrhage is subacute and extracellular methemoglobin is present, then it has a high signal intensity on both T1WI and T2WI. Similarly, joint effusions containing large amounts of proteinaceous material show a high signal intensity on both T1WI and T2WI. Hemosiderin, in contrast, demonstrates low signal intensity with all pulse sequences. Hemosiderin deposits may be found in hemophilia, rheumatoid arthritis, pigmented villonodular synovitis, and synovial hemangioma.

The MRI presentation of *intra-articular loose bodies* varies considerably depending on their tissue composition. Noncalcified chondral loose bodies tend to be of intermediate signal intensity on all SE sequences. Calcified loose bodies are of low signal intensity on all imaging sequences. Meniscal fragments present in similar fashion, but are not evident on plain radiographs. Osteochondromal bodies that contain fat demonstrate high signal intensity on T1WI and intermediate to high signal intensity on T2WI. Loose bodies are often surrounded by a joint effusion of high signal intensity on T2WI.

Intra-articular loose bodies arise from disintegration of the articular surface, transchondral fractures, and synovial metaplasia. Fragmentation of the joint surface can accompany a variety of disease processes including trauma, avascular necrosis, osteoarthritis, pseudogout (calcium pyrophosphate dihydrate crystal deposition or CPPD arthropathy), neuropathic and infectious arthropathies. In these conditions one or several nonuniform loose bodies may be present. In transchondral fractures, including osteochondritis dissecans, a defect in the articular surface at the site of origin is invariably associated with the loose body. Synovial metaplasia occurs in idiopathic and secondary synovial osteochondromatosis. In the idiopathic form, preponderant in young males, a large number of loose bodies of approximately equal size are found in an otherwise normal joint prior to development of secondary degenerative changes. Secondary synovial osteochondromatosis develops in an osteoarthritic joint and usually produces fewer (less than 10) loose bodies of varying size. Both chondrocalcinosis and vacuum phenomenon may project as small linear or globular areas devoid of signals between articular surfaces and should not be confused with small loose bodies. Furthermore, a vacuum phenomenon can only be found in joints without effusions.

Intra-articular synovial hemosiderin deposition results in decreased signal intensity in both T1WI and T2-weighted SE images, and, especially, in GRE images. Hemosiderin deposition is commonly associated with chronic hemarthrosis found with intra-articular injuries, neuropathic arthropathy, hemophilic arthropathy, pigmented villonodular synovitis, and synovial hemangiomas. It is also frequently associated with rheumatoid arthritis and hemochromatosis and less with degenerative joint disease.

A *subchondral lesion* with decreased signal intensity on T1WI and increased signal intensity on T2WI may be cystic or solid. Subchondral cysts are commonly associated with osteoarthritis, pseudogout (CPPD arthropathy), and rheumatoid arthritis. In these conditions they are often multiple and, except in rheumatoid arthritis, have a sclerotic margin presenting as a hypointense rim. A single cystic lesion neighboring a normal joint often represents an *intraosseous ganglion*. Cystic subchondral lesions are also a frequent finding in avascular necrosis where they are often accompanied by bone sclerosis, collapse, and fragmentation. A gouty tophus depicts low signal intensity on T1WI and mixed, low to relatively high, inhomogeneous signal intensity on T2WI. Amyloid deposits typically demonstrate low to intermediate signal intensity on all pulse sequences. Juxta-articular cystic osteomyelitis is often tuberculous or fungal in etiology. In pigmented villonodular synovitis he-

mosiderin-laden macrophages within intra-articular soft-tissue masses produce low signal intensity on all imaging sequences, and pressure erosions or subchondral cysts may be associated. Tumors that primarily originate in the subchondral epiphyseal bone are rare and include chondroblastomas in patients below 30 years of age and clear cell chondrosarcomas in patients over 30 years of age. Neoplasms extending from the metaphyses into the subchondral bone, such as a giant cell tumor, are much more common. In the elderly patient skeletal metastases and multiple myeloma must also be considered in this location.

Table 10.1 Arthritis and arthritis-like conditions

Disease	MRI Findings	Comments
Osteoarthritis (Fig. 10.1)	Inhomogeneous decreased signal intensity of the cartilage in T2WI and GRE images. Thinning of cartilage predominantly occurs in areas subject to excessive pressure (e.g., superolateral aspect of hip, medial compartment of knee). Subchondral sclerosis (signal void on all sequences) is an early and common manifestation adjacent to the degenerative cartilage. Subchondral cysts (geodes) surrounded by a sclerotic rim may develop in areas of cartilagineous degeneration or disappearance. Cysts are commonly multiple, of variable size, and often pyriform in shape. Osteophytosis is often prominent, flattening and deformity of the articular surface are late manifestations. Joint effusions are small, if present.	Primary osteoarthritis commonly involves the interphalangeal joints of the fingers (particularly the distal ones), the first carpometacarpal joints, hips, knees, first metatarsophalangeal joints, and spine. Secondary osteoarthritis may affect any joint depending on the underlying causative mechanism. Synovial membrane alterations including joint effusions are not prominent in osteoarthritis except in *erosive osteoarthritis* of the interphalangeal joints. Signs of synovitis including a sizeable joint effusion should suggest an inflammatory process (e.g., pseudogout) or superimposed infection.

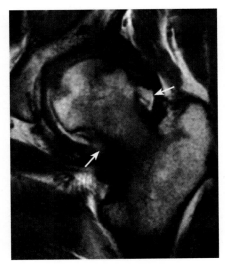

Fig. 10.1 **Osteoarthritis.** Inhomogeneous signal intensity in the femoral head and acetabulum corresponding to sclerosis, geode formations, and osteophytosis containing fatty marrow (arrows) (T1WI, coronal).

Table 10.1 (Cont.) Arthritis and arthritis-like conditions

Disease	MRI Findings	Comments
Rheumatoid arthritis (Figs. 10.2 and 10.2*)	Inflammation and proliferation of synovial tissue (pannus formation) producing joint effusions, marginal erosions, destruction of articular cartilage and subsequently subchondral bone, subchondral cysts, and joint deformities are features demonstrated well by MRI. Acutely inflamed pannus tends to be slightly hyperintense to the joint effusion on T1WI and slightly hypointense on T2WI. Contrast enhancement of the acutely inflamed pannus is rapid and marked, whereas enhancement of synovial fluid is slow (peaking at 30 min or later) and modest, thus facilitating the differentiation of these two conditions. Noninflamed fibrous pannus has a low signal intensity on all pulse sequences and poor contrast enhancement. Similarly, areas with hemosiderin deposition also appear hypointense. Soft-tissue complications associated with rheumatoid arthritis include bursitis, synovial cyst formation, tenosynovitis, and disruption of tendons and ligaments and are well evaluated by MRI.	Most common locations include proximal interphalangeal joints and metacarpal phalangeal joints of hands, wrists, elbows, shoulders, knees and cervical spine. Polyarticular involvement with symmetric distribution is characteristic. *Juvenile rheumatoid arthritis* differs from the adult form in that growth disturbances are associated, loss of joint space and osseous erosions are relatively late manifestations, and periostitis, intra-articular bony ankylosis, epiphyseal compression fractures, and dislocations are common. The synovitis in *seronegative spondyloarthropathies* (*ankylosing spondylitis, enteropathic arthropathy, psoriatic arthritis,* and *Reiter syndrome*) is similar to that of rheumatoid arthritis, but in contrast to the latter, involvement of the sacroiliac joints and spine is early, involvement of the peripheral joints is asymmetric, and new bone formations and bony ankylosis is common.
Gouty arthritis (Fig. 10.3)	Tophi present as soft-tissue masses of low intensity on T1WI and of mixed low and high signal intensity on T2WI. Occasionally regions of very low signal intensity are seen on all pulse sequences, caused by hemosiderin deposition secondary to recurrent hemarthrosis.	MRI may be useful in assessing the full extent of soft-tissue, synovial, cartilaginous, and osseous involvement.
Calcium pyrophosphate dihydrate crystal deposition disease (CPPD, pseudogout) Calcium hydroxyapatite crystal deposition disease (HADD) (Fig. 10.4)	Chondrocalcinosis and synovial, ligamentous, capsular, tendinous, and bursal calcifications are the hallmark of the disease, but are often not appreciated by MRI. They may be best seen on GRE sequences as an irregular signal void due to susceptibility artifacts. Osteochondral changes are similar to osteoarthritis, but signs of synovitis including a sizeable effusion are often associated.	CPPD preferentially affects the joints, whereas HADD has a predilection for the para-articular soft tissues. A combination of CPPD and HADD is not unusual. The shoulder is the most common site of HADD, leading to crystal deposition in the tendinous and bursal structures about this joint. The disease may progress to severe arthritic changes in the glenohumeral joint and complete rotator cuff tear with superior displacement of the humeral head (Milwaukee shoulder syndrome).

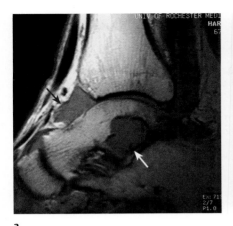

a

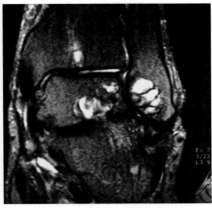

b

Fig. 10.2 Rheumatoid arthritis. a Pannus formation (arrows) of intermediate signal intensity, joint effusion, and erosions in the talus, calcaneus, and anterior tibial malleolus are seen (sagittal PDWI). **b** Pannus and joint effusion depict high signal intensity, and multiple erosions are again seen (coronal T2WI).

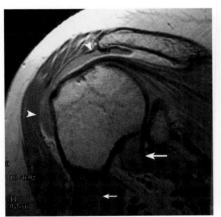

Fig. 10.**2*** **a**

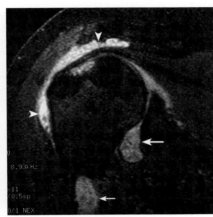

Fig. 10.**2*** **b**

Fig. 10.2* Rheumatoid arthritis. Synovial fluid and pannus formation is seen in the axillary recess of the shoulder joint (long arrow), long biceps tendon sheath (short arrow), and subacromiodeltoid bursa (arrowheads) (**a**: coronal PDWI; **b**: coronal FS T2WI).

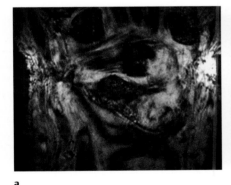

a

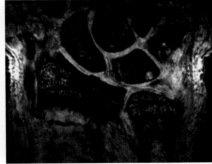

b

Fig. 10.3 Gouty arthritis. Synovial proliferation with heterogeneous high signal intensity consistent with gouty tophi is most conspicuous in the palmar wrist joint capsule (**a**: GRE [T2WI], coronal) and triangular fibrocartilage complex (**b**: GRE [T2WI], coronal). Scapholunate and lunotriquetral ligaments are eroded, and small cysts are seen in several carpal bones.

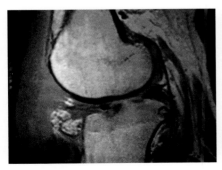

a

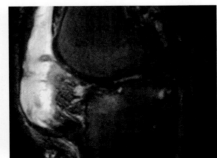

b

Fig. 10.4 CPPD (pseudogout). An inflammatory mass involving the infrapatellar fat pad is associated with a large effusion in the suprapatellar bursa. A small subchondral cyst is seen in the anterior tibia plateau (**a**: PDWI, sagittal; **b**: T2WI, sagittal). Chondrocalcinosis is not appreciated but is evident on plain film radiography.

Table 10.1 (Cont.) Arthritis and arthritis-like conditions

Disease	MRI Findings	Comments
Septic arthritis (Fig. 10.5)	Monoarticular disease with large joint effusion and inflamed edematous synovium that enhances considerably after intravenous administration of Gd-DTPA. Rapid destruction of joint cartilage results in progressive joint space narrowing. Erosion and destruction of the subchondral bone are observed with disease progression. Differentiation of secondary osteomyelitis from reactive bone marrow edema in an early stage may be difficult, since both conditions present with low signal intensity on T1WI and high signal intensity on T2WI. The extent of periarticular inflammation, including possible soft-tissue abscess formation, is well demonstrated.	In acute monoarticular disease joint aspiration is mandatory to diagnose or rule out an infectious etiology. In *tuberculous* (Fig. 10.6) and *fungal arthritis* (Fig. 10.7) the onset is more insidious with symptoms lingering for months, as opposed to days for pyogenic infections, before medical attention is sought. In tuberculous and fungal infections the joint cartilage is affected relatively late in the course of the disease, resulting in relative long preservation of the joint space and subsequent slow and gradual narrowing.
Pigmented villonodular synovitis (Figs. 10.8 and 10.8*)	Lobulated, hypervascular, intra-articular mass associated with hemarthrosis and pressure erosions in about half the cases. T1WI demonstrates a heterogeneous mass with low signal intensity. In T2WI the lesion often has regions of high signal intensity interspersed with foci of low signal intensity. The foci of low signal intensity are caused by fibrosis and hemosiderin deposition and vary considerably from lesion to lesion.	Monoarticular disease typically affecting the large joints (most common knee, but also hip, ankle, elbow, shoulder, and rarely tarsal and carpal joints) of young adults ranging in age from 20 to 50 years. Soft-tissue calcifications are usually not associated and, when present on radiographs, strongly suggest another diagnosis such as *synovial osteochondromatosis* or *synovial sarcoma*. *Localized villonodular synovitis* refers to villonodular synovitis without pigment/hemosiderin deposition.

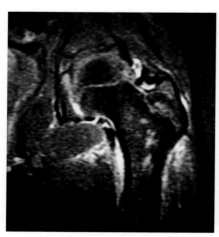

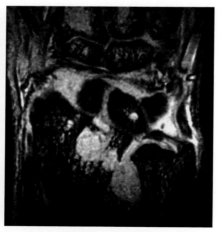

Fig. 10.**5** **Septic arthritis.** Joint effusion in the left hip and hyperintense inflammatory changes in the synovium, adjacent soft tissues, and proximal femur are seen after contrast enhancement (T1WI, FS, +C, coronal).

Fig. 10.**6** **Tuberculous arthritis.** Severe synovial inflammation and joint effusion are seen in the wrist, distal radioulnar joint, and intercarpal joint with erosion of the triangular fibrocartilage complex and the scapholunate and lunotriquetral ligaments (not shown in this image plane) (GRE [T2WI], coronal).

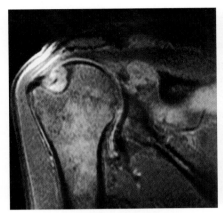

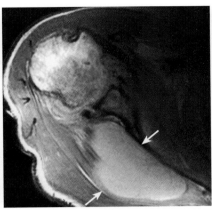

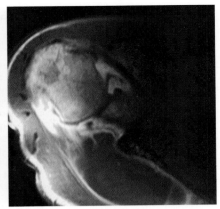

Fig. 10.**7** **Fungal arthritis (*Fusarium solani* arthritis in AIDS).** **a** A hyperintense eroding mass is seen in the superolateral aspect of the humeral head with inflammatory changes in the adjacent supraspinatus tendon and soft tissues as well as in the proximal humerus (T2WI, FS).

Fig. 10.**7 b** Hyperintense inflammatory changes are seen in the humeral head and a large oblong cystic soft-tissue lesion (arrows) (T2WI).

Fig. 10.**7 c** After intravenous Gd-DTPA administration contrast enhancement is seen in the humeral head, adjacent soft tissues, and wall of the cystic lesion (T1WI, FS, +C).

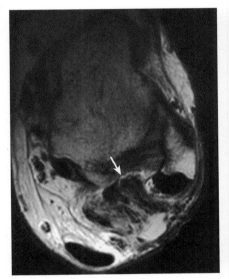

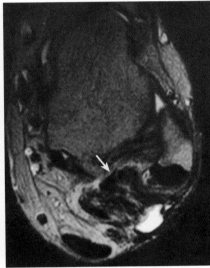

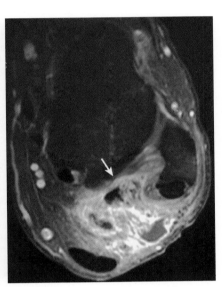

Fig. 10.**8*** **a**

Fig. 10.**8*** **b**

Fig. 10.**8*** **c**

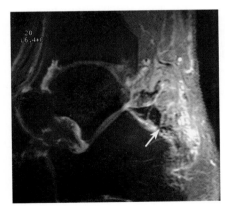

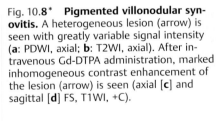

Fig. 10.**8*** **Pigmented villonodular synovitis.** A heterogeneous lesion (arrow) is seen with greatly variable signal intensity (**a**: PDWI, axial; **b**: T2WI, axial). After intravenous Gd-DTPA administration, marked inhomogeneous contrast enhancement of the lesion (arrow) is seen (axial [**c**] and sagittal [**d**] FS, T1WI, +C).

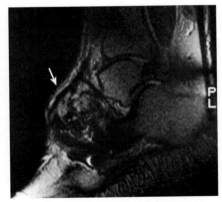

Fig. 10.**8*** **d**

Fig. 10.**8** **Pigmented villonodular synovitis.** A heterogeneous soft-tissue mass (arrow) is seen in the dorsum of the foot with erosion of the adjacent tarsal bones. The hypointense foci within the mass are caused by hemosiderin deposition and fibrosis (T2WI, FS, sagittal).

Table 10.**1** (Cont.) Arthritis and arthritis-like conditions

Disease	MRI Findings	Comments
Osteochondromatosis (synovial) (Fig. 10.9)	Hyperplastic synovium with cartilagenous metaplasia resulting in multiple intra-articular loose bodies of relatively uniform size measuring up to 3 cm with varying degrees of calcification or ossification. Noncalcified cartilaginous bodies are of intermediate to high signal intensity on T1WI and T2WI. Calcified and ossified loose bodies are of low signal intensity on all pulse sequences. They may be better appreciated on T2WI when surrounded by a hyperintense joint effusion. Osteochondral bodies that contain fatty marrow have a high signal intensity on T1WI and intermediate to high signal intensity on T2WI.	Idiopathic form is usually a monoarticular disease of young adults (20–50 years of age) with male predominance (2:1). The knee is the most common location, followed by elbow, hip, shoulder, ankle, and wrist. Pressure erosions are more commonly found in tight joints (e.g. hip). Secondary osteoarthritis is common in late stages. Secondary synovial osteochondromatosis (chondrometaplasia) may develop in any joint with chronic synovitis (e.g. primary osteoarthritis). Loose intra-articular bodies can also be found in any disease associated with disintegration of the articular cartilage and transchondral fractures.
Osteochondritis dissecans and osteochondral fracture (Fig. 10.10)	Purely chondral or osteochondral fractures of the articular surface occur. Osteochondral fracture fragments are of low to intermediate signal intensity on T1WI, slightly brighter on T2WI, and often inhomogeneous due to hemorrhagic and ischemic changes. Bone marrow edema and hemorrhage may be evident in the bone neighboring the loose body. A line of hyperintense fluid on T2WI may separate the fragment from the underlying bone. Loose fragments are completely encircled by the fluid. Cystic changes in the underlying bone also indicate fracture fragment instability. Partially or completely dislodged fracture fragments with corresponding articular cartilage defect are readily identified.	Occurs in adolescents with male predominance (3:1) without history of trauma in up to 50%, or at any age secondary to trauma and ischemia. Common locations include knee (non-weightbearing intercondylar aspect of medial femoral condyle, lateral femoral condyle, and lower medial facet of patella), talus (lateral and medial talar dome), elbow (capitellum), and humeral head. Treatment depends on the staging: stable osteochondritis dissecans with largely intact articular cartilage is usually treated conservatively. A loose in situ fragment may be treated by internal fixation. Partially and completely displaced fragments are resected.
Avascular necrosis (AVN), osteonecrosis of subarticular bone (Fig. 10.11)	In the early stage a segmental, wedge-shaped, or elliptical area of high signal intensity (yellow marrow fat) is demarcated by a band or ring of lower signal intensity on T1WI and higher signal intensity on T2WI. The zone of demarcation in the periphery of the infarct initially consists of hyperemia and edema and later of granulation tissue. Subsequently a "double line sign" may become evident on T2WI, composed of an inner hyperintense band caused by granulation tissue and an outer hypointense band caused by fibrosis and sclerosis. The outer hypointense band may also represent in part a chemical shift artifact. With necrosis the center of the infarct becomes hypointense on T1WI and inhomogeneous on T2WI. Contrast enhancement is initially limited to the periphery of the infarct but with time progresses slowly towards its center due to revascularization and repair. Nonviable necrotic tissue does not enhance. A healed infarct usually appears hypointense on all image sequences due to fibrosis and sclerosis (trabecular thickening). Subchondral fractures may be imminent when a crescent-shaped, hypointense zone is seen on all pulse sequences in the subarticular bone of an otherwise intact joint surface. Gaps of low signal intensity on both T1WI and T2WI images or a subchondral line of high signal intensity on T2WI, representing joint fluid, hemorrhage, or granulation tissue in the fracture cleft may be associated. Focal articular collapse and deformities are evident in more advanced stages. A small joint effusion is a common finding in all stages.	Epiphyses consist mainly of marrow fat cells that are most resistent to ischemia, surviving up to 5 days. In contrast hematopoietic cells die within 6–12 hours and osteocytes within 12–48 hours. Dynamic changes in AVN include loss of blood supply leading to cell death with subsequent cell necrosis, followed by revascularization from the periphery, ingrowth of mesenchymal cells with eventual fibrosis, and bone remodeling. The earliest abnormalities are, however, evident at the infarct periphery, where hyperemia, edema, and hemorrhage are followed by granulation, fibrosis, and new bone formation. These sequential dynamic alterations can easily explain all described MRI changes, taking into account that different pathohistologic stages may overlap in an infarct. AVN is often associated with trauma, sickle cell disease, vasculitis (e.g., lupus erythematosus, rheumatoid arthritis) hypercortisolism (exogenous and endogenous steroids), renal transplantation, irradiation, Gaucher disease, Caisson disease, pancreatitis, and alcoholism.

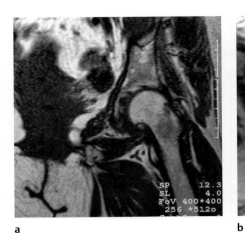

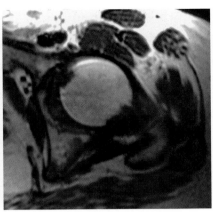

Fig. 10.**9** **Synovial osteochondromatosis.** Numerous small intra-articular loose bodies of varying signal intensity project into the joint space between femoral head and acetabulum (coronal [**a**] and axial [**b**] T1WI).

a

b

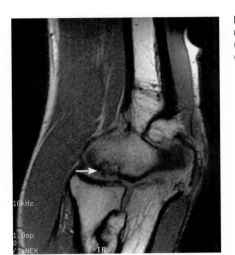

Fig. 10.**10** **Osteochondritis.** A small irregular subchondral fracture fragment (arrow) is seen in the capitellum (PDWI, coronal).

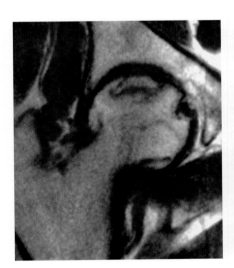

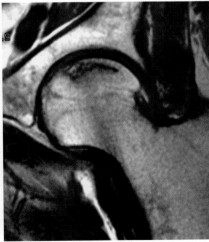

Fig. 10.**11** **Bilateral avascular femur head necrosis.** Demarcation of a hyperintense bony fragment, containing fatty marrow, by a dark band caused by edema and granulation is seen bilaterally (**a** and **b**: T1WI, coronal).

a

b

Table 10.1 (Cont.) Arthritis and arthritis-like conditions

Disease	MRI Findings	Comments
Avascular necrosis (AVN), osteonecrosis of subarticular bone (continued)	*AVN of the lunate (Kienböck disease)* typically occurs at age 20–40 years and may be associated with a short ulna (negative ulnar variance). *Idiopathic AVN of the knee* typically occurs in the weightbearing portion of the medial femoral condyle of an elderly woman.	Plain film staging of femoral AVN: 1) Normal or minimal trabecular mottling, abnormal MRI. 2) Focal osteopenia, sclerosis, and cyst formations. 3) Subchondral lucency ("crescent sign"). 4) Collapse of femoral head. 5) Secondary degenerative changes including the acetabulum. Idiopathic or post-traumatic AVN in the immature skeleton (osteochondrosis) is often associated with an eponym: femoral head (Legg-Calvé-Perthes), patella, inferior pole (Sinding-Larsen-Johansson), tibial tuberosity (Osgood-Schlatter), medial tibial epiphysis (Blount), tarsal navicular (Köhler), metatarsal head (Freiberg), capitulum (Panner), scaphoid (Preiser), phalanges (Thiemann), and vertebral apophyses (Scheuermann).
Transient regional osteoporosis (transient bone marrow edema, transient osteoporosis of the hip) (Fig. 10.12)	Bone marrow edema involving the femoral head, neck, and sometimes intertrochanteric area appears uniformly hypointense on T1WI and hyperintense on T2WI. Occasionally, the edema pattern extends into the acetabulum. A small joint effusion is commonly present. Both uniformity and a more diffuse nature of signal abnormalities differentiate the disorder from AVN. However a small number of patients with typical MRI findings of regional marrow edema will develop AVN at that site.	Self-limited disease, reversible within 2–6 months, most commonly affecting the hip of young and middle-aged adults. In females it often begins in the third trimester of pregnancy with predilection for the left side. Bilateral manifestations or involvement of other joints in the lower extremity occur occasionally. Radiographically a rapidly developing periarticular osteoporosis is evident within a few weeks after onset of symptoms. (DD: AVN). Increased uptake on bone scan is also present. Both *regional migratory osteoporosis* and *reflex sympathetic dystrophy* also present with periarticular bone marrow edema and are probably closely related to transient regional osteoporosis.
Hemophilic arthropathy	Synovial fibrosis and hemosiderin deposition present as hypointense regions intermingled with foci of high signal intensity on T2WI due to synovial inflammation and hemorrhage. Methemoglobin formation may produce hyperintense areas on both T1WI and T2WI. Joint effusions may have variable signal intensities depending on the various blood breakdown products. Cartilage loss is focal or diffuse. Subchondral cystic lesions are prominent and may contain fluid, fresh blood, methemoglobin, hemosiderin, and fibrous material in any combination.	X-linked recessive disorder in males resulting from deficiency of factor VIII (hemophilia A) or IX (hemophilia B, Christmas disease). Abnormalities caused by repeated intra-articular and intraosseous hemorrhages begin during skeletal maturation and result in growth abnormalities (e.g. condylar overgrowth) and arthropathy. Bilateral involvement of large joints is common, but not invariable, with predilection for knee, ankle, and elbow. *Chronic hemarthrosis* leading to synovitis and hemosiderin deposition may also be found in other bleeding disorders including anticoagulant medication, recurrent trauma, neuropathic joint, pigmented villonodular synovitis, and synovial hemangioma. *Juvenile rheumatoid arthritis* most closely resembles hemophilia in larger joints, but can be differentiated from the latter by involvement of the hands, wrists, feet, and spine.
Neuropathic arthropathy (Charcot joint) (Fig. 10.13)	Persistent hemorrhagic joint effusion, articular fragmentation, healing fractures with periosteal thickening and sclerosis, subluxations, and bone resorption are typically associated with decreased signal intensity in the subarticular bone marrow on both T1WI and T2WI. In the diabetic foot decreased signal intensity on T1WI and increased signal intensity on T2WI suggests superimposed osteomyelitis, but an acute neuropathic fracture may present in similar fashion.	Abnormalities are caused by recurrent untreated fractures and dislocations, due to decreased pain sensation, and bone resorption due to sympathetic dysfunction resulting in local hyperemia. *Diabetic foot* is a combination of neuroarthropathy, infection, and vasculitis affecting primarily metatarsophalangeal, tarsometatarsal, and intertarsal joints.

Table 10.**1** (Cont.) Arthritis and arthritis-like conditions

Disease	MRI Findings	Comments
Intra-articular soft-tissue tumors (Fig. 10.14)	*Lipoma arborescens*: irregular fatty proliferation beneath swollen synovial lining associated with joint effusion usually in the knee. *Synovial lipoma*: discrete intra-articular fatty mass. *Synovial hemangioma*: Inhomogeneous hypervascular mass, usually predominantly hypointense on T1WI and hyperintense on T2WI, typically in the knee. Signs of chronic hemarthrosis may be associated. *Intracapsular and capsular chondroma*: partially calcified, often infrapatellar mass with inhomogeneous and variable signal intensity.	*Pigmented villonodular synovitis*: see above in this table. *Synovial osteochondromatosis*: see above in this table. *Synovial chondrosarcoma*: Extremely rare tumor occurring usually in the knee with bizarre calcifications and inhomogeneous signal intensity on MRI. May be secondary to synovial osteochondromatosis. *Synovial sarcoma*: Intra-articular location is rare (<10%). Spotty calcifications in one-third of cases. Inhomogeneous mass, hypointense on T1WI, hyperintense on T2WI.

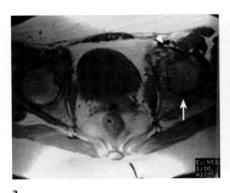
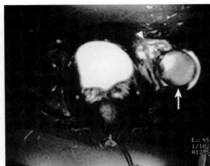

Fig. 10.**12** **Transient bone marrow edema.** Compared with the normal right femoral head, the signal intensity in the left femoral head (arrow) is decreased in (**a**) (PDWI) and markedly increased in (**b**) (T2WI, FS). Note also the left hip joint effusion and the Ewing sarcoma (arrowhead) presenting with heterogeneous signal intensity in the pubic bone.

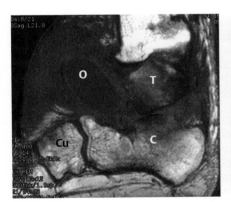
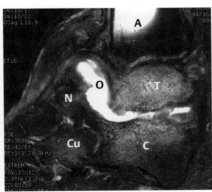

Fig. 10.**13** **Neuropathic arthropathy in syringomyelia.** Severely destroyed subtalar and talonavicular joints with large inhomogeneous joint effusion containing debris and bony fragments are seen. The joint effusion connects with large cystic outpouching (O) anterior of the talonavicular joint surrounded by extensive soft tissue swelling (**a**: T1WI, sagittal; **b**: T2WI, sagittal). A: coil artifact in distal tibia. C: calcaneus. Cu: cuboid. N: navicular bone. T: talus.

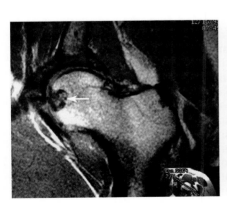
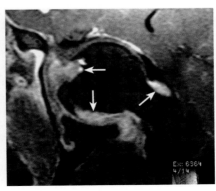

Fig. 10.**14** **Infiltrating synovial neurofibroma.** **a** Poorly defined synovial proliferation with heterogeneous intermediate signal intensity is seen eroding into the femoral head and acetabulum (arrow) (PDWI, coronal). **b** After intravenous Gd-DTPA administration, marked contrast enhancement depicts the full extent of the infiltrating synovial mass (arrows) (T1WI, FS, +C, coronal).

10A Shoulder

Anatomy

The articular surfaces of the glenohumeral joint are covered by hyaline cartilage. A fibrocartilaginous structure, the labrum, is attached to the glenoid rim to increase joint stability. The fibrous joint capsule is reinforced by the tendons of the supraspinatus, infraspinatus, teres minor, and subscapularis, which form the rotator cuff.

Several *bursae* are located in the shoulder area. The most important is the subacromial-subdeltoid bursa, which separates the deltoid muscle, acromion, and coracoclavicular ligament from the rotator cuff. The bursa does not communicate with the glenohumeral joint unless perforation of the cuff has occurred.

The *glenohumeral ligaments* represent thickenings or reinforcements of the anterior joint capsule. A superior, middle, and inferior ligament are discerned, each extending from the anterior glenoid rim near the glenoid labrum to the humeral neck. The subscapular recess (bursa) located between the subscapularis tendon and middle glenohumeral ligament communicates with the shoulder joint through two openings located between this ligament on one side and the superior and inferior glenohumeral ligaments, respectively, on the other side.

The *coracoacromial arch* (Fig. 10.1) consists, from anterior to posterior, of the coracoid process, the coracoacromial ligament, and the acromion. Between this arch and the humeral head pass the rotator cuff, long biceps tendon, subacromial-subdeltoid bursa, and coracohumeral ligament. Congenital and acquired, osseous or soft-tissue abnormalities narrowing this space may all lead to impingement on the rotator cuff.

Rotator Cuff Lesions

The rotator cuff stabilizes the glenohumeral joint. Supraspinatus, infraspinatus, and teres minor muscles contribute between one-third and one-half to abduction and 80% to external rotation in the shoulder joint. The subscapularis muscle is the principal internal rotator of the arm. Impairment of these functions and shoulder pain are commonly associated with rotator cuff pathology. Diseases of the rotator cuff include impingement syndrome, inflammation, degeneration, and partial or complete ruptures.

The *impingement syndrome* is related to the restricted space between the coracoacromial arch above and the humeral head below, compressing the rotator cuff passing through. Sites of impingement include congenital or post-traumatic changes in the coracoid process, thickening and spur formations in the coracoacromial ligament, and especially abnormalities in the acromion. Bony spurs may protrude inferiorly from the undersurface of the anterior acromion or the arthritic acromioclavicular joint. Congenital anomalies of the acromion associated with impingement include an os acromiale (unfused apophysis of the anterior acromion), a decreased acromial slope (angle between inferior surface of acromion and horizontal plane) and a curved (type 2) or hooked (type 3) acromion as opposed to a normal flat undersurface (type 1) (Fig. 10A.**2**). In

these conditions the rotator cuff becomes more severely impinged by the coracoacromial arch, and the chronic irritation caused by arm movements may lead to inflammation of the subacromial bursa and tendons and eventually rotator cuff tear.

Rotator cuff tendinitis is also referred to as rotator cuff tendinosis or tendinopathy, since it is more often caused by degeneration, repeated microtrauma, or ischemia rather than inflammation (Fig. 10A.**3**). On MRI the signal intensity of a normal rotator cuff is low and homogeneous in all sequences. An increased signal intensity within the supraspinatus tendon near its insertion may be, however, observed on short echo time (TE) images (e. g. T1WI and proton density weighted images) in asymptomatic adults. This intermediate intratendinous signal intensity, about 1 cm from the greater tuberosity, fades with increasing TE, that is with T2WI. The explanation for this apparent normal finding is debated and includes artifacts (e.g., "magic angle" phenomenon or partial volume averaging), variations in normal anatomy, or subclinical tendon degeneration. Similar but more extensive MRI findings are indicative of chronic rotator cuff tendinitis (tendinosis). In this condition an increased signal intensity within the tendon is seen on T1WI and proton density weighted images, but is less conspicuous or even absent in T2WI. Histologically these MRI findings correspond to mucoid degeneration and mild inflammation. In acute tendinitis a slight increase in the linear intratendinous signal intensity may be found on T2WI when compared with the T1WI and proton density weighted images. In these cases the inflammatory changes may occasionally extend into the subdeltoid fat plane. A focal high signal intensity similar to fluid in the rotator cuff on T2WI is not compatible with the diagnosis tendinosis and suggests a partial or complete rotator cuff tear.

Calcific tendinitis may occur anywhere in the rotator cuff, but is most often located in the supraspinatus tendon. The diagnosis is made more easily on plain films than MRI. Calcifications are devoid of signal on MRI and may be missed within the low signal intensity tendon on spin-echo (SE) sequences. They may be easier to appreciate on gradient echo (GRE) sequences due to susceptibility artifacts.

Rotator cuff tears are classified as full-thickness or complete tears and partial-thickness or incomplete tears. Full-thickness tears extend from the articular surface to the bursal surface of the cuff, and partial-thickness tears involve either the articular or bursal surface of the cuff or are located within its substance (intratendinous tear). Rotator cuff tears are most often located in the supraspinatus tendon, but they may either extend to or originate in other components of the rotator cuff.

Rotator cuff tears are caused by trauma, attrition, inflammation, ischemia, and impingement. Acute traumatic rotator cuff tears are rare and usually occur in young adults as an isolated injury or in combination with other shoulder injuries such as anterior dislocation causing a subscapularis tendon rupture. Most rotator cuff tears, however, occur spontaneously in patients over 40 years of age with predilection for the dominant arm. In these cases the rotator cuff is weakened by impingement, repetitive stress,

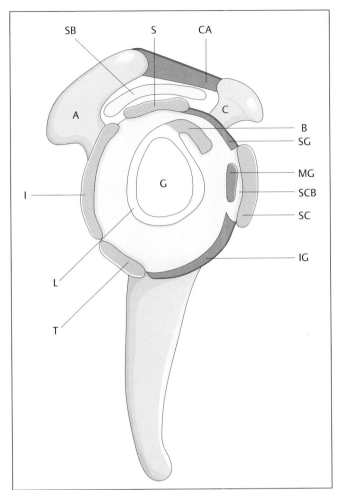

Fig. 10A.**1 Glenohumeral joint and coracoacromial arch.**
A: acromion. B: biceps tendon (long head). C: coracoid process. CA: coracoacromial ligament. G: glenoid fossa (cartilage). I: infraspinatus tendon. IG: inferior glenohumeral ligament. L: glenoid labrum. MG: middle glenohumeral ligament. S: supraspinatus tendon. SB: subacromial-subdeltoid bursa. SC: subscapularis tendon. SCB: subscapularis bursa. SG: superior glenohumeral ligament. T: teres minor tendon.

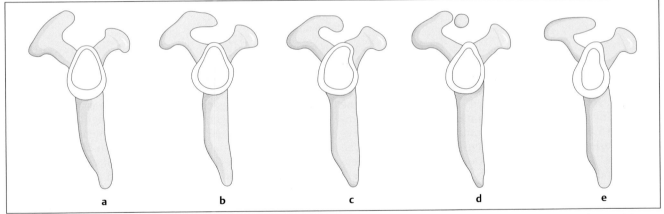

Fig. 10A.**2 Congenital acromial anomalies associated with the impingement syndrome. a** Normal acromion with flat undersurface (type 1). **b** Curved acromion (type 2). **c** Hooked acromion (type 3). **d** Os acromiale. **e** Decreased acromial slope (decreased angle between inferior surface of acromion and horizontal plane).

degeneration, and inflammation such as rheumatoid arthritis and calcium hydroxyapatite crystal deposition disease (HADD, also referred to as *Milwaukee shoulder syndrome).*

The MRI presentation of *partial-thickness tears of the rotator cuff* varies with stage and location of the lesion (Fig. 10A.**4**). An intratendinous tear depicts a region of intermediate signal intensity paralleling the long axis of the tendon in both T1WI and proton density weighted images,

which increases in signal intensity on T2WI. The MRI findings reflect the intratendinous edema and hemorrhage associated with such a tear. However, this condition may be difficult, if not impossible, to differentiate from acute tendinitis, which presents in similar fashion on MRI. Partial-thickness tears can be diagnosed more reliably when an eccentric focal lesion on either side of the tendon increases from intermediate signal intensity on T1WI to high signal intensity on T2WI. Furthermore, small incomplete

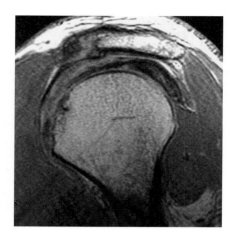

Fig. 10A.**3 Rotator cuff tendinitis.** The signal intensity in the rotator cuff over the humeral head is heterogeneous and slightly increased (sagittal, PDWI). Sequelae of acromioplasty are also evident.

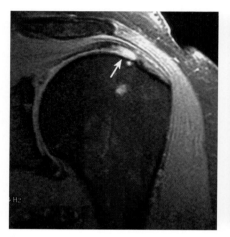

a

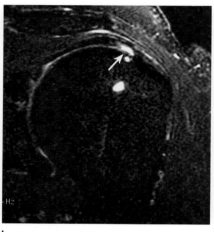

b

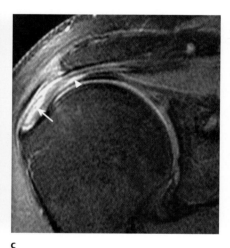

c

Fig. 10A.**4 Partial-thickness tear of rotator cuff.** A focus of increased signal intensity is seen in the supraspinatus tendon (arrow) that does not extend to its

acromial surface (coronal, **a**: PDWI; **b**: T2WI). **c** Longitudinal intratendinous tears are seen in the supraspinatus tendon (arrowhead) and infraspinatus tendon

(arrow) of a second patient (PDWI, coronal).

surface tears characteristically lie perpendicular to the long axis of the tendon. Focal thinning of a tendon combined with MRI findings of chronic tendinitis (intermediate intertendinous signal intensity on all spin echo sequences) is another manifestation of a partial tear. Secondary findings commonly associated with an incomplete rotator cuff tear include obliteration of the subdeltoid or peribursal fat plane and a small to moderate-sized joint effusion.

Complete rotator cuff tears may be classified as small (less than 2 cm), moderate (2–4 cm), large (4–5 cm), and massive (greater than 5 cm). Another classification is based on the number of tendons involved: small–supraspinatus alone is involved; moderate–two tendons are involved; large–three or more tendons are involved. Rotator cuff tears usually begin anteriorly in the supraspinatus tendon near its insertion into the greater tuberosity.

Full-thickness tears are diagnosed by MRI with the demonstration of a complete tendinous defect that is filled with fluid or, less commonly, with granulation tissue (Figs. 10A.**5** and 10A.**6**). In these cases a hyperintense area separating the ruptured tendon is seen. With progressive fibrosis and eventually scarring no discrete tendon defect

may be evident. Instead the tendon appears irregular and thin with inhomogeneous low to intermediate signal intensity on all SE sequences. With complete scarring the ruptured tendon may present as a region of marked focal thinning with low signal intensity on all pulse sequences.

Retraction of the ruptured tendon and muscle is another direct sign of a complete rotator cuff tear. The retracted muscle often assumes a globular shape. Retraction is however only present in large tears and may, if longstanding, eventually be associated with muscle atrophy. Secondary signs of a full-thickness tear of the rotator cuff include a large shoulder joint effusion, fluid in the subacromial-subdeltoid bursa, and diffuse loss of the peribursal and subdeltoid fat plane. Any one of these signs occurring in isolation is, however, not diagnostic for a complete rotator cuff tear. Plain film findings of a chronic rotator cuff tear include narrowing of the acromiohumeral distance to less than 7 mm, reversal of the normal acromial undersurface convexity to concavity, and the development of both small cystic lesions and sclerosis along the undersurface of the acromion and in the greater tuberosity. These findings can also be appreciated with MRI.

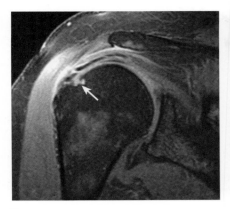
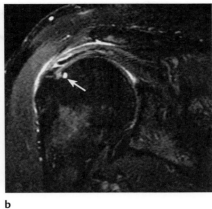

a   b

Fig. 10A.**5   Full-thickness tear of the rotator cuff without retraction.** An irregular increased signal intensity (arrow) is seen involving the entire width of the infraspinatus tendon (coronal, **a**: PDWI; **b**: T2WI).

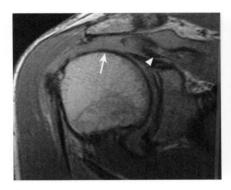
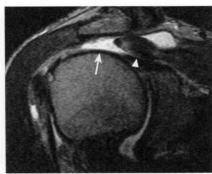

a   b

Fig. 10A.**6   Full-thickness tear of the rotator cuff with retraction.** A large defect filled with fluid is seen in the supraspinatus tendon (arrow). The retracted supraspinatus muscle (arrowhead) assumes an egg-like shape (coronal, **a**: PDWI; **b**: T2WI).

Biceps Tendon Lesions

The tendon of the long head of the biceps muscle originates from the superior portion of the glenoid labrum and glenoid tubercle and extends obliquely across the top of the humeral head into the intertubercular groove. The tendon emerges from the joint at the lower portion of the groove, surrounded by a sheath that directly communicates with the joint. Biceps tendon abnormalities are commonly associated with the impingement syndrome or large rotator cuff tears.

Biceps tendinitis and *tenosynovitis* produce nonspecific MRI findings. Discrete increased intratendinous signal intensity on T1WI and proton density weighted images are observed in chronic tendinitis but may also be present in asymptomatic subjects. A small amount of fluid in the biceps tendon sheath is commonly seen in healthy individuals. Tenosynovitis can only be diagnosed when the biceps tendon is completely surrounded by fluid in the absence of sizeable joint effusion.

Biceps tendon dislocation (Fig. 10A.**7**) may occur as an isolated lesion but more commonly occurs in association with a large anterior rotator cuff tear. On MRI the dislocated, low-signal-intensity tendon is seen medial to the bicipital groove and is best appreciated on axial images.

Biceps tendon rupture (Fig. 10A.**8**) occurs in the elderly patient, usually without a major traumatic incident. Most tendon ruptures occur just distal to its exit from the glenohumeral joint. In this case the intracapsular portion of the tendon lies free in the joint cavity, whereas the extra-articular portion is pulled distally. The biceps tendon is absent from the intertubercular groove, which is usually filled with fluid and only rarely with scar tissue.

Adhesive capsulitis of the glenohumeral joint (frozen shoulder) occurs in the elderly patient either as primary disease or, more often, secondary to trauma and/or shoulder immobilization. A contracted and thickened joint capsule with small or absent subscapular and axillary recesses and multiple intracapsular adhesions with frequent involvement of the biceps tendon and sheath are characteristic, but difficult to diagnose by MRI.

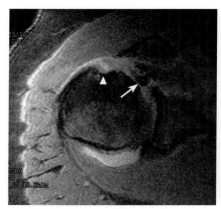 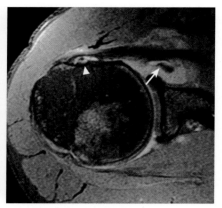

Fig. 10A.**7 Biceps tendon dislocation.** The low-signal-intensity biceps tendon (arrow) is dislocated medially. The bicipital groove (arrowhead) is filled with fluid of the joint effusion (PDWI).

Fig. 10A.**8 Biceps tendon rupture.** The biceps tendon is absent from its normal location in the bicipital groove (arrowhead). The retracted proximal end of the biceps tendon (arrow) is seen in the anterior glenohumeral joint surrounded by the hyperintense joint effusion (PDWI).

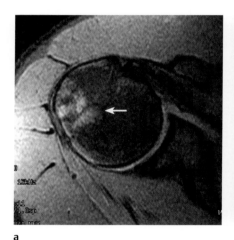 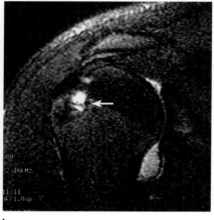

a   **b**

Fig. 10A.**9 Hill-Sachs lesion.** A compression fracture (arrow) in the posterolateral aspect of the humeral head presents with increased signal intensity (**a**: axial, PDWI; **b**: coronal, T2WI, FS).

Shoulder Instability

A shoulder instability is present when the humeral head slips out of its socket during normal activities. It may be the sequelae of a specific traumatic episode, such as a dislocation, or occur with overuse and repetitive microtrauma, as seen in swimmers and athletes who throw. An atraumatic instability without a history of acute or chronic trauma is considerably less common. Shoulder instability can be described by its direction as anterior (more than 90%), posterior (5%), or multidirectional. A special type of inferior subluxation of the humeral head is the drooping shoulder. It is found with a large, usually post-traumatic hemarthrosis or neuromuscular paralysis involving the shoulder region.

Shoulder stability is dependent upon intact glenohumeral osseous structures, glenoid labrum, capsule, and pericapsular soft tissue. Bony abnormalities seen in *anterior instability* include Hill-Sachs and osseous Bankart lesions. A *Hill-Sachs lesion* (Fig. 10A.9) is a posterolateral compression fracture of the humeral head caused by impingement on the anteroinferior rim of the glenoid fossa during dislocation. The lesion appears on MRI as a wedge-shaped defect on the posterolateral aspect of the humeral head. It is evident on axial images at the level of the coracoid process and should not be confused with normal posterolateral flattening of the humeral head seen more distally. An *osseous Bankart lesion* is a defect in the anterior glenoid rim secondary to an avulsion fracture, produced by the dislocating humeral head.

The *glenoid labrum* is a fibrocartilaginous extension of the glenoid rim with low signal intensity on all MRI sequences. It is typically triangular in shape with a sharp or rounded free edge. Rare normal variants difficult to differentiate from labral pathology include cleaved, notched, flat, and even partially absent labra. In the proper clinical setting, however, an absent labrum should unequivocally be considered to be pathologic. A normal cleft that does not traverse the entire length of the labrum is commonly

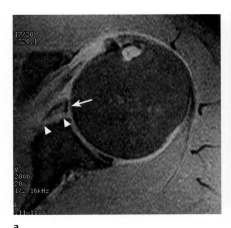
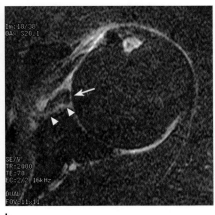

a   b

Fig. 10A.**10** **Fracture of the anteroinferior glenoid labrum.** A tear (arrowheads) in the anteroinferior labrum (arrow) presents with increased signal intensity (**a**: PDWI; **b**: T2WI, FS).

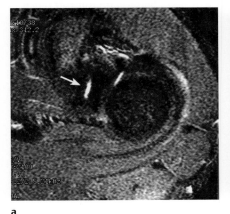
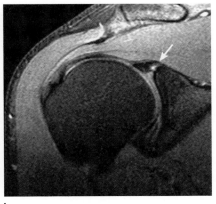

a   b

Fig. 10A.**11** **SLAP lesion (superior labral tear).** A superior glenoid labral tear presents as a hyperintense line (arrow) in (**a**) (axial T2WI, FS) and as hyperintense focus (arrow) in (**b**) (coronal PDWI).

seen between the articular cartilage and the labrum and should not be mistaken for a tear. The proximity of the attachments of the superior and the middle glenohumeral ligaments to the anterior labrum may also mimic a labral tear.

The glenoid labrum is often divided into six quadrants: I, superior; II, anterosuperior; III, anteroinferior; IV, inferior; V, posteroinferior; and VI, posterosuperior. Labral tears occur most often in quadrants I to III. On MRI increased signal intensity within the labrum, but not extending to its surface, represents internal labral degeneration without a tear. Labral cysts are degenerative or post traumatic in nature and more commonly found in the posterior labrum. They appear hypointense on T1WI and hyperintense on T2WI and may extend into the para-articular soft tissue. A labral tear can be diagnosed when the increased signals seen on T1WI and proton density weighted images extend to the surface of the labrum. On T2WI hyperintense fluid is commonly but not always seen in the tear. Labral blunting,

fragmentation, displacement, or absence all indicate a labral tear. The detached labral fragment is sometimes visible as an enlarged, round to ovoid mass of low signal intensity. Fractures of the anteroinferior labrum are commonly associated with anterior dislocations and referred to as *true Bankart lesions* (Fig. 10A.**10**).

A superior labral tear with anterior and posterior extension is termed a SLAP lesion (Fig. 10A.**11**). It involves the biceps tendon anterior to the labrum and may be associated with rotator cuff tears and anterior instability. Four types of SLAP lesions are discerned. Type 1 reveals superior labral degeneration; type 2 a tear in the superior labrum; type 3 a bucket-handle tear in the superior labrum; and type 4 a bucket-handle labral tear extending into the proximal biceps tendon as a longitudinal or split tear. MRI classification of these lesions is, however, often difficult and not always reliable. As anywhere else intermediate signal intensity in the superior labrum suggests degenerative changes and bright signals on T2WI a tear.

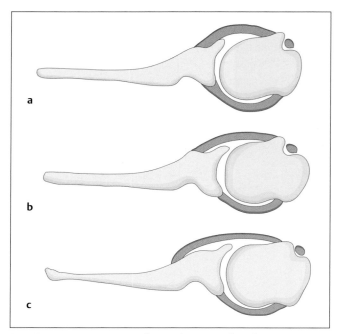

Fig. 10A.12   Anterior capsular insertion on the glenoid.   a Type 1: capsule inserts in or near the glenoid labrum.   **b** Type 2: capsule inserts less than 1 cm medial to the labrum.   **c** Type 3: capsule inserts more than 1 cm medial to the labrum.

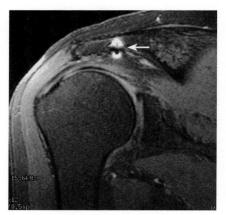

Fig. 10A.13   Surgical rotator cuff repair and acromioplasty. Sequelae of acromioplasty are seen, including a large metallic artifact (arrow) consisting of a tiny focus of signal void surrounded by a larger area of high signal intensity. The increase in signal intensity in the repaired rotator cuff are within normal range and cannot be differentiated from a partial tear under these circumstances (PDWI, coronal).

The fibrous *glenohumeral joint capsule* is reinforced by the tendons of the rotator cuff and in addition anteriorly by the superior, middle, and inferior glenohumeral ligaments. Both rotator cuff tendon and glenohumeral ligaments cannot always be separated by MRI from the capsule that appears as low signal intensity structure on all sequences.

Three types of anterior capsular insertions on the glenoid are differentiated (Fig. 10A.12). Type 1 inserts in or near the glenoid labrum, type 2 less than 1 cm medial to the labrum, and type 3 more than 1 cm medial to the labrum. Types 2 and 3 may be normal variants, but more often result from traumatic avulsion of the capsule (capsular stripping) in anterior dislocations. Regardless of its origin, type 2 and especially type 3 capsules are associated with joint laxity and thus predispose to anterior instability and recurrent dislocations. In these cases the subscapularis tendon forming the anterior rotator cuff is often thinned, redundant, or even torn, resulting eventually in subscapularis muscle atrophy.

Isolated *posterior instability* is uncommon, accounting for only 5% of instabilities. MRI findings are similar to those of anterior instability and include posterior labral and capsular detachments and tears, as well as laxity of the posterior capsule. With posterior dislocations a compression fracture on the anteromedial aspect of the humeral head caused by its impaction or the posterior glenoid rim may be present and is referred to as *reverse Hill-Sachs lesion*. In multidirectional instability a redundant capsule and abnormal anterior, posterior, and inferior labrum may be found.

Postoperative Shoulder

Interpretation of the MRI findings in the postoperative shoulder presents a diagnostic challenge, since normal postoperative changes are often difficult to differentiate from pathologic postoperative conditions. Major complications such as large hematoma formations, soft-tissue infections, and osteomyelitis can be diagnosed and accurately localized.

Acromioplasty is used for treatment of shoulder impingement syndrome and involves resection of the undersurface of the anterior acromion. The procedure may also include partial or complete removal of the coracoacromial ligament, acromioclavicular joint, and distal clavicle. The signal intensity within the remaining portions of the acromion are decreased on both T1WI and T2WI after healing. Low and high signal intensity artifacts related to tiny metallic fragments that break off from burring instruments during surgery are often seen (Fig. 10A.13). These microscopic metallic substances are not visible on radiographs or CT, but are especially pronounced on GRE imaging. Evaluation of the rotator cuff in this condition is more difficult due to distortion of the adjacent soft tissues.

Surgical repair of a rotator cuff tear is usually combined with acromioplasty. A communication between the shoulder and subacromial-subdeltoid bursa may remain after a clinically adequate repair. Furthermore, a partial rotator cuff tear cannot be differentiated from an intact repaired tendon, since a similar increase in signal intensity is found in both conditions on all pulse sequences. In the postoperative shoulder a full-thickness tear can only be reliably diagnosed by MRI, when a discontinuity of the cuff is identified with fluid-like signal intensity within the gap on T2WI.

Many surgical procedures are advocated for the *repair of anterior shoulder instability* and *recurrent dislocations,* including direct repair of labral and capsular lesions (Bankart), shortening of the anterior capsule and subscapularis muscle (Putti-Platt), transfer of the subscapularis tendon from the lesser to the greater tuberosity (Magnuson-Stack), bone grafts to the anterior glenoid and coracoid process, and transfer of the coracoid process to the neck of the scapula (Bristow-Helfet). MRI differentiation of surgical complications and recurrent lesions from postoperative scarring and residual untreated lesions due to the type of repair is usually very difficult, if not impossible.

Entrapment Neuropathies

Suprascapular nerve entrapment occurs most frequently in the suprascapular notch. Patients present with pain, weakness, and atrophy of the supraspinatus and infraspinatus muscle. The entrapment may be caused by scapular and humeral fractures, anterior shoulder dislocation, anomalies of the transverse scapular ligaments and notch, tumors, and ganglia. The latter may be associated with a tear in the glenoid labrum, most commonly located in the posterosuperior quadrant. Such ganglia are also referred to as labral cysts. A more distal entrapment of the suprascapular nerve leads to isolated involvement of the infraspinatus muscle and is often seen in chronic overuse, particularly in baseball pitchers and weightlifters.

The *quadrilateral space syndrome* results from entrapment of the axillary nerve as it passes through a space bounded superiorly by the teres minor muscle, medially by the long head of the triceps muscle, inferiorly by the teres major muscle, and laterally by the surgical neck of the humerus. Clinical findings include skin paresthesias in the distribution of the axillary nerve and weakness of the teres minor and/or deltoid muscles. MRI reveals atrophy with fatty infiltration of the teres minor or deltoid muscle, or both.

10B   Elbow

Anatomy

The elbow consists of three articulations contained within a common joint cavity. These articulations are: 1) humeroulnar, between the trochlea of the humerus and the trochlear notch of the ulna; 2) humeroradial, between the capitulum of the humerus and the facet on the head of the radius; and 3) proximal radioulnar, between the circumference of the radial head and the osseofibrous ring formed by the radial notch of the ulna and the annular ligament. The latter is a thick band of fibrous tissue that attaches to the anterior and posterior margins of the radial notch of the ulna.

A fibrous capsule invests the elbow completely. The anterior and posterior portions of the elbow are relatively thin, whereas the medial and lateral portions are reinforced by collateral ligaments (Figs. 10B.1 and 10B.2). The *medial (ulnar) collateral ligament* has a triangular shape and is composed of the anterior, posterior, and oblique (transverse) parts. The anterior bundle is functionally the most important structure of the medial collateral ligament and extends from the medial epicondyle to the medial aspect of the coronoid process. The posterior bundle of the medial collateral ligament has a fanlike appearance and runs from the medial epicondyle to the medial margin of the olecranon. The oblique (transverse) band of the medial collateral ligament is often only feebly developed and stretches between the olecranon and coronoid processes. Both the posterior and the oblique (transverse) bands of the medial collateral ligament are often difficult to define on MRI. The *lateral (radial) collateral ligament* arises from the lateral epicondyle and inserts into the annular ligament. The most posterior fibers of the lateral collateral ligament, often referred to as the *lateral ulnar collateral ligament*, pass over the annular ligament and insert on the supinator crest of the ulna just below and posterior to the annular ligament insertion.

The *muscles of the elbow* are divided into anterior, posterior, medial, and lateral compartments. The anterior compartment contains the brachialis and biceps muscles. The brachialis lies anterior to the elbow joint and inserts into the ulnar tuberosity. The biceps is superficial to the brachialis and inserts into the radial tuberosity. The posterior compartment contains the triceps and anconeus muscles. The triceps inserts into the proximal olecranon. The anconeus arises from the posterior aspect of the lateral epicondyle and inserts more distally into the olecranon. The medial compartment contains the pronator teres, palmaris longus, and flexors of the wrist and hands, which arise from the medial epicondyle as the common flexor tendon. The lateral compartment contains the supinator, brachioradialis, and the extensors of the wrist and hand, which arise from the lateral epicondyle as the common extensor tendon.

Superficial bursae about the elbow include the olecranon bursa and the medial and lateral epicondylar bursae. Besides the subcutaneous olecranon bursa, two other bursae are occasionally identified in the olecranon region: the intratendinous olecranon bursa within the distal triceps tendon, and the subtendinous olecranon bursa beneath this tendon and immediately above the tip of the olecranon. An inflamed subtendinous bursa can be differentiated from an elbow joint effusion by the absence of fluid in the anterior elbow compartment. Inflamed medial and lateral epicondylar bursae should not be confused with tears in the ulnar and radial collateral ligaments. There is also a large number of deep elbow bursae, but these are rarely inflamed as an isolated event.

Collateral Ligament Lesions

Collateral ligaments are thickenings of the medial and lateral joint capsule of the elbow. Ligamentous injuries and degeneration occur with or without involvement of the overlying flexor tendons medially and extensor tendons laterally. Partial and complete ligamentous tears are associated with both acute trauma and chronic overuse. In the latter condition capsular microtears, hemorrhage, and edema may eventually lead to ligamentous disruption. Injuries to the medial collateral ligament predominate and usually occur in the flexed elbow with valgus stress. This injury is common in athletes who throw and may be associated with lesions in the annular ligament and triceps tendon. Most tears occur in the anterior bundle of the medial collateral ligament. MRI abnormalities of an acutely or chronically injured collateral ligament include laxity, irregularity, poor definition, and increased signal intensity within and around the ligament (Figs. 10B.3 and 10B.4). The regions of increased signal intensity, which are most prominent on T2WI, reflect the presence of hemorrhage and edema. Acute medial collateral ligament tears due to abnormal valgus stress may be accompanied by signs of lateral compression overload such as bone bruises in the capitulum and radial head. In chronic medial collateral injuries, ulnar traction spurs and regions of calcifications or heterotopic bone formations similar to the Pellegrini-Stieda phenomenon in the knee may be evident.

Lateral Epicondylitis

Lateral epicondylitis is caused by inflammation, degeneration, and tearing of the common extensor tendon. The condition is also known as *tennis elbow*, since it occurs as a result of repetitive sports-related microtrauma and chronic overuse. Lateral epicondylitis, however, affects nonathletes even more commonly and occurs more frequently than medial epicondylitis. Although the type of pathologic lesion associated with lateral epicondylitis may vary, partial tearing of the fibers within the extensor tendons (especially the extensor carpi radialis brevis tendon) from their epicondylar attachments is typical. On MRI an increased signal intensity on T1WI, which does not further increase on T2WI, is indicative of tendon degeneration (chronic tendinitis or tendinosis). A higher signal intensity on T2WI

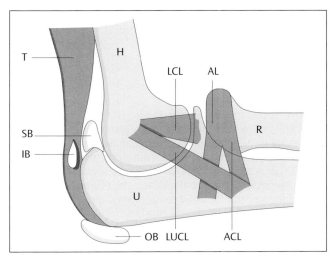

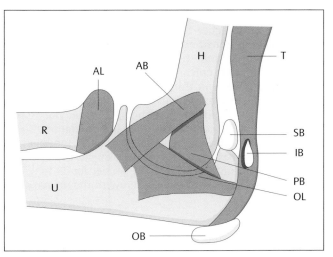

Fig. 10B.**1** **Lateral aspect**

Fig. 10B.**2** **Medial aspect**

Figs. 10B.**1** and 10B.**2** **Ligaments and bursae of the elbow.** AB: anterior bundle of medial collateral ligament. AL: annular ligament. ACL: accessory collateral ligament. H: humerus. IB: intratendinous bursa. LCL: lateral (radial) collateral ligament. LUCL: lateral ulnar collateral ligament. OB: olecranon bursa. OL: oblique (trans-

verse) band of medial collateral ligament. PB: posterior bundle of medial collateral ligament. R: radius. SB: subtendinous bursa. T: triceps tendon. U: ulna.

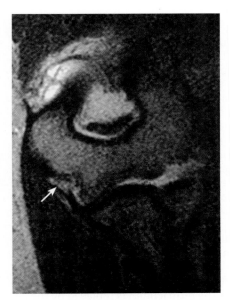

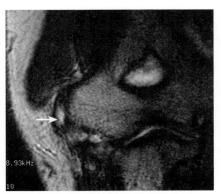

Fig. 10B.**4** **Partial lateral collateral ligament tear.** A focus of increased signal intensity (arrow) is seen in the lateral collateral ligament (T2WI, coronal).

Fig. 10B.**3** **Partial medial collateral ligament tear.** A focus of increased signal intensity is seen in the medial collateral ligament (arrow) associated with an elbow joint effusion (T2WI, coronal).

as compared with T1WI suggests a partial tendon tear or possibly a more acute tendinitis. In these conditions increased signal intensities on T2WI may also be present in the surrounding soft tissues, including the anconeus muscle and lateral epicondyle. Tendon thickening favors tendinitis, and tendon thinning a chronic, partial tendon tear. A complete tear is diagnosed on MRI when a fluid-filled gap separates the tendon from its epicondylar attachment. Surrounding soft-tissue edema and inflammation is usually present. Similar signal alterations in tendons and neighboring muscles may however also be produced by local corticosteroid injections and persist for as long as 1 month. They should not be confused with the primary disorder.

Medial Epicondylitis

Medial epicondylitis is caused by inflammation, degeneration, and tearing of the common flexor tendon that originates from the medial epicondyle. The condition usually occurs with chronic overuse of the flexor-pronator muscle group and occurs in pitchers, golfers, and tennis players who use an exaggerated top spin requiring excessive pronation of the forearm. Tendon pathology and MRI findings are similar to the ones described with the more common lateral epicondylitis.

In the skeletally immature individual the unfused apophysis of the medial epicondyle rather than tendon may fail with chronic overuse of the flexor-pronator muscle group. In the little leaguer's elbow, pain along the medial elbow may be caused by a stress fracture or avulsion of the medial epicondylar apophysis. MRI is able to detect these injuries before complete avulsion occurs by demonstrating soft-tissue and marrow edema about the medial epicondylar apophysis. It may be associated with osteochondrosis of the capitulum (Panner disease) in 5–10-year-old boys, or osteochondritis dissecans (osteochondral fracture) of the capitulum in slightly older children.

Biceps Tendon Lesions

Rupture of the *distal biceps tendon* accounts for less than 5% of all biceps tendon injuries (Fig. 10B.**5**). Tears occur usually in men over 40 years of age as a result of forceful elbow flexion against resistance and are most commonly located at or near the insertion on the radial tuberosity. Proximal retraction of the biceps may be minimal when the bicipital aponeurosis remains intact. As with other tendinous or ligamentous tears, a complete tear demonstrates a gap in the low signal intensity tendon which may be retracted. In partial tears some tendinous fibers remain intact. Alterations in signal intensity depend on the age of the injury, although high signal intensity within the torn tendon and adjacent soft tissue and bone is usually present on T2WI due to edema, hemorrhage, and inflammation.

Chronic tendinitis (tendinosis) in the distal biceps tendon is common and may precede spontaneous tendon rupture. Chronic inflammatory and degenerative changes present with intermediate signal intensity within the tendon on all pulse sequences and may be associated with osseous proliferation at the radial tuberosity and inflammation of the bicipital bursa sandwiched in between tendon and radial tuberosity. Increased intratendinous signal intensity observed only with short echo time (TE) sequences, but

characteristically absent on T2WI, may be caused by the "magic angle" phenomenon and should not be confused with tendon pathology.

Triceps Tendon Lesions

Rupture of the triceps tendon is rare (Fig. 10B.**6**). The avulsion typically occurs at the tendinous attachment in the olecranon. In a majority of patients an avulsion fracture of the olecranon is associated. A complete tear usually presents as an area of high signal intensity separating the hypointense tendon fragments. When the elbow is imaged in extension, an intact triceps tendon may appear lax and redundant. This finding should not be confused with tendon retraction secondary to a complete rupture. Olecranon bursitis may mimic or occasionally accompany a partial triceps tendon tear that is even less common than a complete rupture.

Inflammatory and degenerative changes in the triceps tendon are fairly common, presenting with intermediate intratendinous signal intensity on all pulse sequences. Similar MRI findings, however, may occasionally be observed in a normal distal triceps tendon due to the presence of an intratendinous bursa or, when limited to T1WI and proton density weighted images, due to the "magic angle" phenomenon.

Entrapment Neuropathies

An entrapped or compressed nerve may demonstrate on MRI increased signal intensity on T2WI, focal enlargement in girth, displacement by a space-occupying mass, and subluxation. Displacement and subluxation are, however, not always associated with symptoms.

Of the three major nerves traversing the elbow, the *ulnar nerve* is most frequently affected. The entrapment occurs in the fibro-osseous tunnel posterior to the medial epicondyle of the humerus. The floor of the tunnel is formed by the elbow joint capsule and the posterior and transverse bands of the medial collateral ligament. The roof of the tunnel is formed proximally by the cubital tunnel retinaculum and distally by the flexor carpi ulnaris aponeurosis. The retinaculum may be absent in about 10% of cases, allowing the nerve to dislocate anteriorly over the medial epicondyle during flexion, producing functional neuritis. In another 10% of cases the retinaculum is replaced by the anconeus epitrochlearis muscle causing static compression of the ulnar nerve. Other causes of ulnar nerve compression include thickening of the retinaculum or medial collateral ligament, fractures and osteophytes of the medial epicondyle, soft-tissue tumors (Fig. 10B.**7**), and adhesions.

Compression of the *radial nerve* may occur above the elbow where it passes between the origins of the lateral and medial heads of the triceps muscle and the distal, usually fractured humerus shaft. Compression of the posterior interosseous nerve, a purely motor branch of the radial nerve occurs just distal to the elbow as the nerve passes into the supinator muscle. Causes of this compression neuropathy include dislocations and fractures of the elbow, rheumatoid arthritis, soft-tissue tumors, and traumatic or developmental fibrous bands.

Entrapment of the median nerve occurs most frequently in the wrist as carpal tunnel syndrome. The medial nerve may be compromised in the presence of a supracondylar

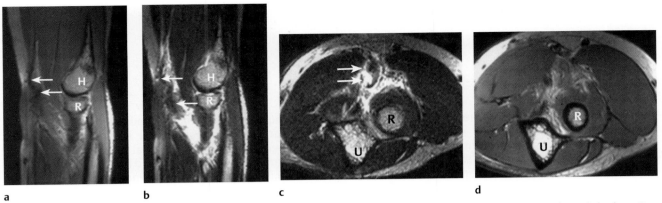

a   b   c   d

Fig. 10B.**5** **Acute distal biceps tendon tear.** A complete rupture of the distal biceps tendon near its insertion into the radial tuberosity associated with an acute hemorrhage is evident. The distal biceps tendon (arrows) appears wavy due to retraction and depicts an irregular contour with thickening of its visualized distal end in **a** (PDWI, sagittal) and **b** (T2WI, sagittal). Note also the hemorrhage between distal biceps tendon and radius in **b** evident as irregular hyperintense zone. The distal biceps tendon (arrows) also appears thickened and contains areas of high signal intensity in **c** (T2WI, axial), the most distal plane of this tendon was visualized. Again a high signal intensity hemorrhage separating the tendon from the radius is evident too. In the subsequent more distal plane in **d** (PDWI, axial) the tendon is no longer visualized (H: humerus, R: radius, U: ulna).

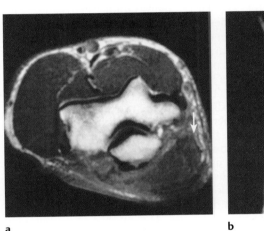

a   b

Fig. 10B.**6** **Triceps tendon tear (old).** **a** An old hematoma (arrows) presenting as low signal intensity mass is seen over the olecranon (T1WI, axial). **b** The ruptured triceps tendon (arrows) is separated from the olecranon by the hematoma (T1WI, sagittal).

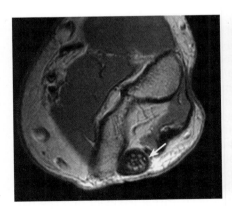
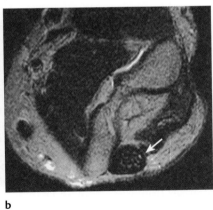

a   b

Fig. 10B.**7** **Fibrolipohamartoma of ulnar nerve.** Ulnar nerve compression was caused by primary ulnar nerve tumor (arrow) causing marked circumferential enlargement of the ulnar nerve (**a**: PDWI; **b**: T2WI).

process arising from the anteromedial surface of the distal humerus and a ligament of Struthers extending from the supracondylar process to the medial epicondyle. Compression of the median nerve or its largest branch, the anterior interosseous nerve occur in the antecubital area frequently secondary to fracture or congenital anomalies.

10C   Wrist and Hand

Anatomy

The distal radius and ulna articulate with the proximal row of carpal bones consisting of scaphoid, lunate, and triquetrium as well as the pisiform within the tendon of the flexor carpi ulnaris. The distal row contains trapezium, trapezoid, capitate, and hamate and articulates with the bases of the metacarpals. The distal radioulnar joint is an L-shaped articulation composed of the sigmoid (ulnar) notch of the distal radius, head of the ulna, and the triangular fibrocartilage.

Carpal ligaments are classified as either extrinsic or intrinsic. Extrinsic ligaments link the carpal bones to radius or ulna. Intrinsic (interosseous or intercarpal) ligaments connect individual carpal bones (Figs. 10C.1–3).

The *palmar (volar) radiocarpal ligament* is a broad fibrous band originating from the entire anterior inferior circumference of the radius including the radial styloid process. The fibers of this ligament run in a medial and distal direction and insert on the anterior surfaces of the scaphoid, lunate, triquetrium, and capitate. The palmar radiocarpal ligament may be subdivided into three components: radioscaphocapitate, radiolunotriquetral, and radioscapholunate ligaments.

The *palmar ulnocarpal ligament* is a thick fascicle that arises from the anterior ulnar styloid process and triangular fibrocartilage and extends laterally and distally to the triquetrum (ulnotriquetral ligament) and lunate (ulnolunate ligament). The *deltoid* (arcuate) *ligament* is a volar intercarpal (intrinsic) ligament arising from the palmar surface of the capitate. It has a V-shape with the ulnar arm extending to the triquetrum and the radial arm extending to the scaphoid. When additional fascicles radiating from the palmar surface of the capitate to other carpal bones are identified, then the ligament may also be referred to as the radial carpal ligament.

The *dorsal radiocarpal ligament* is thinner and functionally less important than the palmar radiocarpal ligament. It is a thickening of the dorsal joint capsule extending from the distal radius and radial styloid process to the scaphoid, lunate, and triquetrum. The radiotriquetral component of this ligament appears to be the most consistent of these structures. The *dorsal ulnocarpal ligament* reinforces the joint capsule between the ulna and triquetrum. Among several intrinsic dorsal carpal ligaments the *triquetroscaphoid* and *triquetrotrapezial fascicles* are most prominent.

The *collateral ligaments* of the wrist are thickenings of the fibrous capsule and functionally are less important than collateral ligaments in other joints such as the knee. The *ulnar collateral ligament* of wrist joint arises from the ulnar styloid and then divides into two fascicles, one of which inserts into the triquetrum with fibers continuing to the hamate and base of the fifth metacarpal bone and the other into the pisiform. The *radial collateral ligament* of wrist joint extends from the tip of the radial styloid to the scaphoid and trapezium.

The two most important intrinsic (interosseous) ligaments are the *scapholunate* and *lunotriquetral ligaments*. These ligaments connect the proximal aspects of the corresponding bones from their palmar to their dorsal surfaces,

thus completely separating the radiocarpal and midcarpal compartments. Three additional interosseous ligaments are found in the distal carpal row connecting the trapezium, trapezoid, capitate, and hamate. These distal interosseous ligaments do not extend from the volar to the dorsal portion of the wrist capsule, explaining the normal communication between the midcarpal and common carpometacarpal compartments of the wrist.

The *triangular fibrocartilage complex* (*TFCC*) is composed of the triangular fibrocartilage (TFC), the meniscus homologue, the ulnar collateral ligament of wrist joint, the dorsal and palmar radioulnar ligaments, and the sheath of the extensor carpi ulnaris tendon. The TFC separates the radiocarpal compartment from the distal radioulnar joint. The TFC is thicker peripherally and may even be fenestrated centrally. This "normal TFC fenestration" is virtually exclusively found in older individuals and therefore most likely represents a degenerative TFC tear in an asymptomatic person. The TFCC arises from the ulnar aspect of the distal radius and inserts on the ulnar head and styloid. As it extends distally, it is joined by fibers of the ulnar collateral ligament, becomes thickened to form the meniscus homologue, and inserts distally into the triquetrum, hamate, and base of the fifth metacarpal. On its volar aspect the TFCC is firmly attached to the triquetrum and lunotriquetral ligament and less strongly to the lunate and ulnolunate ligament. In its dorsal aspect the TFCC is incorporated into the sheath of the extensor carpi ulnaris tendon. The prestyloid recess is a protrusion of the radiocarpal joint between the TFC and meniscus homologue.

The *carpal tunnel* (Fig. 10C.4) is an oval space bounded dorsally, medially, and laterally by the carpal bones and volarly by the *flexor retinaculum*, a strong broad ligament extending from the pisiform and hook of the hamate medially to the scaphoid and trapezium laterally. Running through the carpal tunnel are the median nerve and the tendons of the flexor digitorum superficialis (four) and profundus (four) and the flexor pollicis longus tendon.

The *Guyon's canal* (ulnar tunnel) is a fibro-osseous, semi-rigid, triangular tunnel at the anteromedial aspect of the wrist through which ulnar nerve and artery pass (Fig. 10C.5). The tunnel measures approximately 4 cm in length, extending from the proximal edge of the pisiform to the hook of the hamate. The walls of the canal consist of the pisiform medially and the hook of the hamate laterally. The floor is composed of the flexor retinaculum and the origin of the hypothenar muscles and the roof of the pisohamate ligament, the volar carpal ligament and the palmaris brevis muscle.

The long *flexor tendons* of the fingers and thumb pass through the carpal tunnel invested in synovial sheaths. The four flexor digitorum superficialis tendons proximal to the carpal tunnel are arranged in two rows, with the tendons to the middle and ring finger superficial to the tendons of the index and little finger. In the carpal tunnel, the four tendons of both the flexor digitorum superficialis and profundus are lined up side by side. Exiting the carpal tunnel the flexor digitalis superficialis and profundus tendons are

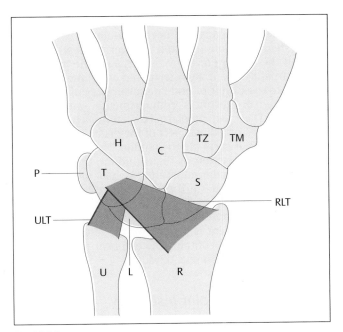

Fig. 10C.**1**

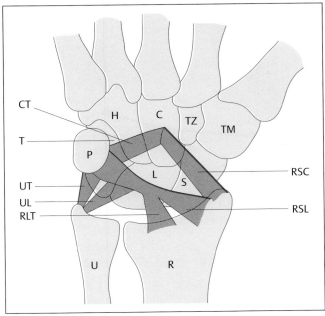

Fig. 10C.**2**

Fig. 10C.**1–3 Ligaments of the wrist.** Dorsal view (Fig. 10C.**1**), palmar view (Fig. 10C.**2**), and coronal section (Fig. 10C.**3**). C: capitate. CT: capitotriquetral ligament. H: hamate. I: interosseous ligaments (distal carpal row). L: lunate. LT: lunotriquetral ligament. M: meniscus homologue. P: pisiform. PR: prestyloid recess. R: radius. RC: radial collateral ligament. RLT: radiolunotriquetral ligament. RSC: radioscaphocapitate ligament. RSL: radioscapholunate ligament. S: scaphoid. SL: scapholunate ligament. T: triquetrum. TFC: triangular fibrocartilage. TM: trapezium. TZ: trapezoid. U: ulna. UC: ulnar collateral ligament. UL: ulnolunate ligament. ULT: ulnolunotriquetral ligament.

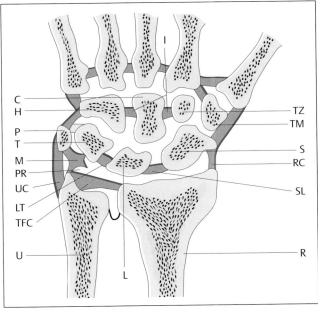

Fig. 10C.**3**

Fig. 10C.**4 Carpal tunnel.**
A: abductor pollicis brevis. AD: abductor digiti minimi. C: capitate. E: extensor digitorum communis tendon. EC: extensor carpi ulnaris. ECB: extensor carpi radialis brevis. ECL: extensor carpi radialis longus. EI: extensor indicis. EM: extensor digiti minimi. EP: extensor pollicis longus. EPB: extensor pollicis brevis. F: flexor retinaculum. FC: flexor carpi radialis. FD: flexor digitorum profundus. FP: flexor pollicis longus. FS: flexor digitorum superficialis. H: hamate. M: median nerve. P: palmaris longus. T: trapezium. TZ: trapezoid. U: ulnar nerve. UA: ulnar artery.

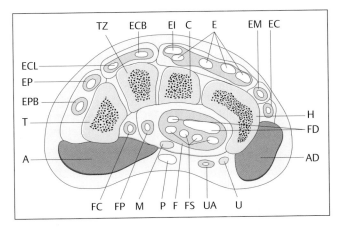

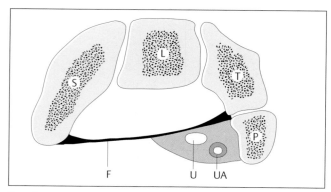

Fig. 10C.5   Guyon's canal (ulnar tunnel).
F: flexor retinaculum. L: lunate. P: pisiform. S: scaphoid. T: triquetrum. U: ulnar nerve. UA: ulnar artery.

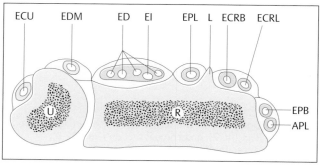

Fig. 10C.6   Extensor compartments of the wrist.
Compartment 1: abductor pollicis longus (APL) and extensor pollicis brevis (EPB). Compartment 2: extensor carpi radialis longus (ECRL) and extensor carpi radialis brevis (ECRB). Compartment 3: extensor pollicis longus (EPL). Compartment 4: extensor digitorum (ED) and extensor indicis (EI). Compartment 5: extensor digiti minimi (EDM). Compartment 6: extensor carpi ulnaris (ECU). L: Lister's tubercle. R: radius. U: ulna.

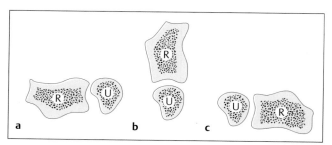

Fig. 10C.7   Normal alignment in the left distal radioulnar joint.   a Supination. The joint is not congruent, but the ulna is centered within the sigmoid notch.   **b** Neutral position, and **c** pronation: in these positions the joint is congruent. R: radius. U: ulna.

invested by the ulnar bursa and fan out in pairs toward their respective digits. In the finger both superficial and deep flexor tendons are enveloped by a common tendon sheath. These tendon sheaths terminate over the metacarpal heads, except for the tendon sheaths of the thumb and little finger that usually communicate with the radial and ulnar bursae, respectively. These two bursae may communicate with each other through an intermediate bursa. The tendons of the flexor digitorum profundus insert on the bases of the distal phalanges 2 to 5, while the tendons of the flexor digitorum superficialis insert on the shafts of

the middle phalanges of these digits after splitting to allow the deep flexor tendons to proceed distally.

The *extensor tendons* invested in synovial sheaths are located on the dorsum of the wrist beneath the superficial dorsal carpal ligament. By interrupted attachments of this ligament to the posterior and lateral surfaces of the radius and ulna, six distinct compartments are created (Fig. 10C.6). The most medial (sixth) compartment is located at the dorsomedial aspect of the distal ulna and contains the extensor carpi ulnaris tendon. The fifth compartment contains the extensor digiti minimi, the fourth the extensor digitorum communis and extensor indicis. Lister's tubercle separates the third compartment containing the extensor pollicis longus from the second compartment containing the extensor carpi radialis longus and brevis. The first compartment is located on the lateral aspect of the distal radius and contains the extensor pollicis brevis and abductor pollicis longus tendons.

Distal Radioulnar Joint Instability

The main stabilizing structure of the distal radioulnar joint is the TFCC. Subluxations and dislocations in this joint are therefore invariably associated with a disruption in the TFCC that may be traumatic, inflammatory, or degenerative in nature. An isolated injury to the TFCC or ulnar styloid fracture is infrequently associated with a distal radioulnar joint dislocation. It occurs much more in combination with radius fracture, e.g. the radius shaft (Galeazzi's fracture) or the radial head (Essex-Lopresti injury).

For diagnosis of a distal radioulnar joint instability the wrist has to be imaged in pronation, neutral position and supination of the forearm. In the normal wrist the articulating surfaces of the distal radius and ulna are congruent in pronation and neutral position, but not in supination due to the normal configuration of the distal ulna (Fig. 10C.7). Furthermore, minimal dorsal subluxation of the ulna in pronation and minimal volar subluxation of the ulna in supination may occur in the normal wrist. Comparison views of the opposite side are therefore helpful for diagnosing minor degrees of instability. The advantage of MRI over CT lies with its ability to demonstrate at the same time TFCC abnormalities commonly associated with distal radioulnar joint instability.

TFCC Lesions

The TFC appears on coronal MRI sections as a triangular low signal intensity structure with the apex attached to the articular cartilage of the radius and the base attached to the ulnar styloid process and fovea at the base of the radial aspect of this process. The ulnar attachment may appear bifurcated, with two bands of lower signal intensity separated by an area of higher signal intensity, or it may be obscured by surrounding loose vascular or fibrofatty tissue of intermediate signal intensity. Joint fluid may collect in the prestyloid recess between the TFC and meniscus homologue and appear as a region of increased signal intensity on T2WI.

Progressive degeneration of the TFC occurs with age and may not be associated with any symptoms. On MRI degenerative changes in the TFC are apparent as regions of intermediate signal intensity, which do not increase in intensity on T2WI or gradient-echo (GRE) images. Degenera-

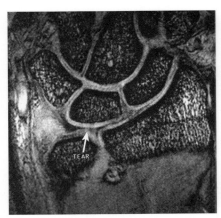

Fig. 10C.**8** **TFC tear.** A focus of increased intensity (arrow) is seen in the central portion of the TFC. Increased signal intensity is also present in the ulnar attachment of the TFC consistent with inflammatory/edematous changes (GRE [T2WI], coronal).

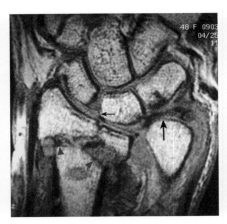

a

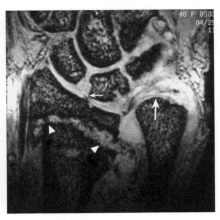

b

Fig. 10C.**9** **TFCC tear.** Extensive increased signal intensity (long arrow) is seen in the TFCC consistent with a complex post-traumatic tear. Widening of the scapholunate distance with complete scapholunate liga-

ment (short arrow) is also evident. Fluid is seen in the distal radius fracture (arrowheads), indicating nonunion. Positive ulnar variance is also present (**a**: PDWI, coronal; **b**: GRE [T2WI], coronal).

tive TFC tears are much more common than traumatic lesions. Degenerative perforations tend to occur in the central region of the TFC where it is thinnest (Fig. 10C.**8**). Traumatic tears of the TFC occur most commonly near its radial attachment (Fig. 10C.**9**). Tears appear as a region of intermediate signal intensity on T1WI and proton density SE images, which increases on T2WI or GRE images. In complete TFC tears the abnormal signal extends from the proximal to the distal articular surface. In partial tears the abnormal signals involve only one TFC surface, commonly the proximal one, particularly in the presence of a positive ulnar variance. TFC tears are often associated with fluid collections in the adjacent joint compartments (radiocarpal and distal radioulnar joints). TFC tears are frequently combined with tears in the lunotriquetral ligament since both structures are firmly attached to each other volarly.

Ulnar Impaction (Abutment) Syndrome

Normally the distal radius and ulna are of equal length (neutral ulnar variance). In negative ulnar variance the ulna is relatively short compared with the radius, which results in an increased force applied to the radial side of the wrist and lunate bone leading to a higher incidence of avascular necrosis of the lunate (Kienböck's disease). In this condition the fibrous TFC is thicker than normal and its perforation uncommon. In positive ulnar variance the ulna is relatively long compared with the radius and may abut the lunate and triquetrum (Fig. 10C.**10**). In this condition the TFC is thinner than normal and therefore more susceptible to degeneration and perforation (ulnar impaction or abutment syndrome). A tear in the lunotriquetral ligament and degenerative changes in the articular surfaces of the distal ulna and lunate are often associated. Sclerosis and cysts are frequently found in the proximal aspect of the lunate and triquetrum near the ulnar abutment. The ulnar impaction (abutment) syndrome has to be distinguished from the *ulnar impingement syndrome* consisting of a short ulna impinging on the radius and causing a painful pseudarthrosis.

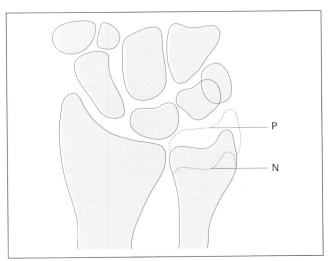

Fig. 10C.**10** **Ulnar variance.** Neutral variance occurs when the carpal surfaces of the radius and ulna are equal. Positive ulnar variance (P) occurs when the ulna is longer than the radius. The condition predisposes to TFC degeneration and tear (ulnar impaction or ulnar abutment syndrome). Negative ulnar variance (N) occurs when the ulna is shorter than the radius. This condition predisposes to avascular necrosis of the lunate (Kienböck's disease).

Carpal Instability and Ligamentous Injury

Both extrinsic and intrinsic ligaments of the wrist contribute to carpal stability, whereas the role of the collateral ligaments in this function is limited. The volar radiocarpal and intercarpal ligaments are most important for stabilization of the carpus.

Carpal instability can be classified into static or dissociative and dynamic or nondissociative types. Imaging of the latter may be difficult and usually requires a functional study, such as fluoroscopy or cine MRI. *Triquetrohamate instability* presents with painful clicking caused by abnormal motion between the triquetrum and hamate. Static instability patterns are evident on conventional radiographs

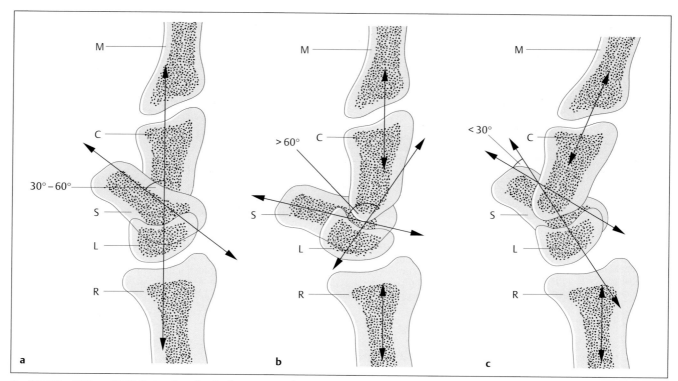

Fig. 10C.11 DISI and VISI (lateral projection). a Normal. A continuous line can be drawn through the longitudinal axis of the capitate, lunate, and radius and this line intersects a second line through the longitudinal axis of the scaphoid at an angle of 30°–60°. **b** DISI. The lunate is flexed towards the back of the hand and the scaphoid is tilted volarly. The longitudinal axis connecting capitate, lunate, and radius is interrupted, and the angle between the lunate and scaphoid axes is greater than 60°. **c** VISI. The lunate is flexed towards the palm, and the angle between the lunate and scaphoid is less than 30°. The longitudinal axis connecting capitate, lunate and radius is again interrupted with dorsal tilt of the capitate.
C: capitate. L: lunate. M: third metacarpal. R: radius. S: scaphoid.

and include *volar, dorsal,* or *ulnar translocation (subluxation) of the carpus* with regard to the distal radius. Instabilities within the proximal carpal row include scapholunate and lunotriquetral dissociations and *scapholunate advanced collapse (SLAC).* Two other major carpal instability patterns are *dorsal (DISI)* and *volar (VISI) intercalated segmental instability* (Fig. 10C.11). In lateral (sagittal) projection the angle between the axes of the scaphoid and lunate ranges from 30° to 60°. In DISI the lunate is tilted dorsally and the scapholunate angle measures more than 60°. In VISI the lunate is tilted volarly and the scapholunate angle measures less than 30°. DISI is often associated with rotary subluxation of the scaphoid (distal pole of scaphoid is tilted towards the palm) and scapholunate dissociation (scapholunate distance at site of ligamentous insertion measures more than 4 mm in frontal projection). In VISI the capitate is often tilted dorsally, resulting in a capitolunate angle of more than 30° (normal, 0°–30°), and lunotriquetral dissociation may also be associated. Scapholunate dissociation and rotary subluxation of the scaphoid represent stage 1 of four sequential stages of dislocations involving the lunate. Stage 2 (perilunate dislocation) represents a dorsal dislocation of the capitate. Stage 3 (midcarpal dislocation) consists of a subluxation of the lunate associated with a dorsal dislocation of the capitate. Stage 4 (lunate dislocation) represents a complete lunate dislocation associated with a dorsal dislocation of the capitate. Extent and severity of the associated injuries to extrinsic and intrinsic wrist ligaments increases correspondingly from stages 1 to 4.

On MRI normal ligaments are of low signal intensity on all pulse sequences. Age-related degeneration may be evident as a region of slightly increased signal intensity on T1WI, which remains unchanged or even decreases on T2WI. A "magic angle" phenomenon may present in similar fashion and must be differentiated. Ligamentous tears may be traumatic, degenerative, or inflammatory in nature. Complete tears appear as distinct areas of discontinuity within a ligament with increased signal intensity, especially on T2WI and GRE images. Severe distortion of an entire ligament including fraying and thinning is also indicative of a complete tear. A partial tear may be diagnosed when there is focal ligamentous thinning or irregularity or a fluid signal pattern involving less than the full ligamentous width.

On MRI the *scapholunate ligament* is consistently visualized and presents as a thin linear or triangular (delta-shaped) structure traversing the space between the proximal scaphoid and lunate. A ligamentous *scapholunate tear* (Fig. 10C.12) may be demonstrated directly or suggested when this ligament is elongated, incomplete, or not seen at all. Widening of the scapholunate distance indicates a more advanced ligamentous injury. The normal *lunotriquetral ligament* has a similar appearance to the scapholunate ligament, but is not consistently visualized by MRI, unless special techniques such as volumetric GRE are used. Depending on the imaging parameters employed, nonvisualization of the lunotriquetral ligament may not be a reliable indicator of an abnormality in this ligament. Otherwise, the diagnostic criteria for a tear in the lunotriquetral ligament are identical to those for the scapholunate ligament (Fig. 10C.13). Fluid is commonly seen in the metacarpal joint with either scapholunate or lunotriquetral ligament tears, but this finding is not specific.

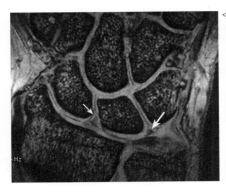

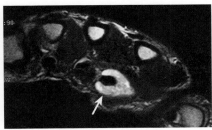

◁ Fig. 10C.**12** **Partial tear scapholunate ligament.** An incomplete hyperintense line (small arrow) is seen in the scapholunate ligament. A complete tear (large arrow) traversing the entire lunotriquetral ligament is also present (GRE [T2WI], coronal).

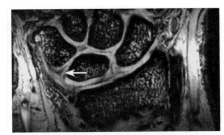

Fig. 10C.**13** **Lunotriquetral ligament tear.** A hyperintense line (arrow) is seen in the lunotriquetral ligament (GRE [T2WI], coronal).

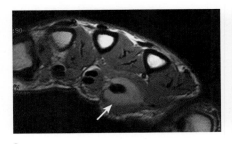

a b

Fig. 10C.**14** **Tenosynovitis.** Fluid collection (arrow) surrounds the paired flexor tendon of the index finger (**a**: PDWI; **b**: T2WI).

MRI evaluation of both the palmar radiocarpal and ulnocarpal ligaments is hampered in conventional planes because of the oblique orientation of these ligaments. If they are not visualized in their entirety, a tear can only reliably be diagnosed when an obvious discontinuity of the ligament with a hyperintense signal intensity within the gap is seen on T2WI. In the functionally most important palmar radiocarpal ligament, tearing commonly occurs at its radial origin. Volumetric GRE sequences and reformatting in oblique planes is required for improved diagnostic accuracy.

Gamekeeper's thumb is an injury to the ulnar collateral ligament of the first carpometacarpophalangeal joint with or without a bony avulsion resulting from a violent abduction of the thumb, most often a skiing accident. On coronal MRI the normal ulnar collateral ligament is evident as a band of low signal intensity. Its distal half is covered by the adductor aponeurosis, often visible as a paper thin band of low signal intensity. A nondisplaced tear of the ulnar collateral ligament appears as discontinuity of the ligament distally without ligamentous retraction. Displacement of the ulnar collateral ligament, also known as Stener lesion, is associated with proximal retraction or folding of the ligament. The proximal margin of the adductor aponeurosis may abut the folded ulnar collateral ligament, appearing as a rounded lesion of low signal intensity, and hereby create a "yo-yo on a string" appearance.

Tendon and Tendon Sheath Lesions

Tendinitis (inflammation or degeneration of the tendon) and *tenosynovitis* (inflammation of the tendon sheath) often occur simultaneously and may affect both the extensor and flexor tendons. De Quervain syndrome refers to tenosynovitis affecting the abductor pollicis longus and extensor pollicis brevis tendon about the styloid process of the radius. Involvement of the extensor carpi ulnaris tendon and sheath at the level of the distal ulna and styloid process is another common manifestation. Tendinitis and tenosynovitis in the flexor tendons occur commonly in or about the carpal tunnel.

On MRI tendinitis (tendinosis) presents with increased signal intensity within the tendon on both T1WI and T2WI. Focal tendon thickening may also be associated. An intratendinous tear cannot be differentiated by MRI from tendinitis. Tendons not aligned parallel to the main magnetic field may demonstrate the "magic angle" phenomenon, where an increased intratendinous signal intensity is only apparent on T1WI and proton density weighted images, but not with T2WI. Tenosynovitis is diagnosed by excessive fluid accumulation within the tendon sheath that may be distended (Fig. 10C.**14**). Suppurative tenosynovitis cannot be differentiated by MRI from noninfectious tenosynovitis, but MRI may be useful in assessing the extent of the disease.

Tendon ruptures occur secondary to trauma, degeneration, chronic inflammation (e.g. rheumatoid arthritis), and infections. Complete ruptures present as tendon discontinuity and fluid accumulation within and around the gap in the tendon. Incomplete ruptures are depicted by MRI as focal tendon thickening or thinning with increased signal intensity, especially on T2WI.

Ganglions (ganglion cysts) are the most common soft-tissue lesion of the hand and wrist. The dorsum of the wrist

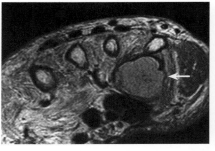

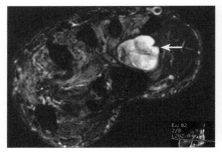

Fig. 10C.15   Ganglion. A large cystic lesion (arrow) is seen between the fifth metacarpal bone and the deep flexor tendons (**a**: spoiled GRE; **b**: T2WI, FS).

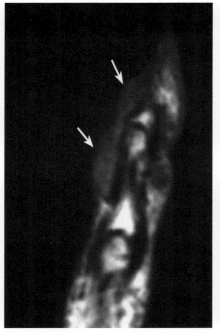

Fig. 10C.16   Giant cell tumor of tendon sheath. An inhomogeneous mass (arrows) isointense to muscle is seen in the index finger (T1WI, sagittal).

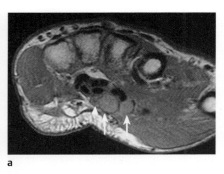

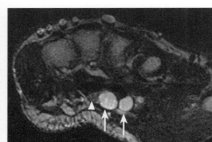

Fig. 10C.17   Carpal tunnel syndrome. A multiloculated ganglion (arrows) abuts the median nerve (arrowhead) (**a**: PDWI; **b**: T2WI).

is the most frequent location. They are intimately related to joints, tendons, and tendon sheaths. On MRI ganglions are isointense or slightly hyperintense relative to muscle on T1WI and proton density weighted images and hyperintense on T2WI. They are well delineated, often lobulated, and may contain fine septa (Fig. 10C.15). The thin wall of the ganglion occasionally enhances after intravenous Gd-DTPA administration.

Giant cell tumor of the tendon sheath (Fig. 10C.16) occurs most frequently in the fingers, but may also be found about the wrist. On MRI the lesion has a low signal intensity on T1WI. Depending on the presence of hemosiderin deposition and/or dense acellular fibrous tissue, the signal intensity of these lesions on T2WI ranges from low to high. Scar tissue around a tendon may also present with low signal intensity on all SE sequences.

Carpal Tunnel Syndrome

The most frequent entrapment syndrome of the median nerve occurs in the carpal tunnel. The syndrome affects the dominant hand or is bilateral in 50% of cases. It occurs more often in women than men, usually between age 35 and 65, and in individuals holding a job requiring repetitive wrist motions (e.g., typists, key punch operators, and grocery store checkers). Other causes include rheumatoid

arthritis and other arthritic and synovial processes, trauma, hemorrhage, benign tumors (e.g., ganglion [Fig. 10C.17], lipoma, hemangioma, or neuroma), amyloidosis, gout, diabetes, myxedema, hypoparathyroidism, acromegaly, pregnancy, and congenital anomalies (small carpal tunnel and muscle anomalies).

The most important MRI finding in patients with carpal tunnel syndrome is an abnormal median nerve. At the level of the pisiform this nerve may be enlarged to a size two to three times that at the level of the distal radius. The enlargement may be segmental or diffuse and is commonly associated with an increased signal intensity in T2WI due to edematous changes.

In cases of chronic carpal tunnel syndrome the median nerve may even show a decrease in signal intensity due to fibrosis and may appear flattened, especially at the level of the hamate. This should not be confused with the change in shape of a normal median nerve as it travels distally: at the level of the distal radius it is round or oval and often becomes more elliptic at the level of the hamate. Contrast enhancement of the abnormal median nerve is either increased due to edema or absent due to ischemia.

Palmar bowing of the flexor retinaculum and signs of flexor tenosynovitis and tendinitis, most commonly resulting from repetitive wrist flexion, are also common MRI findings in carpal tunnel syndrome. Enlargement of the individual tendon sheaths results in increased separation of

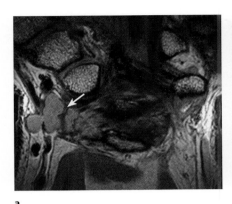 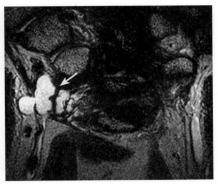

a   **b**

Fig. 10C.**18** **Guyon's canal syndrome.** Compression of the ulnar nerve, as caused by a large multiloculated ganglion (arrow), presenting with intermediate signal intensity in (**a**) (PDWI, coronal) and high signal intensity in (**b**) (T2WI, coronal).

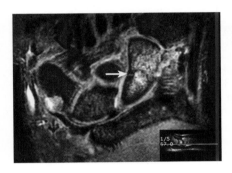

Fig. 10C.**19** **Fibrous nonunion of scaphoid fracture with avascular necrosis of the proximal fragment.** Nine months after trauma the scaphoid fracture line is still evident as a hypointense line (arrow). The proximal fracture fragment is collapsed and demonstrates heterogeneous signal intensity (T2WI, coronal).

the individual tendons. Increased signal intensity secondary to fluid accumulation in the enlarged tendon sheaths is best appreciated on T2WI. Regions of low signal intensity within the carpal tunnel on T2WI may be caused by gout, amyloid, fibrosis, or scarring.

In the postoperative patient, the flexor retinaculum and contents of the carpal tunnel are displaced volarly. In cases of persistent or recurrent carpal tunnel syndrome MRI may reveal incomplete retinacular excision, scar formation at the site of surgery, neuritis of the median nerve, or development of a neuroma, which can occur when the median nerve is cut inadvertently.

Guyon's Canal (Ulnar Tunnel) Syndrome

Causes of entrapment of the ulnar nerve as it traverses through the Guyon's canal include ganglia (Fig. 10C.**18**) and other soft-tissue masses, vascular injury (pseudoaneurysm or thrombosis of the ulnar artery), fractures of the hook of the hamate or pisiform, muscle hypertrophy (e.g. palmaris brevis), anatomic variations (e.g. presence of abductor digiti minimi within the canal), and hypertrophy of the volar (palmar) carpal ligament. In these conditions the entrapped ulnar nerve may appear focally or diffusely enlarged and edematous.

Avascular Necrosis and Fractures of Carpal Bones

Scaphoid fractures are located in the tuberosity, waist, proximal or distal pole of the scaphoid. Occasionally acute scaphoid fractures are difficult to diagnose on plain radiographs. In these instances MRI depicts the low signal density fracture line surrounded by bone marrow edema and hemorrhage. In a bipartite scaphoid two scaphoid ossicles, each containing normal bone marrow without signs of edema or hemorrhage, are linked to each other by a thin fibrous band of low signal intensity on all sequences.

Complications of scaphoid fractures include nonunion and avascular necrosis (Fig. 10C.**19**). A healed scaphoid fracture can unequivocally be diagnosed by MRI when marrow continuity across the fracture site is demonstrated. On the other hand, nonunion of a scaphoid fracture is diagnosed when fluid of high signal intensity on T2WI is shown in the fracture gap. In fibrous nonunion a low signal intensity on both T1WI and T2WI is seen in the fracture defect. However, a fibrous nonunion is difficult, if not impossible, to differentiate from ongoing fracture healing unless comparison MRI examinations are available and neither a change nor progress in fracture healing is evident.

Post-traumatic avascular necrosis of the *proximal scaphoid fracture fragment* is a frequent complication since the major arterial vessels enter through the distal half of the

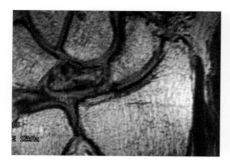
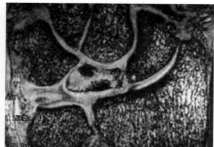

a   b

Fig. 10C.**20** **Kienböck disease. a** An overall inhomogeneous decrease in signal intensity is seen in the lunate (PDWI, coronal). **b** The signal in the lunate is increased and irregular (GRE [T2WI], coronal).

bone. MRI findings in this condition consists of uniform low signal intensity on both T1WI and T2WI in the often collapsed proximal fragment due to fibrosis or sclerosis. An increased signal intensity in T2WI may be seen in an earlier stage of the disease process due to marrow edema. Spontaneous avascular necrosis of the scaphoid is referred to as *Preiser disease.*

Avascular necrosis of the lunate is best known as *Kienböck disease.* It occurs most commonly between age 20 and 40 years and is more common in males. Kienböck disease frequently affects the dominant hand of manual laborers, or a history of trauma may be elicited. A negative ulnar variance is present in the majority of cases.

Radiographic changes are distinctive. Initially the lunate may have a normal architecture and density, but a subtle linear or compression fracture may often be delineated (Stage 1). Subsequently, an increased density of the lunate bone relative to the other carpal bone is noted (stage 2). Eventually the entire lunate may collapse and fragment (stage 3). Complications include scapholunate dissociation and secondary degenerative joint disease (stage 4). The al-

terations in stage 4 are virtually identical to the *SLAC* pattern secondary to trauma with disruption of the scapholunate ligament.

MRI can demonstrate all stages of Kienböck disease (Fig. 10C.**20**), but its value is in diagnosing stage 1 when the radiographic changes are subtle at best and the disease is still reversible with proper treatment such as immobilization. A uniform loss of signal intensity within the lunate on T1WI is the hallmark of the disease. Occasionally the loss of signal intensity on T1WI is focal and preferentially located in the radial half of the lunate. In cases of partial involvement differentiation from lunate cysts, intraosseous ganglia, and osteochondral fractures may be difficult. The signal characteristics of Kienböck disease varies considerably on T2WI depending on the presence of edema, fibrosis, or sclerosis.

Avascular necrosis rarely occurs in the *capitate*. In fractures of the capitate the proximal fracture fragment is susceptible to avascular necrosis since the major blood supply occurs, similar to the scaphoid, from the distal portion of this bone.

10D Hip

Anatomy

The hip is a ball and socket joint. The *acetabulum* is a hemispherical cavity on the lateral aspect of the innominate bone about its center and is directed laterally, downward, and forward. The acetabular articular surface is shaped like an inverted "U" (Fig. 10D.1). The area inside the "U" is filled with fat and the ligament of head of femur (ligamentum teres) extending from the fovea centralis of the head of the femur to each side of the acetabular notch and transverse ligament, respectively. A fibrocartilaginous labrum surrounds the acetabular rim. Inferiorly the labrum is incomplete but connected by the transverse ligament. This ligament has an elliptical configuration and should not be confused with an acetabular labrum tear on MRI. The spherical *head of femur* is covered with articular cartilage, except for a small depressed area located slightly inferiorly and posteriorly to its center, the fovea centralis. A physeal scar separating the epiphysis from the metaphysis in adults may be seen on MRI as a thin black line that varies in length and visibility and should not be confused with an incomplete or healing fracture.

There are numerous bursae in the hip region, of which the iliopsoas and trochanteric bursae are clinically the most important. The *iliopsoas bursa* lies between the iliopsoas muscle and the anteromedial surface of the hip joint. The bursa measures 3–7 cm in length and 2–4 cm in width and communicates with the hip in up to 15% of patients. Clinically iliopsoas bursitis may mimic an arthritic hip disorder. A markedly distended iliopsoas bursa may produce a mass in the ilioinguinal region simulating a hernia, lymphocele, abscess, or hematoma. *Three trochanteric bursae* are recognized, each separating one gluteus muscle or its tendon from the greater trochanter. Trochanteric bursitis is one of the most common bursal inflammations.

Acetabular Labrum Lesions

Abnormalities of the acetabular labrum occur at any age. In *developmental dysplasia of the hip (DDH)* the fibrocartilaginous labrum, normally seen as a triangular structure of low signal intensity, may be slightly everted (type 1: positionally unstable hip), everted and hypertrophied (type 2: partially dislocated hip), or inverted and hypertrophied (type 3: completely dislocated hip). Other potential causes preventing the reduction of a dislocated hip in DDH, which can readily be diagnosed by MRI, include infolding of the joint capsule, invagination of the psoas tendon into the joint, enlargement of the acetabular (pulvinar) fat pad, thickening of the ligament of head of femur, and infolding of the transverse ligament. The precise location of the dislocated cartilaginous femoral head of intermediate signal intensity is easily depicted by MRI, usually in superoposterior location from the dysplastic acetabulum (Fig. 10D.2).

Tears in the acetabular labrum occur not only in infants, but also in young adults and, less commonly, in elderly persons. Labral tears in adults may or may not be associated with dysplastic changes of the acetabulum. Cystic degeneration of the labrum and ganglions in the

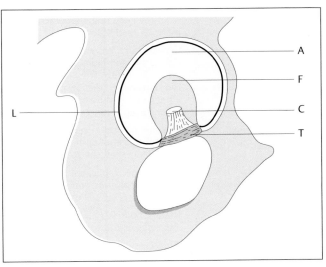

Fig. 10D.**1 Acetabulum.**
A: articular cartilage. C: ligament of head of femur (ligamentum teres). F: acetabular fat (covered by synovial membrane). L: acetabular labrum. T: transverse ligament.

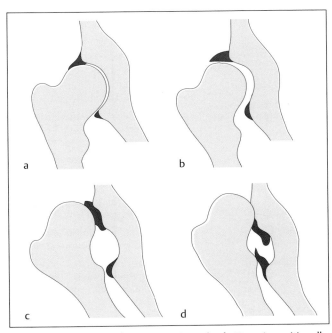

Fig. 10D.**2 Patterns of DDH. a** Normal. **b** Type 1: positionally unstable hip with slightly everted labrum. **c** Type 2: subluxated hip with everted and hypertrophied labrum. Subluxation is easily reduced in flexion. **d** Type 3: dislocated hip with inverted and hypertrophied labrum that impedes reduction.

acetabulum or soft tissues about the labrum may be associated with labral tears and are all well depicted with MRI. Occasionally gas is visible within these intraosseous and para-articular ganglions. Labral abnormalities often lead to a rapidly progressing osteoarthritis of the hip and may be referred to as *acetabular rim syndrome*.

Table 10D.**1** Etiology of AVN of the hip

Disease	Comments
Femoral head dislocation	Posterior dislocations (85%) are invariably associated with either rupture of the ligament of head of femur or avulsion fracture of the femoral head. At a later stage sequelae of a femoral head fracture may mimic AVN. Development of AVN following hip dislocation is caused by compromise of the blood supply deriving from the circumflex femoral artery branches rather than the disruption of the foveal artery within the ligament of head of femur.
Femoral neck fracture	Intracapsular femoral neck fractures result in extensive interruption of blood flow to the femoral head. The only remaining blood supply may be within the ligament of head of femur, provided it was functional prior to fracture. The prevalence of AVN depends on the re-establishment of adequate blood flow from the remaining intact vasculature and the ingrowth of new vessels into the femoral head. Infarcts typically are located in the anterolateral weightbearing segment, but are often more extensive and may even involve the entire femoral head.
Sickle cell disease	Sludging of sickled erythrocytes within the sinusoidal vascular bed results in functional occlusion. If the process becomes sufficiently extensive, infarction occurs. Bilateral involvement and association with metadiaphyseal osteonecrosis (bone infarcts) is common.
Corticosteroid therapy and Cushing disease	Mechanisms implicated in the development of AVN of the femoral head include microscopic fat emboli, steroid-induced osteoporosis with subsequent microfractures, compromise of the sinusoidal blood flow by an increasing fat cell mass, and elevation in intraosseous marrow pressure within the femoral head.
Alcoholism	The alcoholic fatty liver may be associated with chronic fat emboli which may lodge in bone. Similar mechanisms to those for hypercortisolism have also been proposed. Metadiaphyseal infarcts are rare.
Pancreatitis	Fat necrosis in bone presumably results from circulating lipases. Metadiaphyseal infarcts are more common than AVN of the femoral head. Alcoholism may be associated.
Gaucher disease	Sinusoidal blood flow obstruction caused by lipid (glucocerebroside) containing histiocytes packing the sinusoids. Metadiaphyseal infarcts are common.
Caisson disease	Dysbaric AVN results from gas (nitrogen) embolization after rapid decompression. Metadiaphyseal infarcts are common.
Pregnancy	Venous stasis with increased intramedullary pressure secondary to impaired venous drainage caused by the enlarged uterus appears to be the etiologic factor. Transient osteoporosis of the hip, commonly occurring in the third trimester of pregnancy and predominantly affecting the left hip, has to be differentiated.
Radiation therapy	The effect of radiation is dose-dependent and mediated through damage to the vascular bed in the femoral head.
Collagen vascular disease	In rheumatoid arthritis and especially systemic lupus erythematosus AVN of the femoral head is caused by either corticosteroid therapy or vasculitis interrupting the arterial blood supply or both.
Renal transplantation	Corticosteroids and immunosuppressive agents used to control rejection appear to be the major etiologic factors. Underlying metabolic bone changes associated with chronic renal disease may be a contributing factor.
Chemotherapy	Patients with lymphoproliferative disorders are particularly at risk for developing AVN. The marrow packing effect of these disorders associated with tumor necrosis are thought to be responsible in the absence of corticosteroid therapy.
Gout and hyperuricemia	A mechanism for apparent association between gout and AVN is not known. Gout may be secondary to alcoholism or treated lymphoproliferative disease, two conditions with a known predisposition for AVN.
Arthritic hip	Synovitis and joint effusion may result in increased intra-articular pressure leading to an increased intraosseous pressure with venous stasis.
Idiopathic	Early conversion of hematopoietic to fatty marrow in the proximal femur and a prominent physeal scar separating the epiphysis from the metaphysis in the femoral head have both been implicated as risk factors for the development of AVN.

Avascular Necrosis of the Femoral Head

Avascular necrosis (AVN) of the femoral head is caused by an interruption of blood flow to the femoral head. It is frequently associated with osteonecrosis (bone infarcts) in other parts of the skeleton. A variety of disorders are associated with a high incidence of AVN of the femoral head and are summarized in Table 10D.**1**.

MRI represents a very sensitive method for early diagnosis of AVN of the femoral head (Figs. 10D.**3–5**). Early MRI abnormalities depend on the alterations of bone marrow fat cells dying within 2 to 5 days after the ischemic event and the development of a hyperemia response in viable tissue and adjacent to the infarct. The increased vascularity at the interface between viable and necrotic tissue subsequently progresses to inflammation, granulation-tissue formation, fibrosis, and eventually new bone formation. Variations of MRI patterns in AVN are indicative of individual differences in extent, distribution, and age of the infarct as well as the host response. Focal homogeneous or inhomogeneous abnormalities predominate, with at least one component of diminished signal intensity on T1WI. Abnormal femoral head AVN patterns on T1WI include: 1) a well-defined homogeneous area of low signal intensity adjacent to the articular surface; 2) a band of low signal intensity crossing the femoral head; 3) heterogeneous loss of signal intensity in the femoral head containing foci of normal signal intensity; and 4) a ring of low signal intensity

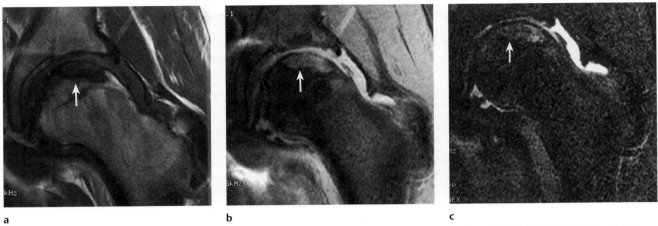

a

b

c

Fig. 10D.**3** **AVN of the hip.** A well-defined area of low (**a**: T1WI), intermediate (**b**: PDWI), and relatively high (**c**: T2WI, FS) signal intensity (arrow) is seen adjacent to the weight-bearing articular surface of the femoral head (coronal planes).

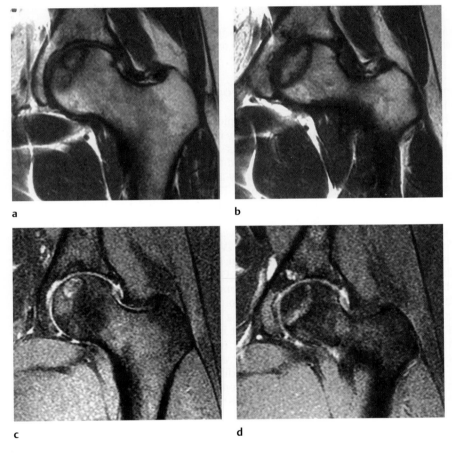

a

b

c

d

Fig. 10D.**4** **AVN of the hip.** A ring (**a**) or band (**b**) of low signal intensity separates a subarticular region of normal signal intensity from the unaffected marrow in the femoral head (T1WI, coronal). **c, d** A "double line" sign is seen at the interface between ischemic and nonischemic bone, consisting of an outer zone of low signal intensity and an inner zone of high signal intensity (T2WI, coronal).

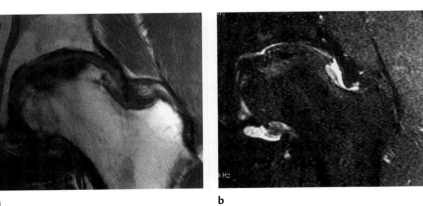

a

b

Fig. 10D.**5** **AVN of the hip.** A collapsed articular surface with fragmentation is seen (**a**: T1WI, coronal; **b**: T2WI, FS, coronal).

Table 10D.2 Staging of AVN of the femoral head

Stage	Clinical symptoms	Radiographic findings	MRI findings	Scintigraphic findings
0	Negative (risk factors present)	Negative	Negative or bone marrow edema pattern	Negative
1	Pain	Negative (occasionally suggestion of minimal mottling)	T1WI: focal, homogeneous or heterogeneous decrease in signal intensity. T2WI: Increased signal intensity at bone-infarct interface.	Decreased flow (early), increased uptake
2	Pain	Patchy osteopenia, sclerosis, and cyst formation	Similar to stage 1. "Double line" sign may be present on T2WI.	Increased uptake
3	Pain	Subchondral lucency (crescent sign)	Crescent-shaped, low signal intensity in subchondral bone on T1WI and T2WI (MRI crescent sign)	Increased uptake
4	Pain and disability	Collapsed or deformed femoral head	Collapsed articular surface or fragmentation of femoral head	Increased uptake
5	Pain and disability	Secondary osteoarthritis with acetabular involvement	Secondary osteoarthritis with acetabular involvement	Increased uptake

surrounding a center of normal signal intensity. A crescent-shaped, hypointense line in the subchondral bone found in both T1WI and T2WI corresponds to the subchondral lucency (crescent sign) of conventional radiography. The most characteristic pattern of involvement is the "double line" appearance, evident on T2WI at the interface between ischemic and nonischemic bone. The "double line" sign consists of a narrower outer zone of low signal intensity, reflecting the presence of fibrosis or bone sclerosis, and a slightly wider inner zone of high signal intensity reflecting granulation tissue formation. A chemical shift artifact may contribute to the "double line" sign also. On T1WI the interface between ischemic and nonischemic bone, evident as a "double line" sign on T2WI, presents as a region of decreased signal intensity. The absence of a "double line" sign, however, by no means excludes an AVN. A large joint effusion is a common but nonspecific finding in hip AVN. Diffusely distributed MRI abnormalities in the femoral head and neck are less common in AVN and are difficult to differentiate from transient osteoporosis of the hip and, occasionally, infection and tumor. Intravenous injection of Gd-DTPA contrast agent is useful in differentiating enhancing viable tissue from nonenhancing necrotic tissue. In a bone marrow edema pattern, such as is found in transient osteoporosis of the hip, the contrast enhancement is homogeneous since nonenhancing necrotic components are absent. Staging of AVN of the femoral head is summarized in Table 10D.2.

Legg-Calvé-Perthes disease is the idiopathic form of AVN of the femoral head affecting preferentially boys between the ages of 4 and 8 years. Bilateral involvement is present in 10% of cases. MRI may depict bone marrow edema as a precursor to Legg-Calvé-Perthes disease. Thickening of the articular cartilage of both acetabulum and femoral head, as well as a variable loss of containment of the femoral head within the acetabulum, are observed in most patients. Complications such as (hypertrophic) synovitis, joint effusion, chondrolysis, growth-plate involvement, and deformity of the femoral head are well assessed by MRI. The bony changes of Legg-Calvé-Perthes disease are similar to acquired AVN of the femoral head discussed above.

Transient Osteoporosis of the Hip

This condition typically occurs in young and middle-aged adults, particularly men. In male patients either hip may be involved, whereas in female patients the disease often begins in the third trimester of pregnancy and the left hip is more frequently affected. The disorder may occasionally involve both hips. The clinical picture includes progressive hip pain over several weeks with subsequent spontaneous regression in 2 to 6 months without permanent sequelae.

On MRI a relatively homogeneous area of decreased signal intensity on T1WI and corresponding area of increased signal intensity on T2WI is found in the femoral head and neck (Fig. 10D.6). Occasionally this bone marrow edema pattern may extend into the intertrochanteric areas or acetabulum. A joint effusion is commonly associated. Radiographically a localized osteoporosis pattern about the hip is present in a majority of cases. To include both osteoporotic and nonosteoporotic cases, the disease is often referred to as *transient bone marrow edema*. The more extensive, diffuse, and relatively homogenous involvement differentiates this disorder from AVN, presenting characteristically as a focal, well-marginated, and inhomogeneous lesion of the femoral head. Some overlap between these two conditions is, however, suggested by the fact that in a minority of cases a bone marrow edema pattern involving the femoral head will progress to unequivocal AVN.

Femoral Neck Fracture

Acute nondisplaced femoral neck fractures and chronic fatigue or insufficiency fractures can at times be difficult to diagnose with conventional radiography. MRI characteristics of a nondisplaced femoral neck fracture include a well-defined linear zone of low signal intensity. This represents the fracture line that is surrounded by marked edema and hemorrhage, presenting on T1WI as a broad and poorly defined zone of low signal intensity and on T2WI as a corresponding region of high signal intensity (Fig. 10D.7).

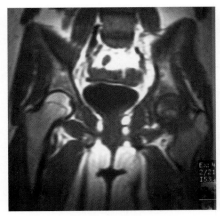

Fig. 10D.**6   Transient osteoporosis of the hip.** Compared with the normal right side, a marked decrease in signal intensity is seen in the left femoral head and neck (T1WI, coronal).

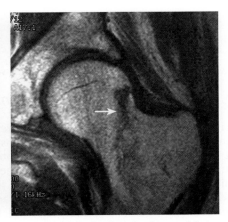

Fig. 10D.**7   Nondisplaced subcapital fracture.** A zone of low signal intensity (arrow) is seen (T1WI, coronal). The fracture was not visible on plain film radiography.

10E Knee

Anatomy

The knee joint is the largest articulation in the human body consisting of three functional compartments: the femoropatellar joint and the medial and lateral femorotibial articulations. The joint surfaces of the femur, tibia, and patella are not congruent. The adjacent articular surfaces of the femur and tibia are more closely fitted together by two crescent-shaped, fibrocartilaginous menisci. The fibrous capsule is reinforced by strong expansions from tendons of muscles surrounding the joints, except anteriorly where the fibrous capsule is absent above and over the patellar surface (Figs. 10E.1 and 2).

The synovial membrane of the knee joint lines the articular capsule, suprapatellar recess (bursa), posterior femoral recesses, and subpopliteal recess. The latter communicates in 10% of adults with the superior tibiofibular joint, a synovial articulation in contrast to the distal tibiofibular joint which is fibrous. The medial and lateral posterior femoral recesses lie behind the posterior portion of each femoral condyle and deep to the corresponding heads of the gastrocnemius muscle. They are separated by a broad synovial fold covering the cruciate ligaments anteriorly and on each side but not posteriorly. Bursae about the knee include anteriorly the prepatellar bursa between the patella and skin (resulting in "housemaid's" knee when inflamed), the subcutaneous infrapatellar bursa between the patellar tendon and skin, the deep infrapatellar bursa between the upper part of the tibia and the patellar tendon, and the pretibial bursa between the tibial tuberosity and skin. Laterally four bursae are commonly present: the lateral gastrocnemius bursa (which sometimes communicates with the knee joint) between the lateral head of the gastrocnemius muscle and joint capsule, the fibular bursa between the lateral (fibular) collateral ligament and tendon of biceps femoris, the fibulopopliteal bursa between the lateral collateral ligament and popliteus tendon, and the previously mentioned subpopliteal recess that may communicate with the fibulopopliteal bursa. Medially located bursae about the knee include the medial gastrocnemius bursa, which often communicates with the knee joint, between the medial head of the gastrocnemius muscle and joint capsule, the anserine bursa between the medial collateral ligament and gracilis, sartorius and semitendinosus tendons, and the bursa semimembranosa between the medial collateral ligament and the semimembranosus tendon.

Synovial plicae are persistent embryonic remnants of septal division of the knee into three compartments (Fig. 10E.3). The suprapatellar plica septates the suprapatellar recess. The infrapatellar plica extends from the intercondylar notch to the infrapatellar (Hoffa) fat pad in front of the anterior cruciate ligament. The medial patellar plica runs vertically along the medial joint capsule adjacent to the medial facet of the patella. On MRI normal plicae appear as thin lines of low signal intensity on all pulse sequences and are only visible in the presence of a joint effusion. Symptoms may only be associated with a markedly thickened medial patellar plica, which may interfere with the normal functioning of the femoropatellar joint.

Meniscal Lesions

Normal menisci are C-shaped fibrocartilaginous structures of low signal intensity on all pulse sequences. They are arbitrarily divided into the anterior horn, body, and posterior horn. Their periphery is attached to the capsule and tibia via the coronary ligaments. The anterior and posterior horns are loosely anchored to the tibial eminence. Except for the peripheral 10% to 30% of the meniscus, which is supplied by the perimeniscal capillary plexus, the adult meniscus is relatively avascular. On sagittal MRI through the body segment the meniscus resembles a bowtie in configuration. This bowtie appearance is normally limited to two consecutive 5-mm thick images, since the average width of the meniscal body (capsular attachment to free inner edge) measures less than 12 mm. On cross section the meniscus has a triangular shape with a sharp central tip. The meniscus may be divided into a circumferential zone (outer one-third) and transverse zone (inner two-thirds). The latter is separated into superior and inferior leaves by the middle perforating collagen bundle, which normally cannot be distinguished from the adjacent meniscal tissue on MRI. The middle perforating bundle demarcates the shear plane of the meniscus. Meniscal degeneration and degenerative tears are most frequently found in that location.

The lateral meniscus has a tight C-shape and covers more of the articular surface of the tibia than the medial meniscus. Its width is relatively constant throughout the entire meniscus. The lateral meniscus has a loose peripheral attachment and, posterolaterally, is separated from the capsule by the popliteus tendon and its sheath. The medial meniscus has a semicircular shape and its width is greater posteriorly than anteriorly. Peripherally, the medial meniscus is firmly attached to the joint capsule, particularly in its midportion, in the region of the medial collateral ligament.

Meniscal tears are more common in the medial than the more mobile lateral meniscus. In the medial meniscus the posterior horn is most frequently affected and the anterior horn the least. In the lateral meniscus tears appear to be preferentially located in the anterior horn. Traumatic and degenerative tears can be distinguished from each other. Traumatic tears usually occur in younger persons as a result of a single traumatic event. They characteristically are vertical tears. Degenerative tears occur more commonly in older persons and in association with osteoarthritis of the knee. Degenerative changes within the meniscus make it more vulnerable to normal stress, eventually leading to a usually horizontal tear.

Meniscal tears can be classified according to their direction as horizontal, vertical, and radial tears. *Horizontal tears* split the meniscus into an upper and lower segment and may be accompanied by a meniscal cyst. *Vertical tears* divide the meniscus into inner and outer segments or separate the meniscus from its capsular attachment. A *radial (transverse) tear* is a special type of vertical tear involving the inner margin (free edge) of the meniscus in perpendicular fashion. When this tear changes its direction within the body of the meniscus by curving either anteriorly or posteriorly, then it is frequently referred to as a *parrot beak*

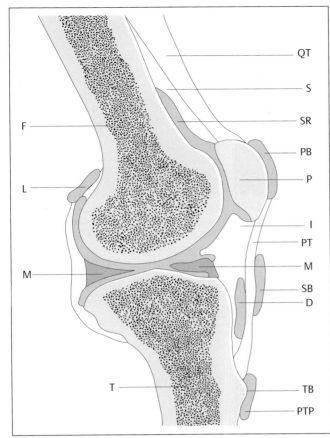

Fig. 10E.**1 Sagittal section through knee** (lateral to midline).
D: deep infrapatellar bursa. F: femur. L: lateral gastrocnemius
bursa. I: infrapatellar fat pad (Hoffa). M: lateral meniscus. P:
patella. PB: prepatellar bursa. PT: patellar ligament (tendon). PTP:
pretibial bursa. QT: quadriceps tendon. S: suprapatellar fat pad.
SB: subcutaneous infrapatellar bursa. SR: suprapatellar recess. T:
tibia. TB: tibial tuberosity.

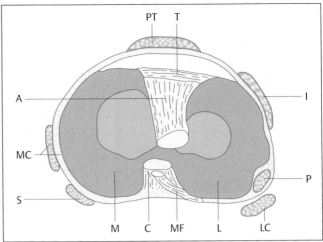

Fig. 10E.**2 Superior view of tibia.**
A: anterior cruciate ligament. C: posterior cruciate ligament. I: iliotibial tract. L: lateral meniscus. LC: lateral (fibular) collateral ligament. M: medial meniscus. MC: medial collateral ligament (superficial and deep band). MF: posterior meniscofemoral ligament
(ligament of Wrisberg). PT: patellar tendon. S: semimembranosus
tendon. T: transverse ligament.

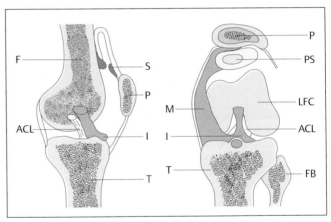

Fig. 10E.**3 Synovial plicae of the knee. a** Lateral
view. **b** Anterior view.
ACL: anterior cruciate ligament. F: femur. FB: fibula. I: infrapatellar
plica. LFC: lateral femoral condyle. M: medial patellar plica. P:
patella. PS: porta to suprapatellar recess T: tibia.

tear or *flap tear*. Radial tears frequently occur in the body of
the lateral meniscus. A *bucket-handle tear* is a longitudinal
vertical tear with a displaced inner fragment, often into the
intercondylar notch. Bucket-handle tears occur normally in the
medial meniscus. *Oblique tears* have features of both
vertical and horizontal tears, while *complex tears* are a
combination of different tears.

The MRI diagnosis of a meniscal tear is based on the alteration of the intrameniscal signal characteristic or the
meniscal morphology, or both. In adults an increased intrameniscal signal intensity represents meniscal
degeneration or intrasubstance tears that may not always
be symptomatic. An MRI grading system divides increased
intrameniscal signals into three grades according to their
configuration and relation to their articular surface (Fig.
10E.**4**). Grade 1 consists of one or several punctate intrameniscal signals not contiguous with an articular surface.
Grade 2 consists of a linear, usually horizontal intrameniscal signal, often originating from the capsular attachment
of the meniscus but without articular extension. Grade 3
consists of a linear intrameniscal signal extending to at
least one articular surface. In adults grade 1 and 2 signal
abnormalities reflect different degrees of meniscal
degeneration without definite tear. In children or adolescents the entire meniscus may be richly vascularized and
account for grade 1 and 2 signals seen in a completely normal meniscus. Grade 3 signal is indicative of a meniscal

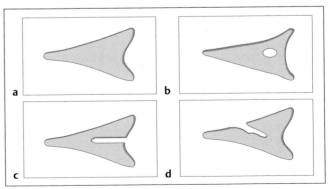

Fig. 10E.**4 MRI grading system of intrameniscal signals. a** Grade 0: meniscus demonstrates uniform low signal intensity. **b** Grade 1: meniscus contains one or several foci of intermediate signal intensity. **c** Grade 2: meniscus contains a
linear region of intermediate signal intensity that does not extend
to an articular surface. **d** Grade 3: meniscus contains a linear or
irregular area of intermediate signal intensity that extends to the
articular surface indicative of a meniscal tear.

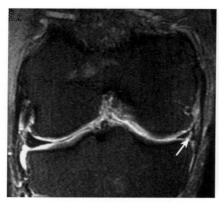

Fig. 10E.**5   Vertical meniscal tear.** A vertical tear (arrow) is seen in the medial meniscus (PDWI, FS, coronal).

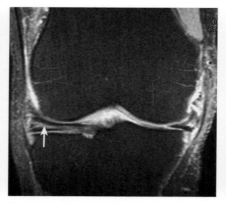

Fig. 10E.**6   Horizontal meniscal tear.** A horizontal tear (arrow) is seen in the medial meniscus (PDWI, FS, coronal).

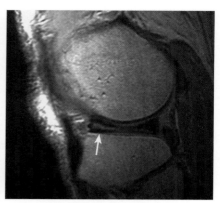

Fig. 10E.**7   Oblique meniscal tear.** An oblique tear (arrow) is seen anteriorly in the lateral meniscus (PDWI, sagittal).

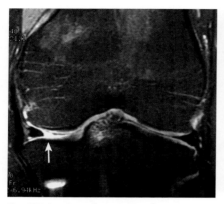

Fig. 10E.**8   Complex meniscal tear.** A complex tear (arrow) is seen in the medial meniscus (PDWI, FS, coronal).

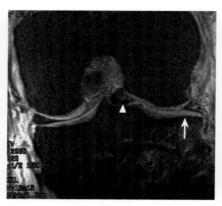

Fig. 10E.**9   Bucket-handle tear.** A tear in the lateral meniscus (arrow), which is too small, is associated with a meniscal fragment (arrowhead) in the intercondylar notch (PDWI, FS, coronal).

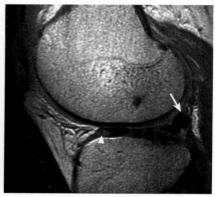

Fig. 10E.**10   Meniscal tear with fragment displacement.** A tear of the anterior horn of the lateral meniscus (arrowhead) is seen. The torn meniscal fragment is posteriorly displaced and flipped over the posterior horn of the lateral meniscus (arrow), which appears markedly increased in size and abnormally shaped (PDWI, sagittal).

tear that macroscopically may or may not extend to an articular surface. The latter occurs in approximately 5% of grade 3 menisci and is referred to as confined intrasubstance cleavage tear. Morphologic alterations of a meniscus indicative of a tear (Figs. 10E.**5–10**) include: partial or complete absence, displacement of a portion, blunting of the inner margin, abrupt change of contour, or focal deformity of the meniscus. Another indicator of meniscal tear is an abnormally small meniscus, even if it has a triangular shape on cross section. MRI findings of a bucket-handle tear include: a foreshortened and truncated or abnormally small meniscus, nonvisualization of the meniscal body (absence of the normal bowtie appearance on peripheral sagittal images), and demonstration of the displaced inner meniscal fragment that is often visible in the intercondylar notch anterior, below, and parallel to the posterior cruciate ligament. In a complex tear of the lateral meniscus the posterior horn may be flipped anteriorly adjacent to the anterior horn, producing a pseudohypertrophy of the anterior horn in the absence of the posterior horn. Meniscal tears should be evaluated with sagittal and coronal planes. Nondisplaced vertical tears, including

radial tears, are usually best visualized in a plane perpendicular to the course of the tear. Horizontal tears of the body are best displayed in the coronal plane and horizontal tears of the anterior and posterior horns in the sagittal plane.

Meniscocapsular separations (Fig. 10E.**11**) or *tears* usually involve the less mobile medial meniscus. Normally there is no fluid between the medial meniscus and the joint capsule. Fluid between the full thickness of the medial meniscus and its capsular attachment is diagnostic of a meniscocapsular separation. However, fluid is normally present in the superior and inferior capsular recesses and should not be confused with a partial meniscocapsular separation. A band of low signal intensity between these two recesses represents the intact meniscal attachment. The occasional presence of fluid in the bursa interposed between capsule and medial collateral ligament should not be mistaken for a meniscocapsular separation either. In the absence of a joint effusion, displacement of the medial meniscus by 5 mm or more from the capsule with uncovering of the tibial articular cartilage is indicative of peripheral detachment but is often difficult to assess.

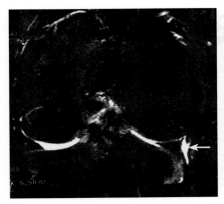

Fig. 10E.11   Meniscocapsular separation. The medial meniscus is separated from the capsule by a fluid-filled gap (arrow) (T2WI, FS, coronal).

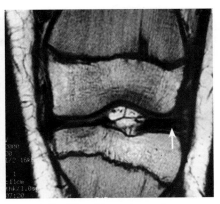

Fig. 10E.12   Discoid meniscus. An enlarged lateral meniscus with bowtie appearance (arrow) is seen (PDWI, coronal).

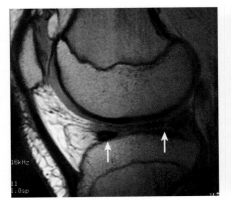

a

Fig. 10E.13   Discoid meniscus with several meniscal tears. An enlarged lateral meniscus (arrows) with several areas of in-

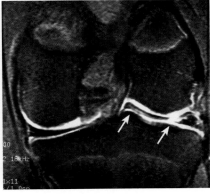

b

creased intrameniscal signal intensity is seen (**a**: PDWI, sagittal; **b**: PDWI, FS, coronal).

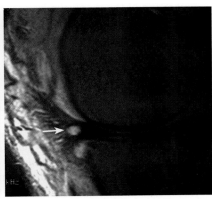

Fig. 10E.14   Meniscal cyst. A small cystic lesion (arrow) is seen in the anterior capsular attachment of the medial meniscus (T2WI, sagittal).

Many pitfalls in overdiagnosing a meniscal tear are well known and must be avoided. The *transverse ligament* overrides the anterior horns of both menisci prior to complete fusion with them and may simulate an oblique tear at these locations. The *meniscofemoral ligament* extends from the posterior horn of the lateral meniscus to the medial condyle of the femur. It consists of the *ligaments of Humphry and Wrisberg* crossing anteriorly or posteriorly of the posterior cruciate ligament, respectively. The relatively high signal intensity caused by the loose connective tissue between either one of these ligaments and the most medial part of the posterior horn of the lateral meniscus may be misinterpreted as a tear. *The popliteal tendon and its sheath* may produce a band of variable thickness and intermediate signal intensity as they course between the posterior horn of the lateral meniscus and the joint capsule. *Fibrillation* or *fraying* of the inner *free edge* of the meniscus produces an increased signal intensity at this location, which does not represent a meniscal tear. Artifacts produced by partial volume imaging or a vacuum phenomenon should not be confused with a meniscal injury either.

A *discoid meniscus* (Figs. 10E.12 and 10E.13) is an enlarged meniscus with a bowtie-like configuration. Lateral discoid menisci are approximately ten times more common than medial discoid menisci and occur in approximately 3% of the population. Most discoid menisci are initially asymptomatic but are prone to tears, degeneration, and cyst formation. On MRI a discoid meniscus should be suspected when a bowtie appearance of the meniscal body is seen on more than two contiguous 5-mm-thick sagittal images. Similarly a discoid meniscus should also be considered when demonstration of the anterior and posterior horn is limited to one or two sagittal slices adjacent to the intercondylar notch. Central tapering seen in the normal meniscus is absent in the discoid meniscus. The height of a discoid meniscus often is increased by 2 mm or more when compared with the opposite normal meniscus.

Meniscal cysts (Fig. 10E.14) are collections of synovial or mucinous fluid in the periphery of a meniscus, presenting as a focal mass or swelling about the joint. They are three to seven times more frequent on the lateral side of the knee and are commonly associated with myxoid degeneration and horizontal cleavage tears of the adjacent meniscus. On

MRI their signal intensity is uniformly low on T1WI and increases on T2WI and gradient echo (GRE) images.

Meniscal ossicles represent foci of ossification within the menisci and should be differentiated from meniscal calcifications (*chondrocalcinosis*), which are much more frequent. Ossicles are frequently associated with meniscal tears, but their etiology is not clear. Ossicles are usually located in the posterior horn of the medial meniscus. They commonly contain fat and thus present with high signal intensity on T1WI.

Evaluation of the *postoperative meniscus* by MRI is difficult since an asymptomatic, surgically repaired meniscus or meniscal remnant may demonstrate both signal and morphologic alterations found with meniscal tears. MRI is unable to distinguish between meniscal healing and retear at least up to 6 months post surgery. Postoperative meniscal fragments adjacent to the site of meniscectomy may be identified, but the relevance of this finding is not clear and requires clinical correlation. After meniscectomy fibrous regeneration of the meniscus may occur within 6 weeks to 3 months. The regenerated meniscus is thinner and narrower than a normal meniscus and demonstrates low to intermediate signal intensity on T1WI, T2WI, and GRE images.

Anterior Cruciate Ligament Injury

The anterior cruciate ligament extends from the posteromedial aspect of the lateral femoral condyle to the anterior intercondylar area, where it inserts just posteromedial to the anterior horn of the medial meniscus. The ligament has an average length of 4 cm and an average width of 11 mm and is broader at its tibial attachment. The anterior cruciate ligament is composed of an anteromedial and posterolateral fiber bundle which often cannot be separated on MRI or gross examination. The main function of the anterior cruciate ligament is to restrain anterior translation of the tibia in the knee. The anterior cruciate ligament also functions as a secondary restraint to internal rotation of the tibia and as minor secondary restraint to varus-valgus angulation at full extension of the knee.

Anterior cruciate ligament tears are most commonly located in the middle portion, followed by tears near the femoral attachment and least of all near its tibial attachment. Injuries to the anterior cruciate ligament occur with forward displacement of the tibia, external and internal rotation of the knee, and varus or valgus stress. Forced valgus in external rotation is the most common mechanism of anterior cruciate ligament injury and is often associated with medial collateral ligament disruption and medial meniscus tear (*O'Donoghue triad*). An anterior cruciate ligament tear secondary to varus stress and external rotation may be associated with an avulsion fracture of the lateral tibial rim at the site of capsular insertion (*Segond fracture*) and a medial or lateral meniscal tear. An avulsion *fracture of Gerdy's tubercle* on the anterolateral aspect of the proximal tibia relates to the iliotibial band insertion.

The anterior cruciate ligament is best evaluated by MRI, when the entire ligament is depicted on a single slice. This is achieved by a sagittal imaging plane with the knee in approximately 15° external rotation. The normal anterior cruciate ligament is seen as a uniform structure of low signal intensity or as one composed of individual fibers of low signal intensity. Individual fibers are identified most frequently at their tibial attachment site. Sometimes a slight inhomogeneous increase in signal intensity is seen in the anterior cruciate ligament near its tibial attachment due to the interposition of fat in the distal fibers.

The proximal anterior cruciate ligament insertion may appear slightly bulbous because of partial volume averaging with the lateral femoral condyle. Overall the signal intensity pattern of the normal anterior cruciate ligament is low, but not as low as that of the posterior cruciate ligament.

On MRI an anterior cruciate ligament tear is diagnosed by alterations in signal intensity, morphology, and the course of the ligament (Fig. 10E.**15**). An increased signal intensity within the anterior cruciate ligament on proton density and T2WI indicates an acute or subacute injury. A cloud-like or amorphous mass of increased signal intensity may be evident within the ligament, reflecting edema or hemorrhage. The absence of intraligamentous edema and hemorrhage, however, does not exclude an acute injury. A complete anterior cruciate ligament tear can be diagnosed when the ligament is either absent (empty notch sign in coronal images) or discontinuous. Disruption of all fibers and an irregular or wavy contour suggests a complete tear also. In sagittal images the completely torn anterior cruciate ligament may appear depressed, with a decreased slope or distal part of the ligament extending almost parallel to the tibial surface. In partial anterior cruciate ligament tear the course of the ligament remains normal or is slightly bowed posteriorly, both intact and disrupted fibers are visualized, and edematous or hemorrhagic changes may be depicted within the ligament. Chronic anterior cruciate ligament tears may also present with posterior bowing, indicating increased laxity of the ligament which also may be attenuated. Scar-tissue formation may result in focal angulation of a completely torn anterior cruciate ligament. False negative diagnoses may result from the formation of scar tissue with adherence of the anterior cruciate ligament to the posterior cruciate ligament simulating a normal course and signal intensity of the anterior cruciate ligament. Foci of myxoid degeneration within the anterior cruciate ligament, partial volume averaging with the lateral femoral condyle and periligamentous or intraligamentous fat should be differentiated from partial anterior cruciate ligament tears to avoid false positive diagnoses.

Secondary signs of an anterior cruciate ligament tear caused by anterior tibial subluxation include buckling (abnormal high arc) of the posterior cruciate ligament producing a "question mark" configuration, undulation and redundancy of the patellar tendon, and the "uncovered lateral meniscus" sign. The latter sign is positive if a vertical line drawn tangentially to the most posterior margin of the lateral tibial plateau intersects any part of the posterior horn of the lateral meniscus. A positive "uncovered lateral meniscus" sign indicates that the lateral meniscus does not subluxate anteriorly with the tibia in an anterior cruciate ligament tear. Bony abnormalities that may be associated with an anterior cruciate ligament tear include: bone bruises in the midportion of the lateral femoral condyle and posterior portion of the lateral tibial plateau and avulsion fractures of the lateral tibial rim (Segond fracture) and posterior margin of the lateral tibial plateau, both related to capsular avulsions of the tibia. Anterior cruciate ligament deficiency also may be caused by avulsion fractures at its sites of insertion. A joint effusion (hemarthrosis) is a common finding associated with anterior cruciate ligament injuries.

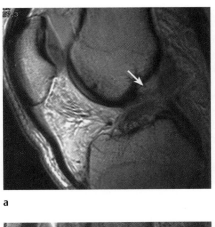

a

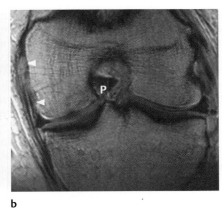

b

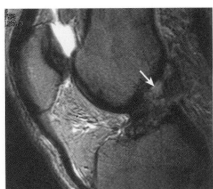

c

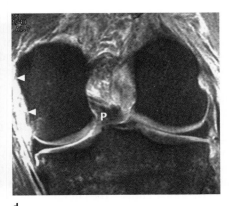

d

Fig. 10E.**15 Anterior cruciate ligament tear.** A complete tear of the anterior cruciate ligament (arrow) is seen in the sagittal images causing complete disruption with increased signal intensity. In the coronal images the anterior cruciate ligament is absent from its normal location ("empty notch sign") and replaced by hemorrhagic fluid. Note the intact posterior cruciate ligament (P) in anatomic position. A tear in the medial collateral ligament (arrowheads) is also evident. (**a**: PDWI, sagittal; **b**: PDWI, coronal; **c**: sagittal T2WI; **d**: coronal T2WI).

MRI evaluation of *anterior cruciate ligament reconstruction* may be hampered by metallic artifacts. Of the many operative techniques employed for the treatment of an anterior cruciate ligament tear, the autogeneous intra-articular reconstruction with a bone-patellar tendon-bone graft has become the most widely used method. Postoperative impingement of the graft may occur in the intercondylar notch causing erosion and possible disruption. A localized fluid collection within or around a graft suggests a tear. The normal graft has a low signal intensity. An increased signal intensity in the intra-articular portion of the graft has been attributed to impingement of the graft by the intercondylar notch. However, regions of increased signal intensity may also be secondary to revascularization and cellular ingrowth in the early postoperative period. Graft inadequacy may also be diagnosed by demonstrating secondary signs of an anterior cruciate ligament instability, such as anterior subluxation of the tibia and buckling of the posterior cruciate ligament. MRI is also an effective method to assess the precise location of the intraosseous tunnels.

Posterior Cruciate Ligament Injury

The posterior cruciate ligament extends from the lateral aspect of the medial femoral condyle to the posterior intercondylar fossa of the tibia. The posterior cruciate ligament is composed of anterolateral and posteromedial bands. It restrains posterior translation of the tibia in the knee, stabilizes the joint against excessive varus and valgus stress, and resists external rotation of the tibia.

Injuries to the posterior cruciate ligament are less frequent than to the anterior cruciate ligament, since it is twice as strong with a larger cross-sectional area and high tensile strength. Tears of the posterior cruciate ligament usually occur in its midsubstance and, less commonly, at its femoral or tibial insertions. Isolated tears of the posterior cruciate ligament are rare. They can be produced by forceful posterior translation of the tibia in a flexed knee (e.g. dashboard injury). More commonly, posterior cruciate ligament tears occur in association with other capsular, ligamentous, or meniscal injuries.

On MRI the posterior cruciate ligament is normally depicted as a band-like structure of low signal intensity. Occasionally in elderly persons regions of intermediate signal intensity are found in the posterior cruciate ligament due to mucoid degeneration. In sagittal images the posterior cruciate ligament has an arcuate shape with the knee in neutral position. The ligament becomes taut in flexion and lax in extension. An abnormal high arc or buckling of the posterior cruciate ligament may indicate anterior tibial subluxation secondary to a tear in the anterior cruciate ligament.

A posterior cruciate ligament tear may be diagnosed by disruption of all or a portion of its fibers. In complete disruption of the posterior cruciate ligament a loss or gap in ligamentous continuity may be evident (Fig. 10E.**16**). Regions of high signal intensity within the ligament on T2WI indicate hemorrhage or edema associated with an acute or subacute tear. Posterior cruciate ligament tears cause less distortion or mass effect than tears in the anterior cruciate ligament. Chronic tears with fibrous scarring demonstrate low to intermediate signal intensity on T1WI and T2WI. Avulsion fractures at the site of posterior cruciate ligament insertions in femur or tibia may depict a bone fragment containing marrow and hemorrhage or edema in the attached ligament.

In the majority of posterior cruciate ligament tears a joint effusion (hemarthrosis) is also present. Other commonly associated abnormalities include anterior cruciate ligament tear (38%), medial collateral ligament tear (23%), lateral collateral ligament tear (6%), medial meniscal tear (32%), lateral meniscal tear (30%), and bone bruise or fracture (36%). Bone marrow abnormalities are particularly characteristic when they are located in the anterior tibia plateau.

Medial Collateral Ligament Injury

The medial collateral ligament is composed of a superficial, deep band. The superficial band, also referred to as the tibial collateral ligament, measures approximately 10 cm in length and extends from the medial femoral epicondyle to the medial aspect of the tibia, approximately 5 cm below the joint line. Its posterior oblique fibers merge with the capsular attachment of the semimembranosus tendon. The joint capsule anterior to the insertion of the superficial band of the medial collateral ligament is reinforced by the pes anserinus composed of the gracilis, sartorius, and semitendinosus tendons. The deep band of the medial collateral ligament (also called deep medial ligament, deep collateral ligament, or middle capsular ligament) reinforces the capsule beneath the superficial band of the medial collateral ligament and is firmly attached to the medial meniscus by its meniscofemoral and meniscotibial components, respectively. The superficial and deep portions of the medial collateral ligament are separated by a bursa that allows movement between the two.

Medial collateral ligament injuries usually occur with excessive valgus force with associated external rotation (clipping injury). Complete medial collateral ligament ruptures may be associated with tears in the anterior cruciate ligament and medial meniscus and contusion or impact fractures in the lateral femoral condyle (typically midportion) and lateral tibia plateau (typically posterior aspect). Medial collateral ligament injuries are commonly graded according to their severity. Grade 1 lesions are sprains without joint instability, Grade 2 lesions are partial medial collateral ligament tears with joint laxity. Grade 3 lesions are complete medial collateral ligament tears with gross instability.

On MRI the medial collateral ligament is best displayed on coronal images and appears as a smooth structure of low signal intensity that extends from the medial femoral epicondyle to the proximal tibial metaphysis. At the level of the joint line the superficial and deep portions of the medial collateral ligament are separated by a bursa and surrounding fat, which should not be mistaken for a localized meniscocapsular separation.

In medial collateral ligament strains (grade 1 lesions) a slight contour irregularity or thickening of the ligament may be evident, but there is no discontinuity of its fibers. Edema and hemorrhage are identified in the soft tissue and subcutaneous fat paralleling the medial collateral ligament. In partial medial collateral ligament tears (grade 2 lesions), discontinuity of some ligamentous fibers or separation of fibers from adjacent cortical bone may be evident. In acute injuries increase in signal intensity, particularly on T2WI, is present within the ligament. Ligamentous attenuation may be found in chronic grade 2 lesions. Complete tears of the medial collateral ligament (grade 3 lesions) are associated with frank discontinuity of all its fibers in the superficial band (Fig. 10E.17). The deep band may or may not be involved.

Total biomechanical failure of the medial collateral ligament is associated with complete disruption of both bands. In the acute stage with hemorrhage and edema within the ligament the signal intensity is relatively low on T1WI and high on T2WI, whereas a subacute intraligamentous hemorrhage presents with a high signal intensity on both T1WI and T2WI. Focal hemorrhage is present at the femoral epicondylar attachment in ligamentous avulsions. A tear of the distal attachment may be associated with a wavy or serpiginous contour. Medial collateral ligament tears may be associated with extensive joint effusions (hemarthrosis) and extravasation of joint fluid.

Inflammation of the bursa within the medial collateral ligament may present with medial joint pain. On MRI a distended bursa with bright signal intensity on T2WI is found. A small amount of fluid in the bursa may, however, be a normal finding and present as a well-defined, elongated collection of fluid extending predominantly inferior to the joint line.

Lateral Collateral Ligament Injury

The lateral (fibular) collateral ligament is part of a complex of supporting structures of the lateral knee. The lateral collateral ligament is a strong rounded cord extending from the lateral femoral epicondyle in a posteroinferior course to its joint insertion with the biceps femoris tendon on the fibular head. The arcuate popliteal ligament is a Y-shaped system of capsular fibers, the stem of which is attached to the head of the fibula. The posterior limb of this ligament arches medially over the popliteus to be attached to the posterior intercondylar area of the tibia. The anterior limb extends to the lateral epicondyle of the femur, where it is connected to the lateral head of the gastrocnemius. All these structures in the posterolateral aspect of the knee are referred to as the arcuate complex and contribute to the integrity of the knee. The iliotibial tract is a reinforced part of the fascia lata, extending along the lateral portion of the knee and inserting in the proximal anterolateral surface of the tibia at Gerdy's tubercle. The iliotibial tract also provides stabilization to the lateral compartment of the knee. The lateral capsular ligament is essentially a capsular thickening. All these lateral supporting structures restrain varus angulation at the knee and external rotation of the tibia.

On MRI the lateral collateral ligament is best visualized on coronal images and appears as a band of low signal intensity. In complete lateral collateral ligament tears a ligamentous discontinuity or avulsion from its bony insertion may be evident and the ligament may demonstrate a wavy contour. Hemorrhage and edema are seen as ligamentous thickening with increased signal intensity on T2WI (Fig. 10E.18). A tear in the distal biceps tendon may be associated with a lateral collateral ligament tear and present on MRI in similar fashion. The iliotibial tract is seen on MRI as a thin band of low signal intensity paralleling the femur. Besides injuries, this structure may also be affected by the *iliotibial tract friction syndrome* presenting in athletes with pain in the lateral aspect of the thigh and knee. MRI may demonstrate edematous changes within and around the iliotibial tract. An avulsion fracture of the iliotibial tract at its insertion in Gerdy's tubercle should not be confused with a Segond fracture, which is an avulsion fracture of the tibial rim at the site of attachment of the lateral capsular liga-

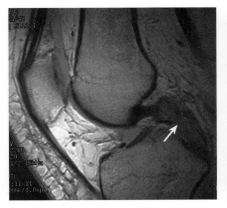
a

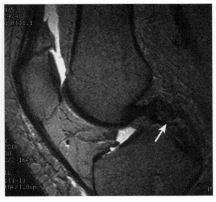
b

Fig. 10E.**16** **Posterior cruciate ligament tear.** A complete tear in the posterior cruciate ligament with disruption of all fibers (arrow) is seen (**a**: PDWI, sagittal; **b**: T2WI, sagittal).

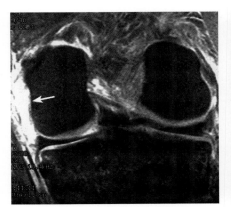

Fig. 10E.**17** **Medial collateral ligament tear.** Complete disruption of all fibers of the medial collateral ligament (arrow) is seen, depicting markedly increased signal intensity (T2WI, FS, coronal).

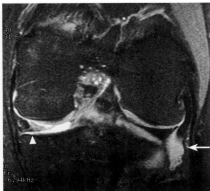

Fig. 10E.**18** **Lateral collateral ligament tear.** Partial disruption of the lateral collateral ligament is seen (arrow), which demonstrates a focal area of increased signal intensity. A complete medial meniscus tear (arrowhead), torn anterior cruciate ligament, and a lateral tibia fracture were also associated (T2WI, FS, coronal).

ment. The location of the Segond fracture is posterior and slightly proximal to Gerdy's tubercle. On MRI the Segond fracture usually presents as localized marrow edema adjacent to the fracture site. The fracture fragment itself often is not visible due to its small size.

Patellar Instability and Lesions

The patella is stabilized by the quadriceps tendon superiorly, patellar tendon (patellar ligament) inferiorly, and the medial and lateral patellar retinacula on each side. Abnormalities in these soft-tissue structures and/or femoropatellar joint result in patellar instability.

In the sagittal plane the patella is in normal position when in semiflexion of the knee the greatest diagonal length of the patella approximately equals the distance between the inferior pole of the patella and the tibial tuberosity (patellar tendon length). In full extension of the knee the patella normally is located higher than in semiflexion. A truly high-riding patella (patella alta) most commonly results from a patellar tendon tear, but is also associated with lateral patellar subluxations, recurrent dislocations, spastic neuromuscular disorders, chondromalacia patellae, and Osgood-Schlatter and Sinding-Larsen-Jo-

hansson disease. A *low-riding patella* (*patella baja* or *profunda*) occurs in quadriceps tendon rupture, but is also found with paralytic neuromuscular disorders, juvenile rheumatoid arthritis, achondroplasia, and following surgical transposition of the tibial tuberosity.

In the axial plane the posterior apex of a normal patella is centered directly above the intercondylar femoral sulcus. The sulcus angle is formed by the highest points of the medial and lateral femoral condyles and the lowest point of the intercondylar sulcus and measures 138° ± 6° (Fig. 10E.**19**). Shallow sulcus angles (larger sulcus angle measurements) predispose to patellar instability. The shape of the normal patella varies from a patella with equal-sized and slightly concave medial and lateral facets to a patella with a totally absent medial facet. A decrease in size of the medial facet and a transition from a concave to a convex articular surface of the medial facet are both associated with an increasing likelihood of patellar instability.

In *patellar instability* lateral subluxation of the patella or signs of the excessive lateral patellar pressure syndrome are evident. Lateral patellar subluxation is diagnosed when the posterior apex of the patella is displaced laterally relative to the intercondylar femoral sulcus and the lateral facet of the patella overhangs the lateral femoral condyle. In *excessive lateral pressure syndrome* the patella is tilted in

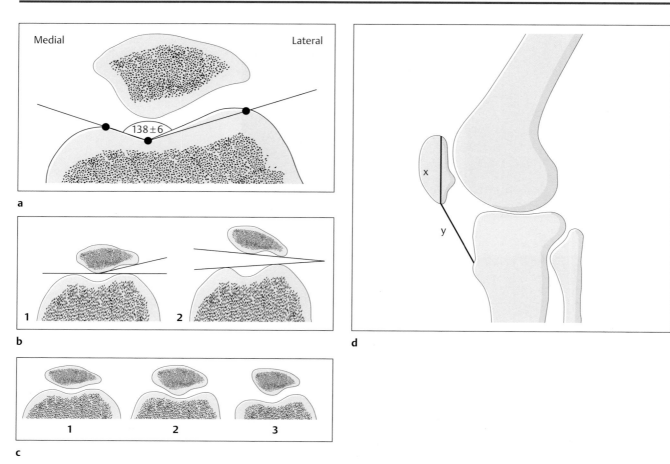

Fig. 10E.**19 Patellar instability assessment. a** In the axial plane the normal sulcus angle formed by lines along the femoral condyles measures 138° ± 6° degrees. Shallow (increased) sulcus angles indicate condylar dysplasia and a tendency for lateral patellar subluxation. Normally the posterior apex of the patella lies centered directly above the intercondylar femoral sulcus or slightly medial to it. **b** Normally an angle formed between a line connecting the anterior femoral condyles and a second line along the lateral facet of the patella opens laterally (1). A lateral patellar tilt consistent with excessive lateral patellar pressure syndrome is diagnosed when the angle of these lines opens medially(2). **c** Ten-dency of lateral patellar subluxation increases with both decreasing size of medial patellar facet and loss of concavity in the articular surface of the medial facet. The original Wiberg patellar classification differentiates between type 1 (medial and lateral facets are equal), type 2 (lateral facet is larger than medial facet, which remains concave), and type 3 (medial facet is small and convex). **d** Patella position: The ratio of patellar tendon length (y) to greatest diagonal length of patella (x) is approximately 1. Patella alta: y/x 1.2. Patella profunda (baja): y/x <0.8. Measurement should be done in flexion between 20° and 70°.

the lateral direction without subluxation. In this condition a line drawn parallel to the articular surface of the lateral patellar facet is horizontal or points downward on the lateral side of the patella. Medial patellar subluxation and dislocation are rare.

The *medial* and *lateral retinacula* are fibrous bands extending from the vastus medialis and lateralis, respectively, to the patella. With MRI they are best visualized on axial images and appear as low density structures. The medial retinaculum appears somewhat thinner than the lateral one and is more frequently torn, reflecting the tendency of the patella to subluxate and dislocate laterally. A torn retinaculum presents as a low-signal-intensity, wavy structure detached from the patella or as a low-density mass adjacent to the patella representing the torn retinaculum or an osteochondral fragment. Hemorrhage and edema may be associated and produce high signal intensity on T2WI (Fig. 10E.**20**).

Partial or complete tears of the quadriceps tendon may result from an acute injury or occur in association with chronic diseases such as rheumatoid arthritis or following corticosteroid therapy. On MRI the normal quadriceps tendon appears as a relatively straight band of low signal intensity measuring approximately 8 mm in the sagittal plane and 35 mm in the coronal plane. On sagittal MRI the normal tendon has a laminated appearance with two, three, or four layers of tissue. Tears of the quadriceps tendon result in partial or complete disruption of its fibers. In complete tears a patella baja and undulating appearance of the patellar tendon is associated. Hemorrhage and edema lead to an increase in signal intensity on T2WI in both partial and complete tears (Fig. 10E.**21**).

Patellar tendon (ligament) tears occur spontaneously, after vigorous exercise, in patellar tendinitis, rheumatoid arthritis, lupus erythematosus, and chronic renal disease. They usually occur at the inferior pole of the patella or, less commonly, at the tibial tuberosity. Complete tears are associated with a patella alta. On MRI the normal patellar tendon presents as a low-signal-intensity structure, but foci of intermediate signal intensity on T1WI and proton

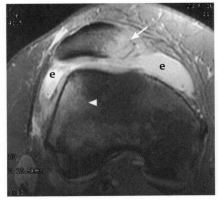

Fig. 10E.**20 Patellar instability with recurrent lateral patellar dislocation.** A large joint effusion (e), bone bruise in the lateral femoral condyle (arrowhead), fractured medial patellar facet (arrow), and hemorrhage in the adjacent medial patellar retinaculum are all sequelae of recurrent lateral patellar dislocations (T2WI, FS, axial).

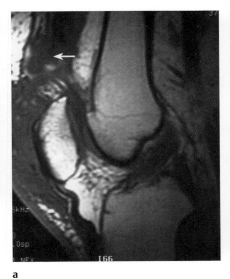

a

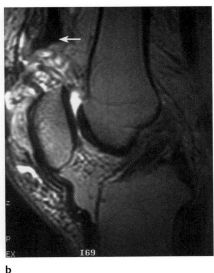

b

Fig. 10E.**21 Quadriceps tendon tear.** Complete rupture of the quadriceps tendon (arrow) is seen. Note also the associated patella baja with undulating patellar tendon (**a**: sagittal, T1WI; **b**: sagittal, T2WI).

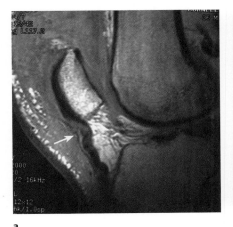

a

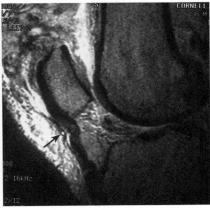

b

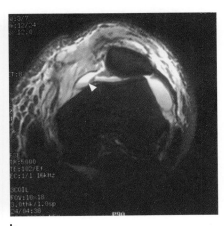

b

Fig. 10E.**22 Patellar tendon (ligament) tear.** Partial patellar tendon tear. Increased signal intensity is seen in the patellar tendon (arrow) at the inferior pole of the

patella (**a**: PDWI, sagittal; **b**: T2WI, sagittal). A tear of the medial retinaculum (arrowhead) and extensive soft-tissue hemorrhage evident as heterogeneous in-

creased signal intensity were associated (**c**: T2WI, FS, axial).

density weighted images are occasionally seen within the patellar tendon, particularly near its tibial insertion. This may be attributed to the "magic angle" phenomenon. Patellar tendon tears may be associated with small avulsions from the inferior pole of the patella or tibial tuberosity, presenting with or without the signal intensity of bone marrow. Other features of patellar tendon injury include foci of increased signal intensity on T1WI within and adjacent to the tendon, fiber disruption, thickening of the tendon, and tendon laxity or retraction (Figs. 10E.**22** and 10E.**23**).

Patellar tendinitis (*jumper's knee*) may be difficult to differentiate from an incomplete patellar tendon rupture. Patellar tendinitis may demonstrate diffuse or focal thickening of the tendon, particularly in its proximal half, and intratendinous areas of intermediate signal intensity on T1WI and high signal intensity on T2WI, which may represent intratendinous tearing.

Osteochondrosis of the distal patellar pole (*Sinding-Larson-Johansson disease*) or tibial tuberosity (*Osgood-Schlat-*

ter disease) occur in adolescence probably secondary to trauma. On MRI focal patellar tendon thickening with or without signs of inflammation and one or several ossicles containing marrow fat may be seen at the sites of patellar tendon insertion in the patella and tibia, respectively. *Osteochondritis dissecans* of the patella usually occurs between the ages of 15 and 20 years and preferentially affects the middle or lower portion of the medial facet of the patella.

Chondromalacia patellae is an idiopathic or post-traumatic softening of the articular cartilage of the patella presenting in adolescents or young adults with retropatellar joint pain. Arthroscopically four grades are distinguished: grade 1 shows cartilage softening; grade 2 shows blister formation; grade 3 shows surface ulceration and fragmentation due to blister ruptures; and grade 4 shows subchondral bone exposure. On MRI grades 1 and 2 cannot be differentiated. Focal areas of articular cartilage swelling with decreased signal intensity on both T1WI and T2WI may be seen. In grade 3 disease irregularities in the articu-

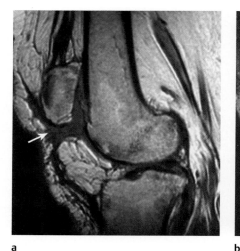
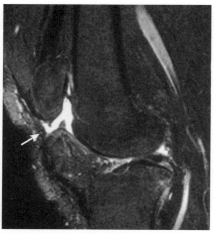

a   b

Fig. 10E.**23** **Complete patellar tendon tear.** Total disruption of the patellar tendon (arrow) is seen at the inferior pole of the patella (**a**: PDWI, sagittal; **b**: T2WI, FS, sagittal).

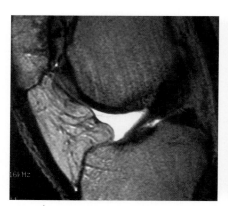
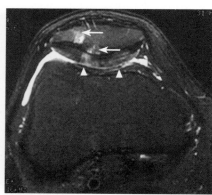

a   b

Fig. 10E.**24** **Chondromalacia patella.** **a** Abnormal heterogeneous signal intensity is evident in the patellar and femoral cartilage of the femoropatellar joint. A hyperintense joint effusion is also seen (T2WI, sagittal). **b** Fluid imbibition of the patellar joint cartilage (arrowheads) and fluid penetration into the subchondral bone (arrow) is seen (T2WI, FS, axial).

lar cartilage with areas of focal thinning may be evident. Imbibed fluid in the surface of the cartilaginous defects may cause an increased signal intensity on T2WI and STIR images. In grade 4 disease frank articular cartilage defects, exposed subchondral bone, and joint fluid penetrating between cartilage and subchondral bone may be evident. Joint effusions are commonly associated. With progression of the disease subchondral sclerosis and secondary osteoarthritic changes in the femoropatellar joint may develop (Fig. 10.24).

Periarticular Synovial Cysts

Numerous bursae exist about the knee which may or may not communicate with the joint. Noncommunicating synovial cysts or bursae are also referred to as ganglions, meniscal cysts or juxta-articular myxomas. The gastrocnemiosemimembranosus bursa located posterior to the medial femoral condyle between the tendons of the gastrocnemius and semimembranosus muscles communicates with the knee joint in up to 50 percent of elderly patients secondary to rupture of the posterior joint capsule. Swelling of this posterior bursa is termed a *Baker cyst*

(see Fig. 9.5, p. 339). Two other popliteal bursae with less frequent joint communication are located beneath the popliteal tendon, and between the medial head of the gastrocnemius and the distal end of the biceps.

Any of these popliteal cysts may enlarge producing a mass with or without pain. Rupture of a cyst is associated with soft tissue extravasation and clinically may simulate thrombophlebitis. MRI is effective in the delineation of intact and ruptured popliteal cysts. The characteristic appearance of a Baker cyst is a well-defined mass of variable size with signal intensity of fluid, located between the tendons of the medial head of the gastrocnemius and semimembranosus muscles.

Bursitis refers to an inflamed bursa presenting as a cystic mass with high signal intensity on T2WI. Commonly involved bursae about the knee involve the prepatellar bursa ("housemaid's" knee) deep infrapatellar bursa (between distal patellar tendon and anterior tibia), anserinus bursa (adjacent to anteromedial tibia) and the suprapatellar recess when completely separated from the knee joint by a suprapatellar plica. Bursitis may either be localized when secondary to chronic stress (e.g. prolonged kneeling in prepatellar bursitis) or part of a generalized inflammatory process such as rheumatoid arthritis and gout.

10F Ankle and Foot

Anatomy

Ligaments of the ankle consist of tibiofibular syndesmosis, medial collateral (deltoid) ligament, and lateral collateral ligaments (Fig. 10F.1). The *tibiofibular syndesmosis* includes the interosseous membrane and the anterior and posterior tibiofibular ligaments. The capsule of the ankle joint is weak anteriorly and posteriorly, but reinforced medially and laterally by the collateral ligaments. Maisonneuve fractures (fractures of medial malleolus and proximal fibula) are associated with syndesmotic injuries.

The *medial collateral ligament* or *deltoid ligament* is composed of three superficial and two deep ligaments. The superficial ligaments originate from the tip of the medial malleolus and extend to the tuberosity of the navicular bone (tibionavicular ligament) to the sustentaculum tali of the calcaneus (tibiocalcaneal ligament) and to the medial tubercle of the talus (superficial tibiotalar ligament). The deep ligaments extend from the anterior and posterior borders of the medial malleolus to the anterior and posterior aspects of the talus (anterior and posterior deep tibiotalar ligaments). Deltoid ligament injuries most commonly occur in association with fibular fractures and syndesmotic injuries.

The *lateral collateral ligaments* of the ankle include three ligaments. The *anterior talofibular ligament* extends from the anterior lateral malleolus to the neck of the talus. The *posterior talofibular ligament* extends horizontally from the posterior lateral malleolus to the lateral tubercle of the talus. The *calcaneofibular ligament* is crossed in its course by the peroneus longus and brevis tendons. The anterior talofibular ligament is the most common to rupture, followed by the posterior talofibular and calcaneofibular ligaments. After an inversion injury to the ankle, visualization of an intact anterior talofibular ligament virtually excludes rupture of any of the other two ligaments.

Tendons in the ankle can be grouped into anterior, medial, lateral, and posterior tendons (Fig. 10F.2). With the exception of the posterior tendons these tendons are all invested in tendon sheaths and about the ankle they change their course from a horizontal to a vertical direction with the help of five different retinacula. The change in direction makes the tendons susceptible to the "magic angle" phenomenon that is greatest when their orientation is at 55° to that of the magnetic field. Under these circumstances an increased signal intensity is seen on T1WI and proton density weighted images and should not be mistaken for intratendinous degeneration.

The *anterior tendon group* from medial to lateral includes the tibialis anterior, extensor hallucis longus, extensor digitorum longus, and peroneus tertius tendons. The *tibialis anterior tendon* has the largest diameter, passes deep to the extensor retinaculum along the anteromedial aspect of the foot, and inserts on the medial cuneiform and first metatarsal. Anterior tibial tendon tears are rare and occur spontaneously in the elderly, usually near the insertion on the first tarsometatarsal joint. Traumatic tears and tendinitis or tenosynovitis are even more unusual and may affect athletes or dancers. The *extensor hallucis longus tendon* runs lateral to the tibialis anterior tendon and inserts into the distal phalanx of the great toe. Acute injuries may be associated with penetrating traumas involving the dorsum of the foot. The *extensor digitorum longus tendon* divides into four slips, each of which inserts into a distal phalanx of one of the four lateral toes. The *peroneus tertius tendon* is extremely variable in size and absent in 5% of the population. When present, it inserts into the fifth metatarsal and may be difficult to separate from the extensor digitorum longus tendon.

The *medial tendon group* from medial to lateral and anterior to posterior, respectively, includes the tibialis posterior, flexor digitorum longus, and flexor hallucis longus tendons. Of the three, the superficially located tibialis posterior tendon is most susceptible to injury. The tendon passes just posterior to the medial malleolus, turns anteriorly below its tip and superficial to the deltoid ligament, and forms broad insertions on the plantar surfaces of the navicular, medial and intermediate cuneiforms, and bases of the second, third, and fourth metatarsals. Occasionally a sesamoid bone, the os tibiale externum, is seen within the tibialis posterior tendon just proximal to its navicular insertion. The os tibiale externum may cause a bulbous enlargement of the tendon and occasionally even contain a small amount of fatty marrow, producing a focus of increased signal intensity that should not be confused with a pathologic process. At the level of the medial malleolus the tendon is about twice as thick as the flexor digitorum longus or flexor hallucis longus tendon. The tibialis posterior tendon is a very important supporting structure of the longitudinal plantar arch. Progressive flat-foot deformity, often referred to as posterior tibial tendon insufficiency and sometimes associated with a painful mass in the medial aspect of the foot, may be the presenting clinical finding in partial or complete tendon tears. Spontaneous ruptures occur in middle-aged and elderly persons, especially females, secondary to chronic tendinopathy resulting from permanent stress on the tendon in supporting the plantar arch. Traumatic tendon ruptures occur in athletes or may be associated with fractures of the medial malleolus, the vicinity of which is the most common location for all tibialis posterior tendon tears. The *flexor digitorum longus tendon* lies posterior to the tibialis posterior tendon, passes medial to the sustentaculum tali, where occasionally it has its own groove, and crosses superficial to the flexor hallucis longus tendon. More distally it divides into four slips which insert into the bases of the distal phalanges of the second to fifth toe. Injuries to this tendon are uncommon. The *flexor hallucis longus tendon* lies posterolateral to the flexor digitorum longus tendon, passes in its own groove beneath the sustentaculum tali, and crosses deep to the flexor digitorum longus tendon to insert on the distal phalanx of the great toe. In approximately 20% of the population there is a normal communication between the ankle joint and the synovial sheath of the flexor hallucis longus tendon, where small amounts of fluid are frequently found. Inflammation and rupture of the flexor hallucis longus tendon occurs in dancers and athletes secondary to excessive plantar flexion of the forefoot, though complete rupture is rare. A *turf toe* (Fig. 10F.3) is a plantar capsular ligament sprain of the first metatarsophalangeal joint (hyperextension injury). It is

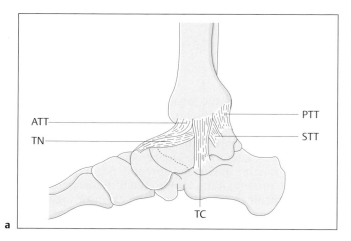

a

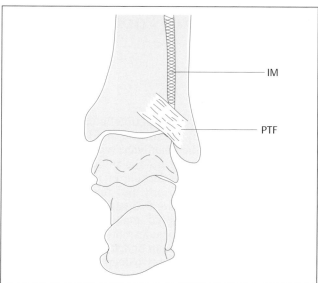

c

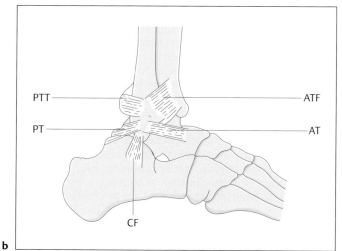

b

Fig. 10F.1 Ankle ligaments. a Medial view. **b** Lateral view. **c** posterior view. The medial collateral (deltoid) ligament consists of the tibionavicular ligament (TN), tibiocalcaneal ligament (TC), superficial tibiotalar ligament (STT), anterior tibiotalar ligament (ATT), and posterior deep tibiotalar ligament (PTT). The lateral collateral ligaments include the anterior talofibular ligament (AT), the posterior talofibular ligament (PT), and calcaneofibular ligament (CF). The tibiofibular syndesmosis consists of the interosseous membrane (IO), anterior tibiofibular ligament (ATF) and posterior tibiofibular ligament (PTF).

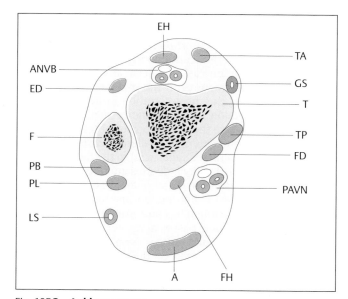

Fig. 10F.2 Ankle anatomy.
A: Achilles tendon. ANVB: Anterior neurovascular bundle. ED: Extensor digitorum longus. F: Fibula. FD: Flexor digitorum longus. FH: Flexor hallucis longus. GS: Greater saphenous vein. LS: Lesser saphenous vein. PB: Peroneus brevis. PL: Peroneus longus. PAVN: Posterior tibial artery and vein and tibial nerve. T: Tibia. TA: Tibialis anterior. TP: Tibialis posterior.

frequently associated with a fractured sesamoid and tenosynovitis of the distal flexor hallucis longus tendon.

The *lateral tendon group* includes the peroneus longus and peroneus brevis tendons. Both tendons descend behind the lateral malleolus in an osseous groove, the peroneus brevis tendon being anterior to the peroneus longus tendon. At the level of the lateral malleolus both tendons share a common synovial sheath and are covered by the superior peroneal retinaculum. At the level of the inferior peroneal retinaculum both tendons are invested in their own tendon sheaths. After curving anteriorly below the lateral malleolus the peroneus brevis tendon runs deep to the peroneus longus tendon along the lateral calcaneus and inserts into the base of the fifth metatarsal. The peroneus longus tendon, covered by a second synovial sheath, crosses the sole of the foot before inserting at the base of the first metatarsal and adjacent medial cuneiform. Peroneal tenosynovitis and tendinitis may be idiopathic, post traumatic, inflammatory, or associated with abnormal foot mechanics (e.g., tarsal coalition or pes planus). Partial and, less commonly, complete tears preferentially occur in the peroneus brevis tendon and may be post traumatic. Peritoneal tendon dislocations occur with violent contraction of the peroneal muscles, leading to disruption of the superior peroneal retinaculum and lateral or anterior dislocations of the peroneal tendons with regard to the lateral malleolus. Congenital anomalies of the lateral malleolus

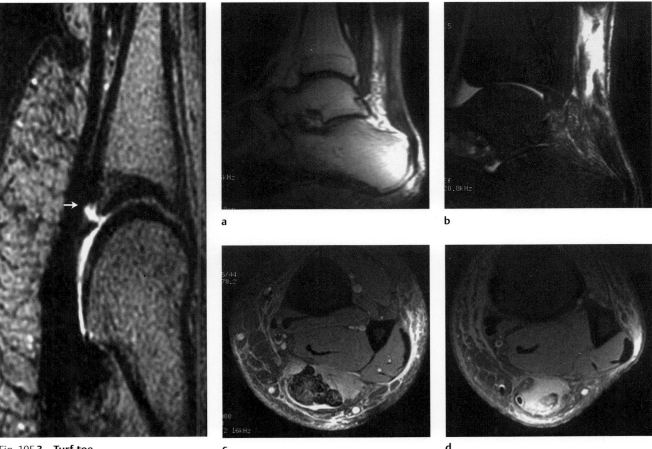

Fig. 10F.**3** **Turf toe.**
A small tear in the plantar capsular ligament (arrow) of the first metatarsophalangeal joint si seen (T2WI, sagittal).

Fig. 10F.**4** **Achilles tendon rupture.**
Complete rupture of the Achilles tendon with surrounding hemorrhage of variable signal intensity is seen (**a**: T1WI, sagittal,

b: T2WI, FS, sagittal **c**: PDWI, FS, axial at origin of Achilles tendon, **d**: PDWI, FS, axial distal to **c**).

(e.g. absence of peroneal tendon groove) and laxity of the retinaculum predispose to recurrent dislocations.

The *posterior tendon group* comprises the Achilles and plantaris tendons. The latter is absent in approximately 10 % of the population. When present, it descends along the medial border of the Achilles tendon and inserts with it into the calcaneus. The *Achilles tendon* is formed by the confluence of the gastrocnemius and soleus tendons and is the largest and strongest tendon in the human body. In the axial plane the normal Achilles tendon appears elliptic with a flattened or mildly concave anterior margin. It should not measure more than 8 mm in diameter in the sagittal plane. The tendon is attached to the posterior surface of the calcaneus at mid level, the retrocalcaneal bursa and an extension of the large pre-Achilles fat pad separating it from the upper part of the posterior calcaneus. In *Haglund syndrome* focal inflammation of the Achilles tendon at its calcaneal insertion and retrocalcaneal bursitis are present.

Tendinitis and peritendinitis of the Achilles tendon commonly develop in athletes secondary to overuse. Complete rupture is five to six times more common in men than women, usually between 30 and 50 years old. The most common location for Achilles tendon disruption is 2–6 cm from its insertion into the calcaneus (Fig. 10F.**4**). In nonathletes with Achilles tendon rupture a predisposing condition such as gout, rheumatoid arthritis, diabetes, chronic renal failure, or corticosteroid injections is usually present.

In addition to partial tendon tearing and tendinitis, thickening of the Achilles tendon is also associated with hyperlipoproteinemia due to intratendinous xanthoma formations, presenting with mixed low and intermediate signal intensity on both T1WI and T2WI.

Tendon Lesions

Normal tendons in the ankle and foot are homogeneous structures of low signal intensity on all MRI sequences, are equal in size on both sides of the body, and have smooth contours and uniform thickness, though they may occasionally become bulbous at their insertion sites. Longitudinal striations within normal tendons may occasionally be observed with advanced imaging techniques such as volumetric gradient echo (GRE) sequences.

Tendon degeneration may present with a focal increased signal intensity within the tendon on all image sequences. Tendon degeneration may be asymptomatic and must be differentiated from the "magic angle" phenomenon, where the focal increase in signal intensity observed on T1WI and proton density weighted images decreases with increasing echo times.

Tendinitis (inflammation of the tendon) presents with an increased signal intensity within the tendon, which is most conspicuous on T2WI (Figs. 10F.**5** and 10F.**6**). This condition

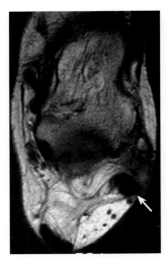

Fig. 10F.**5 Tendinitis.** A thickened peroneus longus tendon (arrow) with slightly increased intratendinous signal intenstiy is seen (PDWI, axial).

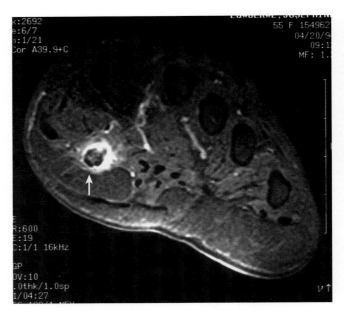

Fig. 10F.**6 Tenosynovitis** and **tendinitis.** After intravenous Gd-DTPA administration increased signal intensity in the flexor hallucis longus tendon with enhancement of the tendon sheath and surrounding soft tissues (arrow) is seen (T1WI, FS, +C, axial).

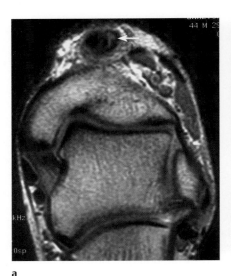

a

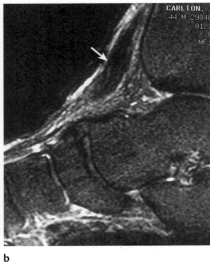

b

Fig. 10F.**7 Partial anterior tibialis tendon tear.** A thickened tendon (arrow) with increased signal intensity is seen (**a**: PDWI, coronal, **b**: T2WI, sagittal).

may be difficult to differentiate from a partial intratendinous tear unless disruption of part of the tendon fibers can be demonstrated. Both tendinitis and partial tendon ruptures may cause tendon thickening and inflammatory or edematous changes in the surrounding tissues. Contour irregularities of the tendon favor a partial tear over tendinitis. *Tendon ruptures* (Fig. 10F.7) may be acute or chronic, and partial or complete. Tendon ruptures occur with acute trauma, chronic overuse, tendon degeneration, tendinitis (e.g., infection, rheumatoid arthritis, systemic lupus erythematosus, gout, hyperparathyroidism, chronic renal failure, diabetes), and long-term steroid therapy. Incomplete tendon tears may be longitudinal within the tendon or transverse involving part of the tendon thickness. Partial tendon tears may also produce a thickened tendon with foci of high signal intensity on T2WI, or the tendon may be markedly attenuated. Complete tendon tears present as a discontinuity of all fibers or a gap filled with fluid, hematoma, or scar tissue depending on the age of the tear. Tendon retraction or a wavy, serpiginous tendon contour may be associated.

Tendon entrapment occurs as late fracture sequelae about the ankle. Both fibrous tissue or callus formation may entrap tendons in close proximity to the fractured bone. Tendon dislocation in the ankle is limited to the peroneus longus and brevis tendons. In this condition both tendons are found laterally or anteriorly with regard to lateral malleolus.

With the exception of the Achilles tendon, all tendons about the ankle are invested in a synovial sheath. Small amounts of tenosynovial fluid may occasionally be normal but a tendon sheath distended by fluid is indicative of tenosynovitis, which may accompany both tendinitis or tendon rupture (Fig. 10F.8).

Ligamentous Injuries

Three MRI planes are required for full evaluation of all ligaments of the ankle. Normal ligaments are thin and of low signal intensity. A slight increase in signal intensity with short echo times (TE) may be caused by the "magic angle"

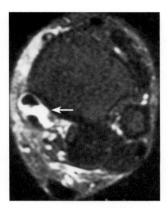

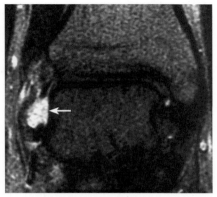

Fig. 10F.**8   Tenosynovitis.** Distended posterior tibialis and flexor digitorum longus tendon sheaths (arrow) are seen (T2WI, axial).

Fig. 10F.**9   Lateral collateral ligament tear.** Increased signal intensity is seen in the anterior talofibular and calcaneofibular ligaments (arrow) (T2WI, coronal).

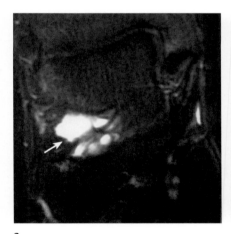

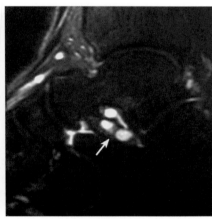

Fig. 10F.**10   Sinus tarsi syndrome.** A multiloculated ganglion with surrounding edematous changes (arrow) presenting with increased signal intensity is seen in the sinus tarsi (T2WI, FS, coronal [**a**] and sagittal [**b**]).

a

b

phenomenon. MRI findings associated with a complete ligamentous tear about the ankle include discontinuity of the ligament and ligamentous laxity or waviness (Fig. 10F.**9**). Attenuation and irregularity of the ligament can be seen in partial tears. In acute tears the gap in the torn ligament appears bright on T2WI due to intervening joint fluid, edema, or hemorrhage. Joint effusion and para-articular hemorrhage or edema indicate an acute injury also. In chronic injuries, ligamentous thickening and irregularities are present without joint effusion and surrounding soft-tissue hemorrhage or edema.

Sinus Tarsi Syndrome

The sinus tarsi is a cone-shaped space filled with fat between the talus and calcaneus anterior of the posterior subtalar joint. The apex of the cone, located posteromedially, represents the tarsal canal, and the expanded anterolateral portion of the cone represents the sinus tarsi. The sinus tarsi syndrome is associated with lateral foot pain,

tenderness, and hindfoot instability due to injury or inflammation of the sinus tarsi including its five ligaments, which are the medial, intermediate, and lateral roots of the inferior extensor retinaculum, the cervical ligament (lateral to the sinus tarsi, extending upwards and medially from the calcaneus to the neck of the talus), and the ligament of the tarsal canal (talocalcaneal interosseous ligament).

On MRI the normal fat of the sinus tarsi is either inflamed and edematous, presenting with decreased signal intensity on T1WI and increased signal intensity on T2WI, or the fat is replaced by fibrosis presenting with decreased signal intensity on all image sequences (Fig. 10F.**10**). The ligaments of the sinus tarsi are poorly visualized since they are also inflamed or poorly contrasted by the fibrosis replacing the fat. Abnormalities of adjacent structures such as the anterior talofibular ligament, calcaneofibular ligament, and tibialis posterior tendon may also be evident.

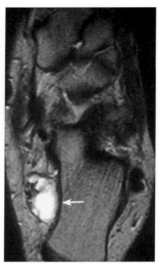

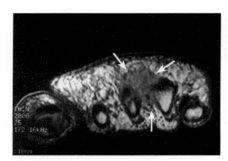

Fig. 10F.**12**   **Morton's neuroma.** A lesion (arrows) of intermediate signal intensity is located between the heads of the third and fourth metatarsals (PDWI, axial).

Fig. 10F.**13**   **Plantar fasciitis.** Increased signal intensity is seen in the plantar fascia (arrows) and adjacent subcutaneous fat (arrowhead) (GRE [T2WI], sagittal).

Fig. 10F.**11**   **Tarsal tunnel syndrome.** A multiloculated ganglion (arrow) located immediately lateral to the posterior tibial nerve branches causes compression neuropathy (T2WI, coronal).

Tarsal Tunnel Syndrome

The tarsal tunnel is located behind and below the medial malleolus. The tarsal tunnel is bound by the flexor retinaculum, medial surface of the talus, sustentaculum tali, and calcaneus. It extends anteriorly to the navicular bone. The resulting fibro-osseous channel allows passage of the posterior tibial nerve, posterior tibial artery and vein, and the tendons of the tibialis posterior, flexor digitorum longus and flexor hallucis longus muscles. The tarsal tunnel syndrome is a compression neuropathy of the posterior tibial nerve or its branches. Post-traumatic changes including scarring after ankle sprain and osseous deformities after calcaneal fractures are the most common cause. Other causes include foot deformities (e.g., tarsal coalition, pes planus, large os trigonum), benign soft-tissue masses (e.g., ganglion, lipoma, schwannomas), and soft-tissue inflammation (e.g. rheumatoid arthritis) (Fig. 10F.**11**). All these bony and soft-tissue abnormalities can impinge on the posterior tibial nerve and are readily detected by MRI.

Morton's Neuroma

Morton's neuroma is a fibrous response of an interdigital plantar nerve to damage caused by mechanical impingement. It occurs most often between the heads of the third and fourth metatarsals, followed by the second and third metatarsals. On MRI Morton's neuroma presents as a mass of low to intermediate signal intensity on both T1WI and T2WI, which may be dumbbell-shaped between metatar-

sal heads (Fig. 10F.**12**). The lesion may be associated with intermetatarsal bursitis. Morton neuromas differ from true neuromas (schwannomas) by their relatively low signal intensity on T2WI.

Plantar Fasciitis

The plantar aponeurosis (fascia) originates from the posteromedial and plantar surface of the calcaneus (medial process of calcaneal tuberosity) and divides anteriorly into five slips, each of which inserts into a proximal phalanx of a toe. Plantar fasciitis is low-grade inflammation of the plantar fascia and perifascial structures secondary to chronic or repetitive trauma resulting in microtears. Heel pain is the presenting clinical symptom.

On MRI the normal plantar fascia presents as a 3–4-mm thin band of uniform low signal intensity. In plantar fasciitis thickening of the plantar fascia by up to 8 mm may be associated with foci of intermediate signal intensity on T1WI and high signal intensity on T2WI (Fig. 10F.**13**). Inflammatory changes in the adjacent subcutaneous tissue and bone marrow edema at the site of calcaneal attachment may also be evident. Occasionally a tear in the plantar fascia can be demonstrated.

Diabetic Foot

The diabetic foot is a combination of vasculitis, infection, and neuropathy. Distinction between these entities is diffi-

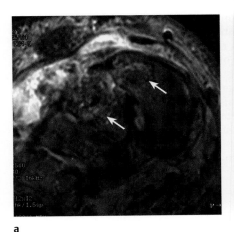
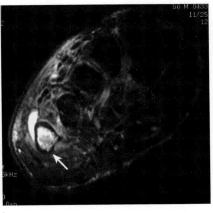

a   b

Fig. 10F.14 Diabetic foot (2 cases).
a An extensive inflammatory process with inhomogeneous high signal intensity in the dorsum of the foot is consistent with cellulitis and abscess formation. The process extends into the adjacent medial and intermediate cuneiforms (arrows) indicative of osteomyelitis (T2WI, FS, axial). **b** High signal intensity is seen in the fifth metatarsal (arrow) consistent with osteomyelitis. The soft tissue dorsal to the fifth metatarsal is also affected as indicated by the comet-shaped focus of high signal intensity representing a small abscess (T2WI, FS, axial).

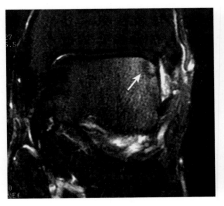
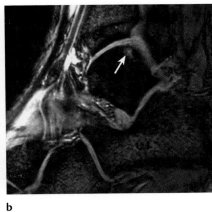

a   b

Fig. 10F.15 Osteochondritis dissecans.
A small osteochondral fracture fragment (arrow) is seen in the lateral talar dome (**a**: T2WI, FS, coronal. **B**: GRE [T2WI], sagittal).

cult with any imaging technique. MRI is extremely valuable in assessing the extent of the disease in soft tissue, bone, and joints, but may not be able to differentiate between different pathologic processes.

In both septic and neuropathic arthropathy articular destruction, bone resorption, secondary sclerosis, and large joint effusions may be present. Subluxation and dislocation favor neuropathic arthropathy. An increased signal intensity on T2WI in the bone marrow adjacent to the involved joint suggests septic arthritis and osteomyelitis, since neuropathic arthropathy usually depicts a hypointense signal intensity in the juxta-articular bone due to fibrosis and sclerosis.

Bone marrow abnormalities in osteonecrosis (avascular necrosis, bone infarcts) and osteomyelitis overlap considerably and largely depend on the stage of the disease. Predominant involvement of only one articular surface in any joint favors avascular necrosis over infection. Bone marrow alterations secondary to osteomyelitis are usually associated with extensive inflammatory changes in the surrounding soft tissues, since osteomyelitis commonly spreads from a contiguous infected neuropathic foot ulcer or abscess and the demonstration of the continuity between primary extrasceletal infective focus and affected bone is virtually diagnostic. In osteonecrosis the disease is largely limited to the bone (Fig. 10F.14). Stress (insufficiency) fractures are not uncommon in the diabetic foot and can be differentiated from osteomyelitis and osteonecrosis when a fracture line is identified, or suspected from their characteristic location in the metatarsals and calcaneus.

Bone Lesions

Tarsal coalition may be osseous, fibrous, or cartilaginous and congenital or acquired. Calcaneonavicular coalition is most common, followed by talocalcaneal and talonavicular coalitions. The first two coalitions account for 90% of primary tarsal coalitions. Tarsal coalitions can usually be diagnosed by plain film radiography, but their accurate delineation often requires CT or MRI. Bony bridging is the hallmark of osseous coalitions. Fibrous coalitions exhibit narrowing of the joint space with hypertrophic irregularities of the articular margins. Cartilaginous coalitions are rare and usually associated with marked narrowing of the involved joint and a cartilaginous bar may be identified.

Stress fractures (fatigue and insufficiency fractures) involve metatarsals (especially the second), calcaneus and, less frequently, the navicular bone. A localized bone contusion is the first MRI finding before the fracture develops. With time the fracture may be evident as a hypointense irregular line surrounded by marrow edema and hyperemia.

Osteochondritis dissecans or *osteochondral fractures* commonly occur in the talar dome (Fig. 10F.15). The middle third of the lateral border and the posterior third of the medial border of the talar dome are the two most common sites of involvement and are affected with equal frequency. The lateral talar dome lesion appears to relate to an inversion injury of the ankle, whereas the medial talar lesion is not invariably considered to be traumatic in pathogenesis. MRI is useful in diagnosing subtle cases of osteochondritis dissecans, in determining precise location and extent of the lesion, and assessing the stability of the subchondral fragment. Reliable signs of lesion stability include demonstration of an intact overlying cartilage and absence of a zone of high signal intensity on T2WI at the interface between the fragment and the talus. High signal intensity, indicative of fluid or granulation tissue, in this zone on T2WI is suggestive of an unstable fragment, whereas fluid encircling the fragment or focal cystic areas beneath the fragment are virtually diagnostic of fragment instability.

Osteonecrosis of the talus is a recognized and disabling complication of talar fractures. Because of its peripheral blood supply the body of the talus is most susceptible to osteonecrosis after a talar neck fracture. The radiographic diagnosis of osteonecrosis is usually delayed for one or several months until osteoporosis of the surrounding viable bone creates a relatively increased density of the talar body or a collapse of the articular surface is evident. MRI is able to diagnose osteonecrosis of the talar body at a much earlier stage by demonstrating alterations of the normal fatty marrow signals in the talar body due to fat cell necrosis. Similarly osteonecrosis of the tarsal navicular bone (Köhler disease) and heads of the metatarsals, most commonly the second (Freiberg disease), are depicted much earlier by MRI than conventional radiography.

10G Temporomandibular Joint

Anatomy

The temporomandibular joint is formed by the condyle of the mandible and the mandibular fossa and articular eminence of the temporal bone (Fig. 10G.1). The major soft-tissue structure of the temporomandibular joint is the articular disk (meniscus); interposed between adjacent osseous elements, it divides the joint into a superior and inferior compartment. The disk is thinned centrally (intermediate zone) and thickened or ridged peripherally. The anterior and posterior ridges are prominent and referred to as anterior and posterior bands. The anterior band is smaller than the posterior band. The circumference of the disk is connected to the fibrous joint capsule and anteriorly to the tendon of the lateral pterygoid muscle. Above, the fibrous capsule attaches to the articular eminence in front, to the lips of the squamotympanic fissure behind, and in between to the circumference of the mandibular fossa; below, the fibrous capsule attaches to the neck of the condylar process of the mandible. The posterior band of the disk is connected to the capsule by the bilaminar zone consisting of fibrovascular and fatty connective tissue.

In closed-mouth position the posterior band of the disk is located in the center of the mandibular fossa and the disk extends anteriorly and inferiorly along the anterior wall of the mandibular fossa. In this position the mandibular condyle is centered in the mandibular fossa so that the apex of the condyle, the posterior band of the disk, and the depth of the mandibular fossa lie in the same coronal plane. With opening of the mouth the condyle rotates on the articular surface of the disk, then the disk-condyle complex translates forward beneath the eminence of the temporal bone.

On MRI the fibrous disk has a uniform low signal intensity on all pulse sequences, except for a slightly increased signal intensity in the central portion of the posterior band on T1WI and proton density weighted images. The posterior disk attachment (bilaminar zone) is seen as two dark lines superior and inferior to a central zone of high signal intensity, which can easily be differentiated from the disk. A normal disk is pliable, adapting its shape to the adjacent articular surfaces. In the sagittal plane the disk has a biconcave (bowtie) appearance, which becomes more pronounced in open-mouth position when the disk is positioned under the articular eminence of the temporal bone.

Internal Derangement

Internal derangement is caused by abnormal disk mobility or disk displacement within the temporomandibular joint and is associated with pain, clicking, and/or limitation of jaw movement, including locking. Disk displacement almost always occurs in an anterior direction and rarely in medial, lateral, or posterior directions. However, it is not unusual for a component of medial or lateral disk displacement to be associated with an anterior disk dislocation.

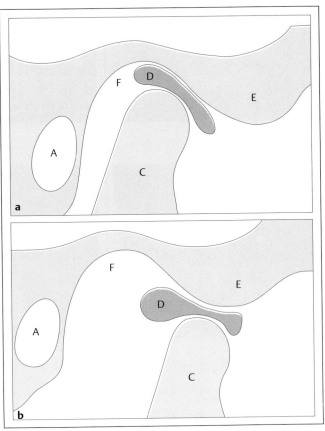

Fig. 10G.**1**   Normal temporomandibular joint in closed-mouth (**a**) and open-mouth (**b**) position.
A: external auditory canal. C: mandibular condyle. D: articular disk. E: articular eminence. F: mandibular fossa.

Anterior disk displacement occurs with and without reduction. *Disk displacement with reduction* (Fig. 10G.**2**) indicates that the disk-condyle relationship normalizes at one point during mouth opening. In other words, the anteriorly moving mandibular condyle recaptures the anteriorly displaced disk. During closing the condyle returns to the mandibular fossa, whereas the disk remains in its displaced anterior position. Clicking is often associated with this condition with both opening and closing of the mouth.

Disk displacement without reduction (Fig. 10G.**3**) indicates that the disk remains displaced with regard to the mandibular condyle in all positions. In this condition opening of the mouth or jaw movement, respectively, is often severely restricted. Deformation of the anteriorly displaced disk varies from minimal thickening of the posterior band or slight buckling of the disk to complete morphologic distortion.

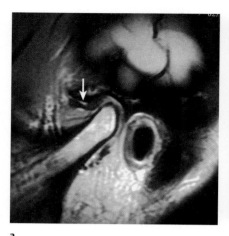
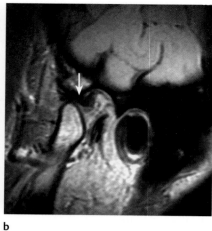

a   **b**

Fig. 10G.**2** **Anterior disk displacement with reduction.** **a** In closed-mouth position the articular disk (arrow) with low signal intensity and biconcave (bowtie) appearance is anteriorly displaced. The mandibular condyle is centered in the mandibular fossa (PDWI, sagittal). **b** In open-mouth position the mandibular condyle, which moved anteriorly, recaptured the anteriorly displaced disk (arrow) with normalization of the anatomic relationship between disk and condyle (PDWI, sagittal).

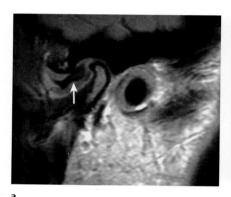
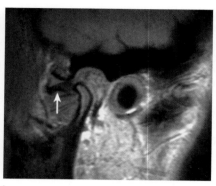

a   **b**

Fig. 10G.**3** **Anterior disk displacement without reduction.** **a** In closed-mouth position the articular disk (arrow) with low signal intensity and biconcave (bowtie) appearance is anteriorly displaced. The mandibular condyle is centered in the mandibular fossa (PDWI, sagittal). **b** In open-mouth position the mandibular condyle, which moved anteriorly, did not recapture the anteriorly displaced disk (arrow), which remains anterior to the condyle (PDWI, sagittal).

MRI allows precise assessment of location and morphology of the disk as well as its relationship to the mandibular condyle in open-mouth and closed-mouth positions. All these factors may be crucial in the selection of the most appropriate conservative or surgical treatment method. On the other hand, MRI is limited in diagnosing perforations in the disk itself or its posterior attachment.

In the *postoperative period* MRI is useful for assessing the location of either the repositioned disk or the synthetic disk implant. Implant complications such as foreign-body granuloma formation with or without bone destruction, avascular necrosis of the mandibular condyle, secondary osteoarthritis, and fractures or disintegration of implants are also well assessed by MRI.

11 Generalized Bone and Bone Marrow Disease

Bone consists of the *mineralized osseous matrix*, the *hematopoietic* or *red marrow*, and the *fatty* or *yellow marrow*. All three constituents of bone contribute to the formation of the magnetic resonance image (MRI). As the relative amounts of these constituents change, the signal intensity of the bone is altered accordingly. The osseous matrix causes a signal void on all imaging sequences. Any disorder associated with an increase in trabecular bone mass, which is evident on radiographs as *osteosclerosis*, presents on MRI with a decreased signal intensity on all image sequences. Such conditions include renal osteodystrophy, sickle cell disease, osteoblastic metastases, myelofibrosis, mastocytosis, fluorosis, and osteopetrosis. In *osteoporosis* the loss of trabecular bone mass and its replacement by fat cells results in an increase in signal intensity, particularly on T1WI.

Important anatomic and compositional differences exist between red and yellow bone marrow. The red marrow contains 40% water, 40% fat, and 20% protein and is richly vascularized, whereas the yellow marrow contains 15% water, 80% fat, and 5% protein and is poorly vascularized.

At birth only red marrow is present. However, *conversion from red to yellow marrow* (Fig. 11.1) begins immediately and occurs first in the terminal phalanges of the hands and feet. Red to yellow marrow conversion progresses from the peripheral to the central parts of the skeleton as a whole and from the diaphyses to the metaphyses in individual bones. Epiphyses and apophyses do not contain any marrow until they ossify. Any red marrow initially contained in these structures undergoes rapid conversion to yellow marrow. Therefore, epiphyses and apophyses contain yellow marrow from early development throughout the entire life, except occasionally in the proximal humeral epiphyses and, even less commonly, in the proximal femoral epiphyses and around the knee, where residual hematopoietic tissue can be found in normal adults.

The *adult bone marrow pattern* is normally present by the end of the third decade of life. At this stage red marrow is predominantly concentrated in the axial skeleton (e.g., vertebra, ribs, sternum, and pelvis) and the proximal appendicular skeleton (e.g., proximal femora and proximal humeri). Yellow marrow dominates the remaining skeleton and is variably admixed in bones containing primarily red marrow. Variations in the adult bone marrow do, however, exist. Islands of hematopoietic tissue may be found in areas dominated by fatty marrow and vice versa. With advancing age the red marrow fraction slowly declines further. Minerals contribute in a negative fashion to the bone marrow signal intensity. Since epiphyses and metaphyses contain a greater amount of trabecular bone than diaphyses, signal intensity at these sites is altered accordingly.

The *MRI appearance of bone marrow* in any bone is dependent on the relative fractions of red and yellow marrow and trabecular bone. Yellow marrow displays signal intensity similar to subcutaneous fat on T1WI and T2WI. Red marrow displays signal intensity lower than that of yellow marrow, but slightly higher than normal muscle and intervertebral disks on T1WI. On T2WI, the signal intensity of

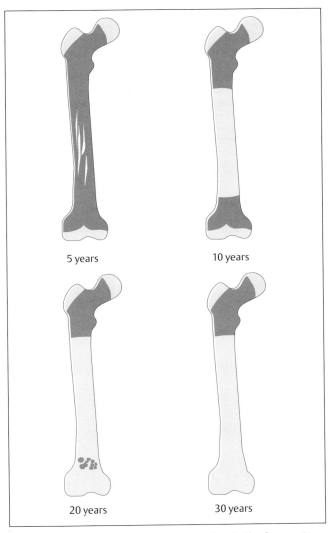

Fig. 11.**1** **Red to yellow marrow conversion in the femur.** Conversion to fatty marrow occurs first in the diaphysis and then progresses to the metaphyses (dark area: red marrow; light area: fatty marrow; numbers indicate age in years).

red marrow increases and approaches that of yellow marrow, but is lower than fluid. With short tau (T1) inversion recovery (STIR) imaging, red marrow signal intensity may even exceed that of yellow marrow, since the signal of fat is nulled making it appear dark on the images. Both STIR and fat suppressed T2-weighted imaging techniques improve detection of most bone marrow lesions.

In the *skull* conversion from red to yellow marrow occurs generally before age 20, but MRI evidence of red marrow may persist in the parietal bones until later in life. In the *vertebral bodies* the red marrow fraction remains relatively high throughout life. The normal age-related conversion of red to yellow marrow in the spine assumes a more focal rather than diffuse pattern. The focal conversion to fatty marrow preferentially occurs in the posterior elements, about the central venous channels and at the periphery of

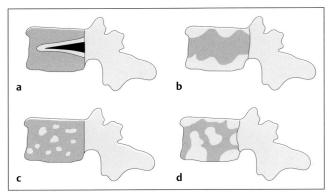

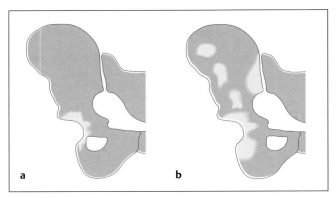

Fig. 11.**2**   **Age-related spine bone marrow pattern.   a** (Pattern 1) Homogeneous red marrow, except for fatty conversion around the central venous plexus.   **b** (Pattern 2) Fatty marrow near endplates and corners of the vertebral body.   **c** (Pattern 3A) Foci of fatty marrow measuring less than 5 mm diffusely distributed throughout the vertebral body.   **d** (Pattern 3B) Foci of fatty marrow measuring more than 5 mm diffusely distributed throughout the vertebral body.

Fig. 11.**3**   **Age-related pelvic bone marrow pattern.   a** Fatty marrow conversion begins before age 5 in the innominate bone.   **b** With age, spotty fatty marrow conversion progresses throughout the pelvis, sparing only the pubic bones. It is usually most pronounced along the sacroiliac joints.

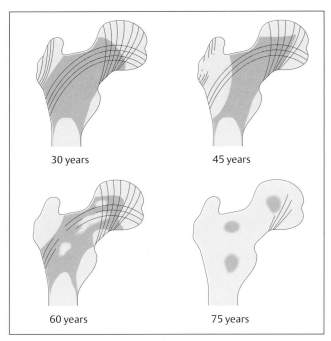

Fig. 11.**4**   **Age-related proximal femur bone marrow pattern.** With increasing age progressive red to yellow marrow conversion is associated with progressive loss of compressive and tensile trabeculae due to increasing osteoporosis (dark area: red marrow; light area: yellow marrow; numbers indicate age in years).

the vertebral bodies, particularly adjacent to the end plates. With degenerative disk disease irregular bands adjacent to the vertebral endplate may be seen, which are either of low signal intensity, representing fibrosis and sclerosis, or of high signal intensity, representing fat. The vertebral endplates with adjacent bone are occasionally hypointense on T1WI and hyperintense on T2WI, consistent with microfractures and inflammation.

Age-related bone marrow pattern in the *spine* and *pelvis* are discerned. In spine pattern 1 (Fig. 11.**2**) the vertebral body has a homogeneous appearance of red marrow, except for linear areas of fatty conversion around the central venous plexus. This pattern predominates in younger

people. In pattern 2 band-like and triangular areas of fatty marrow are found near endplates and corners of the vertebral body. This pattern is seen more commonly in the cervical and lumbar spine with degenerative disk disease. Pattern 3 consists of foci of fatty marrow diffusely distributed throughout the vertebral body measuring less than 5 mm (pattern 3A) or more than 5 mm (pattern 3B) in diameter. This pattern is usually found in patients older than 40 years of age. In the pelvis (Fig. 11.**3**) red to yellow marrow conversion begins before age 5 in the acetabular regions and anterior ilium and progresses with age throughout the pelvis. The marrow becomes heterogeneous, reflecting islands of conversion to fatty marrow. The bone marrow heterogeneity is most pronounced along the sacroiliac joints and least in the pubic bones, where it typically remains homogeneous throughout the entire life.

The *femur* (Fig. 11.**4**) and *humerus* are the only tubular bones which consistently contain red marrow in adulthood. As previously mentioned, conversion of red to yellow marrow occurs in the epiphyses and apophyses almost immediately after their development, although this conversion may not always be complete. In the diametaphyses of these bones red to yellow marrow conversion begins in the mid-diaphyses in early childhood and spreads both distally and proximally. By age 20 the red marrow is usually limited to the proximal metadiaphyses, but islands of red marrow occasionally remain scattered throughout the yellow marrow of the distal femur diametaphyses. These islands have a variety of configurations, ranging from small and circular to large and geographic and must be differentiated from an infiltrative or neoplastic bone marrow process.

Diffuse marrow disorders can be divided into five major categories: 1) myeloid depletion; 2) yellow to red marrow reconversion; 3) marrow infiltration or replacement; 4) marrow edema; and 5) marrow ischemia.

In *myeloid depletion* accelerated replacement of hematopoietic tissue by fatty tissue occurs. On MRI fatty marrow presenting with a high signal intensity on T1WI is depicted in areas where red marrow normally dominates. Myeloid depletion is associated with *radiation therapy*, *chemotherapy*, and *aplastic anemia*.

Reconversion of yellow to red marrow is associated with an increased need for hematopoietic marrow. When the disorder develops in childhood, failure of normal red to yellow conversion occurs. The reconversion in adulthood proceeds in reverse order of the normal conversion process, beginning in the axial skeleton and progressing to the appendical skeleton in a proximal to distal pattern. Causes of reconversion include chronic anemias (e.g., *sickle cell anemia, thalassemia,* and *spherocytosis*), marrow infiltration or replacement disorders (e.g., *leukemia, myeloma, metastases*), and advanced *heart/lung disease*. The process of reconversion is generally symmetric throughout the skeleton, although not necessarily uniform in any particular bone. Osseous expansions, extramedullary hematopoiesis and epiphyseal reconversion are late features of these disorders. The MRI signal pattern and distribution of reconverted red marrow are nonspecific. Differentiation from normal variation in red marrow distribution and neoplastic processes (e.g., metastases, myeloma, and leukemia) can be difficult, since all these conditions display T1 and T2 signal characteristics and distribution patterns similar to normal red marrow.

Marrow infiltration or replacement is caused by a wide variety of disorders, including neoplastic processes, myeloproliferative diseases, inflammatory conditions, lipidoses, and histiocytoses. These disorders may be diffuse, disseminated, or focal. The diffuse form is the most difficult to appreciate on MRI. All disorders have a low signal intensity on T1WI, but their appearance on T2WI is highly variable. *Osteolytic metastases* are hyperintense and *osteoblastic metastases* are hypointense on T2-sequences, whereas the signal intensity of mixed metastases ranges from low to high. Leukemia and lymphoma also have a variable signal intensity, but in many instances they appear isointense to the red marrow and therefore may be difficult to appreciate. Intravenous administration of a gadolinium-based contrast agent may be useful in the differentiation of normal hematopoietic bone marrow from neoplastic or inflammatory processes, since contrast enhancement of normal bone marrow is subtle or absent in adults, but may be marked in young children and pathologic conditions.

Bone marrow edema may be idiopathic (e.g., transient bone marrow edema, reflex sympathetic dystrophy), traumatic, or associated with infection and neoplasm in their periphery. Marrow edema appears homogeneous hypointense on T1WI and hyperintense on T2WI. Conditions presenting or associated with bone marrow edema are regionally limited and often affect only one anatomic site.

Marrow ischemia may result in osteonecrosis or bone infarct. Although usually focal in nature, osteonecrosis may present at multiple sites throughout the skeleton. Osteonecrosis may affect the subarticular (subchondral) bone and is referred to as avascular necrosis, or it may affect the metadiaphyseal regions of the long bones, especially the humerus, femur, and tibia. The appendicular skeleton is much more frequently involved than the axial skeleton, which may reflect the propensity of osteonecrosis to affect the sparsely vascularized fatty marrow in preference to hematopoietic marrow. This concept is supported by the fact that avascular necrosis of the femoral head occurs more frequently in patients with predominantly fatty marrow in the proximal femur than with red marrow. Magnetic resonance imaging is the most sensitive imaging modality to detect osteonecrosis, but controversy exists as to how MRI can detect early bone infarcts. Fat cells die approximately 2 to 5 days following the ischemic event. However, the death of fat cells may not immediately alter their signal intensity. The MRI patterns of bone infarcts depend on location, duration, and stage. The differential diagnosis of generalized bone and bone marrow diseases is discussed in Table 11.**1**.

Table 11.**1** Generalized bone and bone marrow disease

Disease	MRI Findings	Comments
Osteosclerosis (Fig. 11.5)	Diffuse or disseminated areas of decreased signal intensity on all pulse sequences corresponding to the radiographically diffuse or disseminated areas of osteosclerosis.	In renal osteodystrophy, sickle cell disease, osteoblastic metastases, myelofibrosis, mastocytosis (focal or diffuse mast cell proliferation in the bone marrow associated with osteoblastic or, less commonly, osteolytic lesions), fluorosis, osteopetrosis, Paget disease, fibrous dysplasia, and neurofibromatosis.
Hemochromatosis and hemosiderosis (Fig. 11.6)	Iron deposition in the reticuloendothelial system decreases signal intensity, preferentially in the axial (red marrow) skeleton on all image sequences, but may be first apparent on gradient-echo (GRE) imaging. Iron overload in spleen and liver producing decreased signal intensities on all imaging sequences may also be seen.	*Primary* hematochromatosis occurs predominantly in males between 40 and 60 years of age presenting with the classical triad of cirrhosis, skin pigmentation, and diabetes. Iron overload is caused by excessive absorption and retention of iron in liver (hepatocytes), pancreas, heart and pituitary gland. *Hemosiderosis* is much more common and associated with an increased intake and accumulation of iron (e.g., in hemolytic anemias and multiple blood transfusions). Iron overload is primarily located in the reticuloendothelial system (RES) of the spleen, liver (Kupffer cells) and bone marrow. Arthropathy of hemochromatosis is virtually identical to that of pseudogout (calcium pyrophosphate deposition disease, CPPD). In *AIDS* increased amounts of iron in the bone marrow may explain a decreased signal intensity in the vertebral bodies.
Radiation therapy (Figs. 11.7, 11.8)	In the first few weeks mild marrow edema presents with decreased signal intensity on T1WI and increased signal intensity on T2WI. Between weeks 3 and 6 the vertebral marrow becomes either mottled and heterogeneous or displays a central fatty component. Progression to either homogeneous fatty replacement or a pattern of central fat with peripheral zones of lower signal intensity (representing hematopoietic marrow) may subsequently be evident. Marrow abnormalities are limited to the field of radiation and sharply demarcated.	Radiation-induced bone marrow changes depend on the dose and time course. Irradiation may initially cause a mild marrow edema, followed subsequently by a decrease in hematopoietic marrow and compensatory increase in fatty marrow. Full recovery of the hematopoietic marrow following irradiation requires 10 years or longer. *Bone infarction* frequently occurs in the appendicular skeleton and is confined to the field of radiation.
Chemotherapy	In hematologic malignant diseases the affected bone marrow becomes progressively more hyperintense on T1WI, reflecting the decrease in both neoplastic and normal hematopoietic cells. When the remission is stabilized, the bone marrow signal intensity may return to normal due to recovery of the normal hematopoietic cells. Against the background of normal marrow, relapses become evident as focal or diffuse regions of decreased signal intensity on T1WI.	A gradual increase in the fatty bone marrow fraction occurs in both the normal hematopoietic bone marrow and the neoplastic marrow responding to therapy. These changes are usually more obvious in the pathologic bone marrow, where the initial fat fraction is markedly reduced.
Bone marrow transplantation	On T1WI peripheral zones of intermediate signal intensity, representing regenerating hematopoietic cells, and a central zone of high signal intensity, representing fat, are characteristically found in the vertebral bodies. Reciprocal changes are seen on STIR images (hyperintense peripheral and hypointense central zones). Differentiation between repopulation with normal hematopoietic cells and recurrent disease is, however, not possible by MRI.	High dose chemotherapy and/or total body radiotherapy preceding the transplantation results in myeloid (hematopoietic) cell depletion of the bone marrow and its transformation from red to yellow marrow. Approximately 2 weeks after transplantation small islands of regenerating hematopoietic cells are present at biopsy.
Aplastic anemia	Fatty marrow is found in the entire skeleton, including spine and pelvis. Changes are most apparent in areas normally containing red marrow. Small scattered foci of decreased signal intensity on T1WI represent nests of residual hematopoietic marrow.	Uncommon idiopathic or acquired (pharmacological, chemical, or viral exposure) condition characterized by an acellular or hypocellular bone marrow and pancytopenia (anemia, neutropenia, and thrombocytopenia).

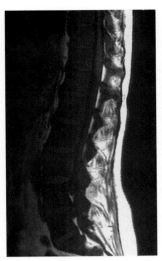

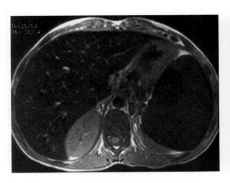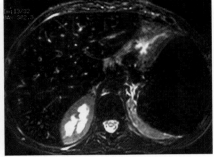

a   b

Fig. 11.**6**   **Hemosiderosis secondary to multiple blood transfusions.** Markedly decreased signal intensity is seen in the spine, grossly enlarged spleen and liver (**a**: PDWI. **b**: T2WI, FS).

Fig. 11.**5**   **Osteosclerosis.** Diffuse decreased signal intensity is seen in the spine caused by osteoblastic breast carcinoma metastases (T1WI, sagittal).

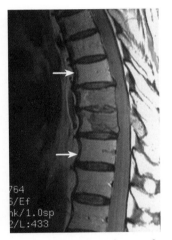

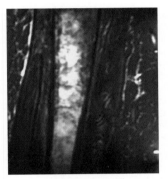

Fig. 11.**8**   **Bone infarct (acute) secondary to radiation of soft-tissue sarcoma.** The marked heterogeneous increased signal intensity in the femur is limited to the radiation field (coronal, STIR).

Fig. 11.**7**   **Radiation therapy for multiple myeloma.** Fatty marrow replacement is seen in the vertebral bodies (arrows) adjacent to two vertebral bodies involved with multiple myeloma (sagittal, T1WI).

Table 11.**1** (Cont.) Generalized bone and bone marrow disease

Disease	MRI Findings	Comments
Sickle cell anemia (Figs. 11.**9**, 11.**10**)	Combination of marrow reconversion and bone infarcts are characteristic. Depending upon the degree of cellularity the red marrow hyperplasia produces a decrease in signal intensity on T1WI that may be equal or slightly lower than muscle, and an increase in signal intensity on T2WI that can exceed fatty marrow. Reconversion to red marrow in the appendicular skeleton progresses from the metaphyses towards the diaphyses and eventually may also involve the epiphyses. The appearance of reconversion progresses from spotty to geographic and eventually diffuse homogeneous involvement. Superimposed acute infarct is evident as areas of intense signal intensity on T2WI, whereas chronic infarcts are hypointense on T2WI, reflecting fibrosis and sclerosis. Hemosiderosis may also contribute in an advanced stage to a loss of signal intensity on all pulse sequences.	Sickle cell disease is characterized by the presence of sickle cell hemoglobin (HbS) and includes sickle cell anemia (HbS-S), sickle cell trait (HbA-S) and diseases in which HbS is combined with another abnormal hemoglobin. The sickle cell trait is present in approximately 7% of North American blacks and sickle cell anemia occurs in approximately 1% of North American blacks. In sickle cell crisis deformation of red blood cells produces vaso-occlusion, ischemia, and necrosis. Osseous pain frequently is related to bone marrow infarction. The *hand-foot syndrome* refers to an infarct in small tubular bones of children between 6 months and 2 years of age. Osteomyelitis (staphylococcus and salmonella) is a frequent complication and difficult to differentiate from infarction.
Thalassemia (Figs. 11.**11** and 11.**11***)	Extensive red marrow hyperplasia and reconversion from fatty to hematopoietic marrow is associated with characteristic bony changes. In the skull widening of the diploic space with thinning of the outer table and severe hair-on-end appearance and sparring of the occiput below the internal protuberance are characteristic. In the chest expansion of the ribs (especially posterior aspects) with thinned cortices and extramedullary hematopoiesis presenting as a paravertebral mass with red marrow signal characteristics are common. In the appendicular skeleton reconverted red marrow, widening of the tubular bones with thinned cortices and Erlenmeyer flask deformities are characteristic. Hemosiderosis decreasing the signal intensity in the bone marrow, spleen, and liver (the latter two are usually enlarged) may also be evident.	Thalassemia major (Cooley anemia, homozygous beta-thalassemia) is characterized by severe anemia and prominent hepatosplenomegaly. The disease becomes manifest in infancy and affects people from Mediterranean descent, especially Italians and Greeks. Thalassemia minor (heterozygous beta-thalassemia) generally is associated with mild clinical findings. *Hereditary spherocytosis* is a hemolytic disease most common in northern Europeans and presents with similar but much less severe bone and marrow changes than thalassemia major. *In iron deficiency anemia* marrow hyperplasia may produce mild skeletal abnormalities, especially in infants and young children.
Polycythemia vera (primary polycythemia)	Partial or complete reconversion of fatty to hematopoietic marrow is evident on T1WI as zones of intermediate to low signal intensity in areas in which fatty marrow is expected. On T2WI the signal intensity of the marrow varies depending on the degree of cellularity and myelofibrosis.	Polycythemia vera is characterized by a benign hyperplasia of all cellular elements in the bone marrow (primarily red blood cells). It usually occurs in middle-aged or elderly patients, predominantly men. Vascular thrombosis and, less often, bleeding are recognized complications. In the later stages of the disease myelofibrosis, myeloid metaplasia, and anemia may develop.
Myelofibrosis (Fig. 11.**12**)	Combination of bone marrow fibrosis and reconversion of fatty to hematopoietic marrow is characteristic. Marrow fibrosis, evident by decreased signal intensity on both T1WI and T2WI may be focal or diffuse and is initially located in the spine, pelvis, and ribs (sites of active hematopoiesis in the adult). Reconversion of fatty to hematopoietic occurs in tubular bones, especially femora, humeri, and tibia, and eventually is followed by marrow fibrosis also. Hepatosplenomegaly is a constant finding and paravertebral extramedullary hematopoiesis may be associated.	Myelofibrosis (myelosclerosis, agnogenic myeloid metaplasia, pseudoleukemia) is characterized by bone marrow fibrosis and sclerosis and extramedullary hematopoiesis. Most affected patients are in the sixth or seventh decade of life. The onset is usually insidious and clinical findings include moderate to severe anemia and splenomegaly. Disease severity can be monitored by serum lactate dehydrogenase (LDH) and cholesterol levels. Radiographically bone sclerosis is evident in approximately half of the patients and most commonly affects spine, pelvis, skull, ribs, and proximal humerus and femur.

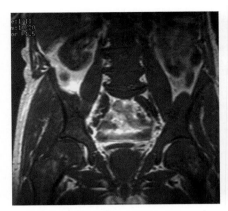

Fig. 11.**9**   **Sickle cell anemia.** Decreased signal intensity due to iron overload is seen in the spine, pelvis, and proximal femora (coronal, T1WI).

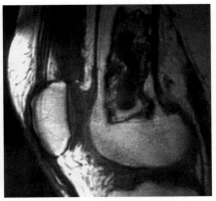

Fig. 11.**10**   **Bone infarct (chronic) in sickle cell anemia.** A large bone infarct is seen in the distal femur metaphysis (sagittal, T1WI).

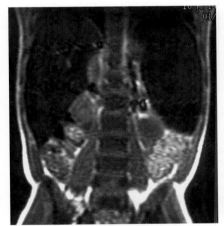

Fig. 11.**11**   **Thalassemia major.** Decreased signal intensity is seen in the axial skeleton and markedly enlarged spleen and liver due to iron overload (coronal, T1WI).

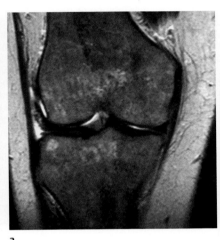

a

Fig. 11.**11***   **Thalassemia minor.** Reconversion of yellow to red marrow is seen in the distal femur and proximal tibia epiphyses,

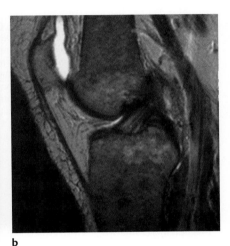

b

producing a characteristic mottled appearance (**a**: coronal, **b**: sagittal, GRE [T2WI]).

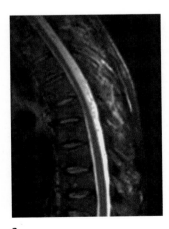

a

Fig. 11.**12**   **Myelofibrosis.** **a** Diffuse decreased signal intensity is seen in the thoracic spine, which has a mottled appearance (T2WI).

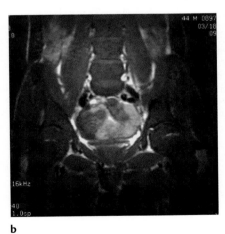

b

b Marked decreased signal intensity is seen in the lumbar spine, pelvis, and both femoral heads and necks, except for both greater trochanters and part of the original physis between femoral head and neck (T1WI).

Table 11.**1** (Cont.) Generalized bone and bone marrow disease

Disease	MRI Findings	Comments
Leukemia (Fig. 11.13)	Leukemic bone marrow infiltrates tend to be diffuse and preferentially located in the red marrow containing bones (axial skeleton in the adults). Patchy infiltrates are less common, except in acute myelogenous leukemia. Leukemic infiltrates present with a decrease in signal intensity on T1WI. Changes in T2WI are more variable and less conspicuous, though an appreciable increase in signal intensity is occasionally evident. Compared with T2WI, STIR sequences improve the visualization of the leukemic process. Response to chemotherapy is evident by an increase in signal intensity on T1WI and eventual return to a normal bone marrow pattern (for additional information see under **Chemotherapy** in this table). *Chloromas* (granulocytic sarcomas) present as single or multiple leukemic mass lesions most commonly associated with acute myelogenous leukemia, especially in children.	Leukemias cannot only be classified in acute and chronic forms, but also according to their phenotypes in myelogenous and lymphoblastic types. Acute leukemias can affect both children and adults. Chronic leukemias usually are diagnosed after age 35. Radiographic bony abnormalities include osteoporosis, radiolucent, and radiodense metaphyseal bands, and osteolytic lesions and are found in 50 to 70% of acute childhood leukemias, occasionally in acute adult leukemia, and rarely in chronic leukemia.
Lymphoma (Fig. 11.14)	Lymphomatous bone marrow infiltration tends to be focal or patchy or, less frequently, diffuse. Infiltrates are hypointense on T1WI and more variable, but usually hyperintense and often inhomogeneous on T2WI. STIR imaging is more sensitive than T2WI in the discrimination of lymphoma from red marrow. In long bones epiphyseal and metaphyseal location with tendency to spread into the nearby joint or soft tissue is not unusual. Magnetic resonance imaging allows differentiation between vertebral, paraspinal, and epidural involvement.	Lymphomas present with lymphadenopathy, splenomegaly, or hepatosplenomegaly. Bony involvement is usually secondary, indicating a tumor stage IV. Primary bone involvement occasionally occurs with non-Hodgkin lymphoma, usually of the histiocytic type. *Non-Hodgkin lymphoma* is three times more common than Hodgkin disease. Radiographically osteolytic or mixed osteolytic-osteoblastic lesions may be evident. *Hodgkin disease* involves primarily the axial skeleton. Osteosclerosis (e.g., ivory vertebra), osteolysis, or a mixed pattern may be present radiographically. *Burkitt lymphoma* is a stem cell lymphoma commonly occurring in children and AIDS patients. Radiographically osteolytic lesions may be found and are particularly characteristic in the facial bones.
Multiple myeloma (Fig. 11.15)	Myelomatous bone marrow involvement tends to be multifocal or patchy, or, less frequently, diffuse. Preferential axial skeleton involvement, often with asymmetric distribution, is common. Focal lesions are hypointense to normal bone marrow on T1WI and hyperintense on T2WI. In diffuse myelomatous involvement the signal intensity in the vertebral bodies approaches that of muscle. On STIR images multiple myeloma is of high signal intensity, occasionally allowing detection of small tumor foci that escape visualization on spin echo sequences. In contrast to the normal bone marrow in the adult considerable contrast enhancement occurs in multiple myeloma. Focal lesions responding to therapy may no longer enhance or demonstrate only peripheral (rim) enhancement. Successfully treated myelomatous lesions may also present as hypointense foci on unenhanced T2WI.	Usually occurs in patients over 40 years old. Laboratory findings include a markedly elevated erythrocyte sedimentation rate, an abnormal IgG or IgA globulin fraction (serum immunoelectrophoresis) in 90%, and Bence-Jones proteinuria in 50% of patients. Radiographically, osteolytic lesions are common in the skull, sternum (pathological fractures), vertebral bodies (often sparing the posterior elements), distal clavicle, acromion, glenoid, and ulnar olecranon. *Waldenström macroglobulinemia* presents clinically, radiographically, and on MRI similar to multiple myeloma, but an abnormal IgM globulin fraction is present on immunoelectrophoresis.

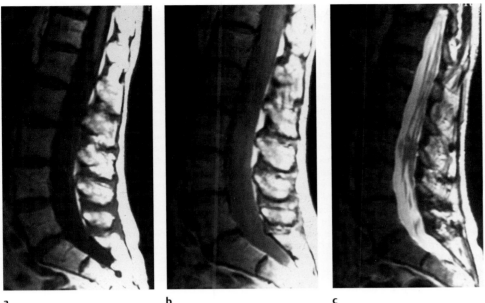

a   b   c

Fig. 11.**13** **Leukemia.** Diffuse involvement of the spine with overall decreased signal intensity is seen (**a**: T1WI. **b**: PDWI, both sagittal). The leukemic leptomeningeal infiltrates are best appreciated in **c** (T2WI, sagittal).

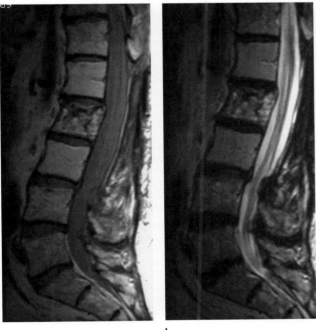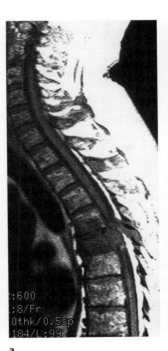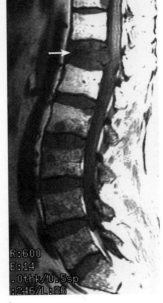

a   b   a   b

Fig. 11.**14** **Non-Hodgkin lymphoma.** Patchy involvement of all vertebral bodies with heterogeneous signal intensity is seen, except in L1 and L3, which depict a homogeneous increased signal intensity due to prior radiation therapy (**a**: sagittal, PDWI. **b**: sagittal, T2WI).

Fig. 11.**15** **Multiple myeloma.** Diffuse involvement of the entire spine, ranging from tiny hypointense foci to complete replacement of an entire vertebral body (arrow) is seen (**a, b**: sagittal, T1WI).

Table 11.1 (Cont.) Generalized bone and bone marrow disease

Disease	MRI Findings	Comments
Metastases (Figs. 11.16, 11.17)	Single or, more commonly, multiple focal lesions with preferential involvement of the axial skeleton usually present with decreased signal intensity on T1WI. Osteolytic metastases are hyperintense on T2WI, but osteoblastic metastases may be isointense or even hypointense to bone marrow. Similarly, successfully treated metastases may appear hypointense on both T1WI and T2WI. A rim of high signal intensity around a lower signal marrow lesion ("halo" sign) on T2WI suggests metastatic disease, whereas a focus of high signal intensity within a lesion of low signal intensity on T1WI ("bull's eye" sign) indicates a fatty marrow island. Melanoma metastases occasionally are hyperintense on T1WI. They have to be differentiated in the hematopoietic marrow from normal fatty deposits which are quite common.	Metastatic bone disease is approximately 100 times more common than a primary bone tumor. Breast, prostate, lung, kidney, and thyroid are the most common primary sites of bony metastases. Breast carcinoma metastases are lytic, mixed, or sclerotic, often extensive, and frequently associated with pathological fractures. Prostatic carcinoma metastases are usually osteoblastic, rarely lytic, and often extensive. Lung carcinoma metastases are usually lytic, occasionally mixed, rarely osteoblastic, and sometimes expansile. Kidney and thyroid carcinoma metastases are invariably lytic, often solitary and expansile. Metastases in children commonly originate from neuroblastoma, Ewing sarcoma, osteosarcoma, and soft-tissue sarcomas.
Gaucher disease	An inhomogeneous or, less commonly, homogeneous decrease in signal intensity in the axial and proximal appendicular skeleton on both T1WI and T2WI is usually present. The patterns suggest marrow replacement by fibrosis and Gaucher cells. Epiphyses are generally spared by the disease itself, but avascular necrosis of the proximal femur epiphyses is a frequent complication. An increase in signal intensity of the bone marrow on T2WI may rarely be caused by the disease itself, but especially when associated with bone pain, indicates a complication such as an acute bone infarct or, less commonly, osteomyelitis. Chronic infarcts demonstrating low signal intensity on both T1WI and T2WI are frequently also found.	Gaucher disease is a rare metabolic disorder leading to the accumulation of abnormal lipids (cerebrosides) in the reticuloendothelial system (RES) (Gaucher cells). Recessive inheritance, hepatosplenomegaly, and deficient acid beta-glucosidase are common to all three types. Type I (chronic nonneuropathic or adult type) is most frequent, occurs in Ashkenazic Jews, becomes manifest in childhood and progressively worsens. Type 2 (acute neuropathic or infantile type) is usually fatal within the first 2 years. Type 3 (subacute neuropathic or juvenile type) is associated with neurological and skeletal manifestations. Radiographically the combination of avascular necrosis of the femoral head, bone infarcts, and cystic lesions in the femur shaft and Erlenmeyer flask deformity of the distal femur is virtually diagnostic. *Niemann-Pick disease* is characterized by widespread accumulation of sphingomyelin in the RES and may present on MRI in a similar fashion.
Osteomyelitis (Fig. 11.18)	Usually solitary, but occasionally multiple or disseminated foci of decreased signal intensity on T1WI and increased signal intensity on T2WI. After intravenous Gd-DTPA diffuse or peripheral (rim) enhancement may be seen.	May be associated with reduced cellular or humoral immunity (e.g., *bacillary angiomatosis in AIDS*). *Chronic recurrent multifocal osteomyelitis (CRMO)* is a subacute or chronic osteomyelitis of unknown cause occurring in childhood, with symmetric involvement at multiple sites.
Osteonecrosis (bone infarct) (Fig. 11.19)	Bone infarcts may be solitary or multiple and are preferentially located in the metadiaphyses of long bones. Acute infarcts appear as circumscribed, usually inhomogeneous areas of low signal intensity on T1WI and of high signal intensity on T2WI owing to edema, hyperemia, and granulation tissue. Subacute infarcts tend to be heterogeneous and characteristically depict a serpiginous outline of low signal intensity on T1WI and of high signal intensity on T2WI. Chronic infarcts demonstrate low signal intensity on both T1WI and T2WI due to fibrosis and calcifications.	Osteonecrosis can be divided into avascular necrosis involving the subarticular bone (see Table 10.1) and bone infarction occurring more frequently in the metadiaphyseal regions of long bones than axial skeleton. Favored anatomical sites include femora, humeri, and tibia. Multiple bone infarcts are common in sickle cell disease, vasculitis (e.g., lupus erythematosus), hypercortisolism, chemotherapy, Gaucher disease, caisson disease, and pancreatitis, and are often associated with avascular necrosis.

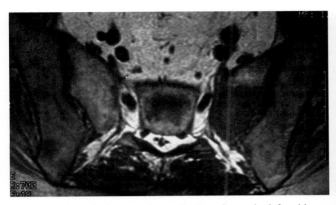

Fig. 11.16 Osteolytic metastases. Scattered, poorly defined hypointense foci are seen in the pelvis and sacrum with the largest lesion being located in the left sacral wing adjacent to the sacro-iliac joint (T1WI, coronal).

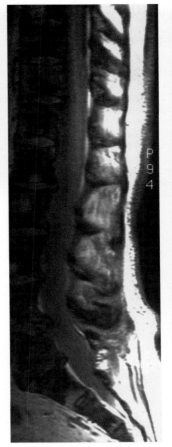

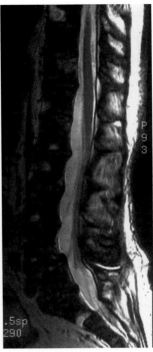

Fig. 11.17 Prostatic carcinoma metastases. An overall decreased signal intensity is seen in the spine, caused by sclerosis with numerous hyperintense foci interspersed (**a**: PDWI; **b**: T2WI, both sagittal).

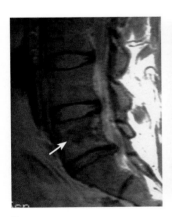

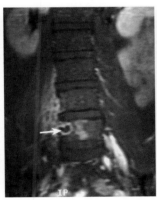

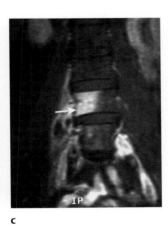

a   b   c

Fig. 11.18 Osteomyelitis (tuberculous in AIDS). a A solitary hypodense lesion (arrow) is seen in L5 (sagittal, PDWI). **b** After intravenous Gd-DTPA administration marked enhancement of the focus in L5 (arrow) and the paravertebral soft-tissue extension is evident (coronal, T1WI, FS, +C). **c** In a more anterior plane a second osteomyelitis focus, not appreciated on precontrast examination, is visualized in L4 (arrow) after contrast enhancement (coronal, T1WI, FS, +C).

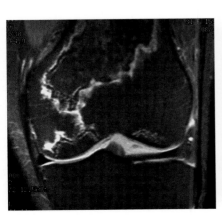

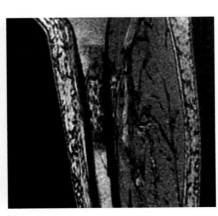

a   b

Fig. 11.19 Osteonecrosis. Bone infarcts in the distal femur with extension into the subchondral bone of the lateral condyle and in the tibia shaft are seen. A small heterogeneous focus of increased signal intensity in the subchondral bone of the medial femur condyle represents early avascular necrosis in that location (**a**: coronal, STIR. **b**: sagittal, spoiled GRE).

Table 11.**1** (Cont.) Generalized bone and bone marrow disease

Disease	MRI Findings	Comments
Reflex sympathetic dystrophy (RSD) (Fig. 11.20)	Bone marrow edema pattern presenting with patchy to uniform decrease in signal intensity on T1WI and corresponding increase in signal intensity on T2WI. Involvement of upper extremity (shoulder-hand syndrome) is more common than lower extremity. It may be bilateral, but then it is much more pronounced on one side. The marrow edema is most severe in the para-articular regions, but its extent is variable. Soft tissue adjacent to the bone marrow involvement may demonstrate signs of edema and/or inflammation.	Reflex sympathetic dystrophy (Sudeck atrophy) is a poorly understood condition that may be initiated by trauma, cerebrovascular and neurological disorders, myocardial infarcts, and malignant neoplasms. Clinical presentation includes stiffness, pain, tenderness, and weakness in an extremity associated with swelling, vasomotor changes, hyperesthesia, and disability. The duration of RSD varies, lasting in some cases for years or even becoming irreversible. Radiographic findings include para-articular osteoporosis and soft-tissue swelling.

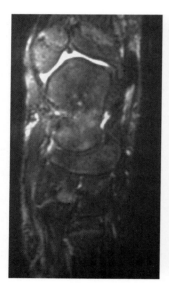
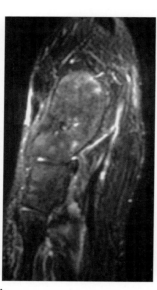
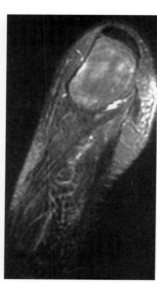

a b c

Fig. 11.**20** **Reflex sympathetic dystrophy (RSD).** Patchy increased signal intensity is seen in the ankle and tarsal bones. Small ankle joint effusion and edematous changes in the surrounding soft tissues is also evident (**a**, **b**, and **c**: T2WI, FS, coronal, 3 different planes from ankle to calcaneus).

12 Localized Bone and Bone Marrow Disease

Conventional radiography remains the primary imaging modality for the evaluation of skeletal lesions. The combination of conventional radiography, which has a high specificity but only an intermediate sensitivity, with radionuclide bone scanning, which has a high sensitivity but only a low specificity, is still the most effective method for detecting and diagnosing bone lesions and differentiating between benign and malignant conditions. Conventional radiography is, however, limited in delineating the intramedullary extent of a bone lesion and even more so in demonstrating soft-tissue involvement.

Although magnetic resonance imaging (MRI) frequently contributes to the characterization of a bony lesion, its greatest value lies in the ability to accurately assess the intramedullary and extraosseous extent of a skeletal lesion. Compared with CT, MRI is superior in the evaluation of bone lesions because of direct multiplanar imaging capability, greater soft-tissue contrast, and improved tissue characterization based on signal behavior on different pulse sequences and relaxation parameters. Computed tomography allows better evaluation of matrix calcification or ossification, cortical violation, and periosteal reactions when compared with MRI.

On MRI most tumors are of low signal intensity on T1WI and of high signal intensity on T2WI. *High signal intensity on T1WI* suggests fat or a subacute hemorrhage. *Low signal intensity on T2WI* may be caused by fibrosis, sclerosis, calcifications, hemosiderin deposition (chronic hemorrhage), flowing blood, gas, and metal artifacts.

Differentiation between a benign and malignant bone lesion is not always possible. Signs of an aggressive or malignant osseous lesion include rapid growth, large size, poor demarcation, cortical violation, soft-tissue extension, and an inhomogeneous signal intensity on T2WI. Signs of a nonaggressive or benign osseous lesion include slow growth, small size, sharp margination, cortical expansion without cortical violation, solid periosteal reaction, no soft-tissue extension, and homogeneous signal intensity on T2WI. However, these MRI features are not infallible and many exceptions occur, indicating the need for histologic confirmation in the appropriate setting.

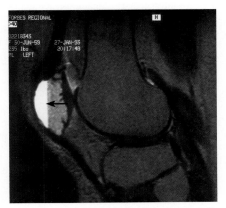

Fig. 12.**1** **Aneurysmal bone cyst in patella.** A fluid-fluid level (arrow) is seen in the expanded patella (T2WI, sagittal).

After *intravenous gadolinium-based contrast medium administration* the normal bone marrow in the adult does not enhance or demonstrates minimal marrow enhancement at best. In young children, however, marked marrow enhancement is sometimes evident. The complete absence of contrast enhancement in a bone lesion indicates benignancy. Enhancement occurs in vascularized benign tumors, malignant tumors, osteomyelitis, inflammation, and granulation tissue. Necrotic centers of neoplasms, infarcts, and abscesses do not enhance, but peripheral enhancement (ring enhancement) occurs in these conditions.

Fluid levels (Fig. 12.**1**) in osseous lesions are most commonly associated with simple (unicameral) and aneurysmal bone cysts, but may occasionally also be found in chondroblastomas, giant cell tumors, and telangiectatic osteosarcomas, whereas both fat-fluid and gas-fluid levels in bone lesions are indicative of acute osteomyelitis. Pneumatocysts are cystic bone lesions containing gas alone or may demonstrate a gas-fluid level. They most commonly are located in the ilium adjacent to the sacroiliac joint. The differential diagnosis of localized bone and bone marrow lesions is discussed in Table 12.**1**.

Table 12.**1** Localized bone and bone marrow lesions

Disease	MRI Findings	Comments
Normal variants	"Bull's-eye" sign: Islands of normal fatty bone marrow presenting on T1WI as areas of high signal intensity surrounded by hematopoietic bone marrow of intermediate signal intensity against the background of fatty marrow. Focal fatty deposits in hematopoietic marrow are common, appearing hyperintense on T1WI and isointense or slightly hyperintense on T2WI.	Hematopoietic marrow islands surrounded by fatty marrow may represent a normal variation or, when more extensive, may be part of a yellow to red marrow reconversion process. They appear hypointense on T1WI and isointense or slightly hypointense on T2WI. They may be difficult to differentiate from neoplastic lesions, unless the latter appear hyperintense on T2WI. A "halo" sign, defined as a rim of high signal intensity about a lesion on T2WI, is indicative of a metastatic lesion.
Subchondral cyst (synovial cyst, geode) (Fig. 12.2)	Single or multiple subchondral lesions measuring up to 3 cm in diameter, usually hypointense on T1WI and hyperintense on T2WI, but greatly variable depending on the composition of the content (synovial fluid, proteinaceous material, loose myxoid, adipose or fibrous tissue, rarely gas). A fibrous or sclerotic capsule may be evident as a peripheral ring void of signals. Communication with an arthritic joint may be seen.	Associated with osteoarthritis (primary and posttraumatic, rheumatoid arthritis, avascular necrosis, and calcium pyrophosphate dihydrate crystal deposition disease (CPPD).
Intraosseous ganglion (Fig. 12.3)	Unilocular or, less commonly multilocular, sharply demarcated juxta-articular lesion presenting with low signal intensity on T1WI and high signal intensity on T2WI. A sclerotic margin may be seen as a thin signalless rim surrounding the lesion. An extraosseous component may be associated. Preferred locations include medial malleolus of tibia, femoral head, acetabulum, and carpal bones. Characteristically the lesion does not communicate with the joint.	Histologically the ganglion contains thick, gelatinous material. A *herniation pit* (Fig. 12.**4**) in the anterolateral surface of the proximal femoral neck is caused by ingrowth of synovial, fibrous, and cartilaginous elements through a perforation in the cortex. It usually measures less than 1 cm in diameter and is stable. It may occasionally enlarge, possibly related to changing mechanics. On MRI a focus of low signal intensity on T1WI and high signal intensity on T2WI consistent with fluid or, less commonly, low signal intensity consistent with fibrous tissue is seen.
Echinococcosis	Complex cystic lesions within bone and adjacent soft tissues with mixed low signal intensity on T1WI and mixed high signal intensity on T2WI due to presence of proteinaceous and cellular debris. Considerable contrast enhancement occurs in capsule and internal septation. Preferred locations include pelvis, vertebral column and adjacent ribs, skull, and long bones.	Caused by *Echinococcus granulosus* (hydatid disease) or, less commonly, *Echinococcus multilocularis*. Cysts may develop in various viscera, particularly the liver and the lungs. Calcification of cyst wall is common, except in lungs. Bone lesions occur in 1 to 2 % of echinococcosis. Radiographically single or multiple expansile cystic lesions containing trabeculation are seen. Cortical violation and soft-tissue mass formation, often with calcifications, may be associated.
Simple (unicameral) bone cyst (Fig. 12.5)	Centrally located, slightly expansile cystic lesion with cortical thinning and low signal intensity on T1WI and high signal intensity on T2WI is characteristic. Preferred locations in children are the metaphyses of long tubular bones (especially humerus and femur) and in adults the calcaneus and ilium of the pelvis. Diaphyseal cysts in long bones are frequently multiloculated. Fluid-fluid levels are common. Gas or gas-fluid levels are occasionally found in pneumatocysts. After intravenous Gd-DTPA administration enhancement of the cyst wall and internal septations occurs.	Radiographically a centrally located osteolytic lesion with cortical thinning and mild osseous expansion is characteristic. In long tubular bones of children the metaphyseal cyst is juxtaposed to the physis and has an elongated shape paralleling the bone axis. Diaphyseal cysts are often large, multiloculated, and expansile. A pathologic fracture is common. The fracture fragment within the cyst drops to the dependent portion of the lesion ("fallen fragment" sign).

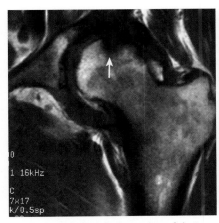

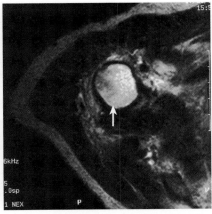

Fig. 12.**2** **Subchondral cyst (geode).** A cystic lesion (arrow) is seen in the subchondral femoral head (T1WI, coronal).

Fig. 12.**3** **Intraosseous ganglion.** A cystic lesion (arrow) is seen in the humeral neck. The irregular, hypointense foci within the lesion were caused by intracystic debris (T2WI).

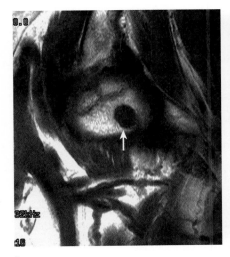

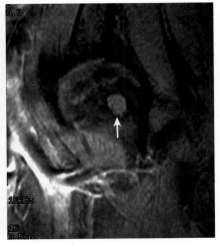

a

b

Fig. 12.**4** **Herniation pit.** A cystic lesion (arrows) is seen in the anterolateral femoral neck, which is characteristic (**a**: T1WI. **b**: T2WI, both sagittal).

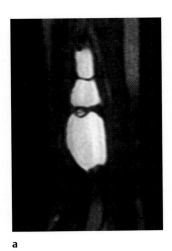

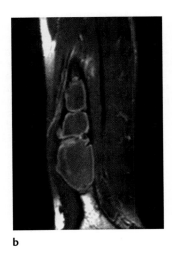

a

b

Fig. 12.**5** **Simple bone cyst.** An expansile, multiloculated, cystic lesion with high signal intensity and thinned cortex is seen in the diaphysis of the humerus in **a**: (T2WI, coronal). After intravenous Gd-DTPA administration enhancement of the cyst wall is evident in **b** (T1WI, +C, coronal).

Table 12.**1** (Cont.) Localized bone and bone marrow lesions

Disease	MRI Findings	Comments
Aneurysmal bone cyst (Figs. 12.6, 12.7**) (see also Fig.** 12.16**)**	An eccentric, expansile and often septated lesion with bubbly appearance is typical in the metaphyses of long tubular bones. Central location with symmetric expansion is more common in the short tubular bones of the hands and feet. In the spine the lesion involves the posterior elements with or without the adjacent vertebral body. The pelvis is another common location. On T1WI the lesion has an inhomogeneous appearance with an overall low signal intensity. Focal areas of higher signal intensity may be caused by methemoglobin. On T2WI the lesion demonstrates multiple cystic compartments, often with diverticular outpouchings, of variable high signal intensity. One or several fluid-fluid levels are commonly present. The lesion may be surrounded by a rim of low signal intensity on all image sequences, corresponding to an osseous shell. An extraosseous extension occasionally may simulate a malignancy. After intravenous Gd-DTPA, variable inhomogeneous contrast enhancement of the lesion is found.	Approximately 80 % of aneurysmal bone cysts are found in patients below age 20. Radiographically an eccentric, osteolytic, occasionally trabeculated lesion in a metaphysis of a long tubular bone represents the classic appearance. Sclerosis at the site where the periosteum is lifted by the lesion ("buttressing") is quite characteristic. Secondary aneurysmal bone cysts are associated with other skeletal lesions including giant cell tumor, chondroblastoma, osteoblastoma, telangiectatic osteosarcoma, malignant fibrous histiocytoma, fibrous dysplasia, and Paget disease.
Epidermoid (inclusion cyst)	Well-marginated, homogeneous or, less frequently, heterogeneous lesion of decreased signal intensity on T1WI and increased signal intensity on T2WI occurring in the skull and terminal phalanges of the hand. In the skull any bone can be affected, but the frontal and parietal bones are the most common locations. Skull lesions usually measure 1 to 5 cm in diameter and may be limited to the diploic space or extend through one or both tables. In the terminal phalanges of the hand the lesion is expansile, causing cortical thinning or destruction, but rarely exceeds 2 cm in diameter.	Usually observed in the second to fourth decades of life. A history of trauma is frequently present, suggesting intraosseous implantation of ectodermal tissue with subsequent development of the epidermoid. In the skull an irregularly shaped button sequestrum is usually present in larger lesions on radiographs and CT. Histologically the cysts are lined with a stratified squamous epithelium supported by a dense fibrous tissue stroma and covered by a hyperkeratotic layer that blends with the debris in the center of the cyst.
Glomus tumor	Well-marginated heterogeneous lesion (salt-and-pepper appearance caused by hypervascularity) occurring in the tuft of a finger or the temporal bone. The lesion is hypointense on T1WI and hyperintense on T2WI, measures usually less than 1 cm in diameter and demonstrates marked contrast enhancement.	Glomus tumors occur in patients of any age, typically are neither palpable nor visible, and present in the fingertips with aching pain and point tenderness. Secondary bone involvement from a soft-tissue glomus tumor is much more common than primary interosseous manifestation, which is limited to the distal phalanx.
Lipoma	Osteolytic lesion often with sclerotic margin demonstrating high signal intensity on T1WI and intermediate to high signal intensity on T2WI. Intratumoral calcifications or ossifications presenting as low density foci may be associated.	Intraosseous lipomas occur most commonly in the metaphyses of the long tubular bones, especially the fibula, femur, and tibia, and in the calcaneus. *Liposarcomas* rarely arise in bone.
Hemangioma	Usually solitary lesion, often with inhomogeneous areas of high signal intensity on both T1WI and T2WI due to fat or methemoglobin accumulation. Extraosseous extension occurs, but typically does not contain fat and thus appears hypointense on T1WI and hyperintense on T2WI. Lesions demonstrate marked contrast enhancement after intravenous Gd-DTPA. Most common sites of involvement are spine and skull.	Usually found in patients over age 40 with female predominance. Radiographically a coarse vertical trabecular pattern ("corduroy" appearance) in the vertebral body is characteristic. In the skull a slightly expansile osteolytic lesion with lattice-like or radiating ("sunburst") pattern is seen. In *cystic angiomatosis* widespread cystic bone lesions appearing hypointense on T1WI, hyperintense or hypointense (when sclerotic) on T2WI, and marked contrast enhancement are frequently associated with visceral involvement.

Table 12.**1** (Cont.) Localized bone and bone marrow lesions

Disease	MRI Findings	Comments
Osteochondroma (Fig. 12.8)	Bony protuberance demonstrating cortical and medullary continuity with parent bone is diagnostic. In the tubular bones osteochondromas characteristically occur in the metaphyses and point away from the nearby articulation. The signal intensity of osteochondromas varies greatly depending on the amount of osseous and cartilaginous tumor tissue present. The mixed signal intensity tends to be low to intermediate on T1WI and intermediate to high on T2WI. The periphery of the lesion is covered by a hyaline cartilage cap of high signal intensity on T2WI. A cartilage cap of 1 cm or less in thickness indicates a benign lesion, whereas a cap thicker than 2 cm is suspicious of malignant transformation. Contrast enhancement in benign osteochondromas is limited to the fibrovascular tissue that may cover the nonenhancing cartilage cap. As a rare complication a bursa may be formed in this tissue and may become inflamed and painful, simulating malignant transformation.	Osteochondromas occur in children and adolescents as a slowly growing painless mass. They are intimately related to the physis and cease to enlarge with fusion of the adjacent growth plates. Rarely, osteochondromas may develop in the adult after injury or trauma. *Hereditary multiple exostoses* present with multiple osteochondromas in the axial and appendicular skeleton.

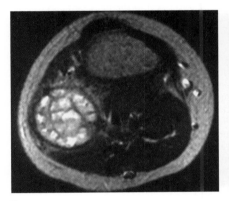
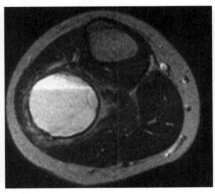
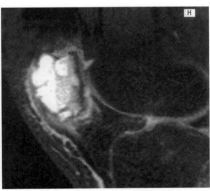

a　　　　　　　　　　**b**

Fig. 12.**6** **Aneurysmal bone cyst.** Markedly expansile lesion in the proximal fibula with trabeculated appearance and multiple small fluid-fluid levels in its superior pole (**a**: T2WI) and a large single fluid-fluid level in its central portion (**b**: T2WI).

Fig. 12.**7** **Aneurysmal bone cyst.** A heterogeneous lesion with multiple small fluid-fluid levels and small outpouchings is seen in the expanded patella (T2WI, FS, sagittal). Same case as Fig. 12.**1**.

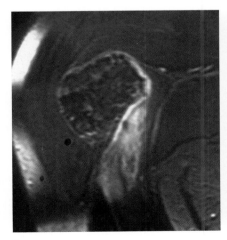
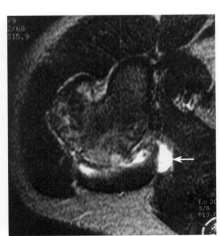

Fig. 12.**8** **Osteochondroma.** **a** A well-defined, heterogeneous lesion is seen originating from the posterolateral aspect of the proximal humerus shaft (coronal, T1WI). **b** The heterogeneous osteochondroma is covered by a layer of hyperintense soft tissue that is most conspicuous on the posterior aspect of the lesion with an inflamed bursa (arrow) posteromedially (axial, T2WI).

a　　　　　　　　　　**b**

Table 12.**1** (Cont.) Localized bone and bone marrow lesions

Disease	MRI Findings	Comments
Enchondroma (Fig. 12.9)	A lobulated intramedullary lesion of low signal intensity on T1WI and high signal intensity on T2WI is found. Small scattered areas of low signal intensity within the hyperintense lesion on T2WI correspond to foci of calcified cartilage and represent a typical finding in enchondroma. Preferred locations are the metaphyses of the long tubular bones and the diaphyses of the short tubular bones in hands and feet.	Enchondromas are usually discovered in the third or fourth decades of life as incidental finding or painless swelling. The presence of pain should arouse suspicion of malignant transformation. Radiographically enchondromas present as well-circumscribed osteolytic lesions with varying degrees of calcifications. *Enchondromatosis* (Ollier disease) is characterized by multiple, asymmetrically distributed enchondromas often in deformed tubular bones and pelvis.
Periosteal (juxtacortical) chondroma (Fig. 12.10)	Soft-tissue mass with erosion of the adjacent cortex and varying degree of periosteal reaction presents with low signal intensity on T1WI and high signal intensity on T2WI. Intratumoral calcified foci are characteristically present and may be appreciated as areas of signal void on T2WI. Moderate inhomogeneous and preferentially peripheral contrast enhancement is typical.	Metaphyses of long tubular bones and hands are most commonly involved. All ages are affected, but the tumor is usually diagnosed under age 30. Slight male predominance.
Chondroblastoma (Fig. 12.11)	Lobulated epiphyseal lesion presenting with low signal intensity on T1WI and variable intermediate signal intensity (hypointense or isointense to fat) on T2WI. The absence of high signal intensity on T2WI may relate to its prominent cellular stroma. Foci of high signal intensity within the lesion on T2WI are caused by hyaline cartilage formation or hemorrhage and foci of low signal intensity due to scattered calcifications. Periosteal thickening and edema in the adjacent bone marrow and soft tissue are relatively frequently associated. These findings should not be confused with tumor extension into these structures.	Benign cartilaginous lesion occurring between age 5 through 25 with slight male predominance. Radiographic features consist of an eccentrically or centrally located osteolytic lesion, often with a thin sclerotic rim, in the epiphysis or apophysis of a long tubular bone. Tumor calcifications are found in less than half of the cases. Approximately 10% of chondroblastomas occur in the hands and feet, with predilection for the talus and calcaneus.
Chondromyxoid fibroma (Fig. 12.12)	Eccentric metaphyseal lesion with cortical expansion, coarse trabeculation, endosteal scalloping, and marginal sclerosis presenting as lobulated mass with low to intermediate signal intensity on T1WI and intermediate to high signal intensity on T2WI. Marked inhomogeneous tumor enhancement is seen after intravenous Gd-DTPA.	Least common benign cartilaginous tumor, usually diagnosed in the second and third decade of life. Predilection for the metaphyses of long tubular bones. Radiographically an eccentric metaphyseal osteolytic lesion with cortical expansion, exuberant endosteal sclerosis, and coarse trabeculation is commonly seen. Destruction of the cortex resulting in a hemispherical osseous defect or "bite" without periosteal reaction is characteristic of larger chondromyxoid fibromas.
Periosteal (juxtacortical) desmoid	Cortical defect in the posteromedial aspect of the distal femur with increased signal intensity in the adjacent soft tissue on T2WI due to inflammation and edema.	Occurs between age 15 and 20 as sequelae of trauma at the adductor magnus tendon insertion. Radiographically a saucer-like defect often associated with sclerosis and periostitis is seen at this site.

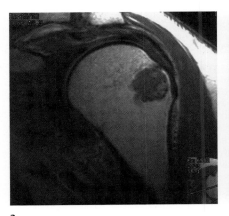

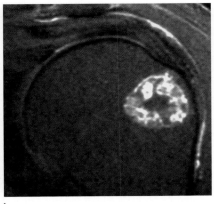

Fig. 12.**9** **Enchondroma.** Well-circumscribed heterogeneous lesion is seen in the humeral neck near the greater tuberosity (**a**: PDWI, coronal. **b**: T2WI, FS, coronal).

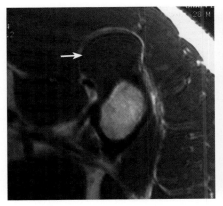

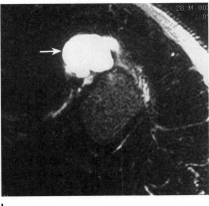

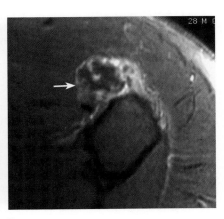

a   **b**   **c**

Fig. 12.**10** **Periosteal chondroma.** A juxtacortical lesion (arrow) is seen in the anterior proximal humoral shaft with homogeneous low signal intensity (isointense to muscle) in **a** (T1WI), and homogeneous high signal intensity in **b** (T2WI). After intravenous Gd-DTPA administration moderate inhomogeneous and mainly peripheral contrast enhancement is seen in **c** (T1WI, FS, +C).

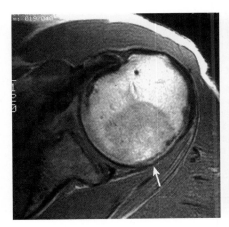

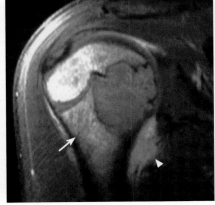

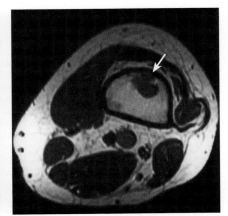

a

Fig. 12.**11** **Chondroblastoma.** **a** A round, slightly inhomogeneous lesion (arrow) is seen in the humeral head (T2WI, axial).

b   The slightly lobulated lesion of intermediate signal intensity in the medial aspect of the humeral head is surrounded by hyperintense bone marrow edema laterally (arrow) and adjacent soft-tissue edema (arrowhead) medially (T2WI, coronal).

Fig. 12.**12** **Chondromyxoid fibroma.** A small, eccentric lesion (arrow) with low signal intensity and suggestion of slight cortical expansion and trabeculation is seen in the anterior distal femur (T1WI).

Table 12.**1** (Cont.) Localized bone and bone marrow lesions

Disease	MRI Findings	Comments
Nonossifying fibroma (Fig. 12.**13**)	Eccentric metadiaphyseal lesion with or without a sclerotic border in the long tubular bones presents with low signal intensity on T1WI and variable signal intensity on T2WI, being typically low, but occasionally intermediate to high depending on the tissue composition and vascularity. With time the lesion may spontaneously disappear or become sclerotic.	Usually an incidental finding in patients under age 20. Smaller lesions are also referred to as *benign fibrous cortical defects*. Radiographically larger lesions may demonstrate cortical thinning and slight expansion and may have an elongated and multi-loculated (bubbly) appearance. *Fibrous histiocytomas* are histologically identical to nonossifying fibromas, but present as slightly more aggressive osteolytic lesion in patients over age 20 without site predilection.
Desmoplastic fibroma	Central, trabeculated, and often slightly expansile lesion of low signal intensity on T1WI and of mixed, low to relatively high signal intensity on T2WI. Preferentially located in the metaphyses of long tubular bones, mandible, and pelvis.	Rare benign neoplasm occurring in the second and third decades of life.
Bone island (enostosis) (Fig. 12.**14**)	Single or multiple intraosseous foci of compact bone present with low signal intensity on all pulse sequences. They are most often located in the spine and pelvis, range in size from a few millimeters to a few centimeters and do not protrude from the cortical surface of the involved bone.	Lesions may slowly increase or decrease in size over years. Radiographically thorny bone spicules radiating from the periphery of the lesion are quite characteristic. Bone scintigraphy is usually negative. In *osteopoikilosis* numerous small sclerotic foci with symmetric distribution are seen in para-articular distribution.
Osteoma	Mass of either uniformly dense compact bone or less dense cancellous bone protruding most commonly from the skull (outer table) and facial bones (especially into paranasal sinuses) presents with low signal intensity on all pulse sequences.	*Gardner syndrome*: Autosomal dominant disease presenting with multiple osteomas, colonic polyposis, and soft-tissue tumors (desmoid tumors and desmoplastic fibrosis).
Osteoid osteoma (Fig. 12.**15**)	The lesion consists of a central nidus surrounded by bone marrow edema, adjacent soft-tissue edema, and reactive sclerosis. The nidus (occasionally more than one) measures less than 2 cm and may be fibrotic or calcified in its center. Depending on the size and the presence of calcification the nidus may not be seen or may be of variable signal intensity, ranging from low to high on T2WI. The diffuse juxta-nidal bone marrow edema and adjacent soft-tissue edema is hypointense on T1WI and hyperintense on T2WI and enhances after contrast administration, whereas the reactive sclerosis is of low signal intensity on both T1WI and T2WI. Depending on its location an osteoid osteoma may be misdiagnosed on MRI as bone island, osteomyelitis, malignant bone tumor, or inflammatory arthritic process.	Occurs in patients between age 7 and 25 with a 3:1 male predominance. Pain is the hallmark of the disease, usually more dramatic at night and ameliorated with aspirin. Bone scintigraphy shows an unusual intense uptake in the center (nidus) of the lesion. Radiographic presentation depends on the location of the lesion: In the cortex of a long tubular bone the nidus, which may not be visible, is surrounded by solid elliptical new bone formation, which may be exuberant. With intra-articular location an inconspicuous small radiolucent focus may be seen, inducing a synovial inflammatory response. In the carpal and tarsal bones a partially or completely calcified lesion without significant reactive sclerosis is characteristic. In the spine an osteosclerotic focus in the posterior elements is the most common presentation.
Osteoblastoma (Fig. 12.**16**)	The lesion shows decreased signal intensity on T1WI, variable signal intensity on T2WI, and marked contrast enhancement after intravenous Gd-DTPA administration. In the long tubular bones an inflammatory reaction in the bone marrow about the tumor and/or nearby soft tissues demonstrates high signal intensity on T2WI, enhances after contrast administration, and, combined with the tumor, should not be mistaken for a malignancy. Actual tumor infiltration into the adjacent soft tissues occurs with a more aggressive variant of osteoblastoma, often referred to as *aggressive (malignant) osteoblastoma*.	Usually found in the second and third decades of life with a 2:1 male predominance. Radiographically a tumor originating from cortical or medullary bone of the diaphysis of a long bone presents as an expansile osteolytic lesion with areas of calcifications or ossifications, bone sclerosis, and often exuberant periosteal reaction. In the spine a well-defined osteolytic lesion that is partially or extensively calcified and arises from the posterior elements is the most common presentation. The size of the nidus (actual lesion size) may be used to differentiate between osteoblastomas (> 2 cm) and osteoid osteomas (< 2 cm).

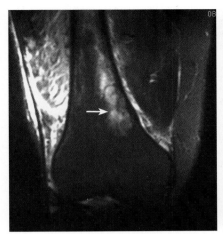

Fig. 12.**13** **Nonossifying fibroma.** An eccentric oblong lesion (arrow) along the medioposterior cortex of the distal femur with heterogeneous intermediate signal intensity is seen (T2WI, FS, coronal). Posttraumatic hemorrhagic changes are present in the vastus lateralis muscle and adjacent soft tissues.

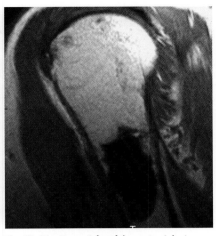

Fig. 12.**14** **Bone island (enostosis).** A large area devoid of signal is seen in the proximal humerus shaft (PDWI, sagittal).

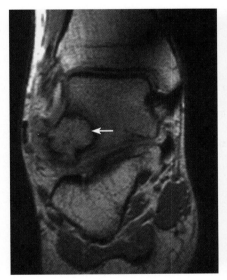

a

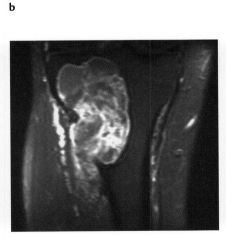

b

Fig. 12.**15** **Osteoid osteoma.** **a** A somewhat irregularly confined nidus (arrow) of intermediate signal intensity in the talus is surrounded by a sclerotic rim devoid of signal (PDWI, coronal). **b** After intravenous Gd-DTPA administration both the nidus and the edema in the adjacent bone marrow and soft tissues enhance considerably (T1WI, FS, +C, coronal).

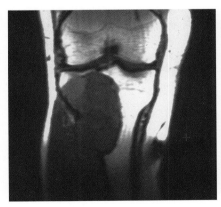

a

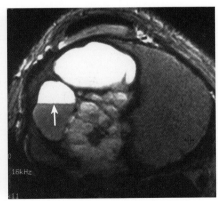

b

c

Fig. 12.**16** **Osteoblastoma with secondary aneurysmal bone cyst.** An eccentric mass with soft-tissue extension is seen in the lateral aspect of the proximal tibia. The osteoblastoma appears hypointense and relatively homogeneous in **a** (T1WI, coronal). After intravenous Gd-DTPA administration considerable heterogeneous contrast enhancement is seen in **b** (T1WI, FS, +C, coronal). A superimposed secondary aneurysmal bone cyst is evident in **c** (T2WI, axial) as two very hyperintense, cystic lesions projecting anterior and lateral of the inhomogeneous osteoblastoma, one demonstrating a fluid-fluid level (arrow).

Table 12.**1** (Cont.) Localized bone and bone marrow lesions

Disease	MRI Findings	Comments
Giant cell tumor (Fig. 12.**17**)	Eccentric, expansile, well-defined lesion, extending from the metaphysis to the subchondral bone, typically presents with an overall low signal intensity on T1WI and high signal intensity on T2WI. However, tumor inhomogeneity with areas of different signal intensity interspersed within the lesion is a frequent finding. Hemosiderin deposition may decrease the signal intensity on all imaging sequences. Fluid-fluid levels and cortical violation with soft-tissue extension occur, but are relatively uncommon. Preferred locations are the epimetaphyses of the long tubular bones (85 %), but pelvis, sacrum, ribs, vertebral bodies, hands, and wrists may also be affected.	Occurs usually in the third and fourth decades of life without gender predilection. Tumor recurrence is not uncommon and malignant giant cell tumors (including malignant transformation) account for about 5 %. Radiographically an eccentric, expansile osteolytic lesion, often with a delicate trabecular pattern ("soap bubble" appearance) in the subchondral bone is characteristic. Sclerosis and periosteal reactions are typically absent. The *giant cell reparative granuloma* has similar histologic features, but with a more benign clinical course and occurs primarily in the facial bones, hands, and feet.
Chordoma (Fig. 12.**18**)	Destructive lesion with osseous expansion and large soft-tissue mass presents with mixed signal intensity, low to intermediate on T1WI, and intermediate to high on T2WI. Internal septation is sometimes evident. Hyperintense foci on T1WI represent subacute hemorrhage (methemoglobin) or possibly proteinaceous material, and hypointense foci on T2WI are caused by hemosiderin, calcifications, or bone fragments. Contrast enhancement is heterogeneous and moderate to marked. Originates from the sacrum and coccyx (60 %), clivus (30 %), and spine, especially C2 (10 %). In the sacrum the tumor grows anteriorly and may contain cystic areas.	Radiographically tumor calcifications are visible in 60 % of sacrococcygeal lesions, in 40 % of spheno-occipital lesions, and 30 % of vertebral lesions. Sacrococcygeal chordomas occur in 40–60-year-old patients with male predominance. Spleno-occipital chordomas are usually diagnosed in 20- to 40-year-old patients without gender predilection. Hematogenous metastases may eventually develop in one-third of cases.
Adamantinoma	Single or multiple, central or eccentric, multilocular, slightly expansile lesions in the diaphysis of the tibia (typically anterior aspect) or rarely, other long tubular bones with low signal intensity on T1WI and high signal intensity on T2WI.	Usually diagnosed in the second through fifth decades of life with slight male predominance. History of trauma is frequent. Local swelling is the major clinical finding.
Ameloblastoma	Multilocular or unilocular lesion with mixed pattern of solid and cystic components usually presents with low signal intensity on T1WI and high signal intensity on T2WI, but occasionally a high signal intensity is observed on T1WI. Contrast enhancement is limited to the solid portions of the tumor. Mandibular location is characteristic, maxillary involvement rare.	Usually diagnosed in the fourth and fifth decades of life without gender predilection. Radiographically a unilocular or multilocular trabeculated lesion with cortical expansion or destruction and occasionally large soft-tissue mass is seen.
Fibrosarcoma (Fig. 12.**19**)	Osteolytic focus of low signal intensity on T1WI and variable, heterogeneous, low to high signal intensity on T2WI, often associated with cortical destruction and soft-tissue mass. May be superimposed on Paget disease, bone infarcts, radiation necrosis, and chronic osteomyelitis.	Rare malignant bone tumor occurring in the third through sixth decades of life without gender predilection. Radiographically an osteolytic lesion with geographic, moth-eaten, or permeative pattern of bone destruction and general lack of both periosteal reaction and osteosclerosis is seen. The lesion may occasionally contain sequestered bone fragments or dystrophic calcifications.

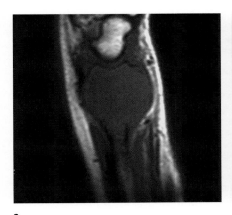

a

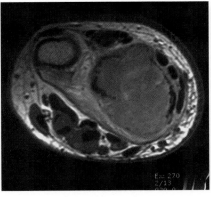

b

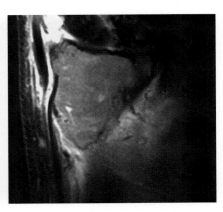

c

Fig. 12.17 Giant cell tumor. a An expansile lesion in the distal radius with homogeneous low signal intensity is seen extending to the subchondral bone (sagittal, T1WI). **b** The lesion appears slightly inhomogeneous, and cortical destruction with soft-tissue extension is seen on its dorsal and particularly palmar aspect (axial, PDWI). **c** After intravenous Gd-DTPA administration moderate inhomogeneous contrast enhancement of the lesion and adjacent soft tissues is seen (coronal, T1WI, FS, +C).

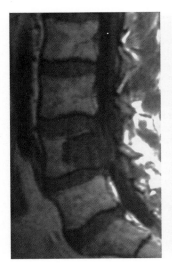

a

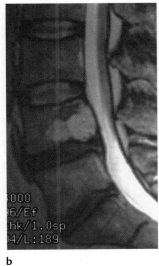

b

Fig. 12.18 Chordoma. A poorly defined, heterogeneous lesion involving the posterior aspect of the L4 vertebral body and protruding into the spinal canal is seen. The lesion appears hypointense in (**a**) (PDWI, sagittal) and hyperintense in (**b**) (T2WI, sagittal).

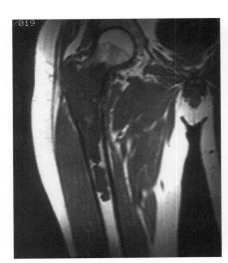

a

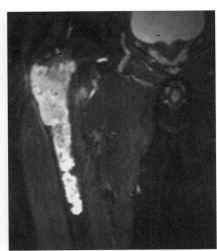

b

Fig. 12.19 Fibrosarcoma. A lesion is seen in the femoral neck and proximal shaft with expansion of the intertrochanteric and subtrochanteric area, where extension into the adjacent soft tissue has also occurred. The lesion is hypointense in (**a**) (T1WI, coronal) and heterogeneous and hyperintense in (**b**) (T2WI, coronal).

Table 12.**1** (Cont.) Localized bone and bone marrow lesions

Disease	MRI Findings	Comments
Malignant fibrous histiocytoma (Fig. 12.20)	Osteolytic lesion with cortical destruction and large soft-tissue mass presents with intermediate signal intensity on T1WI and high signal intensity on T2WI. In the presence of extensive fibromatous stroma the tumor may be hypointense on T2WI. Contrast enhancement is moderate to extensive. Preferred location is the long tubular bone, but any bone can be affected.	Occurs at any age, but the majority are found in the fifth, sixth, and seventh decades of life with slight male predominance. Radiographically an osteolytic lesion with a moth-eaten or permeative pattern, cortical destruction, and absent periosteal reaction is seen. The tumor may be associated with Paget disease, prior radiation therapy, and bone infarcts.
Chondrosarcoma central (Figs. 12.21, 12.22)	Slightly expansile, multilobulated, inhomogeneous, or less commonly homogeneous lesion with low to intermediate signal intensity on T1WI and high signal intensity on T2WI. Areas of decreased signal intensity on T2WI may represent calcified cartilagineous foci. Hemorrhages of different ages may also be found within the tumor. Contrast enhancement occurs in a focal or diffuse fashion and the degree of enhancement may correspond to the degree of malignancy. Cortical breakthrough and soft-tissue mass indicate malignancy. Preferred locations are the metadiaphyses of long bones (particularly femur and humerus), the flat bones (especially pelvis), and the vertebrae.	Occurs usually between age 30 and 60 with male predominance. The tumor arises de novo in the medullary cavity or as a secondary complication of a preexisting enchondroma. Radiographically irregular calcifications (as opposed to punctate, ring, and arc-like calcifications), larger areas of noncalcified tumor matrix, poorly defined osteolysis, poorly defined endosteal erosions, and cortical thickening (even solid) suggest malignancy.
Chondrosarcoma peripheral (Fig. 12.23)	Malignant transformation of a benign osteochondroma is suggested by a bulky cartilaginous cap measuring more than 2 cm in width, a hyperintense cap with inhomogeneous signal intensity (due to areas of calcifications) on T2WI, and contrast enhancement of the cap itself or any other tissue within the lesion below the cap. Inflammation of the tissue surrounding a large bony exostosis may occasionally enhance because of inflammation secondary to friction and is not necessarily associated with malignant transformation. An extraosseous tumor soft-tissue mass has to be differentiated and is diagnostic for malignancy.	Local pain and growth of an osteocartilaginous exostosis in adulthood suggest clinically malignant transformation. Rarely a peripheral chondrosarcoma develops de novo from the periost (juxta-articular chondrosarcoma). Radiographically malignant transformation is suggested by demonstration of scattered and irregular calcifications in the cartilaginous part of the tumor, a large soft-tissue mass, and destruction or pressure erosion of the adjacent bone.
Clear cell chondrosarcoma	Epiphyseal lesion of low signal intensity on T1WI and high signal intensity on T2WI most commonly located in the proximal femur, humerus, and tibia. The hyperintensity of the lesion on T2WI differentiates it from a radiographically identical chondroblastoma, which is hypointense or isointense to fat on this pulse sequence.	Occurs between age 25 and 50 with slight male predominance. Radiographically the slightly expansive epiphyseal lesion depicts poorly to well-defined (sclerotic) margins and central calcifications in approximately one-third of the caces.

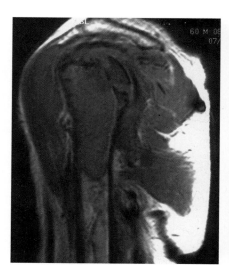
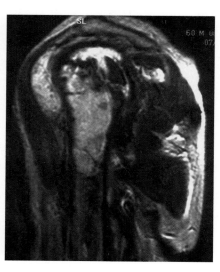

Fig. 12.20 Malignant fibrous histiocytoma. A destructive, heterogeneous mass in the proximal humerus with extension into the shoulder joint and surrounding soft tissue is seen. The mass is isointense to muscle in (**a**) (PDWI, sagittal) and hyperintense in (**b**) (T2WI, sagittal).

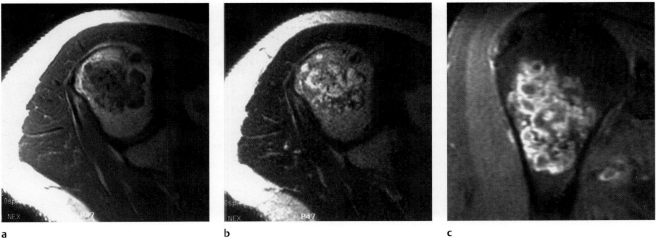

a   b   c

Fig. 12.**21**   **Chondrosarcoma (low grade).** A heterogeneous lesion with scattered small foci of signal void representing intratumoral calcifications is seen in the proximal humerus. The lesion is hypointense in (**a**) (PDWI, axial) and hyperintense in (**b**) (T2WI, axial). After intravenous Gd-DTPA administration inhomogeneous contrast enhancement is evident in (**c**) (T1WI, FS, +C, coronal).

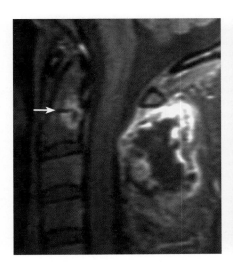
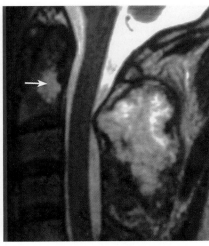

Fig. 12.**22**   **Chondrosarcoma (high grade).** An irregularly shaped mass originating in the posterior elements of C2 seen extending to the posterior aspect of both vertebral body and dens (arrow). The lesion depicts heterogeneous low signal intensity with hyperintense periphery (subacute hemorrhage) in (**a**) (PDWI, sagittal) and heterogeneous increased signal intensity in (**b**) (T2WI, sagittal).

a   b

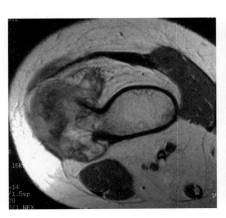
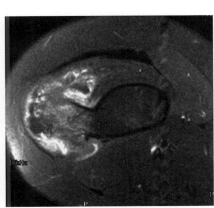

Fig. 12.**23**   **Peripheral chondrosarcoma.** A heterogeneous mass originates from the distal femur with inhomogeneous contrast enhancement (**a**: PDWI). **b**: T1WI, FS, +C.

a   b

Table 12.1 (Cont.) Localized bone and bone marrow lesions

Disease	MRI Findings	Comments
Dedifferentiated chondrosarcoma (Fig. 12.24)	Features of a low grade chondrosarcoma (nonexpansile, hypointense on T1WI, hyperintense on T2WI, with scattered calcifications and poor contrast enhancement) and of a highly anaplastic sarcoma (cortical destruction, large soft-tissue mass, and extensive inhomogeneous contrast enhancement) are found in the same lesion.	The transition between the low-grade chondrosarcoma and the highly anaplastic sarcoma is characteristically sharp. Radiographically the anaplastic component demonstrates a permeative or moth-eaten pattern of bone destruction with large extraosseous soft-tissue mass, usually without calcifications. Occurs in patients over 50 years of age and has a poor prognosis.
Mesenchymal chondrosarcoma (Fig. 12.25)	Features are indistinguishable from a high-grade conventional chondrosarcoma and include a heterogeneous mass with low to intermediate signal intensity on T1WI, high signal intensity on T2WI, cortical destruction, and large extra-osseous soft-tissue component. Contrast enhancement is extensive and inhomogeneous.	Occurs usually between age 20 and 40 and has a poor prognosis. Approximately half of the tumors arise in the soft tissues.
Osteosarcoma (Figs. 12.26, 12.27)	Signal intensity is inhomogeneous and varies greatly. The tumor usually demonstrates an overall low signal intensity on T1WI and a mixed high signal intensity on T2WI. Densely ossified tumors or tumor portions are of low signal intensity on all pulse sequences. Cortical destruction and extraosseous soft-tissue extension is a common finding. The tumor is frequently surrounded by a rim of low signal intensity reflecting the periosteal reaction, which is characteristically interrupted but not always appreciated by MRI. Subacute intratumoral hemorrhage may be evident as areas of increased signal intensity on both T1WI and T2WI. Fluid-fluid levels within the tumor are occasionally seen, especially with telangiectatic osteosarcomas. Intratumoral cystic and necrotic areas appearing hypointense on T1WI and hyperintense on T2WI may be found, especially after radiation therapy or chemotherapy. After intravenous Gd-DTPA administration, the contrast enhancement of the tumor is inhomogeneous and extensive, whereas the peritumoral edema in the bone marrow and adjacent soft tissue enhances more homogeneously and often, but not invariably, somewhat less. On precontrast examination the perineoplastic edema causes a decrease in signal intensity on T1WI and an increase in signal intensity in the affected bone marrow and soft-tissue structures. Preferred locations are the metaphyses of the tubular bones (80 %), particularly femur (40 %), tibia (16 %), and humerus (15 %). Osteosarcomas are relatively infrequent in the fibula, pelvis, mandible, maxilla, and spine and rare in the remaining skeleton.	Conventional osteosarcomas are most common in the second and third decades of life with male predominance. In the elderly, osteosarcomas may be a complication of Paget disease or prior radiation therapy. The radiographic manifestation of *conventional osteosarcomas* depend on tumor localization, extent, and histology. The tumor may be purely osteolytic or purely osteoblastic, but a mixed pattern of osteolysis and sclerosis is most typical. Interrupted periosteal reactions in the form of a Codman triangle or with perpendicular ("sunburst" or "hair-on-end") or laminated ("onion skin") appearance are most characteristic. Cortical destruction and large soft-tissue mass are characteristically associated. *Telangiectatic osteosarcomas* typically present as large expansile osteolytic lesions without significant periosteal reaction and sclerosis. *Small cell osteosarcomas* commonly present as a large predominantly osteolytic lesion extending from the metaphysis to the diaphysis of a long tubular bone associated with interrupted periosteal reaction and large soft-tissue masses. Intraosseous low-grade osteosarcomas typically reveal a purely osteoblastic or mixed blastic and osteolytic lesions without interrupted periosteal reaction in the metaphyses of the femur or tibia. *Gnathic osteosarcomas* present as purely osteoblastic, osteolytic, or mixed lesion of the mandible or maxilla, occur in the middle-aged or elderly and have a relatively benign course. *Intracortical osteosarcoma* is the rarest form of osteosarcoma and occurs as an osteolytic lesion with surrounding sclerosis in the diaphyses of the tibia or femur. *Osteosarcomatosis* refers to simultaneous involvement of more than one skeletal site. It has to be differentiated from a unicentric lesion with distant skeletal metastases.

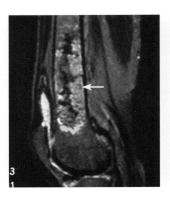
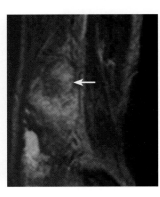

Fig. 12.24 Dedifferentiated chondrosarcoma. A low-grade chondrosarcoma (arrow) in the distal femur shaft shown in (**a**) (T2WI, sagittal) is associated with a large and poorly defined soft-tissue sarcoma (arrow) anterolaterally shown in (**b**) (T2WI, sagittal).

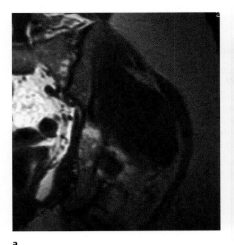

a

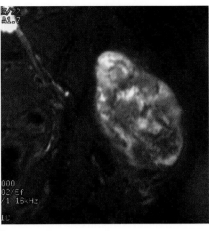

b

Fig. 12.**25** **Mesenchymal chondrosarcoma.** A mass in the left hemipelvis is seen depicting low signal intensity in (**a**) (coronal, T1WI) and heterogeneous high signal intensity in (**b**) (coronal, T2WI).

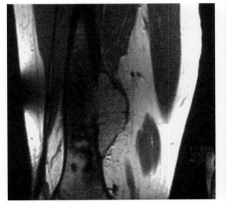

a

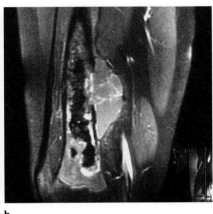

b

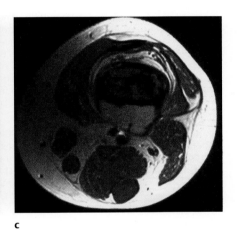

c

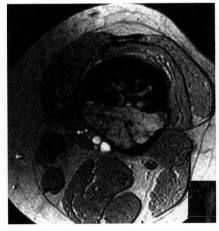

d

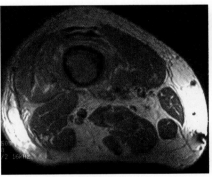

a

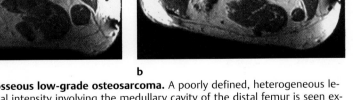

b

Fig. 12.**26** **Osteosarcoma.** Destructive lesion in the distal femur with posterior cortical destruction and a hemorrhagic soft-tissue extension is seen in (**a**). Inhomogeneous, mainly peripheral contrast enhancement is evident in (**b**). The inhomogeneity of the hemorrhagic posterior soft-tissue extension is most conspicuous with the gradient-echo pulse sequence in (**d**) (**a**: sagittal, T1WI. **b**: sagittal, PDWI, +C. **c**: axial, T1WI. **d**: axial, spoiled GRE).

Fig. 23.**27** **Intraosseous low-grade osteosarcoma.** A poorly defined, heterogeneous lesion with low-signal intensity involving the medullary cavity of the distal femur is seen extending into the cortex but not breaking through it (**a**, **b**: PDWI).

Table 12.1 (Cont.) Localized bone and bone marrow lesions

Disease	MRI Findings	Comments
Periosteal osteosarcoma	Oblong inhomogeneous mass with low signal intensity on T1WI, high signal intensity on T2WI, and marked contrast enhancement arising from the diaphyseal surface of a long tubular bone (especially femur and tibia) is most typical.	Radiographically the tumor causes thickening and occasionally saucerization of the adjacent cortex and is often associated with a Codman triangle and radiating or cloud-like osseous proliferations. A *surface high-grade osteosarcoma* originates from the periost with clinical, histologic, and imaging features identical to a conventional osteosarcoma.
Parosteal osteosarcoma (Fig. 12.28)	Well-marginated mass of low signal intensity on all imaging sequences attached to a metaphysis of a long tubular bone, typically without extension into the adjacent bone marrow. The posterior surface of the distal femur is the most characteristic location.	Most common in the third and fourth decades of life with better prognosis than conventional osteosarcomas. Radiographically a large radiodense mass with smooth or irregular margin is attached to the external cortex, which may itself be thickened.
Ewing sarcoma (Fig. 12.29)	Inhomogeneous, poorly defined osseous lesion with decreased signal intensity on T1WI and mixed increased signal intensity on T2WI, cortical destruction, and large soft-tissue mass is the most common presentation. Necrotic and hemorrhagic foci are frequently present. Differentiation between tumor and perineoplastic edema is often difficult, since both demonstrate similar signal intensity and contrast enhancement patterns and the tumor is poorly defined. Preferential locations include the metadiaphyses of long tubular bones, sacrum, and pelvis. Predominantly osteosclerotic lesions are occasionally seen in the spine, pelvis, and ribs, presenting with decreased signal intensity on all pulse sequences.	Usually diagnosed between age 5 and 30 with slight male predominance. Radiographically the lesion depicts a poorly defined osteolysis with a moth-eaten or permeative pattern, cortical violation, interrupted periosteal reaction of the laminated ("onion skin"), or, less commonly, a perpendicular ("sunburst" or "hair-on-end" pattern) and large soft-tissue mass. *Primitive neuroectodermal tumors (PNET)* of bone (Fig. 12.**30**) have similar imaging features, but epiphyseal involvement, pathologic fractures, and distant metastases occur all more frequently when compared with Ewing sarcomas.
Angiosarcoma (hemangio-endo-thelioma) (Fig. 12.31)	Solitary or multifocal, poorly or well demarcated, osteolytic lesions with decreased signal intensity on T1WI, increased signal intensity on T2WI, and marked contrast enhancement. Predilection for the long tubular bones, especially those in the lower extremity, pelvis, and skull.	Occurs commonly in the fourth and fifth decades with male predominance. If multicentric, it may simulate metastases, multiple myeloma, various reticulohistiocytosis, cystic angiomatosis, and cystic osteomyelitis (e.g., tuberculous or fungal). *Hemangiopericytoma* is a borderline malignant tumor with similar imaging feature.
Plasmacytoma (Fig. 12.32)	Expansile osteolytic lesion, with or without trabeculation and cortical violation, presents with low signal intensity on T1WI, high signal intensity on T2WI, and marked contrast enhancement involving the pelvis or spine (especially thoracic and lumbar segments). Collapse of the involved vertebral body or extension into the spinal canal or across the intervertebral disc into the adjacent vertebral body are known complications.	Plasmacytoma may be considered a solitary manifestation of multiple myeloma. In a majority of cases conversion of plasmacytoma to multiple myeloma occurs eventually, as late as 20 years after initial diagnosis. Radiographically plasmacytoma usually presents as expansile, sometimes trabeculated osteolytic lesion measuring up to several centimeters in diameter, but occasionally a purely sclerotic appearance is found that may produce an ivory vertebra in the spine.

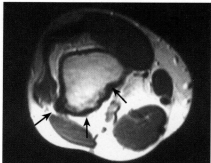

Fig. 12.**28**   **Parosteal osteosarcoma.** Irregular cortical thickening of the enlarged posteromedial aspect of the distal femur (arrows), evident as an undulating band of signal void is contrasted by the fatty marrow in the femur and the adjacent soft-tissue fat (T1WI).

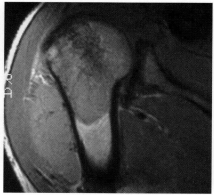
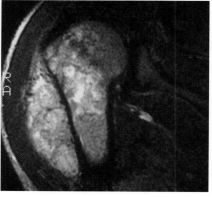

a   b

Fig. 12.**29**   **Ewing sarcoma.** A heterogeneous lesion involving the proximal humerus and extending into the lateral soft tissue is seen. The tumor depicts intermediate signal intensity in (**a**) (PDWI, coronal) and high signal intensity in (**b**) (T2WI, coronal).

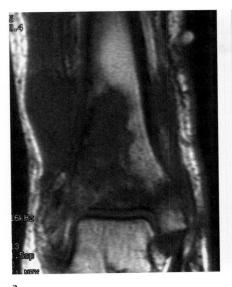

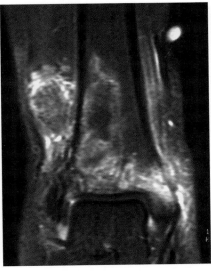

a

b

Fig. 12.30   Primitive neuroectodermal tumor.   a A hypointense destructive lesion is seen in the distal tibia with extension into the lateral soft tissues (T1WI, coronal).   **b** After intravenous Gd-DTPA administration marked inhomogeneous tumor enhancement is seen in the tibia and lateral soft tissues. The enhancement of the soft tissues along the medial tibial border was partly tumorous and partly edematous (T1WI, FS, +C, coronal).

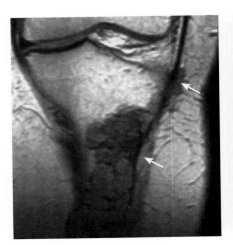

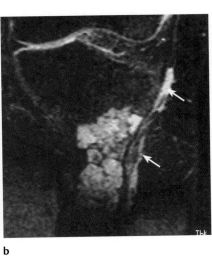

a

b

Fig. 12.31   Angiosarcoma. Poorly defined heterogeneous lesion in the proximal tibia with cortical destruction and soft-tissue extension along the lateral tibial border (arrows). The lesion is hypointense in (**a**) (T1WI, coronal) and hyperintense in (**b**) (T2WI, FS, coronal).

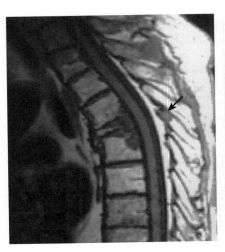

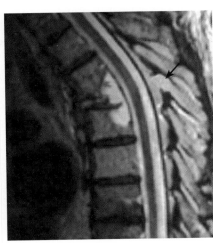

a

b

Fig. 12.32   Plasmacytoma. Fairly homogeneous lesion causing virtually total collapse of T6 and invasion of the posteroinferior aspect of T5 and posterosuperior aspect of T7 is seen. A small tumor focus is also seen in the posterior element of T6 (arrow). The lesion is hypointense in (**a**) (T1WI, sagittal) and hyperintense in (**b**) (T2WI, sagittal).

Table 12.1 (Cont.) Localized bone and bone marrow lesions

Disease	MRI Findings	Comments
Metastases (Figs. 12.33, 12.34)	Solitary or, more commonly, multiple focal lesions with preferential involvement of the axial skeleton, usually presenting with decreased signal intensity on T1WI. Osteolytic metastases are hyperintense on T2WI, but osteoblastic metastases may be isointense or even hypointense. Melanoma metastases occasionally are hyperintense on T1WI. Extraosseous soft-tissue extension is rare, except in ribs. Bony expansion is limited to osteolytic metastases from kidney, thyroid, and lung, and osteoblastic metastases from prostatic carcinoma.	Solitary metastases occur relatively frequently in patients with carcinoma of the kidney and thyroid, but may be encountered with any malignancy.
Lymphoma (Figs. 12.35, 12.36)	Lymphomatous bone marrow infiltration tends to be focal or patchy, or less frequently, diffuse. Infiltrates are hypointense and more variable, but usually hyperintense and often inhomogeneous on T2WI. Short time to inversion recovery (STIR) images are more sensitive than T2WI in the discrimination of lymphoma from red marrow. In long bones epiphyseal and metaphyseal location with a tendency to spread into a nearby joint or soft tissues is not unusual.	Lymphomas present with lymphadenopathy, splenomegaly, or hepatosplenomegaly. Bony involvement is usually secondary indicating a tumor stage IV. Primary bone involvement occasionally occurs with non-Hodgkin lymphoma, usually of the histiocytic type.
Histiocytosis X (Langerhans cell histiocytosis) (Figs. 12.37, 12.38, 12.39)	One or more osteolytic lesions of decreased signal intensity on T1WI and of increased signal intensity on T2WI are seen in the skull, mandible, spine, ribs, and metaphyses or diaphyses of long tubular bones. The lesions are frequently surrounded by a hypointense rim, reflecting marginal sclerosis or periosteal reaction. Cortical violation or destruction and soft-tissue extension may occur. A large and poorly defined soft-tissue mass with inhomogeneous signal intensity may simulate a malignancy or osteomyelitis. Differentiation between the poorly defined soft-tissue component and surrounding edema may be difficult also.	*Eosinophilic granuloma* is the most benign variant usually diagnosed between age 5 and 20. *Hand-Schüller-Christian disease* is characterized by the triad of exophthalmus, diabetes insipidus, and large lytic skull lesions ("geographic skull"). *Letterer-Siwe disease* is the acute disseminated variant in children under age 2. Multiple widespread lytic lesions in the skull may be evident ("raindrop" pattern). Radiographic features of eosinophilic granuloma include lytic skull lesions with beveled edges and button sequestrum and flattened vertebral bodies (vertebra plana).
Amyloidosis	Osteolytic lesions of variable size, low signal intensity on T1WI and low to intermediate signal intensity on T2WI occur most frequently in the proximal humerus and proximal femur. Subchondral amyloid deposition may result in avascular necrosis. Amyloid deposition about the joints of the hand and wrist may lead to an arthropathy simulating rheumatoid arthritis.	*Primary amyloidosis* occurs in patients above age 40 with male predominance. It may be associated with multiple myeloma. *Secondary amyloidosis* is associated with chronic renal disease, rheumatoid arthritis, lupus erythematosus, ulcerative colitis, chronic suppurative disease, and lymphoproliferative disorders.
Brown tumor	Single or multiple, occasionally expansile, well-defined osteolytic lesions of the axial and appendicular skeleton with decreased signal intensity on T1WI and increased signal intensity on T2WI. They subsequently may undergo necrosis and liquefaction, producing cysts. At this stage they will no longer enhance after intravenous Gd-DTPA administration.	Brown tumors are associated with hyperparathyroidism. Other radiographic features of hyperparathyroidism include osteopenia, subperiosteal, endosteal and subchondral resorption, intracortical tunneling, chondrocalcinosis, and para-articular and vascular calcifications. Bone sclerosis is common in secondary hyperparathyroidism.
Hemophilic pseudotumor	The signal intensity pattern is extremely variable and heterogeneous, depending on site of bleeding (intraosseous versus subperiosteal), size of osseous lesion and soft-tissue mass, cortical destruction, periosteal reaction, fibrosis, calcifications, new bone formation, and blood products (methemoglobin and hemosiderin). The signal characteristically reflects the complexity of the lesion with regions of both high and low signal intensity being evident on both T1WI and T2WI. A rim of low signal intensity is consistently seen on all imaging sequences in the periphery of the lesion, probably owing to a fibrous pseudocapsule and/or accumulation of hemosiderin-laden macrophages. Preferred locations are the femur, pelvis, tibia, and small bones of the hands.	Lesions are late sequelae of intramedullary or subperiosteal hemorrhage and occur in fewer than 2% of hemophiliacs. Hemophilic arthropathy, joint contractures, avascular necrosis of the femoral head and talus, spontaneous fractures, and soft-tissue hematomas and pseudotumors may also be evident.

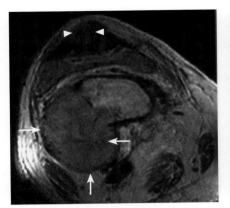

Fig. 12.33 Renal cell carcinoma metastases. A large expansile lesion with intermediate signal intensity is seen in the lateral femoral condyle (arrows). A smaller lesion with the same signal characteristics (arrowheads) originates from the patella (PDWI).

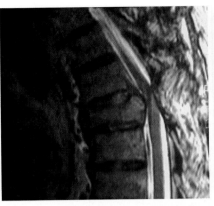

Fig. 12.34 Soft-tissue sarcoma metastasis. Partial compression fracture of T6 and circumferential encroachment of the spinal cord is caused by a lesion that is slightly hyperintense to the bone marrow (T2WI, sagittal).

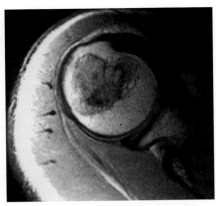

Fig. 12.35 Non-Hodgkin lymphoma (histiocytic type). A heterogeneous lesion of intermediate signal intensity is seen in the humeral head (PDWI).

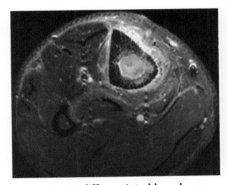

Fig. 12.36 Undifferentiated lymphoma in AIDS. Compared to the normal bone marrow in the fibula, the marrow in the tibia is markedly enhanced after intravenous Gd-DTPA administration. Spread of the bone marrow lymphoma through the Volksmann canal system in the cortex (evident as hyperintense radiating cortical spicules) into the periost and surrounding soft-tissue layers, which are also markedly enhanced, is also evident (T1WI, FS, +C).

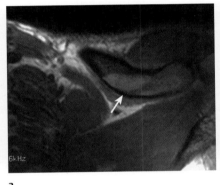

a   b

Fig. 12.37 Histiocytosis X. A relatively well-circumscribed lesion (arrow) is seen in the mid-clavicle (**a**: PDWI, coronal. **b**: T2WI, FS, coronal).

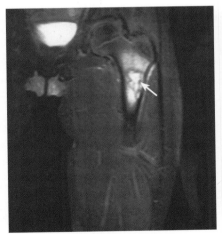

Fig. 12.38 Histiocytosis X. A lesion (arrow) surrounded by marrow edema is seen in the proximal femur diaphysis (T2WI, FS, coronal).

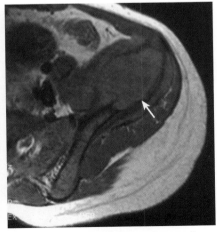

Fig. 12.39 Histiocytosis X. A large soft-tissue mass (arrow) originating in the left iliac wing is seen (PDWI).

Table 12.1 (Cont.) Localized bone and bone marrow lesions

Disease	MRI Findings	Comments
Pigmented villo-nodular synovitis (Fig. 12.40)	Lobulated hypervascular intra-articular mass associated with hemarthrosis and pressure erosions in about half of the cases. T1WI demonstrates a heterogeneous mass with low signal intensity. In T2WI the lesion often has regions of high signal intensity interspersed with foci of low signal intensity or complete signal void. The foci of low signal intensity are caused by fibrosis and intratumoral hemosiderin deposition and may vary considerably between different tumors.	Usually diagnosed in the third through fifth decades of life. Hemorrhagic ("chocolate") joint effusion in the absence of trauma is quite characteristic. Monoarticular involvement of a large joint is typical, affecting, in order of decreasing frequency, the knee, hip, ankle, elbow, shoulder, and tarsal and carpal joints. Radiographically a large eccentric pressure erosion producing a sharply delineated, scalloped defect in an intra-articular bone may mimic a neoplastic lesion.
Osteonecrosis (bone infarct) (Figs. 12.41, 12.42, 12.43)	Bone infarcts are preferentially located in the metadiaphyses of long bones. Acute infarcts appear as circumscribed, usually inhomogeneous areas of low signal intensity on T1WI and of high signal intensity on T2WI owing to edema, hyperemia, and granulation tissue. Subacute infarcts tend to be heterogeneous and characteristically depict a serpiginous outline of low signal intensity on T1WI and of high signal intensity on T2WI. Chronic infarcts demonstrate low signal intensity on both T1WI and T2WI due to fibrosis and calcifications.	Osteonecrosis can be divided into avascular necrosis involving the subarticular bone (see Table 10.1) and bone infarction occurring more frequently in the metadiaphyseal regions of long bones than axial skeleton. Favored anatomic sites include femur, humerus, and tibia. Solitary bone infarcts are frequently diagnosed as an incidental finding.
Radiation therapy (Fig. 12.43, 12.44)	In the first few weeks mild marrow edema presents with decreased signal intensity on T1WI and increased signal intensity on T2WI. Between weeks 3 and 6 the vertebral marrow becomes either mottled and heterogeneous or displays a central fatty component. Progression to either homogeneous fatty replacement or a pattern of central fat with peripheral zones of lower signal intensity (representing hematopoietic marrow) may subsequently be evident. Marrow abnormalities are limited to the field of radiation and are sharply demarcated from the nonirradiated bone . Avascular necrosis and bone infarcts are frequent sequelae in the long bones.	Radiation-induced bone marrow changes depend on the dose and time course. Irradiation may initially cause a mild marrow edema followed by a decrease in hematopoietic marrow and compensatory increase in fatty marrow. Full recovery of the hematopoietic marrow following radiation requires 10 years or longer.

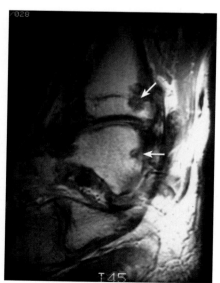

Fig. 12.**40** **Pigmented villonodular synovitis.** A heterogeneous mass with low signal intensity surrounding the ankle and talus is seen. Erosions are seen in the posterior aspect of the distal tibia and talus (arrows). The talar neck and head are largely destroyed (PDWI, sagittal).

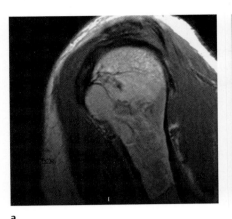

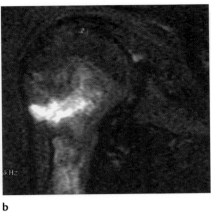

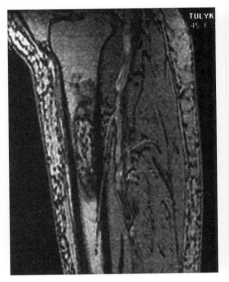

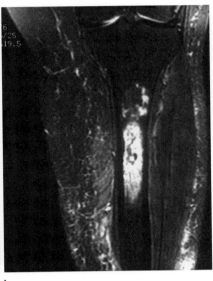

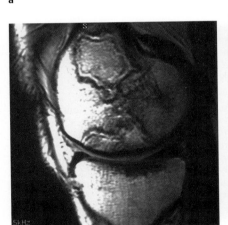

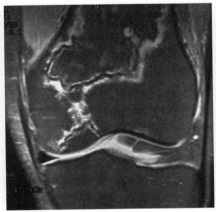

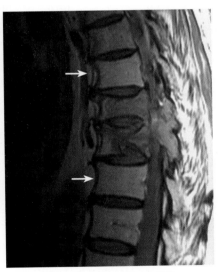

Fig. 12.**41** **Osteonecrosis.** A large heterogeneous lesion with variable signal intensity is seen in the metadiaphysis of the proximal humerus. The involved bone is not expanded and the cortex is intact (**a**: sagittal, PDWI. **b**: coronal, T2WI, FS).

Fig. 12.**42** **Osteonecrosis (acute).** A heterogeneous lesion of variable signal intensity is seen in the diaphysis of the tibia (**a**: spoiled GRE, sagittal. **b**: T2WI, FS, coronal).

Fig. 12.**43** **Osteonecrosis.** An infarct is seen in the distal femur metaphysis extending into the subchondral bone of the medial condyle. The underlying joint cartilage appears intact (**a**: sagittal, PDWI. **b**: coronal, STIR).

Fig. 12.**44** **Radiation-induced fatty marrow conversion.** Following radiation for multiple myeloma involving T10 and T11, a homogeneous increased signal intensity is seen in the neighboring T9 and T12 (arrows) due to radiation-induced conversion of hematopoietic to fatty bone marrow. Signal intensity in T8 and L1 corresponds to normal hematopoietic marrow (PDWI, sagittal).

Table 12.**1** (Cont.) Localized bone and bone marrow lesions

Disease	MRI Findings	Comments
Bone contusion (bone bruise) (Fig. 12.45)	Localized, poorly defined subchondral area of low signal intensity on T1WI and high signal intensity on T2WI and STIR images caused by marrow edema and possibly hemorrhage without an identifiable fracture. Most commonly seen in the knee, where it is frequently associated with ligamentous and meniscal injuries. Resolution of the bone bruise occurs over a period of one to several months.	Trabecular microfractures secondary to compression or impaction. Bone bruises at specific anatomical sites may suggest other associated injuries. For example, a bone bruise of the lateral femoral condyle is frequently associated with medial collateral ligament injury; bone bruises in the lateral femoral condyle and posterolateral portion of the tibial plateau with an anterior cruciate ligament injury; and bone bruises in the lateral femoral condyle anteriorly and medial portion of the patella with lateral patellar dislocation.
Fracture (Fig. 12.46)	Nondisplaced (occult) fractures present on T1WI as a well-defined linear zone of low signal intensity surrounded by a broader and ill-defined zone of less severely decreased signal intensity consistent with marrow edema. On T2WI the fracture line may remain of low signal intensity, but the edematous zone demonstrates high signal intensity. STIR and fat-suppressed T2WI are most sensitive in the detection of these fractures which appear as a broad band of high signal intensity, but the fracture line itself may not be identifiable.	Nondisplaced (occult) fractures which are not detectable by conventional radiography may be further evaluated by bone scintigraphy or MRI. Of the two, MRI appears to be equally sensitive and far more specific in the detection of occult fractures. MRI may be most useful in the diagnosis of suspected occult femoral neck fracture where the scintigraphic diagnosis in an elderly patient may be delayed for 2 to 3 days.
Stress fracture (Fig. 12.47)	Stress fractures appear most typically as a linear zone of low signal intensity surrounded by a broader, poorly defined area of slightly higher, but still hypointense signal intensity on T1WI and as a linear area of low signal intensity surrounded by a broader region of high signal intensity on T2WI. Adjacent soft-tissue edema may also be present.	Stress fractures can be divided into *fatigue fracture*, occurring in normal bone under abnormal stress, and *insufficiency fracture*, occurring in abnormal (usually osteopenic) bone with normal stress. In osteoporosis, such fractures occur in the sacrum, pubic rami, and lower extremities. Sacral insufficiency fractures parallel to the sacroiliac joint (unilaterally or bilaterally) are often combined with a vertical fracture through the body of the sacrum ("H" pattern), and may be associated with pubic fractures resulting in pelvic instability. These fractures are particularly common after steroid and local radiotherapy and should not be confused with neoplastic involvement.
Nonunion (Fig. 12.48)	High signal intensity in the fracture detected on T2WI 6 to 9 months after injury is consistent with the presence of fluid and diagnostic of nonunion. Persistent low signal intensity on T1WI and T2WI at the fracture site indicates fibrosis at this site and, depending on the time course, suggests fibrous union. Bone marrow continuity and bony bridging across the fracture line indicates fracture healing.	Nonunion is the failure of fracture healing during a period of 6 to 9 months after injury. The fracture site remains unstable because of fibrous union or pseudarthrosis (synovium lined cavity with synovial fluid) has developed. In delayed union the fracture healing process is markedly slowed.
Transient bone marrow edema (Fig. 12.49)	Bone marrow edema usually presents with uniformly decreased signal intensity on T1WI and increased signal intensity on T2WI extending from the subchondral bone of a joint into the adjacent metadiaphysis. It may involve one or both articulating bones, and a small joint effusion is frequently present.	Transient bone marrow edema is frequently associated with para-articular osteoporosis. Depending on its location it may be referred to as *transient osteoporosis of the hip* or *regional migratory osteoporosis* when affecting different joints in the lower extremity. *Reflex sympathetic dystrophy (RSD)* may be a related condition, primarily affecting the upper extremities.

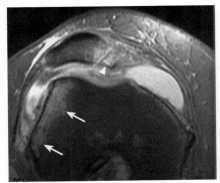

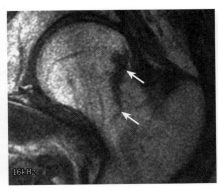

a   **b**

Fig. 12.**45** **Bone contusion (bone bruise).** Increased signal intensity is seen in the lateral femoral condyle (arrows) and medial patellar fracture (arrowhead) following previous lateral patellar dislocation. A large joint effusion is also present (T2WI).

Fig. 12.**46** **Nondisplaced subcapital fracture (not seen on plain radiography).** The fracture (arrows) appears hypointense in (**a**) (T1WI, coronal) and slightly hyperintense in (**b**) (T2WI, FS, coronal).

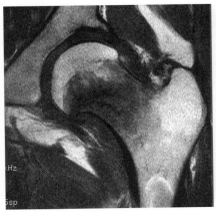

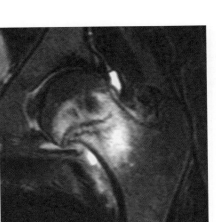

a   **b**

Fig. 12.**47** **Stress fracture.** Two parallel hypodense fracture lines traversing the subcapital area surrounded by bone marrow edema presenting with decreased signal intensity in (**a**) (T1WI, coronal) and increased signal intensity in (**b**) (T2WI, FS, coronal).

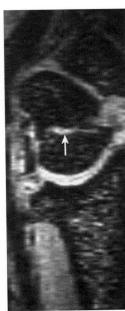

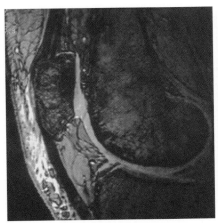

Fig. 12.**49** **Transient bone marrow edema.** Poorly defined areas of increased signal intensity are seen in the distal femur. Radiographically patchy osteopenia was evident (GRE [T2WI], sagittal).

Fig. 12.**48** **Nonunion.** The fracture line in the scaphoid depicts high signal intenstiy consistent with fluid (arrow) 9 months after injury (GRE [T2WI], sagittal).

Table 12.1 (Cont.) Localized bone and bone marrow lesions

Disease	MRI Findings	Comments
Osteomyelitis (acute) (Figs. 12.**50**, 12.**51**, 12.**52**)	Acute osteomyelitis demonstrates low signal intensity on T1WI and high signal intensity on T2WI and particularly STIR images. Additional findings include cortical erosion, periosteal new bone formation, and soft-tissue extension. Differentiation between soft-tissue infection and edema is difficult, since in the acute stage the infection is poorly defined and signal characteristics and contrast enhancement pattern are similar for infection and edema.	Affects all ages, but is commonly found in children, diabetics, and intravenous drug abusers. Occurs by hematogenous route, spread from contiguous infection or direct implantation. Radiographic findings in acute osteomyelitis are delayed for one to three weeks and include localized osteoporosis, bone destruction, and periosteal reaction, usually of the laminated ("onion skin") and, less commonly, of the spiculated ("sunburst" or "hair-on-end") type.
Brodie abscess (Fig. 12.**53**)	A Brodie abscess demonstrates low signal intensity on T1WI and very high signal intensity on T2WI and is outlined by a rim devoid of signal due to sclerotic bone. After intravenous Gd-DTPA administration, marked contrast enhancement occurs in the wall of the abscess. Preferred location is the metaphyses of long bones, especially of the distal tibia.	Most often a staphylococcal infection found in children. Radiographically a lytic, often elongated lesion with sclerotic border is seen. Besides the metaphyses of long bones, the abscess occasionally is found in diaphyseal or epiphyseal location, and in flat or irregular bones including the vertebral bodies. In cortical location it may mimic an osteoid osteoma or stress fracture.
Osteomyelitis (chronic) (Fig. 12.**54**)	In chronic osteomyelitis an active focus of infection appears hypointense on T1WI and hyperintense on T2WI and STIR images and is surrounded by thick sclerotic bone presenting as a rim devoid of signals on all imaging sequences. Additional findings of active chronic osteomyelitis include the demonstration of bone sequestration, sinus tracts, subperiosteal fluid accumulation, periosteal elevation, and contrast enhancement of the infected area. Findings consistent with inactive or healing chronic osteomyelitis include the absence of both contrast enhancement and bone sequestra and the presence of normal marrow fat.	Bone sequestration in osteomyelitis may become evident after 1 month. At that time the sequestrum may be surrounded by granulation tissue and newly formed cortical bone (involucrum). An opening in the involucrum is termed cloaca. Occasionally, intraosseous gas, intracortical fissuring, and fat-fluid (pus) level may be seen. *Epidermoid carcinoma* occurs in 1% of osteomyelitis at the site of a chronically draining sinus and is evident by an enlarging soft-tissue mass eroding the osteomyelitic bone. *Sclerosing osteomyelitis of Garré* presents as localized sclerotic bulge of the cortex or circumferential cortical thickening and sclerosis.

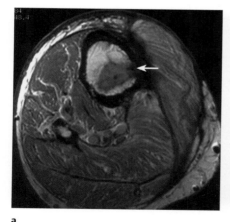
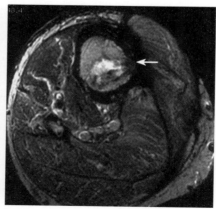

a   b

Fig. 12.**50 Acute osteomyelitis.   a** A heterogeneous focus of decreased signal intensity in **a** (PDWI) and increased signal in **b** (T2WI) is seen in the tibia. The osteomyelitis has broken through the medial tibia cortex (arrow).

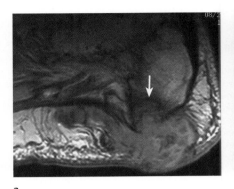

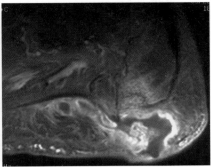

a   b

Fig. 12.**51**   **Calcaneal osteomyelitis secondary to heel pad abscess.   a** An irregular soft-tissue mass in the heel pad with intermediate signal intensity containing several small hypointense foci extends into the calcaneus (arrow) (PDWI, sagittal).   **b** After intravenous Gd-DTPA administration enhancement of the abscess wall and the adjacent calcaneus occurs (T1WI, FS, +C, sagittal).

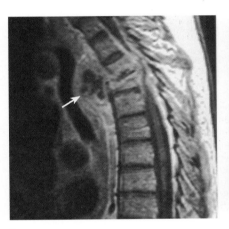

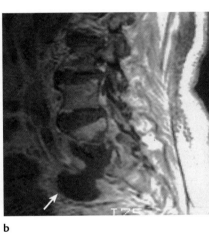

a   b

Fig. 12.**52**   **Spondylitis (two cases).** Destruction of the intervertebral disk and adjacent part of both vertebral bodies is associated with a large anterior soft-tissue abscess (arrow). (**a**: T3/T4 level. **b**: L5/S1 level, both T1WI, sagittal).

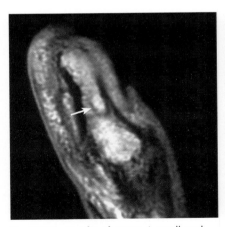

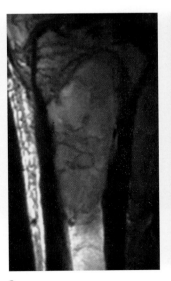

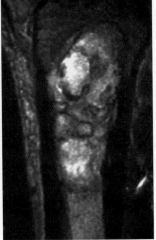

a   b

Fig. 12.**53**   **Brodie abscess.** A small oval hyperintense abscess (arrow) surrounded by a sclerotic rim of low signal intensity is seen in the distal phalanx of the thumb. Increased signal intensity in the remaining distal phalanx indicates surrounding osteomyelitis and edema (T2WI, sagittal).

Fig. 12.**54**   **Chronic osteomyelitis.** A heterogeneous multiloculated lesion is seen in the proximal metadiaphysis of the tibia. The lesion is hypointense to the fatty marrow in **a** (PDWI, coronal) and depicts hyperintense foci in **b** (T2WI, FS, coronal) indicating ongoing active infection.

Table 12.1 (Cont.) Localized bone and bone marrow lesions

Disease	MRI Findings	Comments
Paget disease (Fig. 12.55)	In the inactive phase of Paget disease, MRI findings are identical to plain radiography and include cortical thickening, coarse trabeculation, bone enlargement, reduction in size of the medullary cavity, and bowing deformities. The cortex and thickened trabeculae are devoid of signal. In the long bones, the trabeculae may show a criss-cross pattern separated by fatty marrow or may produce cyst-like areas filled with fat. At times the medullary cavity may appear hypointense on both T1WI and T2WI due to fibrosis and sclerosis. In the active phase of Paget disease, the bone marrow is replaced by fibrovascular tissue, resulting in an inhomogeneous appearance of low signal intensity on T1WI and high signal intensity on T2WI interspersed with thickened trabeculae. Complications such as pathologic fractures, which characteristically have a transverse course, and sarcomatous degeneration are well depicted and easily diagnosed.	Usually an incidental finding in patients over age 40. Polyostotic asymmetric involvement is common, affecting most often pelvis, femur, tibia, spine, skull, scapula, and humerus. Radiographically the pattern of involvement varies from purely osteolytic (e.g., osteoporosis circumscripta in the skull, V-shaped defect in diaphyses of long bones) to purely osteosclerotic (e.g., ivory vertebra). A mixed pattern (e.g., "picture frame" vertebra, "cotton wool" appearance of skull), usually associated with bony enlargement, cortical thickening, and coarse trabeculation is most common. In long bones the disease characteristically extends from an epiphysis to the diaphysis. Bone softening may result in bowing deformities of the long bones, acetabular protrusio, biconcave compression of the vertebral endplates, and basilar invagination.
Fibrous dysplasia (Figs. 12.56, 12.57)	Solitary or multiple, often slightly expansile lesions with uniformly low signal intensity on T1WI. The signal intensity on T2WI varies from low to high, but in the majority of cases is relatively homogeneous. The monostotic form (75%) commonly involves a rib, femur, tibia, humerus, or the mandible, whereas the polyostotic form (25%) frequently involves skull and facial bones, pelvis, spine, and shoulder girdle. In the long bones the lesions are located in the diaphyses or, less commonly, metaphyses. Bowing deformities are frequent in the polyostotic form.	Fibrous dysplasia is usually diagnosed before age 30. Radiographically fibrous dysplasia presents as a slightly expansile osteolytic lesion, often with a sclerotic border. The matrix may, however, also be uniformly dense, partially calcified or ossified, or thick dense bands may be present. *Ossifying fibromas* are closely related to fibrous dysplasia and occur in the facial bones (especially mandible) and tubular bones (especially tibia). In the latter location they are also referred to as *osteofibrous dysplasia* and characteristically involve the anterior cortex of the tibial diaphysis (Fig. 12.58).

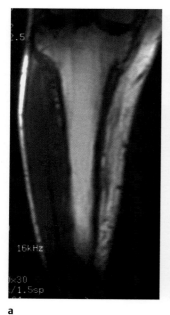 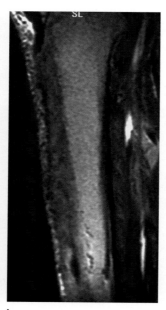

a   **b**

Fig. 12.**55**   **Paget disease.** Enlarged tibia with thickened trabeculae causing hypointense longitudinal streaks in the shaft and a criss-cross pattern in the proximal tibia epiphysis (**a**: coronal, T1WI. **b**:sagittal, T2WI).

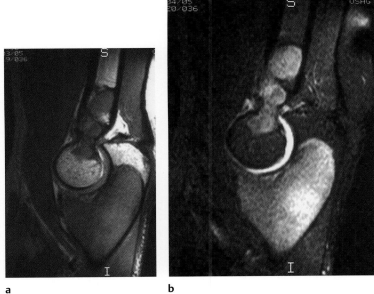

a   b

Fig. 12.**56**   **Fibrous dysplasia.** Enlarged humero-ulnar joint of the elbow with focal homogeneous signal abnormalities. The bone involved, with fibrous dysplasia, presents hypointense in **a** (PDWI, sagittal) and hyperintense in **b** (T2WI, FS, sagittal).

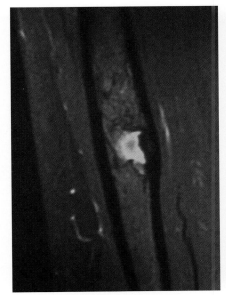

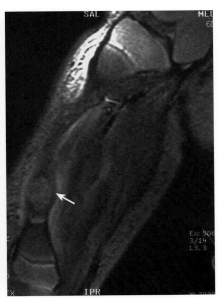

Fig. 12.**57**   **Fibrous dysplasia.** An expanded tibia shaft with heterogeneous signal intensity including a hyperintense focus is seen (T2WI, FS, coronal).

Fig. 12.**58**   **Osteofibrous dysplasia.** A bowed tibia with dysplastic shaft containing an expansile focus of slightly increased signal intensity (arrow) is seen (T2WI, FS, coronal).

Section V   Chest

13 Lungs

Computed tomography (CT), and particularly high-resolution CT, are the image modalities of choice to complement conventional radiography in the evaluation of pulmonary disease. MRI is of limited value for the imaging of pulmonary pathology. Compared with CT, the advantages of MRI in the lungs include multiplanar imaging capability and the ability to display vascular anatomy and blood flow even without the administration of contrast agents. Therefore, the most important indication for pulmonary MRI is the differentiation of normal and pathologic vascular structures from nonvascular pulmonary lesions, especially in patients in whom iodinated contrast agents are contraindicated. Other MRI indications include staging of bronchogenic carcinomas, monitoring their response to treatment, and evaluating tumor recurrence.

Pulmonary thromboembolic disease is diagnosed by the demonstration of intravascular clots and occluded vessels. On spin-echo (SE) sequences pulmonary emboli appear as hyperintense intraluminal lesions of usually medium signal intensity against the background of signal void caused by normal flowing blood. The MRI signal intensity of pulmonary emboli, however, is variable depending on the age of the clot. Pulmonary emboli should not be confused with intraluminal MRI signals caused by slow flow in the pulmonary arteries (e.g. in pulmonary hypertension or proximal to an anatomic or functional vessel occlusion). Gradient-echo (GRE) imaging is sensitive to flow and typically demonstrates pulmonary emboli as low intensity lesions. With optimum technique, visualization of pulmonary emboli is feasible to the level of segmental pulmonary arteries. After intravenous administration of Gd-DTPA, pulmonary emboli appear as hypointense intraluminal defects with little or no contrast enhancement as opposed to primary or secondary neoplastic intravascular processes demonstrating considerable contrast enhancement and a high signal intensity on T2WI on the precontrast MRI.

Chronic pulmonary thromboembolic disease is a relatively uncommon sequela of acute pulmonary thromboembolism in which the emboli become organized and incorporated into the pulmonary arterial walls. These patients develop progressive pulmonary hypertension, which must be differentiated from pulmonary hypertension of other causes because chronic thromboembolic disease is potentially treatable by thromboendarterectomy, provided the central thromboembolic involvement does not extend beyond the lobar arteries.

Pulmonary arterial hypertension may be primary or secondary to a great variety of diseases involving the heart, pulmonary vasculature, or lungs. The underlying pathophysiologic mechanism is an increased pulmonary vascular resistance with elevated pulmonary arterial pressure. The severity of associated anatomic and functional abnormalities demonstrated by MRI is dependent on the severity of the pulmonary hypertension. MRI demonstrates the decreased velocity of pulmonary blood flow in this condition. In healthy subjects intravascular MRI signals are only evident on SE sequences during late diastole when the blood flow is slow. Intraluminal signals during a major portion of the cardiac cycle (e.g., during systole and early diastole) indicates decreased blood velocity. Patients with pulmonary arterial hypertension show a linear correlation between the intensity of the MRI signals in the central pulmonary arteries and the pulmonary vascular resistance. Furthermore, the diameters of the central pulmonary arteries also reflect the pressure within these vessels in pulmonary hypertension. The diameter of a normal main pulmonary artery measures less than 3 cm. A main pulmonary artery diameter of 3 cm and larger associated with bilateral hilar arterial enlargement is indicative of pulmonary hypertension. Right ventricular hypertrophy, frequently with flattening or convexity of the intraventricular septum toward the left ventricular chamber, is usually associated. Pulmonary artery dissection is a rare and usually fatal complication of chronic pulmonary artery hypertension that is readily demonstrated by MRI.

Pulmonary arteriovenous malformations (AVMs) are usually congenital or, less commonly, posttraumatic. They present as round or slightly lobular masses of less than one to several centimeters in diameter on chest radiographs. Identification of feeding and draining vessels is essential to the diagnosis, but often difficult with plain radiography. Occasionally more than one feeding artery and draining vein is present. Approximately one-third of patients have multiple lesions in the lungs, but often only the dominant lesion is evident on chest radiographs. About half of these patients have additional lesions elsewhere, including the skin and mucous membranes. This condition is known as *hereditary hemorrhagic telangiectasis* (*Rendu-Osler-Weber syndrome*). On SE images only the wall of the AVM is usually seen because of the flow-related signal void within the lesion. On GRE images and especially magnetic resonance angiography (MRA) the lesion, including its feeding and draining vessels, are visible as high signal intensity structures.

Pulmonary varix refers to an abnormal tortuosity and dilatation of one or more pulmonary veins. It may be congenital or associated with mitral valve disease. It usually is not recognized until the patient reaches adulthood and most often represents an incidental finding. Radiographically the lesion is apparent as one or more round or oval homogeneous opacities, somewhat lobulated, but well defined, in the medial third of either lung. MRI can display the vascular nature of the lesion and its connection to the left atrium. A pulmonary AVM close to the left atrium may at times be difficult to differentiate.

Bronchopulmonary sequestration is a congenital pulmonary malformation without communication to the bronchial tree. The lesion is usually located in the posterior basal segment of the left or, less commonly, right lower lobe and is almost invariably contiguous with the diaphragm. The radiographic appearance is dependent on the presence or absence of infection. Without infection and subsequent communication with the bronchial tree a homogeneous, sharply defined, lobulated mass is seen radiographically. The cystic nature of the mass caused by blind ending, ectatic bronchi is readily appreciated by MRI. The cysts can be single or multiple and vary in size. When infection has resulted in communication with the bronchial tree, an air-containing cystic mass with or without fluid levels may be evident. The diagnosis of bronchopulmonary sequestration relies on the demonstration of an aberrant systemic artery supplying the sequestered lung. MRI, including MRA, can visualize this aberrant systemic blood supply, most commonly originating from the abdominal aorta or one of its branches. In intralobar sequestrations venous drainage occurs via a pulmonary vein, whereas in the less common extralobar sequestration venous drainage occurs via the systemic venous system (e.g., inferior vena cava, portal system, or azygous and hemiazygos veins).

Other congenital cystic mass lesions in the lungs with characteristic MRI features include bronchogenic cysts and cystic adenomatoid malformations. *Bronchogenic cysts* are solitary, sharply circumscribed, round or oval, homogeneous lesions, which may measure up to several centimeters in diameter and are most commonly located in the central (perihilar) portions of a lower lobe. Communications with the bronchial system eventually may occur after infection. *Cystic adenomatoid malformations* consist of an intralobar mass of disorganized pulmonary tissue with or without gross cyst formation. When present, the cysts usually communicate with the normal airways. The absence of abnormal feeding and draining vessels differentiates this condition from bronchopulmonary sequestration. Acquired fluid-filled structures in the lungs include *cystic bronchiectasis, echinococcal (hydatid) cysts,* and *traumatic lung cysts.* The MRI features of the latter, however, vary depending on the age of the hematoma. Abscesses and malignancies with central necrosis may also present as cystic pulmonary lesions, but their thick and often irregular wall in conjunction with the clinical history differentiates these conditions from other more benign cystic lesions.

Fat-containing focal pulmonary lesions include hamartomas, lipomas, and lipoid pneumonias. Unequivocal demonstration of fat within a pulmonary mass indicates a benign process. However, following intratumoral hemorrhage any pulmonary mass eventually may contain sufficient amounts of methemoglobin to mimic a fat-containing lesion on MRI. In hamartomas focal areas of fat are visible within the tumor in 50% of cases. CT is superior to MRI in diagnosing hamartomas, since characteristic stippled or conglomerate ("popcorn") calcifications present in 30% of cases and are much more readily appreciated. Lipomas rarely originate from the tracheobronchial wall and even more uncommonly from the lung parenchyma itself. Lipoid pneumonias result from the aspiration of instilled oily nose drops and produce chronic airspace consolidations which contain fat density collections that are usually located at the lung bases.

Pulmonary vascular anomalies are well depicted by MRI. *Pulmonary arterial anomalies* include the following conditions: 1) *Absence of the main pulmonary artery.* The right and left main pulmonary arteries are connected to the aorta by a ductus or a single great artery arising from a common semilunar heart valve, invariably in association with a ventricular septal defect (persistent truncus arteriosus). 2) *Proximal interruption or absence of the right or left pulmonary artery.* Vicarious blood flow to the affected hypoplastic lung occurs via markedly hypertrophic bronchial or intercostal arteries or from the innominate or subclavian arteries. 3) *Anomalous origin of the left pulmonary artery from the right.* The aberrant left pulmonary artery passes between the esophagus and trachea in its course to the left hilum ("pulmonary sling"). The intimate relationship of this vessel to the right main bronchus and trachea results in their compression and various obstructive effects on the right or both lungs. 4) *Pulmonary artery stenosis (coarctation).* The pulmonary artery stenoses are usually associated with poststenotic dilatations and may be single or multiple, short or long, peripheral or central, unilateral or bilateral. Cardiovascular anomalies (e.g., infundibular, valvular, or supravalvular stenosis, and atrial septal defect) are commonly associated with central coarctations. 5) *Fistula between right pulmonary artery and left atrium.* Radiographically a round opacity measuring 2 to 3 cm in diameter is seen in the right hemithorax adjacent to the left atrium representing the fistula arising from the otherwise unremarkable right pulmonary artery. 6) *Pulmonary artery dilatation.* Enlargement of the main pulmonary artery occurs in pulmonary arterial hypertension, increased pulmonary flow (left-to-right shunts and high-output states), turbulent pulmonary flow (poststenotic dilatation), and intrinsic abnormalities (aneurysm and idiopathic dilatation). Unilateral left pulmonary artery enlargement suggests poststenotic dilatation, idiopathic dilatation, aneurysm, pulmonary thromboembolism, or surgically produced left-to-right shunts. Unilateral right pulmonary artery enlargement suggests an aneurysm or pulmonary thromboembolism. 7) *Vasculitis and peripheral pulmonary artery aneurysm formation.* Peripheral pulmonary artery narrowing, dilatation, and occlusion combined with aneurysm or pseudoaneurysm formation are evident in polyarteritis nodosa, Takayasu arteritis (chronic inflammatory panarteritis affecting segments of the aorta and its main branches and pulmonary arteries), Behçet syndrome (pulmonary artery aneurysms near hila and venous thromboembolism in patients presenting with aphthous stomatitis, genital ulcerations, uveitis, skin lesions, arthritis, gastrointestinal ulcerations, and central nervous system [CNS] involvement), and intravenous drug addicts (mycotic aneurysms).

Anomalous pulmonary venous return may be total or partial. Total anomalous pulmonary venous return may be classified as supracardiac (to a persistent left superior vena cava and hence to the left innominate vein), cardiac (to the right atrium or coronary sinus), infradiaphragmatic (to portal system), or mixed. The hypogenetic lung (scimitar) syndrome consists of hypoplasia of the right lung and partial anomalous pulmonary venous return via the "scimitar vein" to the inferior vena cava, portal vein, hepatic vein, or right atrium. Absence of the pulmonary artery, systemic arterialization of the lung, pulmonary sequestration, interruption of the inferior vena cava, and/or an accessory right diaphragm are occasionally associated with this condition.

Bronchogenic carcinomas (Fig. 13.1) are classified in squamous cell (epidermoid) carcinomas (35%), adenocarcinomas (35%), small cell carcinomas (20%), large cell carcinomas (8%), adenosquamous carcinomas (1%), carcinoids (0.5%), and bronchial gland carcinomas (0.5%). Squamous cell carcinomas present as endobronchial lesions with airway obstruction (two-thirds) or as peripheral nodules (one-third). Adenocarcinomas present in the great majority of cases as peripheral mass lesions. A subtype of the adenocarcinoma is the bronchioalveolar carcinoma which may present in a diffuse form. Small cell carcinomas commonly present as small lung lesions with large hilar and mediastinal adenopathy. Large cell carcinomas present as large bulky peripheral mass lesions. The tumor-node-metastasis (TNM) staging of bronchogenic carcinomas is shown in Table 13.**1**.

Table 13.1 TNM staging of bronchogenic carcinomas

T0: no evidence of tumor.
T1: tumor less than 3 cm.
T2: tumor more than 3 cm or tumor with visceral pleural invasion or associated with obstructive pneumonia/atelectasis.
T3: tumor less than 2 cm from carina, or invasion of parietal pleura, chest wall, diaphragm, mediastinal pleura, or pericardium.
T4: invasion of carina, heart, great vessels, trachea, esophagus, vertebral body, or malignant effusion.
N0: no lymph node metastases.
N1: peribronchial and/or ipsilateral hilar node involvement.
N2: ipsilateral mediastinal node involvement.
N3: contralateral hilar and/or mediastinal node involvement.
M0: no distant metastases.
M1: distant metastases (bone, adrenals, liver, kidneys, brain, lungs, and others).

Staging (1–3A resectable, 3B-4 nonresectable)
1:   T1–2, N0, M0
2:   T1–2, N1, M0
3A: T3, or T1–3, N2, M0
3B: T1–3, N3, or T4, N0–2, M0
4:   T4, N3, M0, or M1

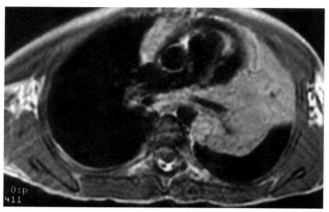

Fig. 13.1 Bronchogenic carcinoma. A large mass with involvement of the ipsilateral hilum and mediastinum and invasion of the adjacent pericardium and chest wall is seen (PDWI).

MRI has no significant role in the diagnosis of bronchogenic carcinomas, but may be valuable in staging the malignancy. Bronchogenic carcinomas present as solitary peripheral or central mass lesions, usually with an irregular or spiculated border. Cavitation occurs in 15 % of cases, most commonly with squamous cell carcinoma. The cavity typically is thick walled with an irregular inner lining. Eccentric calcifications occur in 5 % of cases, but are difficult to appreciate with MRI. Distal airway obstruction presenting as segmental, lobar, or total lung atelectasis and obstructive pneumonitis is found in one-third of the cases. MRI may be helpful in differentiating the central tumor from the obstructive atelectasis and pneumonitis. In the majority of cases the tumor appears hypointense to the obstructive atelectasis on T2WI because of the retained bronchoalveolar secretion in the obstructed lung. After intravenous Gd-DTPA administration, the contrast enhancement of the obstructive atelectasis/pneumonitis tends to be both faster and more extensive than in the tumor.

Endobronchial lesions or circumferential bronchial narrowing or occlusion are commonly evident in central tumors. Similarly, pulmonary vessels may be occluded or contain tumor thrombi. Unilateral hilar adenopathy with or without mediastinal involvement is common and may

be the only manifestation in 5 % of cases, especially in small cell carcinomas. Pleural effusions are present in 10 % of cases and may result from direct pleural invasion by the tumor or from lymphatic obstruction. Localized or diffuse pleural thickening is occasionally found with peripheral tumors. Direct tumor extension into the chest wall, ribs, and spine may also be evident in more advanced cases.

MRI appears to be the most accurate imaging method in assessing preoperatively the *tumor resectability*, i.e. in differentiating between the resectable tumor stage 3A from the nonresectable stage 3B (see Table 13.1). Tumors extending into the chest wall, diaphragm, mediastinal pleura, or pericardium as well as tumors with metastases to the ipsilateral hilar and mediastinal lymph nodes are still considered potentially resectable. On the other hand, tumors involving the heart, great vessels, trachea, esophagus, and carina or with metastases in the contralateral mediastinal or hilar lymph nodes or supraclavicular lymph nodes on either side are considered nonresectable. Tumor invasion of the sternum or spine indicates advanced disease and nonresectability also (Fig. 13.2).

Pancoast tumors (*superior sulcus tumors*) arise from the apex of the lung and have a propensity to invade the apical chest wall with involvement of the rib cage, spine, brachiocephalic vessels, brachial plexus, and cervicothoracic sympathetic chain (Figs. 13.3, 13.4). Depending on the invasion of these structures the patients present with shoulder and arm pain, atrophy of hand muscles, and/or Horner syndrome (enophthalmos, miosis, ptosis, and anhydrosis). The tumors constitute about 3 % of all bronchogenic carcinomas and usually are of the adenocarcinoma or squamous cell carcinoma variety. MRI appears to be the preferred image modality to depict the anatomic relationship of the tumor with contiguous thoracic structures.

Response to treatment and *tumor recurrence* can be evaluated by MRI. Besides reduction in tumor size the development of necrosis within the lung lesion undergoing radiotherapy and/or chemotherapy is also indicative of a beneficial treatment effect. Compared with viable tumors, necrotic tumors are hypointense on T1WI, hyperintense on T2WI, and do not enhance after intravenous Gd-DTPA administration. *Radiation pneumonitis* developing between 1 month and 1 year after treatment, on the other hand, may be difficult to differentiate from tumor progression. Radiation changes are strictly limited to the field of irradiation

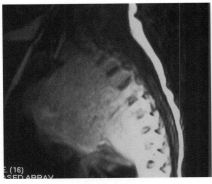

Fig. 13.**2 Nonresectable lung tumor.** Tumor invasion of the spine is evident, indicating nonresectability (PDWI, sagittal).

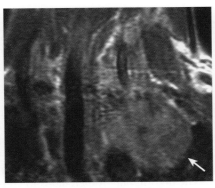

Fig. 13.**3 Pancoast tumor.** A large mass (arrow) in the left pulmonary apex with invasion of the superior pulmonary sulcus is seen (T1WI, coronal).

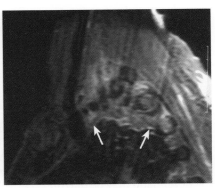

Fig. 13.**4 Pancoast tumor.** A mass in the apex of the right lung with infiltration of the brachial plexus (arrows) is seen after intravenous Gd-DTPA administration (T1WI, FS, +C, sagittal).

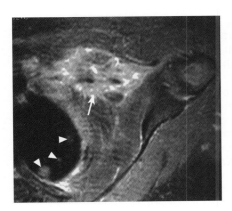

Abb. 13.**5 Breast carcinoma metastases.** Three enhancing pulmonary nodules (arrowheads) are seen.
A large, inhomogeneously enhancing metastasis (arrow) is seen in the left axilla (T1WI, FS, +C).

and do not develop de novo 1 year or later after treatment. On T2WI both active radiation pneumonitis and tumor display a high signal intensity. On gadolinium-enhanced T1WI the radiation pneumonitis tends to demonstrate a higher signal intensity than the tumor, but this difference is of little practical value in differentiating these two conditions.

The transition from radiation pneumonitis to radiation fibrosis is gradual and may be complete after 1 year at the earliest. At this stage MRI can differentiate radiation fibrosis depicting a low signal intensity on both T1WI and T2WI and no contrast enhancement from residual or recurrent tumor demonstrating a high signal intensity on T2WI and significant contrast enhancement.

In *postpneumonectomy* the hemithorax gradually fills with fluid over 3 to 24 weeks and decreases in volume. Subsequently, the fluid may be replaced by connective tissue or the fluid may persist for years. In cases in which the fluid is replaced by the connective tissue the mediastinal shift to the ipsilateral side is more pronounced. A shift of the mediastinum to the contralateral side indicates either a bronchopulmonary fistula with empyema or tumor recurrence. MRI can readily delineate and differentiate between encapsulated empyema and recurrent bronchogenic carcinoma.

Compared with CT, MRI is generally inferior in both detection and characterization of *pulmonary nodules* (Fig. 13.**5**). A possible exception are nodules or mucous plugs close to the hila and in the lung periphery that could be mistaken for pulmonary vessels by CT. The value of MRI in differentiating pulmonary consolidations is limited since, regardless of their pathogenesis, they demonstrate a low signal intensity on T1WI and a high signal intensity on T2WI. A few exceptions do, however, exist: A high signal intensity on T1WI is found in lipoid pneumonias, alveolar proteinosis, and pulmonary infarcts and hematomas containing methemoglobin, whereas a low signal intensity on T2WI is evident in diseases characterized by repetitive episodes of pulmonary hemorrhages, such as pulmonary hemosiderosis and Goodpasture syndrome, owing to the deposition of paramagnetic iron in the lung parenchyma. The increased signal intensity occasionally observed in the latter two conditions may be related to methemoglobin formation.

Differentiation between obstructive and nonobstructive atelectasis may also be feasible with MRI. Obstructive atelectasis occurs when the communication between trachea and lung periphery is obstructed by either an endobronchial lesion or extrinsic compression. The obstructive lesion can often be identified by MRI and the collapsed airless lung parenchyma with a fluid-filled bronchoalveolar system shows a high signal intensity on T2WI as opposed to the low signal intensity of the nonobstructive atelectasis without retained bronchoalveolar secretions.

14 Pleura, Diaphragm, Chest Wall, and Breast

Exudates, transudates, and *sanguinous effusions* cannot be reliably differentiated from each other by MRI. Exudative effusions enhance slightly more than transudative effusions but the difference is too small and the enhancement too little to be of any clinical significance. A chylothorax on the other hand may be diagnosed by MRI by the high signal intensity of lipids on T1WI. A subacute hemothorax of 1 week duration and longer may also present with a high signal intensity on T1WI owing to methemoglobin formation.

On T1-weighted spin-echo (SE) sequences the presence of an exudative or transudative effusion is often difficult to appreciate, since it demonstrates a low signal intensity similar to that of the adjacent lung. The effusion, however, appears hypodense to an adjacent consolidated lung on T1WI. On T2WI the effusion has an increased signal intensity, making the effusion much more easily recognizable. With this imaging sequence the effusion may be difficult to differentiate from consolidated lung.

Pleural fluid initially collects in the most dependent portion of the pleural space, which is posteromedial and caudal to the lung base in supine position. The fluid assumes a crescent or lenticular shape. Small pleural effusions can be differentiated from pleural thickening by their higher signal intensity on T2WI. If necessary, freely mobile fluid can be diagnosed by obtaining images in the prone or lateral decubitus position. Furthermore, after intravenous Gd-DTPA administration, a thickened, inflamed, or neoplastic pleura enhances, whereas purely fibrotic thickening and pleural fluid for practical purposes do not.

Larger pleural effusions extend toward the lateral chest wall and may enter the major fissure, where the fluid tapers medially and produces a characteristic "beak" appearance. A large pleural effusion compresses the lower lobe and displaces it anteriorly, giving the appearance that the collapsed lower lobe floats on the pleural fluid. The airless posterior edge of the lower lobe may be mistaken for the diaphragm with pleural fluid posteriorly and apparent peritoneal fluid anteriorly. Similarly, inversion of a hemidiaphragm by a massive pleural effusion may simulate intraabdominal fluid. However, the correct diagnosis can easily be made by analyzing both fluid collection and lower lobe, as well as their relationship in sequential, more cephalad axial images.

Both pleural effusion and ascites present as arcuate or semilunar fluid collections displacing liver and spleen away from the adjacent chest walls. Differentiation of these fluid collections is possible by MRI using a variety of different criteria. Fluid outside (peripheral to) the diaphragm is pleural, whereas fluid inside the diaphragm is peritoneal. Pleural fluid may surround the lung, while peritoneal fluid may be surrounded by the lung bases. In the posterior costophrenic angle, a pleural fluid collection is posterior to the diaphragm and causes anterolateral displacement of the crus. Posterior peritoneal fluid is anterior to the diaphragm. Pleural fluid gradually decreases in size on more caudal axial images, whereas peritoneal fluid increases in size and progressively extends lateral to the liver and spleen on more caudal images. Fluid seen posterior to the liver is within the pleural space, since the peritoneum does not extend into this region because the bare area of the liver is devoid of peritoneal covering and is attached to the posterior diaphragm.

Unilateral or bilateral pleural effusions not associated with any other signs of intrathoracic disease are most often *tuberculous* in young patients and *neoplastic* in the elderly. Neoplastic effusions are found with *metastases, lymphoma,* and *leukemia* and in the Meigs-Salmon syndrome (nonmalignant pleural effusions and ascites with benign or malignant ovarian tumors, or occasionally with uterine leiomyoma). Besides tuberculosis, viral and mycoplasma infections may present with pleural effusions as the sole finding. Of the connective-tissue disorders, both *rheumatoid disease* and *systemic lupus erythematosus* (primary and drug-induced) may present with pleural effusions as the only intrathoracic manifestation. *Congestive heart failure* is the most common cause of pleural effusions but cardiomegaly and signs of cardiac decompensation are usually associated. In *Dressler syndrome,* effusions usually develop 2 to 4 weeks after myocardial infarct or cardiac surgery (*postpericardiotomy syndrome*), but may occasionally occur months or even years after the causative episode. *Pulmonary thromboembolic disease* presenting with pleural effusions as sole manifestation is highly unusual.

Traumatic and *postsurgical pleural effusions* are common, but history and associated findings are usually diagnostic. Patients with *asbestos exposure* occasionally present with pleural effusion alone. A variety of abdominal diseases such as *pancreatitis, subphrenic abscess, ascites of any cause, renal failure,* and *liver cirrhosis* are frequently associated with pleural effusions, but the primary cause is usually obvious by MRI in these conditions. *Myxedema, familial Mediterranean fever (familial paroxysmal polyserositis),* and *primary lymphedema* are rare inherited conditions presenting with pleural effusions as the only intrathoracic abnormality.

Empyema is a purulent pleural infection usually secondary to a bacterial pneumonia. Other less frequent extrapulmonary sources include bacteremia, subphrenic abscess, spondylitis, thoracotomy, and penetrating chest trauma. An empyema has to be differentiated from a *parapneumonic effusion,* which is an uninfected (sympathetic) serous exudate in pneumonias and resolves spontaneously. It results from increased permeability of the inflamed visceral pleura. Pulmonary infections which frequently extend beyond the pleural space into the chest wall include *actinomycosis* and *nocardiosis,* and occasionally *tuberculosis, blastomycosis,* and *coccidioidomycosis.*

A *loculated empyema* (Fig. 14.1) has a lenticular shape conforming to the pleural space. It is sharply demarcated from the pulmonary parenchyma and forms obtuse angles with the chest wall. The neighboring lung is compressed by a large empyema, resulting in gradual displacement and bowing of the adjacent pulmonary vessels and bronchi. The wall of the empyema consists of the inflamed visceral and parietal pleura and is relatively thin, smooth, and of uniform thickness. After intravenous contrast Gd-DTPA administration, the wall of the empyema enhances so that on T1WI the visceral and parietal pleura layers separated by pus become clearly visible ("split pleura sign"). The shape of an empyema as well as the length of any possibly contained air-fluid level characteristically change when the patient is moved to the prone or decubitus position. In an organizing empyema the walls may become thickened and eventually calcified. Demonstration of fluid collections within the thickened pleural peel, even at this stage, suggests that the infection is still ongoing and active.

An empyema has to be differentiated from a peripheral lung abscess abutting the pleural surface. A *lung abscess* tends to be spherical without change in shape and with equidimensional air-fluid levels when the patient is imaged in different planes. The wall of a lung abscess is irregular and poorly defined and may contain several areas of cavitation. The lesion characteristically forms an acute angle with the chest wall. Pulmonary vessels and bronchi appear to enter the abscess rather than being displaced by it. After intravenous Gd-DTPA administration, the irregularly enhanced periphery contrasts with the nonenhanced necrotic center.

Pleural thickening is caused by fibrosis and neoplasia. Pleural fibrosis is a common sequela of *hemothorax, empyema*, and *exposure to asbestos* and *talc*. In all these conditions, focal to extensive pleural calcifications are frequent, and with the exception of asbestos and talc inhalation, the pleural fibrosis predominantly affects the visceral pleura. Other less common causes of nonneoplastic pleural thickening include *fungal diseases, rheumatoid disease, radiation therapy, organizing pleural effusions* of other causes, *sarcoidosis*, and *splenosis* (posttraumatic implantation of splenic tissue on the left pleura). Neoplastic pleural thickening is associated with *mesotheliomas* (benign and malignant), *metastasis, lymphoma*, and local invasion from *bronchogenic carcinomas* (especially *Pancoast tumors*) and *malignant thymomas*.

Extensive pleural thickening caused by either fibrosis or neoplasia may result in encasement of the lung, causing restriction and loss of volume. In fibrosis the pleural thickening appears uniform and a layer of extrapleural fat often becomes visible separating the parietal pleura, which may be calcified, from the rib cage. With neoplastic lung encasement (e.g., in malignant mesothelioma or metastases) the pleural thickening is irregular and often nodular and the extrapleural fat is invaded by tumor.

Asbestos-related pleural disease is almost invariably bilateral. Pleural plaques (smooth focal thickening of the parietal pleura) are characteristically located adjacent to the inner surfaces of the sixth to tenth ribs posteriorly and laterally, whereas the pleura between these ribs is often not affected ("skip lesions"). Diffuse, more or less uniform thickening in the lower hemithoraces is another slightly less frequent manifestation. Focal visceral pleural fibrosis also occurs and may cause interlobular fissural thickening. Calcifications are common, but difficult to appreciate with MRI. They range from punctate, nodular, and linear densities to complete encirclement of the lower portions of the lung. Pleural plaques with or without calcifications frequently occur in the diaphragmatic pleura, but typically spare the costophrenic angles. Mediastinal and paravertebral plaques are also a common finding.

Benign (fibrous) mesotheliomas usually arise from the visceral pleura. They present as a localized, sharply defined soft-tissue mass, sometimes with slightly lobulated margins, ranging from 2 to 14 cm in diameter. Occasionally the lesion is pedunculated. Larger lesions may undergo malignant degeneration in up to one-third of the cases. Benign

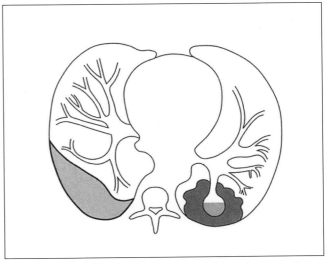

Fig. 14.1 Differentiation between loculated empyema and lung abscess. The empyema (right lung base) has an elliptical shape, well-defined, smooth, uniform walls ("split pleura"), obtuse angles with the chest wall, and displaced vessels. The lung abscess (left lung base) has a spherical shape, one or more cavities usually with air-fluid levels, poorly defined irregular wall, acute angles with the chest wall, and vessels entering the lesion.

mesotheliomas demonstrate a low signal intensity on T1WI and a medium to high signal intensity on T2WI. Larger lesions have an inhomogeneous appearance and irregular contrast enhancement due to necrosis, hemorrhage, cyst formations, and calcifications. A small pleural effusion is occasionally associated.

Malignant mesotheliomas are highly malignant lesions with an extremely poor prognosis. The majority of cases occur in patients with asbestos exposure. The neoplasm presents as a diffuse nodular or plaque-like pleural thickening that eventually encases the entire lung. Hemorrhagic pleural effusions are commonly associated and may mask the irregular nodular pleural thickening caused by malignancy. MRI obtained in different positions (e.g., prone or lateral decubitus) may be useful to separate pleural fluid from mesothelioma. Large effusions associated with mesothelioma are frequently not associated with a significant mediastinal shift to the contralateral side, probably because of tumor encasement of the affected hemithorax. On MRI malignant mesotheliomas appear as heterogeneous lesions with low to medium signal intensity on T1WI and medium to high signal intensity on T2WI. After intravenous Gd-DTPA administration the lesions demonstrate significant but inhomogeneous contrast enhancement differentiating the tumor from asbestos-related pleural thickening and loculated pleural fluid collections. The tumor spreads by local invasion into the fissures and adjacent structures such as ipsilateral lung, mediastinum, pericardium, diaphragm, lateral chest wall, and contralateral hemithorax. Hematogenous metastases are less common.

Pleural metastases (Fig. 14.2) presenting with nodular pleural thickening and effusions are often indistinguishable from malignant mesothelioma. Bilateral involvement, and the absence of asbestos-related pleural disease and pulmonary asbestosis favor metastatic disease. Besides *bronchogenic carcinoma* (especially *Pancoast tumor*) and *malignant thymoma*, both of which invade the pleura by contiguous spread, hematogenous pleural metastases

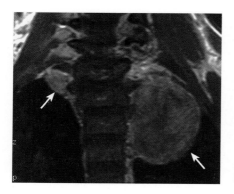

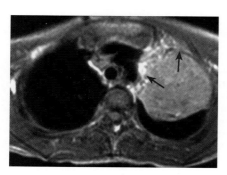

Fig. 14.2 Pleural metastases. Bilateral pleural lesions (arrows) are seen (T1WI, coronal). Diffuse, predominantly osteoblastic metastases in the spine presenting with low signal intensity are also present (metastatic breast carcinoma).

Fig. 14.3 Pulmonary sarcoma metastases. A mass in the left upper lobe with infiltration of the adjacent mediastinum and anterior chest wall (arrows) is seen (PDWI).

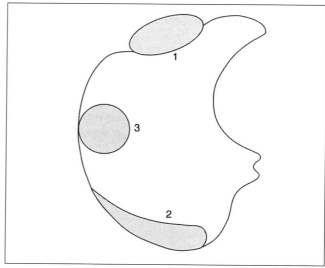

Fig. 14.4 Differentiation between extrapleural, pleural, and subpleural lesions. An extrapleural lesion (1) tends to form obtuse angles with the chest wall by displacing the overlying pleura centrally. A pleural lesion (2) forms either an obtuse angle with the chest wall, when the lesion remains confined between the two pleural layers, or an acute angle, when the lesion protrudes into the lung parenchyma. A subpleural (peripheral lung) lesion (3) tends to form acute angles with the chest wall.

most frequently originate from *carcinoma* of the *breast, kidney, ovary,* and *gastrointestinal tract. Pleural lymphoma* may present as a localized, broad-based pleural mass, usually associated with pleural effusion, but is rarely the initial manifestation of the disease.

An *apical pleural cap* may be caused by a variety of conditions. *Pleural fluid* tends to accumulate over the pulmonary apex in the supine position. Apical pleural thickening without extension into the chest wall most often results from *chronic tuberculosis* (usually bilateral, but often asymmetric) or from *healed empyema, old hemothorax,* or *sequela of radiation therapy.* A soft-tissue mass in the apical chest wall with involvement of the brachiocephalic vessels and plexus and/or invasion of the adjacent ribs and vertebral bodies indicates a malignant lesion. The most common superior sulcus malignancy is a *Pancoast tumor* (Fig. 14.3) but *metastases* (e.g., from breast carcinoma and, less commonly, lymphoma) can present in a similar fashion (Fig. 14.3*). Benign tumors are rare and may be of neural (e.g., schwannoma and neurofibroma) or mesenchymal origin (e.g., fibroma, desmoid, and lipoma). Hematomas and hemorrhages in the superior sulcus are associated with rib, clavicle, and spine fractures, are secondary to aortic and great vessel rupture, or are iatrogenic (catheter perforation). Both *upper lobe atelectasis* and *normal variants* such as excessive periapical fat and *vascular anomalies* (e.g., elongation or dilatation of the subclavian artery) may simulate an apical mass lesion on plain radiography, but can easily be diagnosed by MRI because of their characteristic features.

Extrapleural lesions (Fig. 14.4) commonly originate from the ribs and intercostal soft tissues, including vessels and nerves. These lesions displace the overlying parietal and visceral pleura centrally, thereby forming an obtuse angle between the lesion and the chest wall. Rib involvement further supports the extrapleural nature of the lesion (Fig. 14.5). Rib lesions are most commonly caused by traumatic,

neoplastic, and infectious processes and do not differ in their presentation from other skeletal locations. Common rib lesions include *healing fractures, metastases, multiple myeloma, osteomyelitis* (bacterial, tuberculous, fungal), and *benign conditions* such as fibrous dysplasia, bone cyst, enchondroma, osteochondroma, eosinophilic granuloma, brown tumor, and extramedullary hematopoiesis.

The diaphragm is a large, dome-shaped muscle that incompletely divides the thorax from the abdomen. The diaphragmatic crura are tendinous structures arising from the anterolateral surface of the upper lumbar spine. The right crus is larger and longer than the left crus and originates from the first three lumbar vertebral bodies, whereas the left crus arises from the first two lumbar vertebrae. The diaphragmatic crura may have a nodular appearance that should not be mistaken for enlarged retrocrural lymph nodes. Normally these nodes are quite small and do not exceed 6 mm in cross-sectional diameter.

Diaphragmatic hernias may be congenital or acquired. Hiatal hernia (herniation of the stomach through the esophageal hiatus) is by far the most common type and does not require MRI for diagnosis. *Bochdalek hernias* are commonly left-sided and occur anywhere along the posterior costodiaphragmatic margin. They tend to be rather large and may contain omental or retroperitoneal fat, bowel, spleen, liver, kidney, stomach, and pancreas. *Morgagni hernias* occur through an anteromedial parasternal defect and contain liver, omentum, or bowel. They are rare and usually right sided, tend to be small, and may be associated with a pericardial defect.

Traumatic diaphragmatic hernias are found with both blunt and penetrating trauma, but may be asymptomatic for months and even years. Over 90% are located on the left side, usually in the central or posterior portion of the diaphragm. Omentum, stomach, bowel, spleen, and kidney may all herniate through the ruptured diaphragm. Strangulation is a common complication.

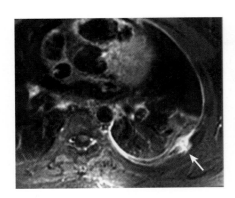

Fig. 14.5 Extra-pleural lesion. An enhancing lesion (arrow) originating from the intercostal nerve is seen infiltrating the adjacent rib, pleura, and lung (Askin tumor) (T1WI, FS, +C).

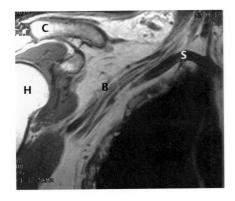

Fig. 14.6 Normal brachial plexus. B: brachial plexus. C: clavicle. H: humerus. S: subclavian artery (T1WI, coronal).

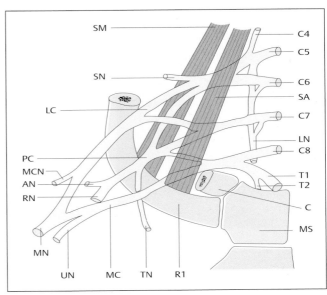

Fig. 14.7 Brachial plexus.
AN: axillary nerve. C: clavicle. C4-C8: ventral rami of these cervical spinal nerves. LC: lateral cord. LN: long thoracic nerve. MC: medial cord. MCN: musculocutaneous nerve. MN: median nerve. MS: manubrium sterni. PC: posterior cord. R1: first rib. RN: radial nerve. SA: scalenus anterior muscle. SM: scalenus medius muscle. SN: suprascapular nerve. T1, T2: ventral rami of T1 and T2 spinal nerves. TN: thoracodorsal nerve. UN: ulnar nerve.

A *diaphragmatic eventration* is caused by a congenitally weak diaphragm with cephalad displacement of the corresponding abdominal content. The eventration occurs more frequently on the right side, where it involves the anteromedial portion of the diaphragm. In this case the liver is displaced cephalad and should not be confused with a peripheral pulmonary or pleural mass. On the left side the eventration usually involves the entire hemidiaphragm and mimics diaphragmatic paralysis. Because of its dome-shape the diaphragm is often inadequately visualized on axial images. Demonstration of diaphragmatic and juxtadiaphragmatic abnormalities and their relationship to the diaphragm may require imaging in the sagittal and/or coronal planes. Kinematic MRI studies can be used to differentiate between diaphragmatic paralysis and eventration, but fluoroscopy remains the method of choice for this purpose.

Because of both superb contrast resolution and multiplanar imaging capability, MRI is the method of choice to visualize lesions in the brachial plexus and axillary space. The *brachial plexus* (Figs. 14.6 and 14.7) is formed by the union of the anterior rami of the lower four cervical nerves (C5 to C8) and of the first thoracic nerve (T1) with variable contributions of C4 and T2. The C5 and C6 roots form the upper, C7 the middle, and C8 and T1 the lower trunks of the brachial plexus. In the lower neck the upper and middle trunks lie above and the lower trunk posterior to the subclavian artery. Just above or behind the medial half of the clavicle the three trunks split into anterior and posterior divisions. The anterior divisions of the upper and middle trunks form the lateral cord. The anterior division of the lower trunk continues as medial cord. The posterior divisions of all three trunks unite to form the posterior cord. In the axilla the cords of the brachial plexus are closely grouped around the axillary artery and the designations "medial," "lateral," and "posterior" indicate the relationships of the cords to this vessel as it passes behind the pectoralis minor muscle.

The *axillary space* is bordered by the pectoralis major and minor muscles anteriorly; the latissimus dorsi, teres major, and subscapularis muscles posteriorly; the chest wall and serratus anterior muscle medially; and the coracobrachialis and biceps muscles laterally. When the patient is scanned with the arms above the head, the axilla is open laterally and an artifactual space becomes visible beneath the trapezius muscle at the level of the thoracic and lower cervical spine. This compartment has been termed *subtrapezial space*.

The axilla contains the axillary artery and vein, branches of the brachial plexus, and a large number of lymph nodes all embedded in fat. The axillary vein lies anteriorly and caudad to the axillary artery, whereas the brachial plexus is located cephalad and posterior to the artery. Axillary lymph nodes normally measure up to 1 cm in diameter, but occasionally slightly larger lymph nodes are found in healthy subjects. Lymph nodes measuring between 1.5 and 2 cm suggest inflammation (reactive hyperplasia) or early neoplastic disease, whereas lymph nodes exceeding 2 cm in diameter are indicative of metastatic or lymphomatous disease (Figs. 14.8–14.12). Both axillary and parasternal (internal mammary) lymph nodes are the primary regional nodes of breast carcinomas and are exquisitely evaluated by MRI.

Primary neoplasms of the chest wall, other than skin and breast lesions, are usually of mesenchymal origin. The MRI presentation of these tumors does not differ from other locations and is discussed in Table 9.2. *Lipomas* (Fig. 14.13 are the most common chest wall tumors and because of their signal characteristics can unequivocally be diagnosed by MRI. They may extend between ribs into the subpleural space and assume a dumbbell configuration. Another frequent, benign chest wall lesion is the intramuscular *hemangioma* presenting on T1WI as a poorly marginated, heterogeneous lesion isointense to skeletal muscle interspersed with areas of increased signal intensity. On T2WI the intramuscular hemangioma appears well marginated

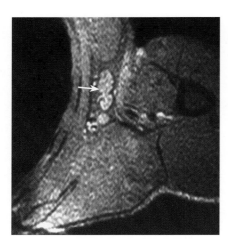

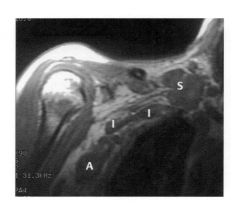

Fig. 14.**8** **Reactive lymph node hyperplasia in AIDS.** Benign lymph node enlargement (arrow) is seen in the axilla (GRE [T2WI]).

Fig. 14.**9** **Non-Hodgkin lymphoma.** Markedly enlarged supraclavicular (S) and axillary (A) lymph nodes are seen, whereas the infraclavicular (I) lymph nodes are only borderline enlarged. Lymphomatous involvement of the proximal humerus with hypointense lesions is also evident (T1WI, coronal).

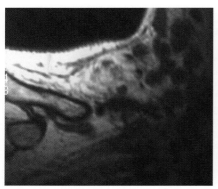

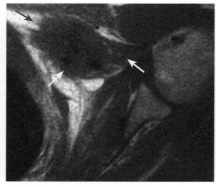

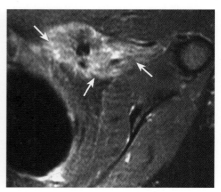

Fig. 14.**10** **Supraclavicular lymph node metastases from breast carcinoma.** Supraclavicular and cervical lymph node metastases are evident as multiple ovoid to round hypointense foci (T1WI, coronal).

Fig. 14.**11** **Axillary lymph node metastases from breast carcinoma.** **a** A large hypointense mass (arrows), isointense to muscle, is outlined by the fat in the axilla (T1WI).

Fig. 14.**11 b** After intravenous Gd-DTPA administration, marked enhancement (arrow) occurs in the axillary mass (T1WI, FS, +C).

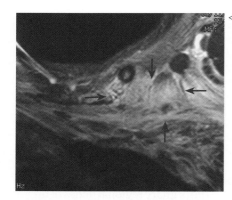

◁ Fig. 14.**12** **Breast carcinoma metastasis following irradiation therapy.** A markedly enhancing mass (arrows) is seen involving the brachial plexus. It could not be determined from this examination if the neurologic symptoms in this patient were caused by radiation-induced inflammation or remaining tumor activity (T1WI, FS, +C, coronal).

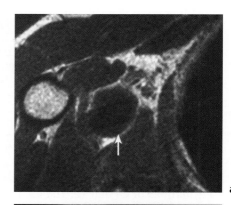

a

◁ Fig. 14.**13** **Lipoma.** A large hyperintense lesion (L) is seen with compression of the brachial plexus from above (T1WI, coronal).

Fig. 14.**14** **Brachial plexus cyst.** A cystic ▷ lesion (arrow) presenting with low signal intensity and absent contrast enhancement is seen in (**a**) (T1WI, +C) and high signal intensity in (**b**) (T2WI).

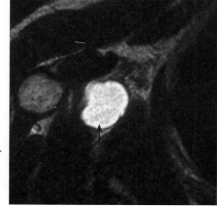

b

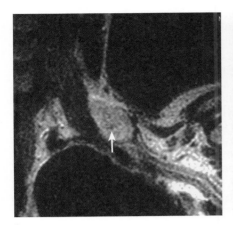

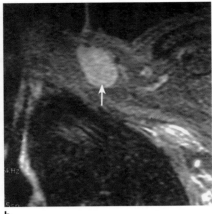

Fig. 14.**15   Brachial plexus schwannoma.**
An avoid lesion (arrow) originating in the
brachial plexus is seen. The lesion depicts
high signal intensity in **a** (GRE [T2WI],
coronal) and marked contrast enhancement in **b** (T1WI, FS, +C, coronal).

a   **b**

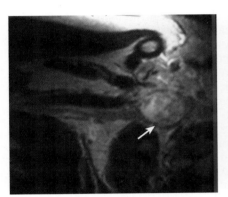

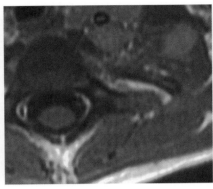

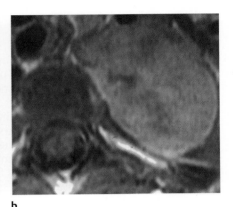

Fig. 14.**16   Brachial plexus schwannoma.**
A globular, well-defined, heterogeneous
mass (arrow) is seen originating from the
brachial plexus (T2WI, coronal).

a

Fig. 14.**17   Neurofibromatosis with
malignant transformation.   a** Multiple
well-defined neurofibromas demonstrate
homogeneous intermediate signal intensity
after intravenous Gd-DTPA administration
(T1WI, +C).

b

b   (caudad to **a**) A larger mass with inhomogeneous contrast enhancement represents a neurofibrosarcoma (T1WI, +C).

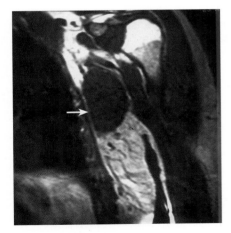

Fig. 14.**18   Fibrosarcoma.** A homogeneous lesion (arrow) of low signal intensity in the lateral chest wall is seen (T1WI,
coronal).

Cysts and *nerve sheath tumors* (schwannomas and neurofibromas) may originate from the brachial plexus (Figs.
14.**14**–14.**17**).

Liposarcomas are the most frequent malignant chest wall
tumor and can be differentiated by MRI from a benign
lipoma by the demonstration of inhomogeneous nonfatty
elements. Other primary malignancies of the chest wall include malignant *fibrous histiocytomas, fibrosarcomas*
(Fig. 14.**18**), and *rhabdomyosarcomas*. These sarcomas typically present as large masses with heterogeneous appearance with low signal intensity on T1WI and medium to
high signal intensity on T2WI. Their contrast enhancement
is irregular, or, in the case of central hemorrhage and
necrosis, limited to the periphery of the lesion. Secondary
chest wall malignancies such as metastases and lymphoma
are, however, much more common than primary sarcomas.

Two rare mass lesions exclusively limited to the chest
wall deserve special mention. The benign *elastofibroma* is a
slowly growing, fibroelastic pseudotumor resulting from
mechanical friction between the inferior tip of the scapula
and chest wall. On both T1WI and T2WI the often lenticu-
lar-shaped lesion is isointense to skeletal muscle, inter-
laced with areas of high signal intensity similar to that of
fat. Partial enhancement of the lesion is evident after intravenous Gd-DTPA administration. The highly malignant
Askin tumor (Fig. 14.**19**) is a neuroectodermal small cell
tumor arising probably from the intercostal nerves in
young caucasian females. It is frequently associated with

and hyperintense as compared with subcutaneous fat.
Desmoids tend to occur in the shoulder region and demonstrate a great variability of MRI characteristics being often
inhomogeneous and isointense to fat on T2WI and isointense to muscle on T1WI. Less commonly desmoids demonstrate low signal intensity on both T1WI and T2WI.

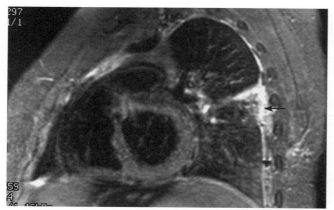

Fig. 14.19   Askin tumor. A poorly defined and inhomogeneously enhancing lesion (arrow) in the posterior chest wall is seen after intravenous Gd-DTPA administration (T1WI, FS, +C, sagittal). Same case as in Fig. 14.**5**.

rib destruction and pleural effusion. On MRI the well-defined heterogeneous mass appears hypointense on T1WI and hyperintense on T2WI with inhomogeneous contrast enhancement.

MRI may supplement mammography in patients with mammographically dense breasts, scars, and silicone implants. Normal glands and ductal tissue have a similar to slightly higher signal intensity than muscle on all pulse sequences and cannot be differentiated from periglandular fibrosis. In *fibrocystic disease* an excess of periglandular fibrous tissue and cysts presenting as well-defined lesions with uniformly high signal intensity on T2WI are seen. *Noncalcified fibroadenomas* are well-marginated, homogeneous lesions with low signal intensity on T1WI and low or high signal intensity on T2WI. *Calcified fibroadenomas* frequently appear heterogeneous and are of low signal intensity on both T1WI and T2WI. *Breast carcinomas* (Fig. 14.20) typically are inhomogeneous lesions with spiculated or irregular borders and demonstrate a low signal intensity on T1WI and a low to high signal intensity on T2WI.

Differentiation between benign and malignant breast lesions by MRI is limited. Signs of a benign lesion include a well-defined, lobular contour, internal septation and lack of contrast enhancement. Spiculated or irregular borders and peripheral or rim enhancement suggest malignancy. After intravenous administration of Gd-DTPA, carcinomas consistently enhance, whereas many benign lesions that can be confused with carcinomas on mammograms, such as cysts, scars, and fat necrosis, do not enhance. In the postoperative (e.g., post biopsy or lumpectomy) or irradiated breast, however, contrast enhancement may persist up to 1 year after treatment. Other benign conditions such as fibroadenomas and fibrocystic disease often enhance, but their enhancement in dynamic imaging is slower than in carcinomas. Diffuse enhancement of normal glandular tissue sometimes occurs in premenopausal women.

In contrast to mammography, breast implants do not impair MRI for cancer detection. Furthermore, MRI appears to be the method of choice to evaluate the integrity of *silicone implants*. Normally a capsule consisting of a layer of fibrous tissue forms around the implant depicting high signal intensity in both T1WI and T2WI. In an intracapsular rupture (Fig. 14.21) the silicone does not leak outside the capsule after the breakdown of the implant shell. An extracapsular rupture (Fig. 14.22) is diagnosed by the demonstration of silicone gel outside the confines of the fibrous capsule. In intracapsular rupture multiple delicate curvilinear lines are evident within the implant ("linguine" sign). These lines represent the collapsed implant shell suspended in the silicone gel and must be differentiated from normally occurring radial folds, which are thicker and fewer and do not extend completely across the implant. Occasionally, a small collection of silicone gel may be seen within a radial fold outside the implant shell ("teardrop" sign). Besides implant rupture, leakage of silicone gel may also occur through an intact shell and is often referred to as gel "bleed." Extracapsular free silicone is usually but not invariably associated with a rupture of the implant shell. Silicone-specific MRI pulse sequences are usually required to differentiate extracapsular free silicone from normal breast tissue or small mass lesions.

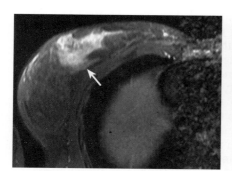

Fig. 14.20   Breast carcinoma. An irregular, spiculated lesion (arrow) with marked contrast enhancement is seen in the breast after intravenous administration of Gd-DTPA (T1WI, FS, +C).

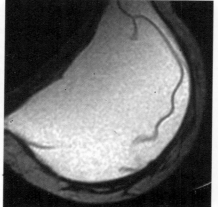

Fig. 14.21   Intracapsular rupture of silicone breast implant. Delicate curvilinear lines ("linguine" sign) within the silicone implant are diagnostic (T2WI).

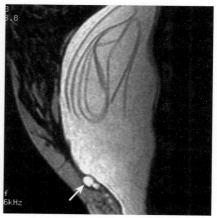

Fig. 14.22   Extracapsular and intracapsular rupture of silicone breast implant. Besides the intracapsular implant rupture evident by the "linguine" sign, a small collection of silicone (arrow) is seen outside the fibrous capsule indicative of extracapsular rupture (T2WI).

15 Heart and Mediastinum

Continued technical advancements and concomitant improvement in image quality have broadened the spectrum of clinical application in mediastinal MRI; in particular, its ability to image in multiple planes and its sensitivity to blood flow yield information not readily available with other modalities. Helical CT scanning remains the primary modality for the evaluation of mediastinal disease, although MRI will likely surpass it in the assessment of vascular pathology. MRI is also reserved for patients who cannot tolerate iodinated contrast and for patient-specific problem solving.

The mediastinum is commonly divided into anterior, middle, and posterior compartments (Fig. **15.1**). Occasionally, the superior mediastinum is also included to describe the area superior to the level of the aortic arch. These divisions are arbitrary and are not delineated by true anatomic boundaries. The anterior mediastinum refers to the space between the sternum and the anterior pericardium. The thymus is anterior to the ascending aorta and distal superior vena cava. In children and adolescents, the thymus is homogeneous, slightly hyperintense to muscle on T1-weighted sequences and approximates fat signal on T2-weighted sequences. The shape of the gland is variable with distinct right and left lobes or a fused triangular configuration. With advancing age, there is progressive fatty infiltration of the thymus. The total thickness of the gland should not exceed 1.8 cm in patients below 20 years and 1.3 cm in older patients. Thymic enlargement may accompany hyperthyroidism or occur as a rebound phenomenon after steroid treatment or chemotherapy. In addition to the thymus, the anterior mediastinum contains the internal mammary vessels, lymph nodes, and brachiocephalic veins. The posterior mediastinum extends from the posterior pericardium to the posterior thoracic wall. It includes the esophagus, descending aorta, azygous and hemiazygous veins, and thoracic duct. The middle mediastinum encompasses all of the space between the anterior and posterior compartments. The pericardium, heart, ascending aorta and aortic arch, proximal great vessels, trachea, and lymph nodes reside within the middle mediastinum. In the craniocaudal dimension the mediastinum extends from the thoracic inlet to the level of the diaphragm. The pulmonary hilum is a roughly wedged-shaped area where the structures that form the root of the lung enter and exit. The bronchi lie most posteriorly in each hilum with the pulmonary arteries anterior to them. Bronchial vessels, nerve plexuses, lymphatics, and lymph nodes are also present. The hila can be considered extensions of the middle mediastinum. Since this compartmentalization of the mediastinum is arbitrary and since many disease processes may involve more than one compartment, the disease processes in this chapter are listed in the same table to avoid repetition. The disease processes are grouped according to the location in which they tend to occur so that processes most commonly observed in the anterior mediastinum appear first, followed by middle and then posterior mediastinum.

Cystic or partially cystic lesions are common in the mediastinum. The signal characteristics of cysts are depend-

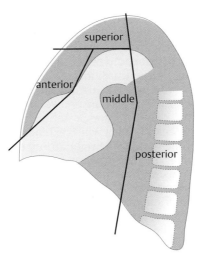

Fig. 15.**1**
Schematic diagram of divisions of the mediastinum.

ent on their contents. Most cysts contain serous fluid, which mimics the signal of water. On T1WI serous cysts are homogenous with low signal intensity relative to muscle; on T2WI they have uniform high signal intensity approximating that of water. Some cystic lesions may contain higher amounts of protein, which alters the signal characteristics such that on T1WI the lesions have higher signal intensity, usually proportionate to the percentage or type of proteinaceous material. These protein-containing cysts have decreasing signal intensity on T2WI.

The presence of hemorrhage will also modify the MR appearance of lesions. Furthermore, the signal characteristics of hemorrhage change with time. In general, hyperacute hemorrhage is low on T1WI and high on T2WI. Subacute hemorrhage is high on T1WI and either high or low on T2WI. Fluid–fluid levels resulting from hematocrit effect can occasionally be observed. Chronic hemorrhage (hemosiderin) is low on T1WI and T2WI. Commonly lesions may bleed intermittently and various stages of maturation will be present in the same lesion creating a heterogenous appearance. In addition, larger lesions may evolve in a circumferential pattern with the perimeter of the lesion having a more chronic appearance and the most central portions appearing more acute.

MRI is now widely applicable to cardiovascular imaging. Spin echo (SE) and gradient recall-echo (GRE) sequences, along with MR angiographic techniques, allow multiplanar anatomic visualization. Functional information can also be obtained with cine imaging and fast GRE sequences, which enable assessment of contractility and regional wall motion. Cardiac and respiratory gating are essential in reducing motion artifacts. Valvular function, shunts, and other flow-related issues can be examined with velocity-encoded techniques.

The pericardium is normally between 1 mm and 2 mm in thickness. Physiologic pericardial fluid is often present, with about 25 ml being average. This fluid is typically seen in the retroaortic pericardial recess as a sickle-shaped collection dorsal to the root of the aorta. Physiologic pericardial fluid can also be observed at the auricle of the right atrium and at the apex of the heart. Subepicardial fat of variable amount surrounds the perimeter of the heart. Fluid in excess of 50 ml is termed pericardial effusion. Pericardial serous transudate can occur in the setting of congestive heart failure, hypoalbuminemia, or after radiation therapy. Lymph in the pericardium may be secondary to neoplasm, cardiothoracic surgery, or obstruction of the hilum or superior vena cava. Fibrous exudate in the pericardium occurs in infections, uremia, collagen vascular diseases, and hypersensitivity conditions. Pericardial collections containing blood products may be seen after surgery or catheterization, trauma, coagulopathy, or secondary to a neoplasm involving the heart or pericardium.

Within the middle mediastinum, the heart is positioned toward the left hemithorax. The right atrium and ventricle are anterior, while the left chambers are posterior. The right atrium forms the right heart border, which extends to the right of the midline of the thorax. The right atrium receives blood from the superior vena cava at its superoposterior margin and from the inferior vena cava and coronary sinus at its inferoposterior margin. As the interatrial septum is obliquely oriented, the left atrium lies posterior to the right atrium and forms the majority of the base of the heart between the right and left mainstem bronchi and anterior to the esophagus. The normal left atrium is 4 cm in diameter. The four pulmonary veins deliver blood to the left atrium.

The right ventricle is the most anterior chamber and is immediately posterior to the sternum. Blood enters the right ventricle from the right atrium via the tricuspid valve. There are most commonly three papillary muscles in the right ventricle, which anchor the *chordae tendinae* to the tricuspid valvular cusps. In cross section the right ventricular chamber is crescent-shaped with a normal transverse diameter of 3.5 cm and wall thickness of 0.5 cm. The right ventricle pumps blood to the lungs through the pulmonic valve and into the main pulmonary artery, which is normally up to 2.8 cm in diameter in adults. The interventricular septum forms the posterior wall of the right ventricle and the anterior wall of the left ventricle. There are two components to the septum. Toward the cardiac apex is the thicker, muscular *pars muscularis*, while the thin, membranous *pars membranacea* abuts the atrioventricular valves. The left ventricle dominates the diaphragmatic surface of the heart (a small fraction anteriorly is occupied by the right ventricle) and cardiac apex. The left atrium communicates with the left ventricle via the mitral valve. In the left ventricle, there are usually two papillary muscles to which the mitral *chordae tendinae* adhere. The left ventricular myocardium is the thickest of the four cardiac chambers. Normal end-diastolic wall thickness is 1.0 cm. The chamber extends to the cardiac apex and is conical, which in cross section is approximately circular with a normal diameter of 4.5 cm. The left ventricle pumps blood into the aorta and systemic circulation through the aortic valve. The cusps of the aortic valve overlie the sinuses of Valsalva from where the coronary arteries originate.

The aorta is the outflow tract of the left ventricle. As it exits the pericardium it ascends and curves posteriorly and superiorly to form the arch of the aorta, where it gives rise to the innominate, left common carotid, and left subclavian arteries. Of note, the *ligamentum arteriosum* bridges the inferior surface of the aortic arch and the superior aspect of the left main pulmonary artery. The descending thoracic aorta continues from the distal arch where it lies along the left margin of the vertebral column in the posterior mediastinum and gradually shifts toward the midline as it reaches the diaphragmatic hiatus. The diameter of the thoracic aorta should not be greater than 4 cm. Pathologic conditions affecting the aorta and great vessels can be examined with standard sequences with phase contrast. MR angiographic techniques with dynamic Gd-DTPA injection rival conventional angiography in imaging aneurysms, dissections, and thrombi.

Cardiac neoplasms are rare. When they are discovered, approximately 80% are benign lesions. The overwhelming majority of malignant neoplasms are accounted for by metastases, with primary cardiac malignancies being extremely rare.

Table 15.**1** Mediastinal and hilar lesions

Disease	MRI Findings	Comments
Developmental		
Bronchogenic cyst	Rounded, sharply circumscribed with thin walls. Signal characteristics similar to water, low on T1WI and high on T2WI. Characteristically located beneath the carina, protruding to the right.	Most common in the middle mediastinum, may occur in the posterior and occasionally in the anterior mediastinum.
Pericardial cyst	Round, smoothly marginated with thin walls. Most common to the right in either the anterior or middle mediastinum. May change shape with patient positioning.	Usually asymptomatic. Differentiated from lipoma and cardiac fat pad by water signal characteristics.
Lymphangioma, cystic (hygroma) (Fig. 15.2)	Thin walled, occasionally with septations. Lobulated contour. Low signal on T1WI and high on T2WI. Occurs most often in the anterior, but also in the middle or posterior, mediastinum.	3–10 % extend to the mediastinum from the cervical or axillary region. 90 % present before the age of two.
Neurenteric cyst, gastroenteric cyst	Posterior mediastinal mass with thin walls. An air–fluid level may be present if there is communication with the gastrointestinal tract.	Spinal anomalies are associated.
Thoracic meningocele	Sharply circumscribed paraspinal posterior mediastinal mass. Can be solitary, bilateral, or multiple. Signal characteristics identical to cerebrospinal fluid (CSF).	Most occur in the lower lumber spine and manifest after birth. Occult meningoceles manifest later in life. Widening of the spinal canal and vertebral erosion are often associated. Lateral thoracic meningocele is associated with *neurofibromatosis type 1*.

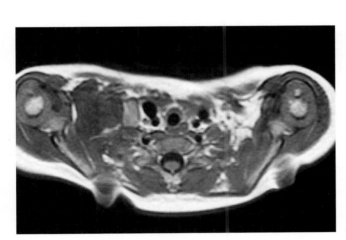

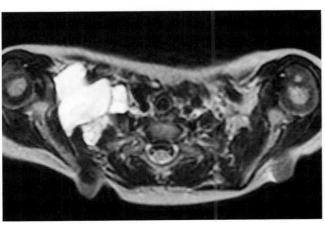

Fig. 15.**2** **Cystic lymphangioma (hygroma).** A lobulated mass in the right superior mediastinum with signal characteristics of serous fluid, uniformly low signal intensity on T1WI and high on T2WI. Note the thin septation evident on the T2WI. (**a**: axial T1WI; **b**: axial T2WI.)

a

b

Table 15.1 (Cont.) Mediastinal and hilar lesions

Disease	MRI Findings	Comments
Thymic neoplasms		
Thymic hyperplasia and thymic rebound hyperplasia	Diffuse symmetric enlargement of the thymus gland. The anteroposterior dimension of the gland is increased with preservation of the normal shape of the gland. Signal characteristics are the same as for a normal gland.	Hyperplasia of the thymus can be associated with *hyperthyroidism*, *Addison disease*, and *myasthenia gravis*. Rebound hyperplasia occurs in children and adolescents recovering from severe illness, after treatment for Cushing disease or after chemotherapy. While it may simulate a neoplasm, the condition resolves spontaneously.
Lipoma	Well-defined lesion with signal characteristics identical to fat, occasionally with thin low-signal fibrous septations. Smooth, lobulated contours. Does not enhance significantly after contrast.	Lipoma is a benign proliferation of adipocytes. It can occur in any mediastinal compartment. *Liposarcoma* of the mediastinum is extremely rare. When it occurs, it is more often in the posterior mediastinum.
Thymolipoma	Lobulated mass of fat that contains layers of soft (thymic) tissue in an undulated pattern. Cysts are not a feature. Does not compress adjacent structures.	Thymolipoma is a benign anterior mediastinal lesion.
Thymic cyst (Fig. 15.3)	Unilocular or multilocular thin-walled anterior mediastinal lesion. High signal on T2WI, low on T1WI. Increased T1WI signal if proteinaceous material or blood products are present.	Usually congenital, but may be inflammatory or neoplastic. Occurs in patients with Hodgkin disease secondary to initial involvement or after radiation therapy. Persistence of the cyst after therapy can occur and does not necessarily represent residual or recurrent disease.
Thymoma	Noninvasive (benign) thymoma is a well-defined lobulated mass. Isointense to muscle on T1WI, approaches fat signal (increased) on T2WI. Invasive (malignant) thymoma (35%) has similar signal characteristics, although it may be heterogeneous. Pleural or pericardial deposits indicate malignancy.	Typically in adults above age 40. Of patients with thymoma, 30% have myasthenia gravis. 10–15% of patients with *myasthenia gravis*, 10% with *hypogammaglobulinemia*, and 50% with *red cell aplasia* have thymoma. *Thymic carcinoid* is radiographically indistinguishable from thymoma. *Thymic carcinoma* is a large anterior mediastinal mass, often with central necrosis, that commonly invades adjacent structures. *Thymic Hodgkin lymphoma* may be difficult to distinguish histologically from thymoma. The presence of chest wall invasion and lymphadenopathy suggests lymphoma.
Germ cell neoplasms		
Teratoma (Fig. 15.4)	Benign teratoma is a well-defined anterior or middle mediastinal mass. Cysts are common, a few tumors are totally solid. Fat is present in 50%. Fat–fluid levels can also be seen. Calcification or ossification is common and may be seen as signal voids. Malignant teratoma has irregular margins, infiltrates mediastinal fat, vessels, and airways. Its thick capsule typically enhances.	The most common mediastinal germ cell tumor. Most are asymptomatic and mature (solid), others are cystic (dermoid cyst), immature, and malignant and thus termed teratocarcinomas. Mixed benign and malignant tumors occur. Occasionally seen in posterior mediastinum.
Seminoma	Large, sharply demarcated mass in the middle or anterior mediastinum. Homogenous on T1WI and T2WI with slight enhancement. Occasionally with relatively small cystic areas.	Male predilection, peak incidence in the third decade. Associated with elevated LDH (80%), b-HCG (15%). Highly radiosensitive.
Nonseminomatous germ cell tumors (embryonal carcinoma, endodermal sinus tumor, choriocarcinoma)	Heterogeneous mass on T1WI and T2WI, often with patchy enhancement. High signal areas on T1WI can be fat and/or blood products and necrosis.	Male predominance, typically in second through fourth decades. Embryonal cell and endodermal sinus tumors associated with elevated alpha feto protein (80%). Increased b-HCG with choriocarcinoma. Mixed tumors occur.

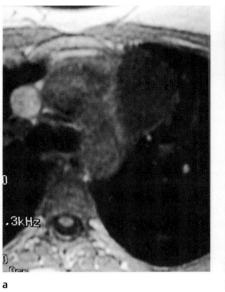

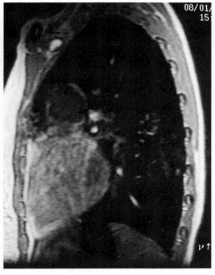

a

b

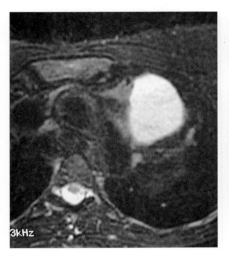

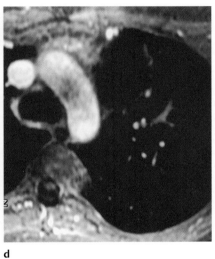

c

d

Fig. 15.**3** **Thymic cyst.** A sharply demarcated, rounded lesion with homogenous low signal on T1WI and high signal intensity on T2WI is seen in the anterior mediastinum abutting the left lateral aspect of the thymus. There is no enhancement after Gd-contrast administration. (**a**: axial T1WI; **b**: sagittal T1WI; **c**: axial T2WI; **d**: T1WI, FS, with contrast enhancement.)

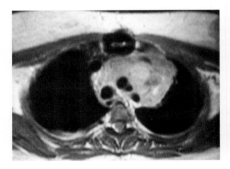

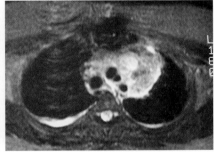

a

b

Fig. 15.**4** **Teratoma.** A heterogenous lobulated mass in the anterior mediastinum (**a**: axial T1WI; **b**: axial T2WI).

Table 15.**1** (Cont.) Mediastinal and hilar lesions

Disease	MRI Findings	Comments
Thyroid and para-thyroid tumors		
Thyroid goiter	Mass in continuity with the cervical thyroid gland. May compress vascular structures and deviate the trachea. Signal characteristics are that of normal thyroid tissue. Cystic areas often present.	Approximately 10% of all mediastinal masses with 75–80% in the anterior mediastinum and 20–25% in the posterior mediastinum.
Intrathoracic thyroid carcinoma	Necrosis is present in over 50% and lymphadenopathy in 75%. Malignant lesions are extremely variable being either hypointense, isointense, or hyperintense to normal thyroid on T1WI and hyperintense or heterogeneous on T2WI.	Benign lesions are equally variable in their imaging appearance, therefore MRI applications include defining the extent of the tumor and involvement of adjacent structures. *Papillary* thyroid carcinoma is the most common type. It spreads locally via lymphatics. *Follicular* thyroid carcinoma occurs in adults and disseminates hematogenously. *Anaplastic* thyroid carcinoma is most often seen in the sixth or seventh decade of life as a rapidly enlarging neck mass. *Medullary* thyroid carcinoma is associated with multiple endocrine neoplasia (MEN) type IIb.
Ectopic parathyroid gland	Round or ovoid 1–2-cm diameter mass that appears similar to a lymph node. Isointense or slightly hypointense to muscle on T1WI and hyperintense on T2WI, although signal characteristics are variable.	Common ectopic locations in the mediastinum include the tracheoesophageal groove, upper and anterior mediastinum in the thymic bed, and the paraesophageal region. Octreotide scintigraphy in combination with MRI can be useful for definitive diagnosis and localization of parathyroid adenomas.
Other primary tumors and tumor-like lesions		
Lymphoma (Fig. 15.5)	Bilateral assymetric enlargement of mediastinal lymph nodes, occasionally several centimeters in diameter, which can coalesce into a large mass. Untreated lymphoma is homogeneous and isointense to muscle on T1WI. On T2WI it can be homogeneously hyperintense (approximating fat signal) or heterogeneous with areas of high and low signal intensity. After therapy, involved nodes may become hypointense to muscle or heterogeneous. Signal voids from calcifications are seen in treated disease, but these can be difficult to detect in lymph nodes.	Mediastinal involvement is more common in Hodgkin disease (50%) than in non-Hodgkin lymphoma (20%). Cervical and upper anterior mediastinal nodes are more often involved in Hodgkin lymphoma.
Leukemia	Usually symmetric, modest enlargement of mediastinal and bronchopulmonary nodes.	Lymphadenopathy occurs more often with lymphocytic than myelocytic leukemia and may be associated with pleural effusion and pulmonary parenchymal disease.
Metastatic lymph node enlargement	Can present as a large, coalescent mass lesion, but lymph nodes greater than 1 cm are considered abnormal. Enhancement, particularly for renal, thyroid, and choriocarcinoma can be pronounced.	Commonly from bronchogenic carcinoma. Other common primaries are head and neck tumors, breast, renal, and melanoma. Lymph node enlargement is a nonspecific finding and may also be caused by infectious and inflammatory processes.
Esophageal neoplasms (Fig. 15.6)	Polypoid masses are common, but infiltatring and superficial spreading (varicoid) forms also occur. Tumors are typically isointense to esophageal muscle on T1WI and are variable on T2WI, thus eccentric wall thickening greater than 3–5 mm suggests a neoplasm. Luminal obstruction with dilatation of the esophagus develops with more advanced tumors. In such cases, debris often fills the prestenotic lumen.	*Squamous cell carcinomas* make up the vast majority (80–90%) of malignant esophageal tumors. *Adenocarcinoma* of the esophagus tends to arise near the gastroesophageal junction and is associated with *Barret's esophagus*. *Leiomyoma* is a smoothly marginated submucosal or subserosal mass. It can project intraluminally. Central necrosis and ulceration is common with larger tumors. Will enhance with Gd-contrast. *Leiomyosarcoma* is rare and cannot be reliably distinguished from leiomyomas. *Esophageal diverticulum* can mimic a cyst and may have an air–fluid level.

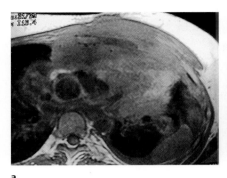

a

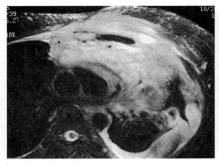

b

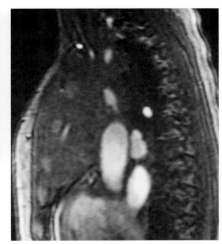

c

Fig. 15.**5**   **T cell lymphoma.** A large homogenous mass with intermediate signal intensity on T1WI and intermediate to high signal intensity on T2WI, with ill-defined borders arising within the anterior mediastinum. The tumor has invaded the chest wall musculature and adjacent ribs. (**a**: axial T1WI; **b**: axial T2WI; **c**: sagittal T1WI, FS, with contrast enhancement.)

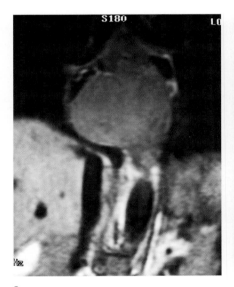

a

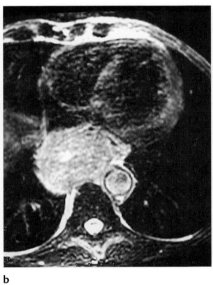

b

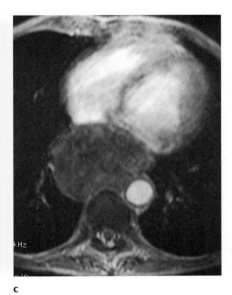

c

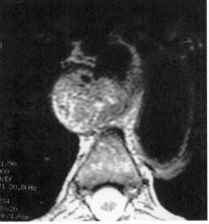

d

Fig. 15.**6**   **Squamous cell carcinoma of the esophagus.** A roughly spherical mass originating from the distal esophagus. The mass does not enhance significantly with contrast. Note that in (**d**), at the level of the aortic arch, the esophageal lumen is dilated and filled with debris due to distal obstruction. (**a**: coronal T1WI; **b**: axial T2WI; **c**: spoiled gradient-recall-echo (GRE) T1WI with contrast enhancement, axial; **d**: axial T2WI.)

Table 15.**1** (Cont.) Mediastinal and hilar lesions

Disease	MRI Findings	Comments
Neurogenic tumors (Fig. 15.7)	Paravertebral well-defined mass. May enhance uniformly. Central necrosis is a feature of larger masses. Neural foramen may be dilated. Destruction of adjacent bone suggests malignancy. Ganglion tumors are generally oriented parallel to the spine in the axis of the sympathetic chain, while nerve sheath tumors tend to be rounded masses.	Neurofibromas and schwannomas are seen in young adults, sympathicoblastomas occur in children. All occur in the posterior mediastinum except the rare paraganglionoma. Hypertensive crisis with an associated mediastinal mass is suggestive of the extremely rare mediastinal pheochromocytoma.
Inflammation		
Pancreatic pseudocyst	Cystic lesion with thick, enhancing walls. May contain debris or fluid–fluid levels, particularly if hemorrhage is present. Most often extends from the abdomen through the diaphragmatic hiatus.	Evidence of pancreatitis may be present within the abdomen.
Sarcoidosis	Characteristic pattern of lymphadenopathy in the upper paratracheal and hilar chains. Large conglomerates may occur.	In the absence of pulmonary parenchymal changes, lymphoma should be considered.
Tuberculosis	In the acute phase paratracheal and tracheobronchial nodes may be assymetrically enlarged and demonstrate central necrosis with high signal on T2WI with peripheral rim enhancement after Gd-contrast administration. Confluent masses are seen later in the course of the disease.	Characteristic pulmonary parenchymal changes are present in the majority of cases.
Cardiovascular		
Aortic aneurysm (Fig. 15.8)	Fusiform or saccular dilatation of the aorta. Thrombus may be seen.	Conditions commonly associated with aneurysm include atherosclerosis, cystic medial necrosis (including Marfan's disease), syphilis, trauma, and mycotic infection. An aneursym just distal to the origin of the left subclavian artery is usually related to prior trauma.

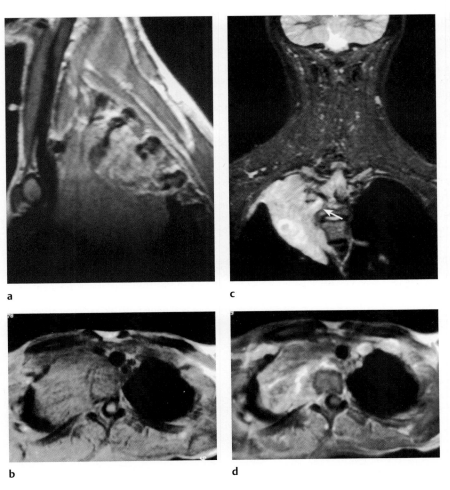

a

c

b

d

Fig. 15.**7** **Plexiform neurofibroma.** A large mass with low to intermediate signal intensity on T1WI, high signal intensity on T2WI, and heterogenous enhancement in the posterior mediastinum. Note extension though the right neural foramen (**c**, arrow). (**a**: sagittal T1WI; **b**: axial T1WI; **c**: coronal T2WI; **d**: axial T1WI with contrast enhancement.)

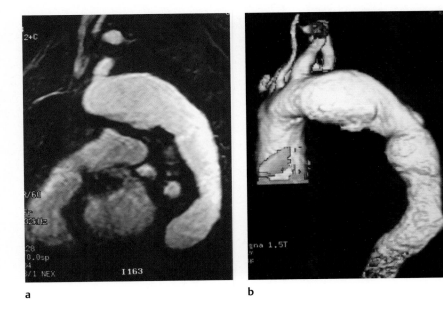

a

b

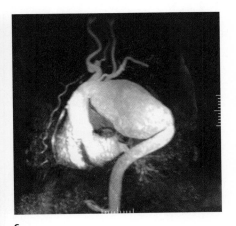

c

Fig. 15.**8** **Thoracic aortic aneurysm.** A fusiform aneurysm of the aortic arch posterior to the origin of the left subclavian artery. An example of a much larger aneurysm is shown in (**c**). (**a**: T1WI spoiled GRE with contrast enhancement, sagittal; **b**: 3D reconstruction T1WI spoiled GRE postcontrast images; **c**: T1WI spoiled GRE with contrast enhancement, sagittal.)

Table 15.1 (Cont.) Mediastinal and hilar lesions

Disease	MRI Findings	Comments
Aortic dissection (Fig. 15.9)	Visualization of an intimal flap is diagnostic. Dilatation of the aorta may or may not be present. The false lumen more commonly has slower flow and/or thrombus.	In general, Stanford type A (DeBakey I and II) involves the ascending aorta and requires surgical treatment. Stanford type B (DeBakey III) affects the descending aorta and is medically managed.
Penetrating aortic ulcer	Tear of the aortic wall in a region of ulcerated atherosclerotic plaque.	Most commonly occurs in the descending aorta. Clinical symptoms may mimic aortic dissection.
Aortic pseudo-aneurysm (Fig. 15.10)	Usually a focal, saccular outpouching of the aorta. Mediastinal hemorrhage is often present in acute cases. Most are discovered arising from the isthmus of the aortic arch at the level of the *ligamentum arteriosum*. Much less commonly occurs at the aortic root or at the level of the diaphragmatic hiatus. Chronic cases may contain thrombus and/or calcification.	Trauma is the most common cause. In the acute setting, conventional angiography or CT are the preferred diagnostic modalities. Concurrent injury to the great vessels is seen in 5% of cases. The risk of spontaneous rupture persists in chronic cases, which may be discovered incidentally after a remote injury.
Stenosis of thoracic aortic branch arteries (Fig. 15.11)	Smooth or irregular narrowing of an artery origin typically at or near the ostium, but segmental narrowing along the course of a vessel is very common. Focal or segmental regions of dilatation may be seen with vasculitis.	The most common cause is atherosclerosis. Vasculitis, including *Takayasu disease* and *Giant cell arteritis*, are rare causes that may affect the great vessels and the aorta. *Fibromuscular dysplasia* is most commonly seen in females and may affect the carotid and intracerebral arteries.

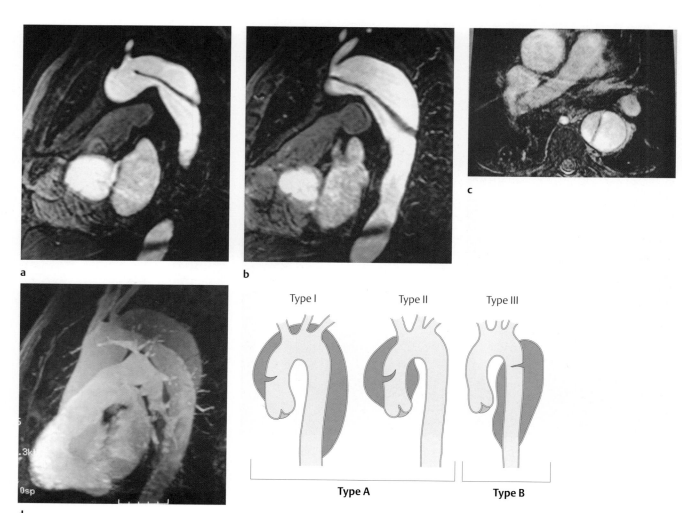

Fig. 15.9 Aortic dissection. Stanford type A (Debakey type 1) dissection of the thoracic aorta. The thin intimal flap divides the true and false lumens. Note the slight hypointensity in the more posteriorly located false lumen in the maximum intensity projection due to slightly slower flow (**d**). **e** Schematic of the Stanford (A, B) and DeBakey (I–III) classifications. (**a, b**: T1WI spoiled GRE with contrast enhancement, sagittal; **c**: T1WI spoiled GRE with contrast enhancement, axial; **d**: maximum intensity projection T1WI spoiled GRE with contrast.)

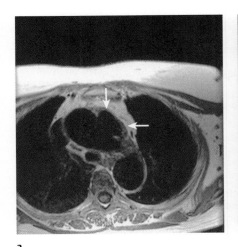

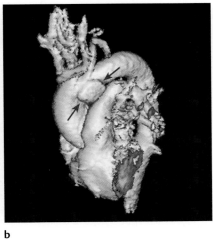

a

b

Fig. 15.**10** **Aortic pseudoaneurysm.** An eccentric outpouching of the aortic isthmus at the level of the ligamentum arteriosum. (**a**: axial T1WI: **b**: 3D reconstruction T1WI spoiled GRE, postcontrast.)

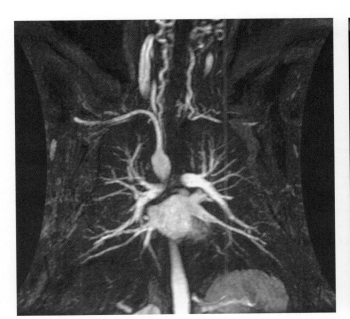

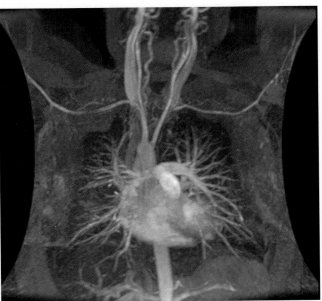

a

b

Fig. 15.**11** **Takayasu arteritis.** The proximal left subclavian artery is occluded. Note that the mid and distal left subclavian artery is reconstituted via collateral flow from the left vertebral artery.

(**a**: T1WI spoiled GRE with contrast enhancement, coronal; **b**: maximum intensity projection T1WI spoiled GRE with contrast enhancement.)

Table 15.1 (Cont.) Mediastinal and hilar lesions

Disease	MRI Findings	Comments
Dilatation of the pulmonary artery (Fig. 15.12)	The pulmonary trunk is dilated.	Common causes include cor pulmonale and congenital pulmonary valvular stenosis. Pulmonary trunk diameter greater than 28 mm predicts pulmonary hypertension.
Pulmonary artery aneurysm	Fusiform or saccular dilatation of the pulmonary artery. May be solitary or multiple.	Seen in the setting of mycotic aneursym, pulmonary hypertension, valvular stenosis, cystic medial necrosis (*Marfan disease*, *Ehlers–Danlos*), arteritis (*Takayasu arteritis* and *polyarteritis nodosa*), and rarely with *Behçet syndrome*.
Pulmonary embolus (Fig. 15.13)	Thrombus in the pulmonary arterial system. Subacute thrombus is hyperintense on T1WI and T2WI due to the presence of methemoglobin. Chronic thrombus, containing hemosiderin, has low signal intensity on T1WI and T2WI.	Risk factors include immobility, recent surgery, and hypercoaguable states with the source usually being deep venous thrombosis in the lower extremities. May precipitate pulmonary hypertension. Nuclear medicine ventilation–perfusion scans and CT are preferred modalities for diagnosis.
Superior vena cava dilatation	Enlarged in the right middle mediastinum.	Secondary to elevated central venous pressure, compression and/or obstruction by a mass, or occlusion by thrombus.
Azygous or hemiazygous vein dilatation	Unusually large vessel at the normal posterior mediastinal location or the corresponding vessel.	Usually an incidental finding; may signify elevated central venous pressure. Azygous continuation of the inferior vena cava will also produce dilatation.
Esophageal varices (Fig. 15.14)	Well-defined tubular or lobulated lesions in the esophageal wall. Signal voids may be apparent on spin echo (SE) sequences or high signal on gradient echo (GRE) sequences, if there is sufficient flow. Prominent enhancement with Gd-DTPA administration.	Most commonly occur in the setting of portal hypertension.
Vascular anomaly	Vessel in an abnormal location.	See Table 15.2 for the most common vascular anomalies.
Trauma		
Mediastinal hemorrhage or hematoma	The appearance of hemorrhage changes with time. This is often complicated by the fact that some lesions will bleed intermittently. Many hematomas are therefore of heterogeneous signal intensity. Hyperacute hemorrhage is low on T1WI and high on T2WI. Acute hemorrhage is low on T1WI and T2WI. Subacute hemorrhage is high on T1WI and may be either high or low on T2WI. Chronic hemorrhage (hemosiderin) is low on T1WI and T2WI.	Associated with trauma, surgery, aortic dissection or leaking aneursym. Common in the upper mediastinum, can be focal or diffuse.
Fracture of vertebra with hematoma	Paravertebral hematoma associated with vertebral fracture(s).	Most occur in the setting of trauma, but occasionally may be seen with pathologic fracture. The thoracic aorta must be scrutinized to exclude concurrent vascular injury.
Miscellaneous		
Morgagni hernia	Anteromedial diaphragmatic hernia, typically at the cardiophrenic angle. May contain omental fat, transverse colon, and liver. More common on the right.	Congenital diaphragmatic defect. Associated with chromosomal abnormalities and/or developmental anomalies. Tends to present in older children.
Bochdalek hernia	Posterolateral diaphragmatic hernia, usually in a paravertebral location. More common on the left, 15 % are bilateral. Omental fat, bowel, and spleen may herniate into the thorax.	85–90 % of congenital diaphragmatic hernias. Tend to be large and can be a source of respiratory distress in the neonate.

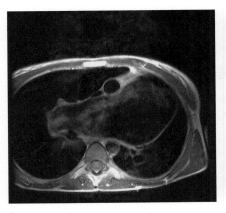
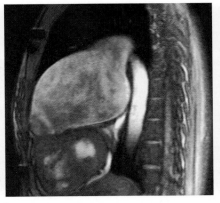
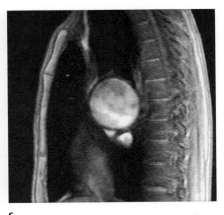

a   b   c

Fig. 15.**12** **Pulmonary arterial hypertension.** Massive dilatation of the pulmonary arteries (**b**: left; **c**: right). (**a**: axial T1WI; **b, c**: T1WI spoiled GRE with contrast, sagittal.)

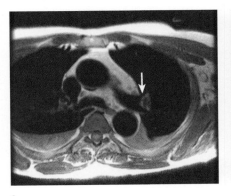
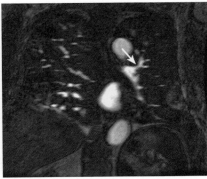
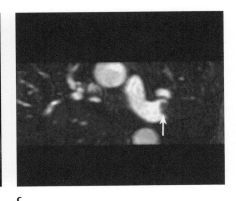

a   b   c

Fig. 15.**13** **Pulmonary embolus.** An embolus is seen in the left main pulmonary artery (arrows). (**a**: double IR, axial; **b**: T1WI spoiled GRE with contrast enhancement, coronal; **c**: T1WI spoiled GRE with contrast enhancement, axial.)

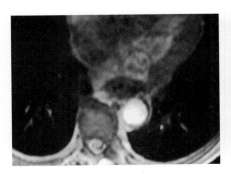
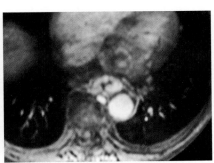

Fig. 15.**14** **Esophageal varices.** **a** During the early phase of the contrast bolus the lobulated thick esophageal wall has intermediate signal intensity. **b** Later in the venous phase the variceal veins enhance prominently. (**a, b**: T1WI spoiled GRE with contrast enhancement, axial.)

a   b

Table 15.1 (Cont.) Mediastinal and hilar lesions

Disease	MRI Findings	Comments
Hiatal hernia (Fig. 15.15)	Air and/or fluid containing mass contiguous with the esophagus and gastric fundus.	Common in elderly and obese patients. Perigastric fat may herniate without the stomach.
Diaphragmatic rupture (Fig. 15.16)	Marked elevation of the hemidiaphragm with herniation of intra-abdominal contents into the thorax. While a tear may be difficult to detect, occasionally absence of the diaphragm will be noted.	May result from blunt or penetrating trauma. The majority are not recognized acutely.
Megaesophagus	The luminal diameter of the esophagus is greater than 10 mm and contains an air–fluid level and or debris. Wall thickness greater than 3 mm when distended.	Causes of megaesophagus include *achalasia*, *Chagas disease*, and *scleroderma*. Malignancies arising at the gastroesophageal junction may mimic this condition.
Extramedullary hematopoeisis	Rounded or ovoid paravertebral masses. Approximates red marrow signal, which is intermediate on T1WI and T2WI though slightly higher than muscle. Occasionally, T1WI signal may be higher due to greater fat content.	Most commonly occurs in congenital hemolytic anemias, such as *hereditary spherocytosis*, *thalasemia*, and *sickle cell anemia*. Pleural-based lesions also occur.

Table 15.2 Aortic and venous anomalies of the mediastinum

Disease	MRI Findings	Comments
Aortic coarctation	Prominent ascending aorta associated with abrupt narrowing of the descending aorta. The stenosis can be focal or segmental. The focal (juxtaductal) form is typically located at the level of the ductus arteriosus. The segmental (tubular hypoplasia) form originates just distal to the left subclavian artery and extends to the level of the ductus. Collateral vessels may be visualized.	Occurs in less that 1% of childbirths. May cause congestive heart failure in the neonatal period. The segmental form is commonly associated with cardiac anomalies. Rib notching generally not seen until after age 6. Focal coarctation is occasionally an incidental finding in adults.
Double aortic arch	The arches may compress both sides of the trachea, usually more on the right side. The right and left arches each give rise to one subclavian and one carotid artery. The arches join posteriorly to form a single descending aorta, which may be on the left (75%) or right side of the chest.	The aortic arches form a ring that encloses the trachea and esophagus. The right arch is usually larger and courses posterior to the trachea and esophagus to join the left arch. The majority are asymptomatic but may cause stridor, dyspnea, or recurrent pneumonia.
Left aortic arch (aberrant right subclavian artery) (Fig. 15.17)	Vessel behind the esophagus in contiguity with the right aberrant subclavian artery, which is seen on the right posterior aspect of the trachea.	The most common anomaly of the aortic arch, with an incidence of 0.4–2%. The right subclavian artery arises as the last branch of the aortic arch and crosses the mediastinum from left to right behind the trachea and esophagus. May cause dysphagia.

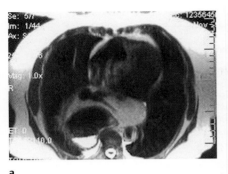

a

Fig. 15.**15** **Hiatal hernia.** A large hernia is seen through the esophageal hiatus containing perigastric fat and the majority of the stomach. (**a**: axial T1WI; **b**: coronal T1WI; **c**: coronal T2WI.)

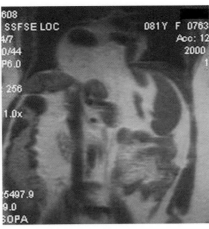

b

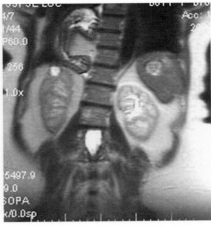

c

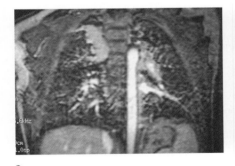

a

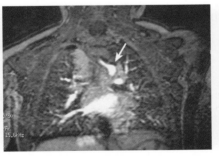

b

Fig. 15.**16** **Diaphragmatic rupture.** The stomach, loops of small bowel, and splenic flexure have herniated into the left hemithorax. (**a**: coronal T1WI; **b** sagittal T1WI.)

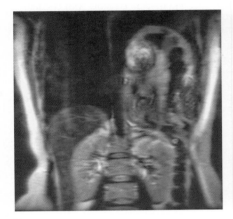

a

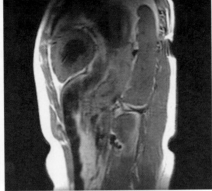

b

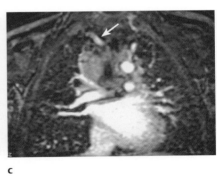

c

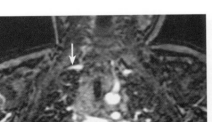

d

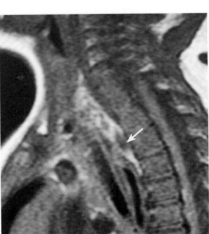

e

Fig. 15.**17** **Left aortic arch with aberrant right subclavian artery.** Serial coronal images demonstrate the aberrant vessel arising from the aortic arch (**b**, arrow) and coursing laterally to the right (**c, d** with arrows). The aberrant right subclavian artery passes posterior to the esophagus and impresses upon its posterior wall (**e**, arrow). (**a–d**: T1WI spoiled GRE with contrast enhancement, coronal; **e**: sagittal T1WI.)

Table 15.2 Aortic and venous anomalies of the mediastinum

Disease	MRI Findings	Comments
Right aortic arch with aberrant left subclavian artery (Fig. 15.18)	The left common carotid artery arises as the first branch of the aorta. The left subclavian artery arises as the last branch and courses in the retropharyngeal location.	Common anomaly, associated with congenital heart disease in 5–12%. The left subclavian artery may arise from the aortic diverticulum of Kommerel, which is an embryologic remnant of the left aortic arch. The ductus or ligamentum arteriosus completes a vascular ring, which is most often asymptomatic.
Right aortic arch with mirror-image branching	The left innominate artery originates as the first branch of the aorta.	Congenital heart disease; tetralogy of Fallot is present in over 90% of cases.
Circumflex right aortic arch (left descending aorta)	Transversely oriented right aortic arch causes impression of the posterior trachea and descends on the left side.	MRI easily discriminates this variant from double aortic arch, which can have a similar appearance on plain radiographs.
Persistent left superior vena cava	Persistent left anterior and common cardinal vein, which drains via the coronary sinus into the right atrium. In 80% the right superior vena cava is also present.	The most common anomaly of the systemic venous return to the heart, with an incidence of 0.3% in normal patients and 4.4% in patients with congenital heart disease. Increased incidence in asplenia syndrome.
Azygos continuation of the inferior vena cava	Dilated azygos and hemiazygos veins in their paravertebral course associated with nonvisualization of the intrathoracic inferior vena cava.	Anomaly with multiple variants. Systemic venous return to the heart is via azygos and hemiazygos veins. Hepatic veins drain independently by a venous confluence into the right atrium. Often associated with cardiac anomaly, abnormal situs, and asplenia or polysplenia.

Table 15.3 Abnormal pericardium

Disease	MRI Findings	Comments
Congenital		
Pericardial defect (Fig. 15.19)	Most defects are partial, though total absence does occur. Partial defects commonly involve the left pericardium over the atrial appendage and left pulmonary artery (70%), which results in interposition of lung parenchyma between the ascending aorta and the pulmonary artery. The heart may be rotated to the left. In the case of a defect in the diaphragmatic pericardium, the lung will be interposed between the heart and diaphragm; very rarely abdominal organs may herniate into the pericardial sac.	A rare anomaly, usually an incidental finding. One-third of cases are associated with other anomalies including atrial septal defect, patent ductus arteriosus, bronchogenic cyst, pulmonary sequestration, mitral stenosis, and tetralogy of Fallot.
Pericardial cyst, pericardial diverticulum	Cystic thin-walled lesion, more common on the right. Diverticula are differentiated from cysts by their communication with the pericardial sac, but are otherwise similar in appearance.	Usually asymptomatic. Often evaluated as a mediastinal contour abnormality at the cardiophrenic angle discovered on chest X-ray.

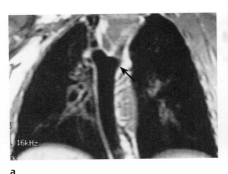
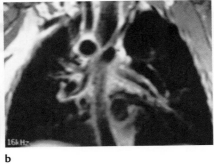

a

b

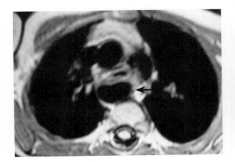
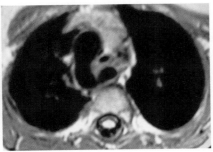

c

d

Fig. 15.**18** **Right aortic arch with aberrant left subclavian artery.** The right-sided thoracic aorta has an eccentric bulge at its left lateral aspect, the diverticulum of Kommerel (arrow). The aberrant left subclavian artery originates at this diverticulum. (**a, b**: coronal T1WI; **c, d**: axial T1WI.)

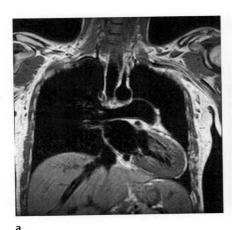
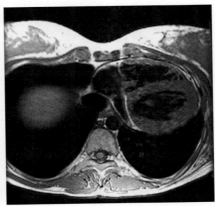

a

b

Fig. 15.**19** **Congenital absence of the pericardium.** The left pericardium is absent, hence the heart is shifted to the left. (**a**: coronal T1WI: **b**: axial T1WI.)

Table 15.**3** (Cont.) Abnormal pericardium

Disease	MRI Findings	Comments
Fluid collections		
Pericardial effusion	Small effusions initially are observed along the dorsal convexity of the heart. Larger effusions may encircle the heart completely. Transudative effusions are low on T1WI and high on T2WI, while exudative effusions are high on T1WI and low on T2WI. Loculation may occur with exudative effusions or chronic transudative effusions.	Causes include acute idiopathic pericarditis, infectious pericarditis (most commonly viral or tuberculosis), acute myocardial infarction, collagen vascular disease, uremia, and neoplasms.
Pericarditis, constrictive pericarditis (Fig. 15.20)	Focal or circumferential thickening (5–20 mm) of the pericardium. The pericardium typically enhances after Gd-contrast administration. Can be associated with an exudative effusion. In constrictive pericarditis the atria are dilated with decreased right ventricular diameter and lengthening of the chamber, creating a characteristic tubular configuration.	All purulent, hemorrhagic, and serofibrinous types of pericardial effusion may transform into constrictive pericarditis. Radiation therapy can also induce pericarditis. Asbestosis is a rare cause.
Cardiac tamponade	Large pericardial fluid collection of acute onset, most often traumatic in origin with blood filling the pericardial sac, which compresses the right atrium and ventricle.	Cardiac tamponade is a surgical emergency. Elevated intrapericardial pressure decreases diastolic filling, which precipitates circulatory collapse.
Neoplasms		
Pericardial metastases, pericardial tumors (Figs. 15.21–15.23)	Irregular mass of variable signal intensity often accompanied by a pericardial effusion, which is exudative or hemorrhagic.	Tumors commonly metastasizing to the pericardium include breast, lung, lymphoma, leukemia, and melanoma. Primary pericardial neoplasms are rare and are seen much more infrequently than metastases. Mesothelioma, teratoma, angiosarcoma, and lipoma may arise from the pericardium.

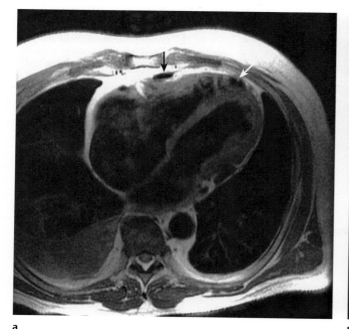
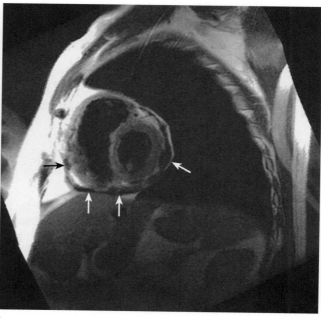

a b

Fig. 15.**20** **Constrictive pericarditis.** Plaque-like low signal foci of calcification are scattered throughout the pericardium, particularly along the posterior and diaphragmatic surfaces (arrows). (**a**: double IR, axial; **b**: double IR, sagittal.)

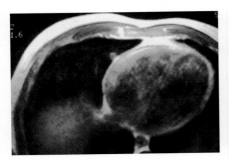
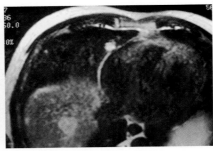

a
b

Fig. 15.**21**   **Pericardial metastasis.** A small nodule adheres to the right lateral aspect of the pericardium in a patient with hepatoma. Note the lesion in the dome of the liver in (**b**). (**a**: axial T1WI; **b**: axial T2WI.)

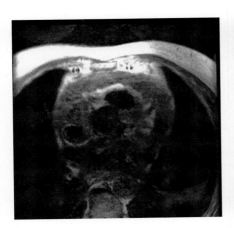
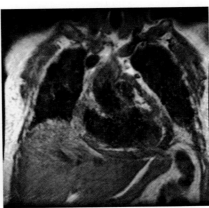

a
b

Fig. 15.**22**   **Primary pericardial mesothelioma.** A thickened, irregularly marginated band of tumor encases the entire pericardium. (**a**: axial T1WI; **b**: coronal T1WI.)

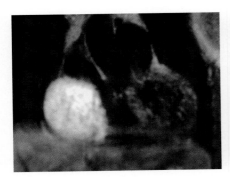
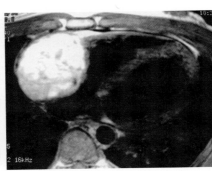

a
b

Fig. 15.**23**   **Pericardial hemangioma, cavernous subtype.** A smoothly marginated, hyperintense lesion originating from the right lateral aspect of the pericardium exerts considerable mass effect on the right atrium. (**a**: coronal T2WI; **b**: axial T2WI.)

Table 15.4 Abnormal heart

Disease	MRI Findings	Comments
Congenital		
Atrial septal defect (Fig. 15.24)	Discontinuity of the atrial septum. *Ostium secundum* defects occur at the fossa ovalis. *Ostium primum* defects occur distal to the fossa ovalis adjacent to the atrioventricular valves. The *sinus venosus* defect lies between the superior vena cava and left atrium.	Ostium secundum defects are the most common type (60–70%). Atrial septal defects may be an isolated phenomenon or part of a spectrum of congenital abnormalities.
Ventricular septal defect (Fig. 15.25)	Membranous defects make up the majority (75%) and consist of an opening just below the crista supraventricularis in the right ventricle, which corresponds to an area just below the right and posterior aortic valve cusps in the left ventricle. Muscular (10%), posterior (10%), and conal defects (5%) also occur.	Ventricular septal defects may be a solitary abnormality or occur with other anomalies such as *tetrology of Fallot, truncus arteriosus, atrioventricular canal,* and *trisomies 13, 18, 21.*
Right ventricular dysplasia (Fig. 15.26)	Focal infiltration of the right ventricular wall with fat or fibrous tissue. Cine imaging may demonstrate focal right ventricular dyskinesis in the affected myocardium.	Usually presents with recurrent ventricular tachycardia. This condition is associated with an inheritance pattern, but may also be sporadic.
Acquired conditions		
Ventricular aneursym (true aneursym), ventricular pseudo-aneursym (false aneurysm) (Fig. 15.27)	Occur in the left ventricle. True ventricular aneurysm is a focal, eccentric dilatation of thinned myocardium often in an anteroapical or inferoposterior location. Cine images may demonstrate paradoxical wall motion with expansion of the aneursym during systolic chamber contraction or it may be akinetic. In ventricular pseudoaneurysm the underlying myocardium is absent, and the overlying pericardium bridges the myocardial defect. These typically occur in a posterolateral location. The communication between a pseudoaneurysm and the ventricular chamber is often proportionately small with the diameter of the defect being less than half that of the aneurysm.	Ventricular aneursym is a sequela of myocardial infarction. Generally, true aneurysms carry a relatively low risk for rupture. Pseudoaneurysms are most commonly the results of myocardial infarction, but may also develop after trauma. These lesions have a high risk of rupture.
Myocardial infarction	Focal regions of ventricular wall thinning, which are akinetic on cine images, represent prior myocardial infarction with scarring. This region may be isointense or hypointense to normal myocardium. Acute myocardial infarction may exhibit increased signal intensity on T2WI relative to normal myocardium. The affected segment is typically akinetic.	Myocardial ischemia may cause focal hypokinesis, dyskinesis, or akinesis. Occasionally, prior hemorrhagic infarctions have residual hemosiderin deposits with low signal intensity on all sequences.
Dilated cardiomyopathy	Left ventricular enlargement and often with right ventricular chamber enlargement with normal or decreased wall thickness. In general, functional imaging demonstrates decreased ventricular ejection fraction.	Causes include ischemic heart disease, infection (most commonly viral), alcohol abuse, drug induced, post partum, and collagen vascular diseases such as systemic lupus erythematosis.

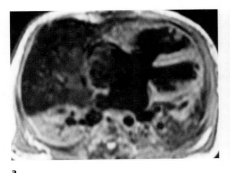

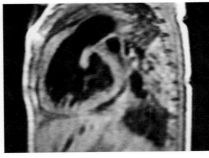

a
b

Fig. 15.**24** **Complete atrioventricular canal.** Atrial and ventricular septal defects are the hallmarks of this anomaly. In this case, an ostium primum defect and membranous ventricular septal defect are present. (**a**: axial T1WI; **b**: sagittal T1WI.)

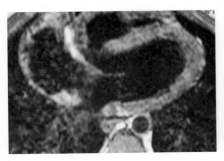

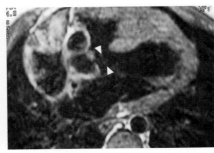

a
b

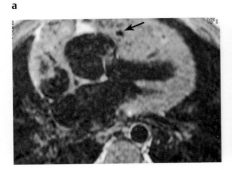

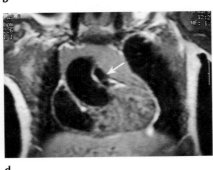

c
d

Fig. 15.**25** **Tetrology of Fallot.** There are four findings seen with this malformation: right ventricular hypertrophy, ventricular septal defect (**b**, arrowheads), pulmonary outflow tract stenosis (**c, d**, arrows), and an overriding aorta. Severe pulmonary outflow stenosis is present in this case. (**a–c**: axial T1WI; **d**: coronal T1WI.)

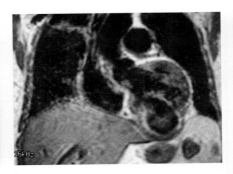

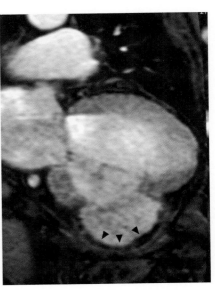

a

b

Fig. 15.**26** **Right ventricular dysplasia.** An irregular region of fatty tissue (arrow) in the anterior wall of the right ventricle (axial T1W1).

Fig. 15.**27** **Left ventricular pseudo-aneurysm.** A large eccentric bulge in the contour of the left ventricle abutting the diaphragm. Note the cresentic layer of low signal thrombus (arrowheads) within the pseudoaneurysm in (**b**). (**a**: coronal T1WI; **b**: T1WI with contrast enhancment.)

Table 15.4 (Cont.) Abnormal heart

Disease	MRI Findings	Comments
Hypertrophic cardiomyopathy (Figs. 15.28, 15.29)	Left ventricular wall thickening, which may be concentric or localized to the ventricular septum either diffusely or focally. The septum may bulge into the chamber and create outflow obstruction. Cine images commonly demonstrate left ventricular diastolic dysfunction.	Most often idiopathic. *Idiopathic hypertrophic subaortic stenosis* may be familial and typically involves focal hypertrophy of the ventricular septum.
Restrictive cardiomyopathy	The pericardium must have normal thickness (less than 5 mm). Myocardial wall thickness may be normal or increased. The atria may be enlarged along with dilatation of the inferior vena cava and hepatic veins. Ejection fraction and wall motion are decreased on functional imaging.	MRI often differentiates this condition from constrictive pericarditis, which shares similar derangements in cardiac function. Restrictive cardiomyopathy is relatively uncommon; etiologies include *amyloidosis*, glycogen storage diseases, and *hemochromatosis*.
Intracardiac thrombus (Fig. 15.27b)	Mural or pedunculated mass attached to the chamber wall or within a ventricular aneursym. Atrial thrombi tend to develop in the atrial appendage or along the superoposterior aspect of the chamber. Imaging characteristics are variable; in general, high signal on T1WI and T2WI for subacute thrombus and low signal on T1WI and T2WI for chronic thrombus, but many are heterogeneous. No enhancement with Gd-contrast.	Thrombi most commonly occur in conditions that reduce blood flow such as dilated cardiomyopathy, myocardial infarction, and atrial fibrillation.
Neoplasm		
Myxoma (Fig. 15.30)	Lobulated lesion arising from the endocardium. May be pedunculated and prolapse through a valve. Classic location is at the fossa ovalis of the left atrium, but may be seen in any chamber. Signal intensity similar to myocardium on both T1WI and T2WI. Occasionally may have a cystic component.	The most common primary cardiac neoplasm. Usually occurs in adults.
Papillary fibroelastoma	Subendocardial lesion most commonly seen on a valve. Usually 2–10 mm diameter. Low signal intensity on T1WI and T2WI.	Right-sided lesions are more often observed in children; left-sided lesions are more common in adults.
Hemangioma	Usually a well-defined lesion, but can also have poorly defined margins. Can occur within any chamber wall. On T1WI cardiac hemangiomas are isointense to myocardium and on T2WI are hyperintense.	Often incidental, but may be arrhythmogenic.

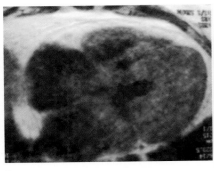
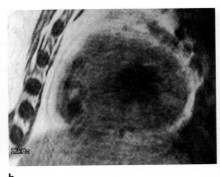

a
b

Fig. 15.**28** **Left ventricular hypertrophy.** There is marked, concentric thickening of the left ventricular myocardium. (**a**: axial T1WI; **b**: sagittal T1WI.)

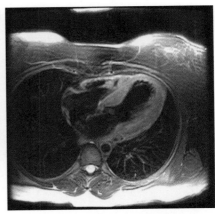

Fig. 15.**29** **Idiopathic hypertrophic suba-ortic stenosis.** Eccentric thickening of the subvalvular ventricular septum bulging into the lumen of the left ventricle (axial T1WI).

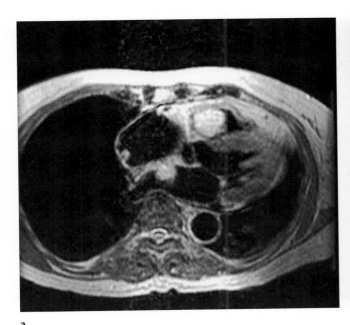

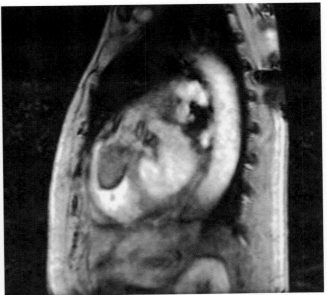

a

b

Fig. 15.**30** **Myxoma.** Pedunculated right atrial mass has herniated through the tricuspid valve into the right ventricle. The stalk is well demonstrated in image (**c**) (arrow). A lipoma is incidentally noted in the atrial septum. (**a**: double IR, axial; **b**: T1WI spoiled GRE with contrast enhancement, sagittal; **c**: double IR, sagittal.)

c

Table 15.4 (Cont.) Abnormal heart

Disease	MRI Findings	Comments
Lipoma (Fig. 15.31)	Well-defined lesion that typically occurs on the epicardial surface of the heart. Signal characteristics identical to fat, as discussed in Table 15.1.	Usually an incidental finding.
Fibroma	Well-circumscribed lesion often with a thin, low signal pseudocapsule. Most common in the left ventricle. Variable on T1WI, but most often isointense to myocardium. Low signal intensity on T2WI is characteristic.	Can be seen at any age. May present with arrhythmia or congestive heart failure.
Metastasis (Fig. 15.32)	Variable signal characteristics depending on the primary tumor.	Cardiac involvement either by direct invasion or metastasis occurs in approximately 5–10% of all malignancies. Melanoma, breast, and lung are the most common.
Sarcomas (angiosarcoma, rhabdomyosarcoma, malignant fibrous histiocytoma)	Irregular heterogeneous mass with ill-defined margins that may be intramural or, when large, protrude into the chamber lumen. Areas of necrosis and/or hemorrhage may be present. Angiosarcoma enhances markedly after Gd-contrast administration.	The vast majority of primary malignant cardiac tumors are sarcomas. Primary cardiac lymphoma is extremely rare and may present as a solitary mass or with multiple foci.
Rhabdomyoma	Myocardial lesion that may protrude into the chamber at any location. May be multiple.	Most common primary cardiac neoplasm in children. Associated with *tuberous sclerosis*.
Hamartoma	Well-demarcated lesion hypointense to myocardium on T1WI and on T2WI. With Gd-contrast adminstation may become isointense to myocardium.	Extremely rare tumor. Usually seen in the pediatric population, but does present in adulthood. Arrhythmogenic.
Miscellaneous		
Abscess	Most commonly a thick-walled cystic lesion, but may be ill defined; often with central necrosis. The wall has low signal on T1WI, variable on T2WI with enhancement after Gd-contrast administration. The signal intensity of abscesses varies with general approximation of muscle signal on T1WI and high signal on T2WI.	May develop as complication of bacterial endocarditis or surgery and commonly involves the perivalvular regions or ventricular septum. *Tuberculous abscess* is an infrequent complication of tuberculous pericarditis or direct invasion from an adjacent lymph node.
Bacterial endocarditis	Irregular, nodular, sometimes pedunculated masses attached to a valvular leaflet.	The classic clinical triad is fever, heart murmur, and positive blood cultures. Infection may spread to the adjacent myocardium and create an abscess. The majority of cases have an underlying valvular abnormality. Increased risk in intravenous drug abusers.
Hematoma	Variable signal characteristics. See Table 15.1 for discussion.	May be the result of trauma or iatrogenic.
Sarcoidosis	Often multifocal, nodular myocardial lesions that do not distort the chamber contours. Iso to hypointense to myocardium on T1WI and high signal intensity on T2WI.	A rare manifestation of this disease, usually presenting with arrhythmias. Sarcoid granulomas in the myocardium over time will transform to areas of scarring similar in appearance to old myocardial infarction.
Rheumatoid arthritis	Nodules may be intramural or project into the chamber lumen. Typically lesions are up to 1 cm in diameter.	Nodules are almost always accompanied by musculoskeletal involvement with rheumatoid arthritis.
Amyloidosis	Diffuse or rarely patchy areas infiltrating into the myocardium with signal intensity between myocardium and fibrous tissue on all sequences. Morphologically may mimic hypertrophic cardiomyopathy; however, systolic ejection fraction is decreased with amyloidosis.	Deposition of fibrinous protein amyloid in various locations of the body. May be idiopathic, occur secondary to chronic infection/inflammation or *multiple myeloma*.
Hemochromatosis	Diffuse or patchy low signal on T1WI and T2WI in the myocardium due to the accumulation of iron. GRE sequences will accentuate regions of deposition.	May be caused by primary (idiopathic) hemochromatosis, multiple transfusions, or hemolytic anemias. Cardiac involvement is not seen in the absence of hepatic abnormalities.

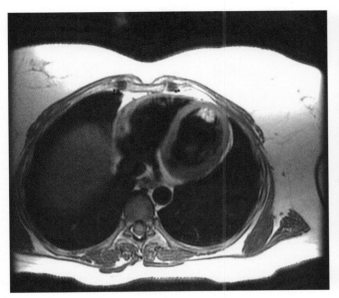

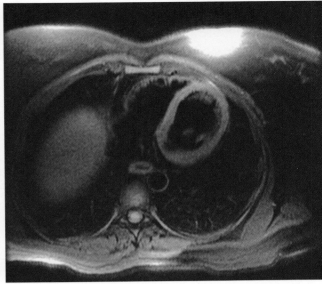

a

b

Fig. 15.**31** **Cardiac lipoma.** A well-defined lesion with signal characteristics identical to fat arising from the endocardium at the left ventricular apex. (**a**: double IR, axial; **b**: double IR, FS, axial.)

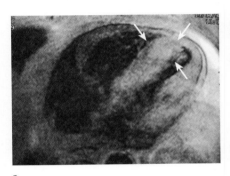

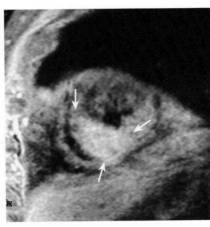

a

b

Fig. 15.**32** **Metastasis to the ventricular septum.** A nodular lesion (arrows), slightly hyperintense to myocardium, is seen in the muscular portion of the ventricular septum in a patient with cholangiocarcinoma. (**a**: axial T1WI; **b**: sagittal T1WI).

Section VI

Abdomen and Pelvis

16 Liver

The liver is the largest organ of the body with an average volume of 1350–1500 ml. The liver is covered by peritoneum except for the gallbladder bed, the porta hepatis, parts surrounding the inferior vena cava, and the posterior surface to the right of the inferior vena cava called the "bare area" which is in direct contact with the diaphragm. The liver is divided into a larger right and a smaller left hepatic lobe, each of which is composed of two segments. The *right lobe* is divided into anterior and posterior segments, and the *left lobe* into medial and lateral segments (Fig. 16.1). The *caudate lobe* is a separate, much smaller lobe located on the posteroinferior aspect of the liver between the right and left liver lobe. The caudate lobe is bordered on its right side by the inferior vena cava and on its left side by the fissure of the ligamentum venosum. The caudate lobe derives its arterial blood supply from both the right and left hepatic arteries and has venous drainage directly into the inferior vena cava. The papillary process of the caudate lobe often projects downward in front of the celiac artery and may sometime simulate an extrinsic mass.

The right and left hepatic lobes are separated by the middle hepatic vein superiorly and the gallbladder fossa inferiorly. The right hepatic vein divides the right hepatic lobe into an anterior and posterior segment. The medial and lateral segments of the left hepatic lobe are separated by the left hepatic vein superiorly and the fissure for the ligamentum teres inferiorly. Each of these four main segments may be subdivided into superior and inferior parts. These subsegments are surgically resectable, since they take the arterial, portal, venous, and ductal anatomy of the liver into account (Fig. 16.2).

Three anatomic fissures may be visualized in the liver: 1) for the gallbladder (interlobar fissure); 2) for the ligamentum teres; and 3) for the ligamentum venosum (Fig. 16.3). *The fissure for the gallbladder (interlobar fissure)* is an incomplete fissure in the plane of the gallbladder fossa separating the right and left hepatic lobe. The *fissure for the ligamentum teres* is a cleft of variable depth forming the left boundary of the *quadrate lobe*, which is part of the medial segment of the left hepatic lobe. The quadrate lobe is bounded on the right by the gallbladder fossa and posteriorly by the porta hepatis. The *fissure for the ligamentum venosum* has a transverse orientation and separates the caudate lobe from the lateral segment of the left hepatic lobe. Occasionally a *right inferior accessory fissure,* extending horizontally from the gallbladder fossa to the right lateroinferior margin of the liver, is also evident. This fissure should not be confused with an "accessory" fissure sometimes found in the elderly, which is created in the right hepatic lobe by scalloping of the diaphragm.

Intrahepatic portal triads contain branches of the hepatic artery, portal vein, and biliary system. These structures are located in the central portion of the hepatic segments. Hepatic veins are located between segments and are not accompanied by other structures.

The basic sequences for the evaluation of the liver include T1WI and T2WI and dynamic gadolinium-chelate-enhanced images. On T1WI the normal liver is relatively bright compared with the darker spleen, whereas on T2WI the liver is relatively dark to the brighter spleen. Gadolinium causes shortening of T1 resulting in enhancement in T1WI.

Gadolinium chelates such as Gd-DTPA have the same pharmacokinetic properties as the iodinated water-soluble contrast agents. After intravenous injection they are rapidly distributed over the extracellular space (combined vascular and interstitial space) where they obtain an equilibrium within two minutes. Hepatic lesions derive their blood supply exclusively from the hepatic arterial system, whereas the normal liver receives only 20% of its blood from the hepatic artery and 80% from the portal vein. Therefore, in the arterial phase immediately after an intravenous bolus of Gd-DTPA, hypervascular lesions initially enhance more than the surrounding liver parenchyma when the contrast material has reached the liver only by the arterial route but not yet by the portal venous route. However, compared with the liver parenchyma the vast majority of focal hepatic lesions enhance overall less and more slowly and their contrast material washout is also delayed. Hence in the portal phase, when the contrast agent has reached the liver by both the arterial and portal route, such lesions appear hypointense. But this differential enhancement between liver and lesion rapidly decreases with time, especially after a contrast material equilibrium between the intravascular and interstitial space is attained (approximately 2 minutes after a bolus injection).

Focal hepatic lesions tend to be hypointense on T1WI and hyperintense on T2WI. The differential diagnosis of a *hyperintense hepatic focus on T1WI* should include, besides focal fatty infiltration and a fat-containing tumor, hepatocellular carcinoma, melanoma, hemorrhagic lesion, thrombosed portal vein, and lesions in a hemosiderotic liver with an overall decreased signal intensity due to iron overload. Regenerating hepatic nodules commonly present as hypointense lesions on T2WI. Tumors with very high signal intensity on T2WI simulating a hepatic cyst include hemangiomas, cystic metastases, and cystadenocarcinomas. A *hypointense fibrous central scar* may be associated with focal nodular hyperplasia, hepatic adenomas, hemangiomas, and fibrolamellar hepatocellular carcinomas. In focal nodular hyperplasia, however, the central scar frequently depicts high signal intensity on T2WI due to an abundance of abnormal blood vessels and edema. A *hypointense fibrotic capsule* or *pseudocapsule*, respectively, may be depicted in hepatic adenomas and hepatocellular carcinomas. On T2WI a ring sign is occasionally found in these conditions, comprising an inner hypointense fibrous layer and an outer hyperintense layer consisting of compressed blood vessels and bile ducts.

MRI is the imaging modality of choice to evaluate both *fatty infiltration* and iron deposition in the liver. Fat (primarily triglyceride) may accumulate within the hepatocytes in obesity, diabetes, malnutrition, and after exposure to ethanol and a variety of other chemical toxins. Fatty changes may be diffuse, patchy, or focal. On CT a hypodense hepatic focus is likely to represent focal fatty infil-

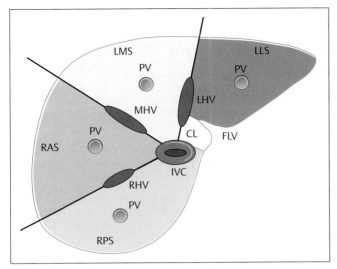

Fig. 16.**1** **Hepatic segmental anatomy.** The hepatic veins provide landmarks for the functional segmental liver anatomy.
CL: caudate lobe. LLS: lateral segment left lobe. LMS: medial segment left lobe. RAS: anterior segment right lobe. RPS: posterior segment right lobe.
Vascular structures: IVC: inferior vena cava. LHV: left hepatic vein. MHV: middle hepatic vein. RHV: right hepatic vein. PV: intrahepatic portal vein branches.
FLV: fissure of the ligamentum venosum.

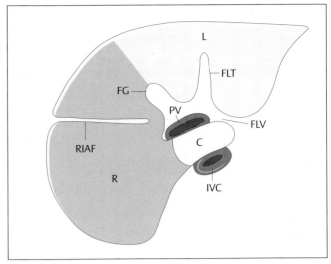

Fig. 16.**3** **Hepatic fissures.**
FG: fissure for gallbladder (interlobar fissure). FLT: fissure for ligamentum teres. FLV: fissure for ligamentum venosum. RIAF: right inferior accessory fissure. IVC: inferior vena cava. PV: portal vein and right portal vein branch. C: caudate lobe (white). L: left hepatic lobe (light gray). R: right hepatic lobe (dark gray).

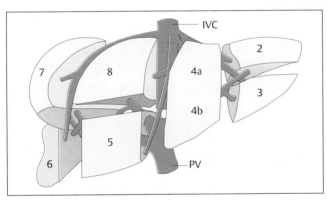

Fig. 16.**2** **Functional subdivision of liver segments.**
1: caudate lobe (not shown). 2: left lateral superior subsegment. 3: left lateral inferior subsegment. 4a: left medial superior subsegment. 4b: left medial inferior subsegment. 5: right anterior inferior subsegment. 6: right posterior inferior subsegment. 7: right posterior superior subsegment. 8: right anterior superior subsegment. IVC: inferior vena cava. PV: portal vein.

tration if, on MRI, the lesion has a slightly increased signal intensity on T1WI and appears normal on T2WI because of its relative insensitivity to fat. Fat-suppression (FS) techniques may furthermore be used for corroboration of the correct diagnosis. Nonfatty hepatic areas depicting high signal intensity on T1WI may be associated with hemorrhage or deposition of melanin, copper, amyloid, and proteinaceous material, but again fat saturation techniques should allow differentiation between these causes and lipid-containing lesions.

Increased hepatic iron deposition is associated with both idiopathic (primary) and secondary hemochromatosis, hemosiderosis (e.g., hemolytic anemias and transfusional iron overload), and cirrhosis. Iron deposition lowers the signal intensity especially on T2WI. In all conditions in which the iron is primarily deposited in the reticuloendothelial system the spleen is affected to a greater extent than the liver. In primary (idiopathic) hemochromatosis the iron is deposited in the hepatocytes and not in the reticuloendothelial system (Kupffer cells) of the liver and thus the spleen is not affected.

The differential diagnosis of focal liver lesions is discussed in Table 16.**1** and the differential diagnosis of diffuse liver disease in Table 16.**2**.

Table 16.1 Focal liver lesions

Disease	MRI Findings	Comments
Hepatic cyst (Fig. 16.4)	Sharply delineated, homogeneous round or oval lesion with low signal intensity on T1WI, very high signal intensity on T2WI, and no enhancement of either its content or the wall after intravenous Gd-DTPA. Rarely cysts are hemorrhagic or contain proteinaceous material and may depict an increased signal intensity on T1WI and a decreased signal intensity on T2WI or a fluid–fluid level. Cysts are frequently multiple. Occasionally closely grouped cysts may mimic a multicystic mass.	Solitary or multiple, usually congenital lesions with an incidence of approximately 2.5% in the Western population and a 4:1 female predominance. A higher incidence is found in Asian women. In both *polycystic kidney disease* (Fig. 16.5) and *von Hippel–Lindau disease* multiple hepatic cysts are usually also present. *Foregut cysts* are located near the anterosuperior margin of the liver and, because of their mucin content, are isointense or hyperintense on T1WI and hyperintense on T2WI. Cysts presenting with irregular inner margins, septations, or even minimal late contrast enhancement should raise the possibility of cystic neoplasms.
Echinococcal disease (Figs. 16.6 and 16.7)	May be indistinguishable from a simple hepatic cyst. Frequently the cyst is complex and septated with mixed low signal intensity on T1WI and mixed high signal intensity on T2WI due to the presence of proteinaceous material and cellular debris. Cyst wall and septa, but not the cyst content itself, may enhance after intravenous Gd-DTPA. Septation is caused by daughter cysts, arranged peripherally within the main lesion. Satellite cysts located outside the main lesion are not uncommon. Complications include cyst rupture into the biliary system with subsequent obstructive jaundice.	*Echinococcus granulosus (cysticus)* is the causative organism of *hydatid disease* endemic in the Mediterranean, Middle East, South America, Australia, New Zealand, Baltic border countries, and Africa. Cyst wall consists of three layers: 1) pericyst (formed by the host); 2) exocyst (chitinous outer cyst membrane); and 3) endocyst (inner lining of syncytial cells). Calcification of the cyst wall is common and well appreciated by CT. *Echinococcus alveolaris (multilocularis)* is a less common but more aggressive form of echinococcal disease.
Caroli disease	Dilated intrahepatic bile ducts with beaded appearance or multiple cystic structures converging toward the porta hepatis are characteristic. Sludge and calculi may form in dilated ducts.	Autosomal recessive condition presenting with segmental saccular dilatation of intrahepatic bile ducts. Medullary sponge kidney is associated in 80% of cases, infantile polycystic kidney disease occasionally. Complications include pyogenic cholangitis and intrahepatic abscesses.

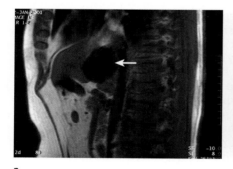
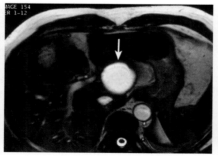
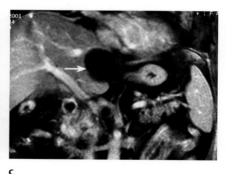

a   **b**   **c**

Fig. 16.4   Hepatic cyst. Sharply delineated, homogeneous, round lesion (arrow) with low signal intensity in (**a**) (T1WI, sagittal), very high signal intensity in (**b**) (T2WI [GRE], axial), and absent contrast enhancement in (**c**) (coronal T1WI, FS, +C).

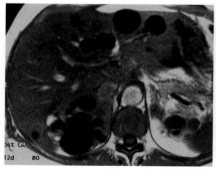
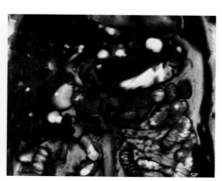

a   **b**

Fig. 16.5   Multiple hepatic cysts in polycystic kidney disease (autosomal dominant or adult type). Multiple sharply delineated cysts are seen in the liver and both kidneys in (**a**) (spoiled GRE, axial) and (**b**) (T2WI [GRE], coronal).

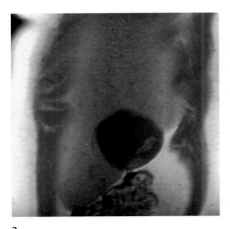

a

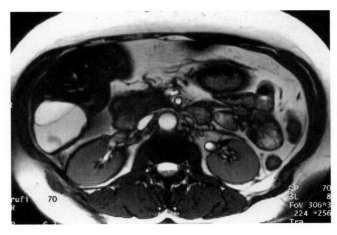

c

Fig. 16.**6**   **Hydatid disease *(Echinococcus granulosus).*** A septated cyst with mixed signal intensity and detached membranaceous material in the posterior segment of the right hepatic lobe depicts an overall low signal intensity in (**a**) (sagittal T1WI) and a very high signal intensity in (**b**) and (**c**) (sagittal and axial T2WI [GRE]).

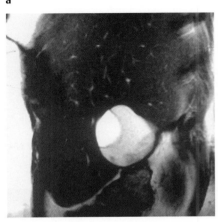

b

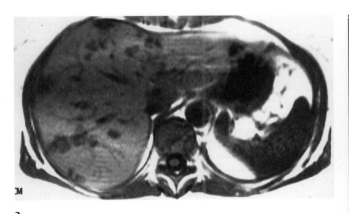

a

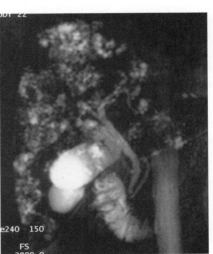

c

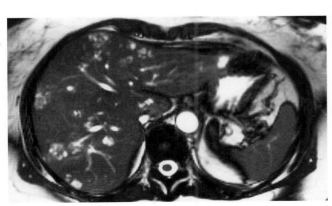

b

Fig. 16.**7**   ***Echinococcus alveolaris.*** Multiple small lesions are seen scattered throughout the liver. Each individual lesion consists of a cluster of tiny cysts giving it a heterogeneous appearance with low signal intensity in (**a**) (T1WI) and high signal intensity in (**b**) (T2WI [GRE]) and (**c**) (magnetic resonance cholangiography [MRCP]).

Table 16.1 (Cont.) Focal liver lesions

Disease	MRI Findings	Comments
Choledochal cyst	Most common presentation is a cystic dilatation of common bile duct, but may occasionally be associated with cystic dilatation of intrahepatic bile ducts.	In children and young adults presenting with jaundice, abdominal pain, and palpable mass. Common in Asia (especially in Japan). Increased risk of cholangiocarcinoma.
Intrahepatic extension of pancreatic pseudocyst	Round or tubular intrahepatic cystic mass; the latter may mimic a localized dilated intrahepatic bile duct.	Complication of pancreatitis.
Hemangioma (Figs. 16.8–16.10)	Lesion with well-defined lobular border depicting low signal intensity on T1WI and high signal intensity on T2WI. After intravenous Gd-DTPA injection a peripheral nodular enhancement pattern is characteristic, with centripetal progression to eventually uniform high signal intensity within 10 minutes with or without persistent central scar. A peripheral discontinuous ring of nodule immediately after Gd-DTPA is virtually diagnostic. A uniform enhancement pattern *immediately* after Gd-DTPA administration is often found in small (<2 cm) hemangiomas and is indistinguishable from hypervascular metastases or a small hepatocellular carcinoma.	Hemangiomas are the most common benign hepatic tumors occurring in approximately 5% of the population with female predominance. They are usually small, asymptomatic, and discovered incidentally, but may enlarge during pregnancy or estrogen administration. Giant hemangiomas (>5 cm) are uncommon but may be symptomatic due to hemorrhage or thrombosis. The vast majority of hepatic hemangiomas are of the cavernous type. Capillary hemangiomas are very rare in the liver. In *cystic angiomatosis* (Fig. 16.11) extensive hemangiomatous and/or lymphangiomatous lesions in one or multiple tissue planes (e.g., bone, muscle, subcutaneous fat, viscera) are evident. The diagnosis is usually made in the first three decades of life.

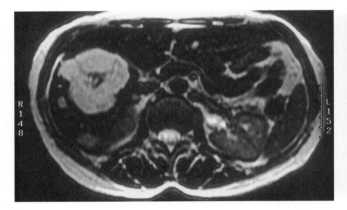

a

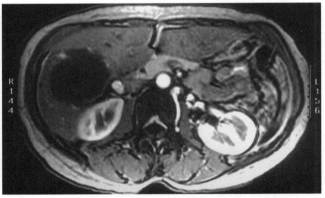

b

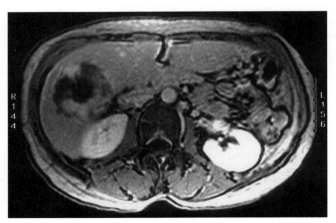

c

Fig. 16.8 **Hemangioma.** A large, slightly lobulated lesion with very high signal intensity and hypointense central scar is seen in (**a**) (T2WI). After intravenous Gd-DTPA administration a diagnostic peripheral nodular enhancement pattern with centripetal progression within the hypointense lesion is seen in (**b**) and (**c**) (T1WI, +C; arterial and portal phase, respectively).

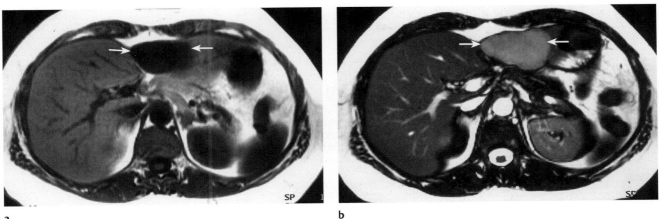

a **b**

Fig. 16.**9** **Hemangioma.** A large lesion (arrows) is seen in the lateral segment of the left hepatic lobe with low signal intensity in (**a**) (T1WI) and high signal intensity in (**b**) (T2WI [GRE]).

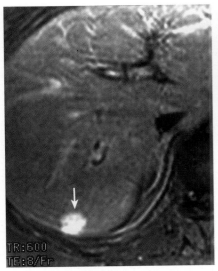

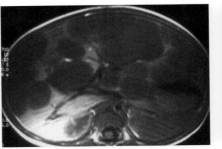 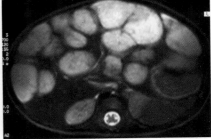

a **b**

Fig. 16.**11** **Cystic angiomatosis.** Multiple, different sized and shaped, slightly heterogeneous lesions are evident throughout the enlarged liver. They appear hypointense in (**a**) (T1WI) and hyperintense in (**b**) (T2WI).

Fig. 16.**10** **Hemangioma.** A small peripheral liver lesion (arrow) with immediate uniform contrast enhancement is seen after intravenous Gd-DTPA administration (T1WI, FS, +C).

Table 16.1 (Cont.) Focal liver lesions

Disease	MRI Findings	Comments
Focal nodular hyperplasia (Figs. 16.12 and 16.13)	Lobulated, isointense to slightly hypointense lesion on T1WI and isointense to slightly hyperintense mass on T2WI. A central scar with higher or, less commonly, lower signal intensity may be observed on T2WI depending on the prevalence of blood vessels, edema, or fibrous tissue. Peripherally radiating septa containing large vascular channels and bile ducts may also be evident. After intravenous Gd-DTPA administration an immediate intense uniform blush, usually fading within 1 minute, to near isointensity is characteristic. The central scar may appear hypointense immediately after intravenous Gd-DTPA and gradually enhance to hyperintensity with time. Early vigorous and homogeneous enhancement of the central scar is another common presentation.	Relatively rare benign hepatic neoplasm, usually asymptomatic, most commonly occurring in young females (75%). Association with oral contraceptives is questionable. Focal nodular hyperplasia is composed of hepatocytes, Kupffer cells, and bile ducts and frequently possesses a central scar. Twenty percent are multiple. The lesion is pedunculated in about 10% of cases. A normal or increased 99mTc sulfur colloid scan is found in 70%. No malignant potential. Intratumoral hemorrhage is very rare.
Hepatic adenoma (Figs. 16.14 and 16.15)	Slightly hypointense to mildly hyperintense lesion on T1WI and slightly hyperintense on T2WI or near isointense with liver on all imaging sequences. A capsule may be seen as a peripheral zone of low signal intensity on both T1WI and T2WI. Tumors may also depict a mixed high signal intensity on both T1WI and T2WI due to the presence of hemorrhage or, less commonly, fat. Contrast enhancement of the lesion varies but is usually moderate.	Ninety percent are found in young women using oral contraceptives, but adenomas are overall less common than focal nodular hyperplasia. Histologically they are composed of hepatocytes but no Kupffer cells (always cold on 99mTc sulfur colloid scans) and may contain fat. Large areas of necrosis and hemorrhage may also be found within the tumor and are a frequent cause of pain. *Hepatic adenomatosis.* Multiple focal hepatic lesions with the appearance of multiple adenomas.

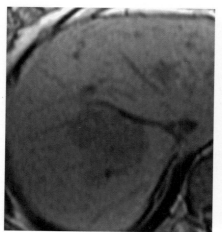

a

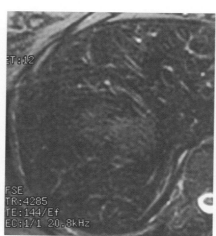

b

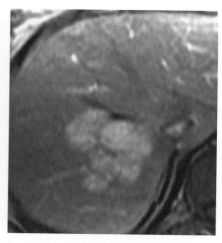

c

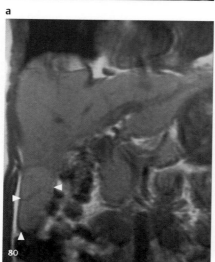

d

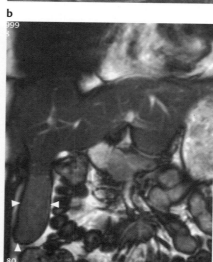

e

Fig. 16.**12 Focal nodular hyperplasia** (two patients). In the first patient a lobulated right hepatic mass is seen that is slightly hypointense on T1WI (**a**), minimally hyperintense on T2WI (**b**), and markedly enhanced immediately after intravenous Gd-DTPA administration (arterial phase) in (**c**) (T1WI, FS, +C). In the second patient a pedunculated lesion (arrowheads) originating from the right hepatic lobe is seen in (**d**) (coronal T1WI) and (**e**) (coronal T2WI [GRE]).

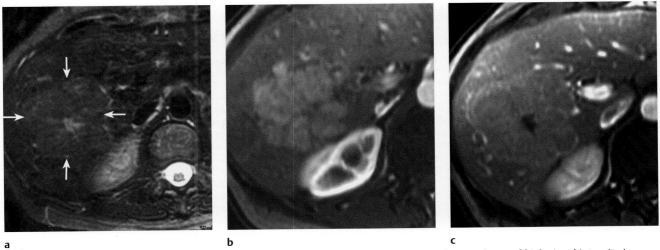

a   b   c

Fig. 16.**13   Focal nodular hyperplasia.** A lobulated, slightly hyperintense lesion (arrows) with central scar of high signal intensity is seen in the right hepatic lobe in (**a**) (T2WI, FS). Dynamic contrast enhancement depicts an immediate, marked blush in the arterial phase in (**b**) (T1WI, FS, +C). After 60 seconds the blush has rapidly faded and a central hypointense scar becomes visible in (**c**) (T1WI, FS, +C).

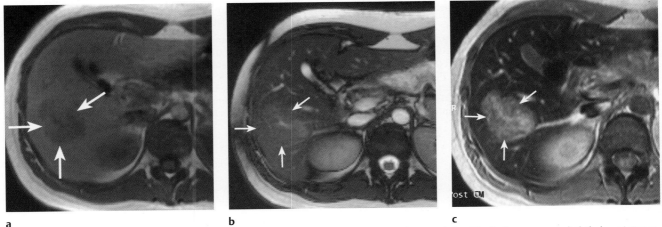

a   b   c

Fig. 16.**14   Hepatic adenoma.** A heterogeneous lesion (arrows) is seen in the right hepatic lobe. The lesion appears slightly hypointense in (**a**) (T1WI), slightly hyperintense in (**b**) (T2WI [GRE]), and depicts inhomogeneous contrast enhancement in (**c**) (T1WI, +C).

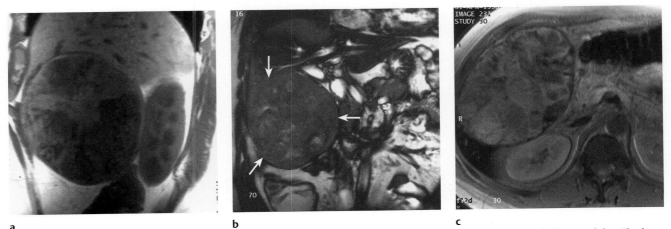

a   b   c

Fig. 16.**15   Hepatic adenoma.** A large, well-demarcated (encapsulated), heterogeneous lesion is seen in the right hepatic lobe. The lesion is hypointense to the liver in (**a**) (T1WI, sagittal), slightly hyperintense (arrows) in (**b**) (T2WI [GRE], coronal), and shows moderate inhomogeneous contrast enhancement in (**c**) (T1WI, FS, +C, axial).

Table 16.**1** (Cont.) Focal liver lesions

Disease	MRI Findings	Comments
Nodular regeneration in cirrhosis (Figs. 16.16 and 16.17)	Multiple nodular lesions of variable signal intensity; usually hyperintense on T1WI and often hypointense on T2WI relative to an inflamed, damaged liver or, less commonly, hyperintense relative to a fibrotic liver. In 25 % of cases iron accumulation in regenerative nodules is greater than in the surrounding liver parenchyma, contributing to their lower signal intensity. After intravenous Gd-DTPA administration, regenerative nodules usually enhance less than the surrounding liver parenchyma.	A micronodular pattern (1–5 mm) is commonly associated with alcoholism, whereas a macronodular pattern (up to several centimeters) is usually a late sequelae of hepatitis B or C. In the absence of inflammatory changes the cirrhotic liver may depict an overall decrease in signal intensity on both T1WI and T2WI. The liver atrophy commonly affects the right lobe and medial segment of the left lobe most, while the lateral segment of the left lobe and the caudate lobe frequently undergo hypertrophy. *Dysplastic nodules (adenomatous hyperplasia)* are large regenerative nodules with dysplastic histologic features. The majority of these lesions will eventually become malignant. They tend to be hyperintense on T1WI, isointense to slightly hypointense on T2WI, and enhance similar to the liver.
Mesenchymal hamartoma (Fig. 16.18)	Mixed solid and cystic mass. Predominantly cystic lesions depict varying signal intensity on T1WI, depending on the protein concentration of the cystic content, and marked hyperintensity on T2WI. Predominantly mesenchymal (fibrous) lesions are hypointense on T1WI and T2WI. Solid tumors may enhance considerably after intravenous Gd-DTPA administration.	Rare developmental lesions with cysts ranging from a few millimeters up to 14 cm. Presents as enlarging hepatic mass ranging from 5 to 30 cm in the first two decades of life (peak age 1–2 years) with 2:1 male predominance. *Hepatic lipomas* are rare tumors presenting as discrete areas of fat with or without septation. They are usually associated with renal angiomyolipomas.
Biliary cystadenoma	Multilocular cystic lesion measuring between 2 and 35 cm in diameter with varying signal intensity on T1WI and T2WI depending on both protein and blood content of the cysts, which may depict papillary excrescences and mural nodules. After intravenous Gd-DTPA administration, cyst walls and internal septa may enhance.	Rare benign multilocular cystic tumor originating from intrahepatic bile ducts in 85 %. Occurs predominantly in Caucasians over 30 years of age (peak: fifth decade) with 4:1 female predominance. May recur or develop into a *malignant cystadenocarcinoma* that cannot be differentiated by MRI from its benign counterpart.

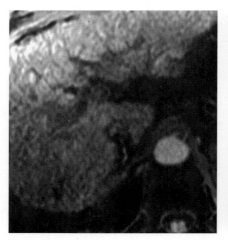

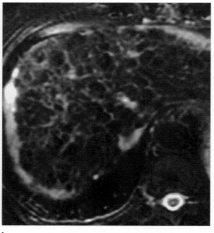

a   b

Fig. 16.**16 Nodular regeneration in cirrhosis.** Multiple different-sized nodules are seen in a cirrhotic liver and appear slightly hyperintense in (**a**) (spoiled GRE) and hypointense in (**b**) (T2WI, FS). The overall decreased signal intensity in (**b**) is caused by considerable iron deposition in the cirrhotic liver and, to even a greater extent, in the regenerative nodules.

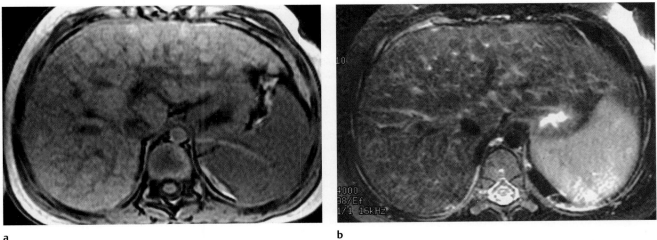

a   **b**

Fig. 16.**17   Nodular regeneration in hepatorenal tyrosinemia** (congenital enzyme defect presenting with hepatocellular degeneration and Fanconi syndrome). Multiple regeneration nodules are seen throughout the liver and appear hyperintense in (**a**) (T1WI) and slightly hypointense in (**b**) (T2WI, FS).

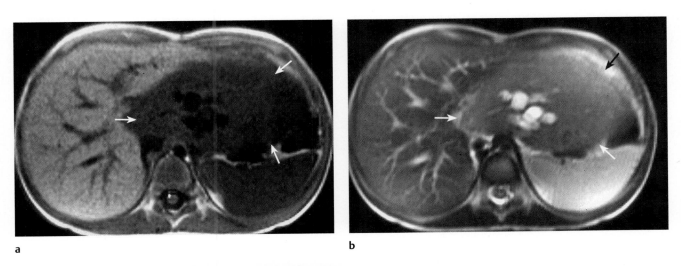

a   **b**

Fig. 16.**18   Mesenchymal hamartoma.** A predominantly solid lesion (arrows) with central cystic component is evident in the enlarged left liver lobe. The lesion is hypointense in (**a**) (T1WI), slightly hyperintense in (**b**) (T2WI), and, with the exception of its cystic component, enhances considerably after intravenous Gd-DTPA administration in (**c**) (T1WI, FS, +C).

c

Table 16.1 (Cont.) Focal liver lesions

Disease	MRI Findings	Comments
Hepatocellular carcinoma (Figs. 16.19–16.22)	Solitary or less common multifocal or diffuse lesions, often arising in a previously damaged liver. Signal intensity may vary from hypointense to hyperintense on both T1WI and T2WI. Most common appearance is a low signal intensity on T1WI and moderately high signal intensity on T2WI. Smaller lesions may be hyperintense on T1WI due to the presence of fat. A well-defined, hypointense, fibrous pseudocapsule or a ring sign on T2WI consisting of an inner hypointense fibrous layer and an outer hyperintense layer (compressed blood vessels and bile ducts) may be seen. Demonstration of tumor invasion into the portal vein (35%) and/or hepatic veins (15%) helps to differentiate hepatocellular carcinoma from other hepatic malignancies. Contrast enhancement in larger lesions is typically inhomogeneous. The degree of enhancement is variable and ranges from peripheral to diffuse. DD: An inhomogeneous diffuse enhancement pattern is uncommon in hepatic metastases.	Most common primary visceral malignancy in the world with an incidence of 5–20% in Southeast Asia, including Japan and sub-Saharan Africa. In the Western hemisphere, however, the incidence is less than 1%. Peak age is the sixth and seventh decade (lower in high incidence areas) with a male predominance of 3:1. Risk factors include cirrhosis, chronic hepatitis B and C, carcinogens (aflatoxin, sex hormones, thorotrast) and metabolic diseases (hemochromatosis, Wilson disease, alpha-1-antitrypsin deficiency, galactosemia type I, glycogen storage disease). Metastases to lung, adrenals, lymph nodes, and bone are frequent. Elevated alpha-feto-protein (75–90%) differentiates hepatocellular carcinoma from cholangiocarcinoma.

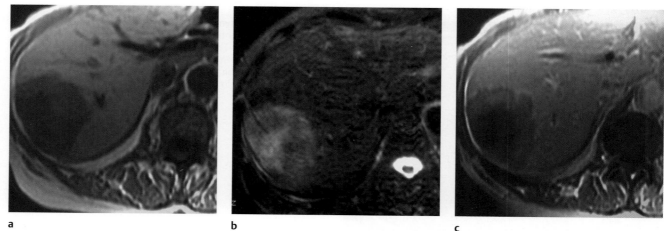

a   b   c

Fig. 16.**19** **Hepatocellular carcinoma.** A large mass lesion with necrotic center is seen in the right hepatic lobe depicting low signal intensity in (**a**) (T1WI), high signal intensity especially of the necrotic areas in (**b**) (T2WI, FS), and moderate peripheral contrast enhancement in (**c**) (T1WI, +C).

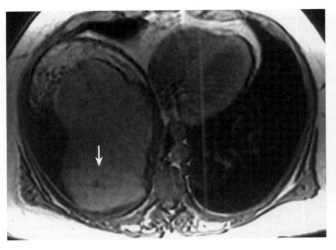

a

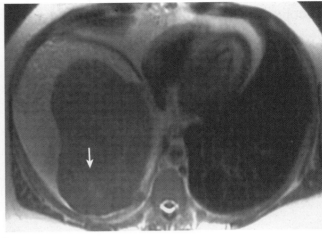

b

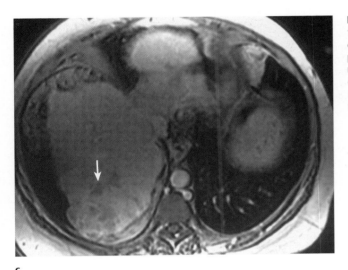

c

Fig. 16.**20** **Hepatocellular carcinoma in cirrhosis.** A poorly defined lesion (arrow) is seen in the shrunken cirrhotic liver that is cephalad displaced due to eventration of the right hemidiaphragm. The lesion appears hyperintense in (**a**) (T1WI) and minimally hyperintense in (**b**) (T2WI). Diffuse inhomogeneous contrast enhancement is seen in (**c**) (T1WI, +C). A markedly enlarged spleen is also evident with decreased signal intensity due to hemosiderin deposition.

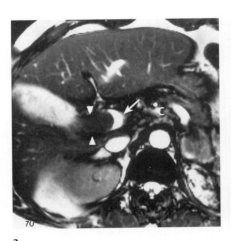

a

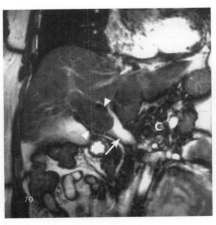

b

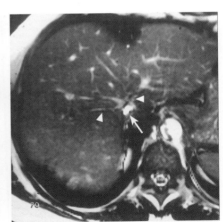

Fig. 16.**22** **Hepatocellular carcinoma.** Invasion of the right hepatic vein including tributaries (arrowheads) and inferior vena cava (arrow) by the tumor is evident (T2WI [GRE]).

Fig. 16.**21** **Hepatocellular carcinoma.** Invasion of the portal vein (arrow) by a tumor thrombus (arrowheads) is evident. Multiple portosystemic venous collaterals (C) are also evident (**a**: axial; **b**: coronal, both T2WI [GRE]).

Table 16.**1** (Cont.) Focal liver lesions

Disease	MRI Findings	Comments
Fibrolamellar hepato-cellular carcinoma (Fig. 16.23)	Solitary homogeneous lesion that is mildly hypo-intense on T1WI and slightly hyperintense on T2WI. A hypointense central scar, often with a radiating appearance, is evident on both T1WI and T2WI in approximately half of the cases. After intravenous Gd-DTPA the lesion enhances diffusely with the ex-ception of the central scar.	Compared to the (regular) hepatocellular carci-noma the fibrolamellar variety occurs in younger patients (10–30 years old) without underlying risk factors, equal sex distribution, and negative alpha-fetoprotein. Central calcifications are appreciated by CT in approximately one-third of the patients.
Metastases (Figs. 16.24–16.26)	Usually multiple round or oval lesions with indis-tinct or sharp border. Hypointense on T1WI and isointense to markedly hyperintense on T2WI. High signal intensity on T1WI may be found in hemor-rhagic and melanoma metastases. A central coagu-lation necrosis, often associated with colorectal car-cinomas, may depict low signal intensity on T2WI. After intravenous Gd-DTPA administration, a pe-ripheral ring enhancement may be found with sub-sequent central progression and occasionally simul-taneous peripheral contrast wash-out. In contrast to hemangiomas, the ring enhancement in hyper-vascular metastases is uniform in thickness and depicts a jagged or serrated, rather than a nodular inner margin. Small hypervascular metastases and hemangiomas may both enhance rapidly in a uni-form fashion, but the contrast wash-out is delayed from the hemangiomas.	More than 20 times more common than all pri-mary liver malignancies combined. Common sites of origin are the colon (42 %), stomach (23 %), pan-creas (21 %), breast (14 %), and lungs (13 %). *Hypervascular* liver metastases originate from kid-ney, colon, gonads, endocrine tumors, breast, melanoma, and sarcoma. *Hemorrhagic* liver metastases originate from colon, kidney, thyroid, breast, melanoma, and choriocarci-noma. *Cystic* liver metastases originate from colon, ovary, lung, carcinoid, melanoma, and sarcoma.

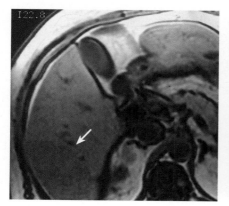
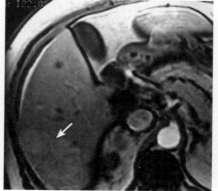
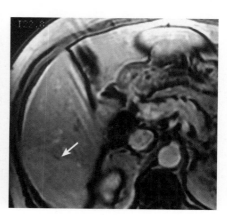

a b c

Fig. 16.**23** **Fibrolamellar hepatocellular carcinoma.** A hypointense, homogeneous lesion (arrow) is seen in the right liver lobe in (**a**) (T1WI). Contrast enhancement in the arterial phase is slightly heterogeneous (**b**) (T1WI, +C) and becomes more homogeneous with time (**c**) (T1WI, +C). No definite central scar is identified in this case.

aphaelLiver   **503**

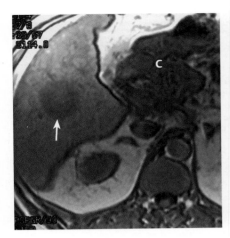

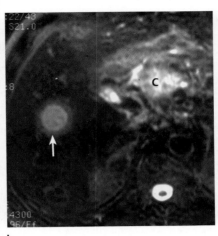

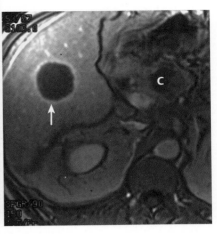

a

Fig. 16.**24** **Pancreatic carcinoma metastasis.** A solitary necrotic metastasis (arrow) is seen in the right hepatic lobe. Signal characteristics of the primary pan-

b

creatic carcinoma (C) and liver metastasis are similar and depict low signal intensity in (**a**) (T1WI) and high signal intensity in (**b**) (T2WI, FS).   **c** Peripheral ring enhance-

c

ment of the hepatic metastasis is evident after Gd-DTPA administration (T1WI, FS, +C).

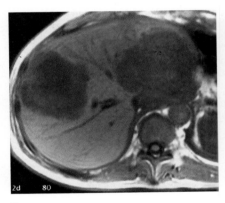

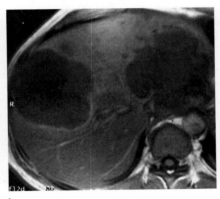

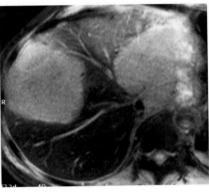

a

Fig. 16.**25**   **Colon carcinoma metastases.** Two large hypointense lesions are seen in the liver in (**a**) (T1WI). After intravenous

b

administration of Gd-DTPA contrast enhancement progresses from a thin peripheral ring in (**b**) (T1WI, FS, +C) to eventually

c

complete homogeneous enhancement of the entire lesions in (**c**) (T1WI, FS, +C).

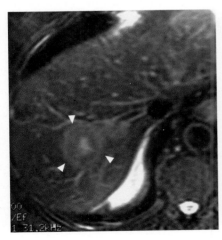

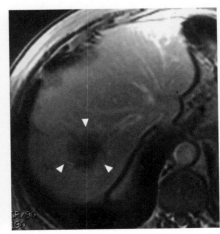

Fig. 16.**26**   **Rectal carcinoma metastasis.** **a** A solitary lesion (arrowheads) is seen with markedly hyperintense center due to tumor necrosis and slightly increased signal intensity in its periphery due to compressed surrounding hepatic tissue and mild edema. (T2WI, FS).   **b** After intravenous injection of Gd-DTPA, contrast enhancement is limited to the tumor periphery (T1WI, FS, +C). Several smaller metastases with similar signal characteristics are seen in the anterolateral liver margin.

a

b

Table 16.**1** (Cont.) Focal liver lesions

Disease	MRI Findings	Comments
Lymphoma **(Fig.** 16.**27)**	Focal lesions are hypointense on T1WI and isointense to minimally hyperintense on T2WI. After intravenous Gd-DTPA administration poor contrast enhancement of the lesion is common, which may be associated with peripheral ring enhancement. Other lesions may enhance similar to the surrounding liver parenchyma and thus remain isointense even with dynamic imaging.	Primary hepatic lymphoma is rare and presents as a solid solitary mass. Secondary lymphoma is common (over 50% at autopsy) and presents usually as a diffuse infiltrative process without alteration of the hepatic architecture or, less commonly, as focal nodular lesions.
Angiosarcoma	Multinodular lesions or, less commonly, large solitary mass, often with central necrosis and/or hemorrhage. Presenting as heterogeneous lesions with low signal intensity on T1WI, high signal intensity on T2WI, and considerable, preferentially peripheral enhancement after intravenous Gd-DTPA administration.	Represents approximately 1% of primary liver neoplasms. Occurs usually after the age of 50 with a 4:1 male predominance. Associated with hemochromatosis, neurofibromatosis, and exposure to polyvinyl chloride, arsenic, or thorotrast with a latent period of up to 30 years. *Fibrosarcoma, malignant fibrous histiocytoma, and leiomyosarcoma* are less common.
Cholangiocarcinoma (intrahepatic) **(Figs.** 16.**28** and 16.**29)**	Large heterogeneous mass, measuring up to 20 cm in diameter. Hypointense on T1WI and hyperintense on T2WI, often with a large central area of hypointensity due to fibrosis. Contrast enhancement after intravenous Gd-DTPA administration is variable, but usually poor or absent. Satellite nodules are found in about half of the cases.	Represents approximately 10% of primary liver neoplasms. Peak age is the sixth decade with male predominance. A diffuse sclerosing cholangitic cholangiocarcinoma is extremely difficult if not impossible to differentiate from sclerosing cholangitis by MRI.
Hepatoblastoma **(Figs.** 16.**30** and 16.**31)**	Large inhomogeneous mass, commonly in the right liver lobe, with low signal intensity and hyperintense foci (hemorrhage) on T1WI and high signal intensity with hypointense (fibrous) bands on T2WI. After intravenous Gd-DTPA administration, peripheral tumor enhancement is typical. Multifocal lesions or diffuse replacement of the liver parenchyma are less common manifestations.	In children, usually below 3 years of age, with 2:1 male predominance. May be associated with markedly elevated alpha-feto-protein (one-fifth of cases) and occasionally hemihypertrophy (Beckwith–Wiedemann syndrome) *Embryonal sarcoma* presents in children and adolescents as large intrahepatic mass with hemorrhagic and necrotic foci.
Extrahepatic tumor	Direct invasion of the liver by malignancies originating in the adrenal, kidney, gallbladder, and stomach.	Extrahepatic epicenter of lesion may be the clue to the correct diagnosis of the lesion's origin.

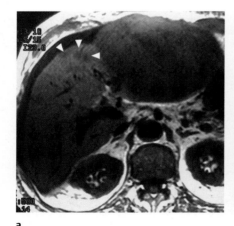

a

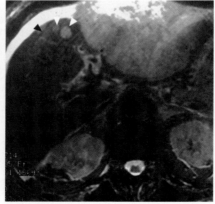

b

Fig. 16.**27** **Hepatic lymphoma.** A large mass is seen involving the entire left hepatic lobe. Several small nodules (arrowheads) of similar signal characteristics are evident in the anterior aspect of the adjacent right hepatic lobe. The lymphoma has a homogeneous low signal intensity in (**a**) (T1WI) and a more heterogeneous high signal intensity in (**b**) (T2WI). Only minimal peripheral contrast enhancement was evident after intravenous Gd-DTPA administration (not shown).

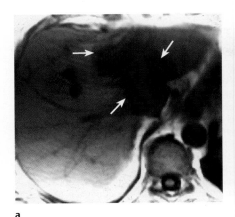

a

Fig. 16.**28** **Cholangiocarcinoma.** **a** A relatively poorly defined, hypointense mass (arrows) is evident in the left hepatic lobe (T1WI).

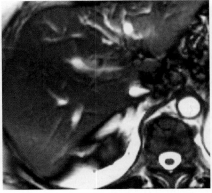

b

b Dilatation of the corresponding peripheral bile ducts secondary to more central obstruction by the slightly hyperintense mass is better appreciated (T2WI [GRE]).

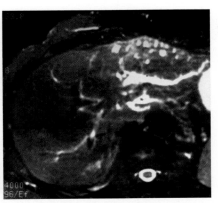

Fig. 16.**29** **Cholangiocarcinoma.** Massive dilatation of the left intrahepatic bile ducts is seen. The signal intensity of the left hepatic lobe is increased overall due to edema. The actual tumor mass could not be identified (T2WI, FS).

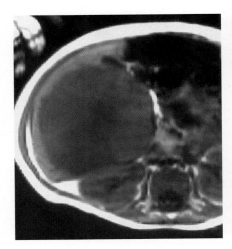

a

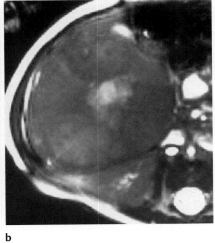

b

Fig. 16.**30** **Hepatoblastoma.** A large mass is seen replacing virtually the entire right hepatic lobe except for a small peripheral rim. The heterogeneous mass depicts overall low signal intensity in (**a**) (T1WI) and intermediate to high signal intensity in (**b**) (T2WI).

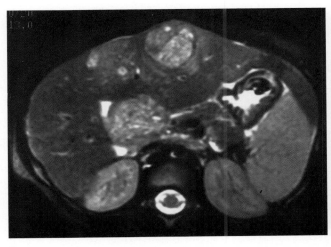

a

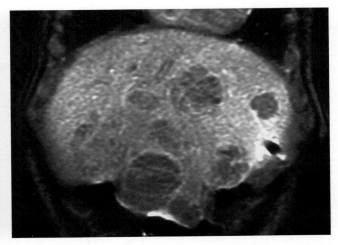

b

Fig. 16.**31** **Multifocal hepatoblastoma.** **a** Multiple heterogeneous nodules with high signal intensity are seen in the liver (T2WI, FS, axial). **b** After intravenous Gd-DTPA administration thin peripheral ring enhancement is seen in all nodules (T1WI, FS, +C, coronal).

Table 16.1 (Cont.) Focal liver lesions

Disease	MRI Findings	Comments
Hepatic abscess (Figs. 16.**32** and 16.**33**)	Solitary or multiple, often slightly heterogeneous, cystic lesions with low signal intensity on T1WI and high signal intensity on T2WI. Lesions may be septated, producing a multilocular appearance. 20–30% contain gas, producing a signal void. After intravenous Gd-DTPA administration an enhanced abscess wall is characteristic and found in almost 90% of cases. This wall enhancement may be surrounded by a hypointense zone on T1WI in about 20% due to edema in the periphery of the abscess ("double-target sign"). Several abscesses within the same anatomic liver segment suggests a biliary origin ("cluster sign").	*Pyogenic abscesses* (88%) are caused by *E. coli*, aerobic streptococci, *Staphylococcus aureus*, and anaerobes. May be solitary or multiple and usually are associated with ascending cholangitis, portal phlebitis (secondary to appendicitis, diverticulitis, or colitis), trauma, or surgery. *Amebic abscess* (10%) is caused by *Entamoeba histolytica* spreading from colon to liver via the portal system. It is usually solitary (75%), located in the right liver lobe, and does not contain gas unless a hepatobronchial or hepatoenteric fistula is present. Invasion of the right hemidiaphragm with development of an empyema is common. *Fungal abscesses* (2%) are most frequently caused by *Candida albicans* or, less commonly, by *Aspergillus fumigatus* in immunocompromised patients. They are usually multiple, less than 1 cm in diameter, and peripheral (subcapsular). Similar microabscesses are occasionally also caused by *Pneumocystis carinii* and atypical mycobacterial infections, especially in AIDS.
Hepatic trauma (Figs. 16.**34** and 16.**35**)	In the first few hours following trauma the intrahepatic hemorrhage/hematoma appears hypointense on T1WI and hyperintense on T2WI. Subsequent intracellular deoxyhemoglobin and methemoglobin formation progressively decreases the signal intensity on T2WI in the first few days. After a few days redistribution of the methemoglobin from the lysed red blood cells into the extracellular space begins, resulting in increased signal intensity primarily on T1WI and to a lesser extent on T2WI. The process begins in the periphery of the hematoma and extends inward over time. After a few weeks phagocytes begin to invade the hematoma, metabolize the hemoglobin breakdown products, and store the iron in the form of ferritin and hemosiderin; this produces signal loss in the periphery of the hematoma that is most pronounced on T2WI but is also seen to a lesser degree on T1WI. Therefore two concentric rings, an inner bright one and an outer dark one, may be identified on both T1WI and T2WI.	*Laceration*: irregular cleft or stellate lesion which may extend to the liver periphery. *Intrahepatic hematoma*: a round, oval, or irregularly shaped lesion without enhancement or with rim enhancement. Tracking of blood along the portal radicles may also be evident. *Subcapsular hematoma*: well-marginated, crescent-shaped or lenticular-shaped lesion contained by the liver capsule. *Bilioma* (bile pseudocyst): crescent or ovoid cystic lesion within or immediately adjacent to the liver secondary to traumatic or iatrogenic rupture of the biliary system. *Liver resection*: Serous fluid collection (*seroma*) may develop at the site of liver segmentectomy. May grow for weeks and then gradually subside unless it becomes infected. *Periportal edema* ("periportal collar") is a common finding in the normal *liver transplant*. True transplant complications may be vascular (stenosis, most commonly at anastomotic sites, thrombosis, and pseudoaneurysm formation), biliary (strictures, extrinsic compressions, and leaks), or parenchymal (rejection, infarction, and infection).

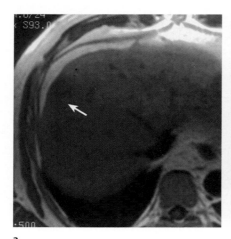
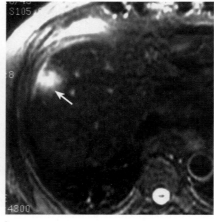
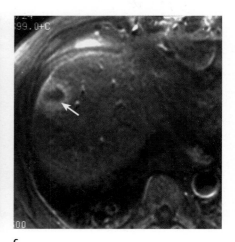

a

b

c

Fig. 16.32 Hepatic abscess *(E. coli)*. A peripheral lesion (arrow) is seen in the anterior segment of the right hepatic lobe. The lesion appears hypointense in (**a**) (T1WI) and slightly inhomogeneous and markedly hyperintense in (**b**) (T2WI, FS). **c** After intravenous Gd-DTPA administration enhancement of the abscess wall is evident (T1WI, FS, +C).

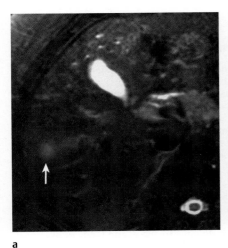

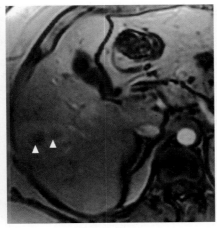

Fig. 16.**33** **Hepatic abscess.** **a** A band-like area of increased signal intensity is evident with a small cyst-like focus on its lateral end (arrow) (T2WI, FS). **b** After intravenous Gd-DTPA administration an irregular, peripheral enhancement is seen surrounding two small hypointense foci of liquefaction (arrowheads) (T1WI, FS, +C). The second more medially located and smaller abscess is not appreciated on the precontrast examination.

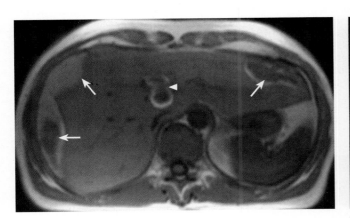

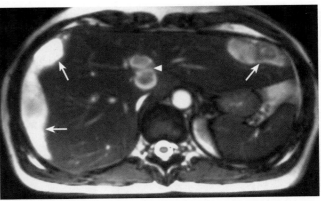

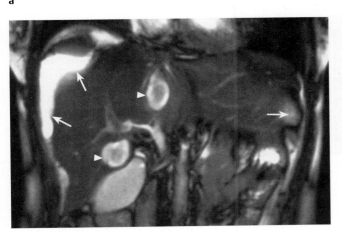

Fig. 16.**34** **Subcapsular and intrahepatic hematomas.** The subacute subcapsular hematomas (arrows) and intrahepatic hematomas (arrowheads) present as slightly to markedly hyperintense lesions with or without low signal intensity centers in all pulse sequences (**a**) (T1WI, axial), (**b**) (T2WI [GRE], axial), and (**c**) (T2WI [GRE], coronal). The high signal periphery is due to extracellular methemoglobin formation. The low signal intensity centers of the hematomas are caused by methemoglobin and deoxyhemoglobin within intact red blood cells. Note the similar signal characteristic of all hematomas, though the degree of hematoma maturation as judged by the peripheral extracellular methemoglobin formation varies from lesion to lesion.

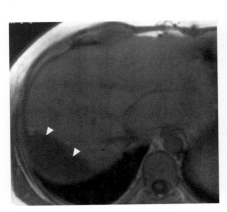

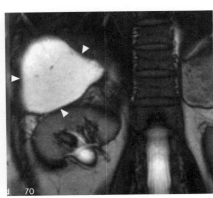

Fig. 16.**35** **Bilioma.** A uniform, hypointense, crescent-shaped, subcapsular lesion (arrowheads) is evident in the posterior segment of the right hepatic lobe (**a**: T1WI, axial). The large bilioma (arrowheads) depicts very high signal intensity in (**b**) (T2WI, coronal) and causes caudad displacement and medial rotation of the upper pole of the right kidney.

Table 16.1 (Cont.) Focal liver lesions

Disease	MRI Findings	Comments
Focal fatty infiltration (Fig. 16.36)	Single or multiple, nodular to lobulated lesions of varying size with higher signal intensity than the normal liver parenchyma on both T1WI and T2WI. However the difference in signal intensity to normal hepatic parenchyma is often relatively small, especially on T2WI, and FS techniques are usually required to corroborate the diagnosis. Absent contrast enhancement and mass effect (no bulging of liver contour and undisplaced vessels and bile ducts) are characteristic.	Focal fatty infiltration must be differentiated from tumors containing fat, such as hepatic adenomas and hepatocellular carcinomas. Regenerative nodules also may contain fat. Truly lipomatous tumors are uncommon in the liver. *Focal confluent fibrosis* (Fig. 16.37) refers to a severely damaged and scarred liver area with abnormal signal intensity that may resemble a focal mass.
Portal vein thrombosis (Fig. 16.38)	Discrete wedge-shaped regions of increased signal intensity are seen on both T2WI and Gd-DTPA-enhanced images with lobar or segmental portal vein obstruction. The increased enhancement distal to the obstructed portal vein branch reflects the increased hepatic arterial supply. At a later stage segmental hepatic atrophy may be found with compensatory hypertrophy of the nonaffected liver. A bland thrombus usually has a similar signal intensity on T1WI and T2WI, may appear relatively bright in the subacute stage due to methemoglobin formation, and has variable signal intensity in the chronic stage.	Portal obstruction may be caused by bland thrombus, tumor thrombus, or extrinsic compression. The signal intensity of a tumor thrombus corresponds to the primary lesion and tends to be higher on T2WI. The tumor thrombus may also enhance after intravenous Gd-DTPA administration. Tumor thrombosis of the intrahepatic portal system is commonly associated with hepatocellular carcinoma. Extrinsic compression of portal vein branches is most often caused by malignant tumors of any etiology. Liver infarction due to hepatic artery occlusion is rare.

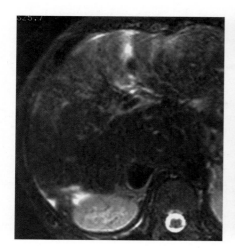

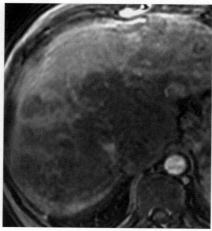

a

b

Fig. 16.36 Focal fatty infiltration. Decreased signal intensity is seen in the enlarged caudate lobe and the adjacent posterior segment of the right hepatic lobe caused by fatty infiltration (**a**: T2WI, FS). Contrast enhancement of this area is decreased when compared with the anterior segment of the right hepatic lobe and left hepatic lobe. The enhancement of the left hepatic lobe in particular appears inhomogeneous and nodular due to chronic hepatitis and early alcoholic cirrhosis (**b**: T1WI, FS, +C).

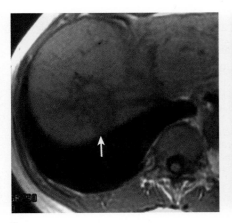

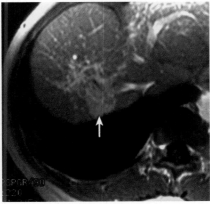

Fig. 16.**37** **Focal confluent fibrosis.** An irregular-shaped focus (arrow) is seen in the right hepatic lobe appearing hypointense in (**a**) (T1WI) and hyperintense in (**b**) (T2WI [GRE]).

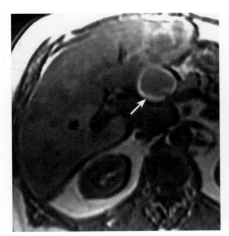

a

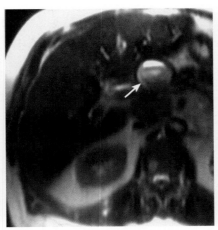

b

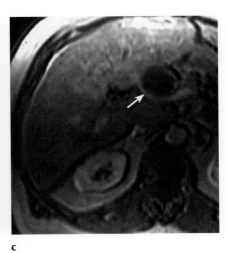

c

Fig. 16.**38** **Portal vein thrombosis with infarction of the left hepatic lobe and diffuse metastatic disease.** A dilated portal vein (arrow) is seen, almost completely occluded by a large central thrombus. The thrombus is of intermediate signal intensity in (**a**) (spoiled GRE) and (**b**) (T2WI [GRE]) and does not enhance after intravenous Gd-DTPA in (**c**) (T1WI, FS, +C). Compared with the relatively little affected posterior segment of the right hepatic lobe and caudate lobe, the signal intensity of the left lobe is increased overall in (**a**) and (**b**), and more enhanced in (**c**). Multiple small metastases originating from a rectal carcinoma are also seen scattered throughout the liver.

Table 16.1 (Cont.) Focal liver lesions

Disease	MRI Findings	Comments
Budd–Chiari syndrome (hepatic vein thrombosis) (Fig. 16.39)	Thrombosed or absent hepatic veins and intrahepatic collaterals often present as multiple comma-shaped flow voids which may be seen on T1WI and T2WI. In the acute stage the peripheral liver enhances less than the central liver. In the chronic stage the hypertrophied central portion of the liver, including the caudate lobe, may enhance less than the atrophied liver periphery and thus mimic a focal mass. Regional differences in signal intensity are frequent and may be caused by a combination of congestion, atrophy, hypertrophy, and/or iron deposition.	Obstruction of the hepatic venous outflow results in portal hypertension, ascites, and progressive hepatic failure. Hepatic venous outflow obstruction may be incomplete or segmental. Chronic hepatic venous obstruction produces hepatic ischemia leading to development of nodular regenerative hyperplasia. The nodules vary in size and typically depict a high signal intensity on T1WI and intermediate to low signal intensity on T2WI.
Radiation injury	Sharply defined edematous region of decreased signal intensity on T1WI and increased signal intensity on T2WI corresponding to the radiation port. After intravenous Gd-DTPA administration, increased enhancement is found in the radiation-damaged liver. In fatty liver disease, the fat may be reduced in the radiation port.	May develop within weeks up to 6 months after a radiation of 35 Gy or more. The radiation damage may resolve or progress to fibrosis.

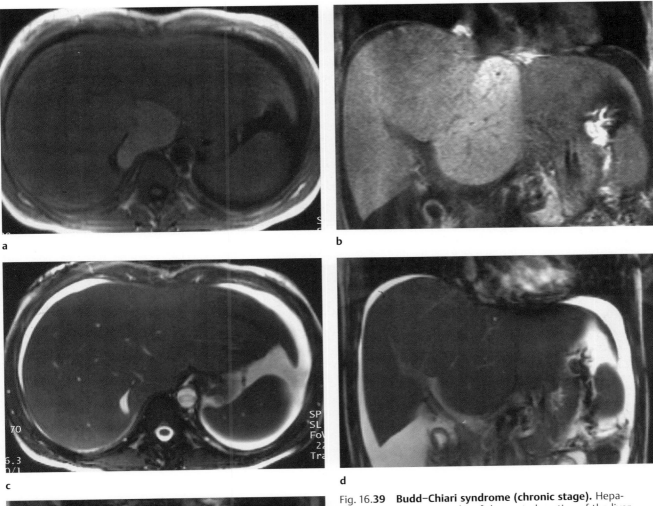

a

b

c

d

Fig. 16.**39**   **Budd–Chiari syndrome (chronic stage).** Hepatomegaly with hypertrophy of the central portion of the liver, including the quadrate and caudate lobes, is seen. Ascites is present. Normal hepatic veins are absent. Intrahepatic collaterals present as tiny linear or comma-shaped flow voids in (**a**) (spoiled GRE, axial) and (**b**) (T1WI, coronal) or as corresponding hyperintense structures in (**c**) (T2WI [GRE], axial) and (**d**) (T2WI [GRE], coronal).   **e** Extrinsic compression of the intrahepatic portion of the inferior vena cava (arrow) by the enlarged liver with prestenotic dilatation is seen (T2WI [GRE], coronal).

e

Table 16.2 Diffuse liver disease

Disease	MRI Findings	Comments
Fatty liver (Fig. 16.40)	Diffuse fatty infiltration usually is associated with hepatomegaly and may present with only slightly increased signal intensity on T1WI and appear normal on T2WI. FS techniques may be required to diagnose the fat accumulation. Lack of mass effect is characteristic. Hepatic architecture is preserved in areas of fatty infiltration. Fat-spared areas in diffuse fatty infiltration may depict round or, when bordering a fissure, straight margins and are preferentially located anterior to the portal vein bifurcation (quadrate lobe) and around the gallbladder bed.	Fat (primarily triglyceride) accumulation in hepatocytes is most commonly associated with obesity or alcohol abuse. Other causes include diabetes mellitus, steroids, debilitation, protein malnutrition, parenteral hyperalimentation, hepatitis, chemotherapy, and various hepatotoxins. Liver function tests are frequently normal. Both the appearance and resolution of fat may occur within 1 week.
Cirrhosis (Figs. 16.41–16.43)	Small liver with nodular surface and relative sparing or even hypertrophy of both the lateral segment of the left lobe and the caudate lobe is commonly found. On the other hand, the anterior segment of the right lobe and the medial segment of the left lobe tend to be most severely affected and atrophied. In an early stage the liver may be enlarged. Multiple regenerative nodules ranging in size from a few millimeters to several centimeters are characteristic and commonly hyperintense on T1WI and hypointense on T2WI. After intravenous Gd-DTPA administration, they typically enhance less than the surrounding liver parenchyma. Siderotic regenerative nodules, which accumulate iron more than the surrounding hepatic parenchyma, may also be present. Occasionally tiny peribiliary cysts are also found. Portosystemic venous collaterals, ascites, and splenomegaly are characteristic associated findings.	Cirrhosis is characterized by diffuse parenchymal destruction, fibrosis, and nodular regeneration. Etiology may be toxic (e.g., alcohol, drugs), infectious (e.g., viral hepatitis, schistosomiasis), biliary obstructive (e.g., biliary cirrhosis, sclerosing cholangiopathy), vascular (e.g., hepatic veno-occlusive disease), nutritional, and hereditary (e.g., hemochromatosis, Wilson disease, alpha-1-antitrypsin deficiency). Micronodular cirrhosis (1–5 mm) is commonly due to alcoholism, and macronodular cirrhosis (up to several centimeters) due to hepatitis. Hepatocellular carcinoma occurs in 10% of patients with cirrhosis and is best diagnosed during the arterial phase of a dynamic contrast-enhanced MRI. *Nodular regenerative hyperplasia* refers to noncirrhotic portal hypertension caused by diffuse small vessel disease. Predisposing conditions include polycythemia vera, Budd–Chiari syndrome, and collagen vascular diseases. Areas of the liver with decreased blood flow atrophy, whereas those with adequate flow enlarge and form nodules.

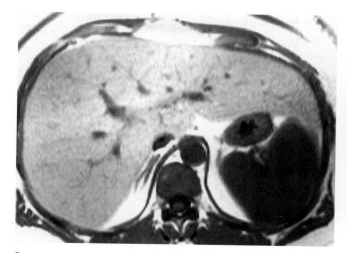

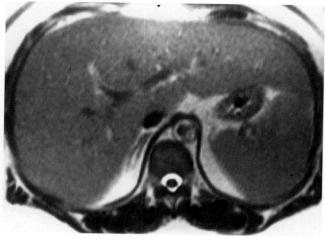

a

b

Fig. 16.**40** **Fatty liver.** Diffuse increased signal intensity is seen in the enlarged liver in (**a**) (T1WI). In (**b**) the signal intensity of the fatty liver is similar to the normal spleen (T2WI). The most effective technique to diagnose fatty liver is a comparison of in-phase (water + fat) and out-of-phase (water − fat) images, where a markedly decreased signal intensity of the fatty liver is found with the latter technique (not performed in this patient).

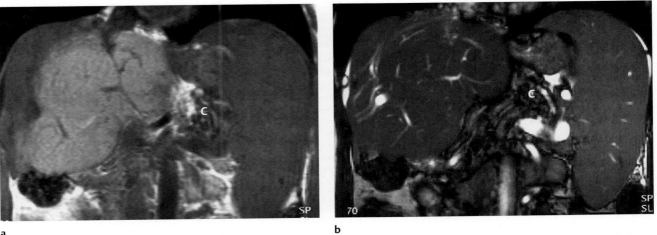

a b

Fig. 16.**41** **Cirrhosis (micronodular).** A small liver is seen with scarred surface and marked hypertrophy of its central portion including the caudate lobe. Splenomegaly and portal hypertension evident by the porto-systemic venous collaterals (C) are also present (**a**: T1WI, coronal; **b**: T2WI [GRE], coronal).

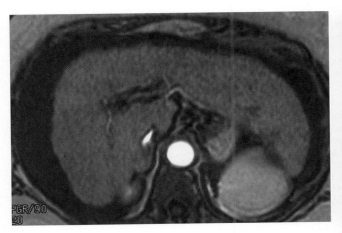

a

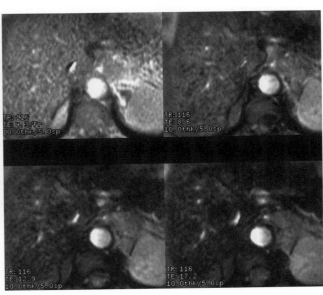

b

Fig. 16.**42** **Cirrhosis with siderotic regenerative nodules.**
a A shrunken liver surrounded by ascites is seen (spoiled GRE).
b The tiny siderotic nodules are best appreciated as low signal intensity foci on progressively T2-weighted GRE images.

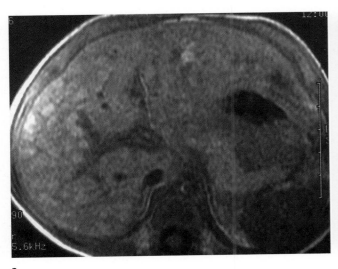

a

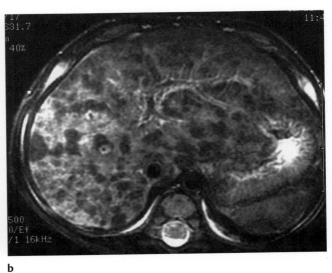

b

Fig. 16.**43** **Nodular regenerative hyperplasia in polycythemia vera.** Multiple nodules are evident that are hyperintensive in (**a**) (T1WI) and hypointensive in (**b**) (T2WI, FS).

Table 16.2 (Cont.) Diffuse liver disease

Disease	MRI Findings	Comments
Hepatic iron overload (Figs. 16.44 and 16.45)	Iron deposition lowers signal intensity, especially on T2WI. The skeletal muscle is an ideal reference tissue for assessing decreased hepatic signal intensity, since the normal liver is more intense on all pulse sequences and the skeletal muscle is not affected by iron overload. In *idiopathic (primary) hemochromatosis* decreased signal intensity of both liver and pancreas, but not spleen, is typically found since the excessively absorbed dietary iron is accumulated in parenchymal cells (e.g. hepatocytes) and not in the reticuloendothelial system. In patients requiring *multiple blood transfusions* the iron accumulates primarily within the reticuloendothelial system of the liver (Kupffer cells), spleen, and bone marrow. In *hemolytic anemias* without blood transfusions the hepatic iron load may be normal (e.g. sickle cell anemia) or increased (e.g. *thalassemia major* due to increased absorption of oral iron).	*Idiopathic (primary) hemochromatosis* is an autosomal recessive disorder caused by excessive absorption and retention of dietary iron in the parenchymal cells of the liver, pancreas, heart, and pituitary gland. The onset of clinical manifestations is usually delayed to the age of 40 to 60 years. The most important clinical symptoms include hepatomegaly (90%), skin pigmentation (90%), arthropathy (50%), and diabetes mellitus (30%). Iron deposition in the reticuloendothelial system (e.g. following multiple blood transfusions) is relatively harmless (*hemosiderosis*). After saturation of the storage capacity of the reticuloendothelial system (usually >40 units of blood or 10 g of iron) the iron begins to accumulate in parenchymal cells of organs characteristically involved with primary hemochromatosis, resulting in similar clinical symptoms (*secondary hemochromatosis*).
Wilson disease (hepato-lenticular degeneration)	Chronic hepatitis or cirrhosis with hyperintense lesions on T1WI and hypointense nodules on T2WI. The hypointense nodules on T2WI may be surrounded by hyperintense inflamed septa. Pancreas is normal (DD: idiopathic hemochromatosis).	Autosomal recessive disease with excessive copper retention due to impaired biliary excretion. Presents in children and young adults with green Kayser–Fleischer corneal ring (diagnostic), jaundice, portal hypertension, and neurologic (extrapyramidal) symptoms.
Diffuse hepato-cellular carcinoma (Fig. 16.46)	Advanced diffuse hepatocellular carcinoma is commonly hypointense on T1WI and hyperintense on T2WI, similar to metastases. After intravenous Gd-DTPA administration, hepatocellular carcinoma is usually hyperintense to the liver in the arterial phase (prior to the contrast agent reaching the liver by the portal vein), hypointense to the liver in the portal phase, and often isointense to the surrounding liver on delayed images. Portal invasion is a common associated finding.	Diffuse hepatocellular carcinoma is usually associated with chronic liver disease such as cirrhosis, chronic active hepatitis, or hemochromatosis.

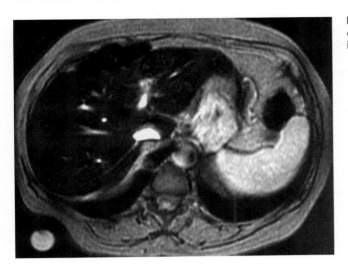

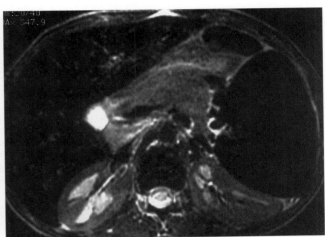

Fig. 16.**44** **Idiopathic (primary) hemochromatosis.** Markedly decreased signal intensity is seen in the liver, whereas the signal intensity in both spleen and vertebra is normal (T2WI [GRE]).

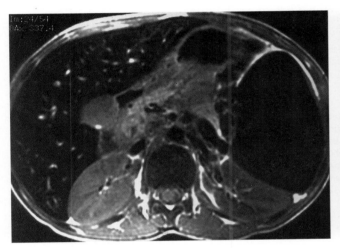

a

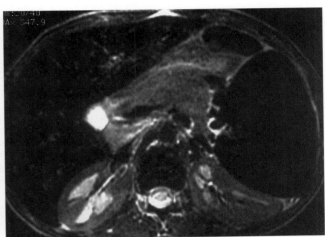

b

Fig. 16.**45** **Hemosiderosis (iron overload caused by multiple blood transfusions in sickle cell disease).** Markedly decreased signal intensity is seen in the liver, enlarged spleen, and visualized vertebra, whereas the signal intensity in the pancreas is normal (**a**: T1WI; **b**: T2WI, FS).

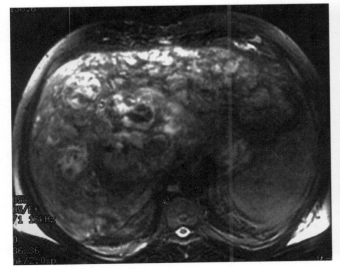

a

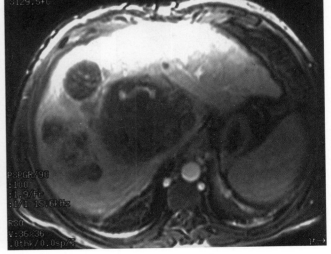

b

Fig. 16.**46** **Multifocal hepatocellular carcinoma in cirrhosis.** A heterogeneous liver with multiple different-sized nodules is seen in (**a**) (T2WI [GRE]). After contrast enhancement the multiple hypointense hepatoma nodules in the periphery of the right lobe and the large mass involving the caudate lobe are more readily appreciated (**b**: T1WI, +C). Occlusion of the inferior vena cava, with numerous collaterals in the anterior abdominal wall, is also evident.

Table 16.2 (Cont.) Diffuse liver disease

Disease	MRI Findings	Comments
Diffuse metastatic disease (Figs. 16.47 and 16.48)	Multiple well to poorly defined foci, often with similar signal intensity to that of the spleen on T1WI and T2WI. Central necrosis may increase signal intensity on T2WI. Compared with diffuse hepatocellular carcinoma, early ring-like contrast enhancement is more common in metastatic disease, whereas vascular invasion is unusual.	Colorectal carcinoma metastases may develop coagulative necrosis centrally, which may be nearly isointense to the liver on T2WI. Endocrine tumor metastases can have extremely high signal intensity on T2WI, mimicking hemangiomas or cysts. Melanoma metastases may be hyperintense on T1WI and hypointense on T2WI. Peritoneal spread to the liver (e.g. from ovarian carcinoma) preferentially involves the liver periphery.
Diffuse lymphoma	Often isointense to the liver, or similar to diffuse metastatic disease. Presents with poorly defined foci that are hypointense on T1WI and hyperintense on T2WI.	More common with secondary involvement by non-Hodgkin lymphoma than Hodgkin disease. Generalized lymphadenopathy and splenomegaly are commonly associated.
Sarcoidosis	Multiple granulomas, usually smaller than 1 cm in diameter, with low signal intensity on both T1WI and T2WI. Contrast enhancement is only minimal and delayed. Rarely an increased signal intensity of the diffusely involved liver is seen on T2WI when compared with the normal spleen (liver-spleen "intensity flip-flop").	Focal involvement of the liver is less common.
Amyloidosis	Hepatomegaly with diffuse increase in signal intensity on T1WI (similar to subcutaneous fat) and normal signal intensity on T2WI.	MRI findings in hepatic amyloidosis and fatty infiltration are similar and require FS techniques for their differentiation. Associated splenic involvement in amyloidosis may depict decreased signal intensity on both T1WI and T2WI.
Schistosomiasis (Fig. 16.49)	Hepatosplenomegaly and portal hypertension (porto systemic-venous collaterals) secondary to periportal fibrosis. Presents as wall thickening (fibrotic collar) around the portal vein radicles or diffuse micronodular pattern with low signal intensity on both T1WI and T2WI. Ascites is usually not present (DD: liver cirrhosis).	Worldwide major cause of portal hypertension with over 200 million people affected. Three types: 1) *Schistosoma hematobium* (Africa, Mediterranean, Southwest Asia) 2) *Schistosoma mansoni* (Africa, Arabic peninsula, Caribbean, West Indies, South America) 3) *Schistosoma japonicum* (China, Japan, Philippines).
Diffuse biliary disease	See Table 17.1.	

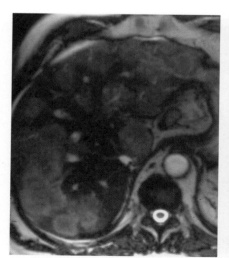
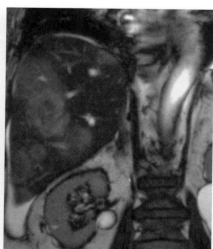

Fig. 16.**47** **Diffuse colonic carcinoma metastases.** Multiple, partially confluent, hyperintense metastases with lower signal intensity centers, presumably due to coagulative necrosis, are noted throughout the liver (**a**: T2WI [GRE], axial; **b**: T2WI [GRE], coronal).

a   b

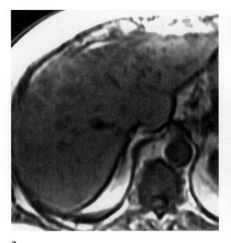

a

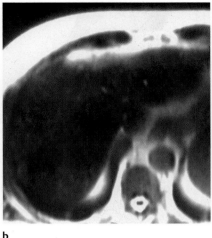

b

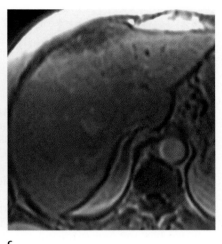

c

Fig. 16.**48** **Diffuse rectal carcinoma metastases.** Multiple hepatic metastases are scattered throughout the liver. They are best appreciated as hypointense foci in (**a**) (T1WI), and relatively poorly visualized as slightly hyperintense foci in (**b**) (T2WI) and after contrast enhancement in (**c**) (T1WI, FS, +C).

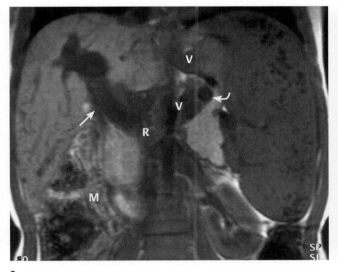

a

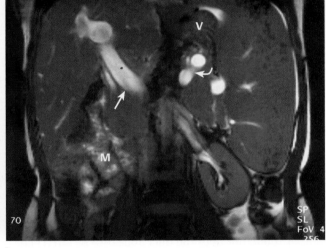

b

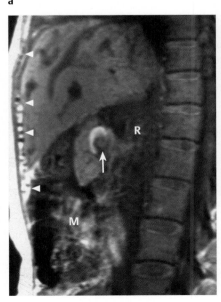

c

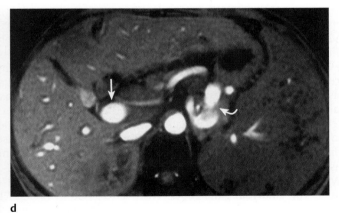

d

Fig. 16.**49** **Schistosomiasis.** Signs of portal hypertension are evident and include: marked splenomegaly, dilated portal vein (arrow) and splenic vein (curved arrow), gastroesophageal varices (V), retroperitoneal collaterals (R), mesenteric collaterals (M), and subcutaneous collaterals in the anterior abdominal wall (arrowheads) presenting with corkscrew or beaded appearance. The numerous small hypointense foci in the spleen represent granulomas. The liver size and texture are within normal limits. Note, however, the low signal intensity rings or collars surrounding many hyperintense peripheral portal vein radicles, best appreciated in the right hepatic lobe in (**d**), indicating thickening of their walls by periportal fibrosis. (**a**: T1WI, coronal; **b**: T2WI [GRE], coronal; **c**: spoiled GRE, sagittal; **d**: T2WI [GRE], axial).

17 Biliary Tract

Ultrasonography remains the imaging modality of choice for the evaluation of the biliary system. CT and MRI complement this technique in selected cases. Magnetic resonance cholangiopancreatography (MRCP) is a new noninvasive imaging modality that enables visualization of biliary and pancreatic ducts comparable to percutaneous transhepatic cholangiography (PTHC) and endoscopic cholangiopancreatography (ERCP), although at the moment with a lower spatial resolution. It is based on the concept that bile and pancreatic duct fluid are static and have long T2 relaxation times. Therefore, on T2WI these ducts display a high signal intensity and can easily be differentiated from vascular structures containing flowing blood with shorter T2 times and rapid dephasing.

Dilatation of the *biliary system* occurs most frequently as the result of obstruction. Normal intrahepatic ducts measure less than 3 mm in diameter. They are usually not visualized on conventional MR pulse sequences designed to evaluate the liver. Dilated intrahepatic ducts are visualized as multiple branching tubular, round, or oval structures converging toward the porta hepatis. The common hepatic duct is formed by confluence of the right and left hepatic ducts in the porta hepatis. Normally the common hepatic duct measures 3 to 6 mm in diameter and is located anterior to the portal vein and lateral to the hepatic artery. The cystic duct with the characteristic spiral valves of Heister arises from the neck of the gallbladder and joins the common hepatic duct to form the common bile duct. A diameter of the common bile duct in excess of 8 mm is indicative of biliary obstruction. Patients who underwent cholecystectomy years ago sometimes have a common bile duct diameter in excess of 8 mm without obstruction. However, in these patients the cross section of the duct is neither round nor does the duct appear to be stretched.

The *gallbladder* is a piriform sac partly contained in a fossa on the inferior surface of the right hepatic lobe. The gallbladder bile depicts a high signal intensity similar to other fluids on T2WI and varies on T1WI from hypointense (unconcentrated bile) to hyperintense (concentrated bile) with regard to the liver. Occasionally the bile exhibits a gradient with the concentrated bile layering dependently. The gallbladder may be anomalously located intrahepatically, suprahepatically, or even retrorenally. Duplication of the gallbladder occurs but is rare. The gallbladder wall measures 1 to 2 mm when distended and seen in profile. *Gallbladder wall thickening* is usually due to acute or chronic cholecystitis and less commonly due to gallbladder wall edema (e.g., hypoalbuminemia), neoplasm, liver dysfunction, and ascites. An *enlarged gallbladder* with a diameter in excess of 5 cm suggests cystic or common bile duct obstruction due to cholelithiasis or tumor, but may also be found with gallbladder hydrops or empyema, diabetes, and prolonged fasting.

Gallstones are frequently diagnosed in routine MRI as a round or faceted foci of low or absent signal intensity surrounded by hyperintense bile on T2WI. Biliary calculi must be differentiated from intraluminal tumors, sludge, blood clots, parasites (e.g., *Ascaris* and liver flukes), and air bubbles.

Obstruction of the extrahepatic biliary system produces prestenotic dilatation. Abrupt termination of a dilated common bile duct in the absence of a calculus suggests a malignancy, whereas gradual tapering of the dilated duct favors a benign stricture or nonobstructing extrinsic compression (e.g., pancreatitis). *Ampullary tumors* are benign (adenomas) or malignant (carcinomas) lesions originating from the glandular epithelium of the ampulla of Vater, causing early ductal obstruction. They present with intermittent jaundice and at the time of diagnosis usually measure less than 3 cm in diameter. They may be associated with familial polyposis coli or the Gardner syndrome (colonic polyposis, osteomas, and a variety of soft-tissue tumors, including desmoids). They are different from *periampullary tumors* such as pancreatic carcinoma, cholangiocarcinoma of the distal common bile duct, and benign or malignant duodenal wall tumors.

Extrinsic, right-sided compression of the common hepatic duct caused by a gallstone impacted in the cystic duct associated with chronic inflammation is referred to as *Mirrizzi syndrome*. Obstruction at the porta hepatis often is secondary to a cholangiocarcinoma arising from the confluence of the hepatic ducts (*Klatskin tumor*), but other malignancies can produce a similar appearance.

Multiple intrahepatic and/or *extrahepatic ductal stenoses* often associated with intervening saccular dilatations are seen in sclerosing cholangitis as well as in cholangitis associated with AIDS or liver transplants. Multiple saccular dilations exclusively limited to the intrahepatic ducts are found in Caroli disease, congenital hepatic fibrosis, and suppurative cholangitis with tiny saccular abscesses.

Gas in the biliary system is usually secondary to operative procedures such as sphincterotomy and biliary-intestinal anastomosis. Other less common causes include gallstone fistula, choledochoenteric fistula secondary to a malignant neoplasm, emphysematous cholecystitis and cholangitis, surgical instrumentation (e.g., ERCP), or an incompetent sphincter of Oddi.

The differential diagnosis of bile duct disease is discussed in Table 17.1, and the differential diagnosis of gallbladder disease in Table 17.2.

Table 17.**1** Bile duct disease

Disease	MRI Findings	Comments
Choledochal cyst (Figs. 17.1–17.3)	Developmental cystic dilatation of the common bile duct measuring up to 15 cm in diameter. Expanded classification includes additional cystic disorders of the extrahepatic/intrahepatic bile ducts. Type 1: Fusiform dilatation of the common bile duct with or without common hepatic duct dilatation. Type 2: Saccular or diverticulum-like outpouching from common bile duct. Type 3: Choledochocele Type 4a: Multiple intrahepatic and extrahepatic bile duct cysts. Type 4b: Multiple extrahepatic bile duct cysts. Type 5: Single or multiple intrahepatic bile duct cysts (including Caroli disease).	Choledochal cysts (types 1 and 2) characteristically present in children and young adults with jaundice, abdominal pain and palpable mass. Most common in Asia (Japan). Complications include cholelithiasis, pancreatitis, cholangitis, and malignant transformation in 10 % of patients. Direct cholangiography or HIDA scan demonstrates direct communication(s) of the cyst(s) with biliary system. DD: Pancreatic pseudocyst, hepatic cyst, enteric duplication cyst, spontaneous loculated bilioma, and other noncommunicating fluid collections.

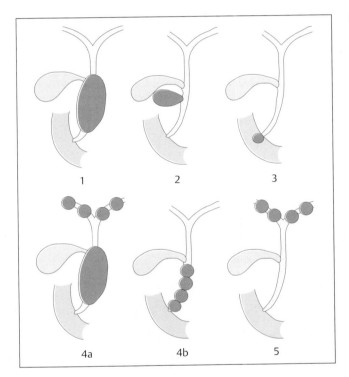

Fig. 17.**1** **Classification of congenital biliary cysts.**
1. Choledochal cyst. 2. Diverticulum of extrahepatic duct. 3. Choledochocele. 4. Multiple segmental cysts (4a. intrahepatic and extrahepatic; 4b. extrahepatic only). 5. Intrahepatic cysts only (Caroli disease).

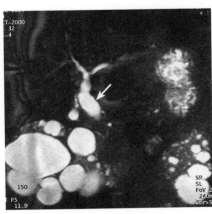

Fig. 17.**2** **Choledochal cyst (type 1).** Fusiform dilatation of the common hepatic and common bile duct (arrow) is seen associated with adult polycystic kidney disease (MRCP).

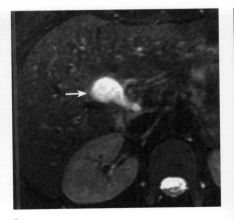

a

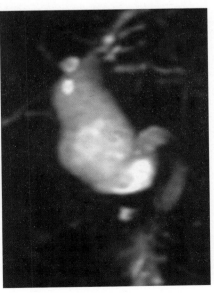

b

Fig. 17.**3** **Choledochal cyst (type 1).** Multiple small gallstones are seen throughout the cyst (arrow) in both (**a**) (T2WI, FS, axial) and (**b**) (MRCP).

Table 17.1 Bile duct disease

Disease	MRI Findings	Comments
Choledochocele	Small cystic mass in the medial wall or lumen of the second portion of the duodenum caused by dilatation of the distal/intramural portion of the common bile duct with herniation into the duodenum. May contain stones or sludge.	Congenital or acquired (secondary to stone passage, stenosis, and inflammation). Also referred to as type 3 choledochal cyst or diverticulum of common bile duct. Direct or magnetic resonance cholangiography (MRC) depicting the sac-like dilatation of the intramural common bile duct segment is diagnostic.
Caroli disease	Irregular saccular dilatation of the intrahepatic bile ducts appearing hypointense on T1WI and hyperintense on T2WI. (DD: Polycystic liver disease, where cysts do not connect with intrahepatic bile ducts). Extrahepatic bile ducts may be dilated.	Autosomal recessive disease associated with medullary sponge kidney (80%), infantile polycystic kidney disease, and increased risk of cholangiocarcinoma. Complications include bile stasis with recurrent cholangitis, biliary calculi, liver abscesses, and septicemia.
Congenital hepatic fibrosis	Ectasia of peripheral biliary radicles ("lollipop-tree") associated with portal hypertension and hepatosplenomegaly.	Congenital cirrhosis with rapid, fatal progression. DD: Caroli disease which is not associated with cirrhosis and portal hypertension.
Cholangiocarcinoma (extrahepatic) (Figs. 17.4–17.7)	Obstructing soft-tissue mass of variable size arising from an extrahepatic bile duct or abruptly obstructing stricture of varying length without appreciable mass are common presentations. Marked dilatation of the intrahepatic ducts without dilatation of the extrahepatic biliary system is quite characteristic. An associated prestenotic extrahepatic bile duct dilatation, however, is not uncommon either. Contrast enhancement of the lesion is variable.	Presenting commonly in the sixth and seventh decades of life with gradual onset of fluctuating painless jaundice. Predisposing conditions include inflammatory bowel disease (especially ulcerative colitis), sclerosing cholangitis, liver flukes, and choledochal cysts. A *Klatskin tumor* is a cholangiocarcinoma originating in the confluence of the hepatic ducts.

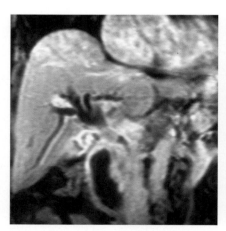

a

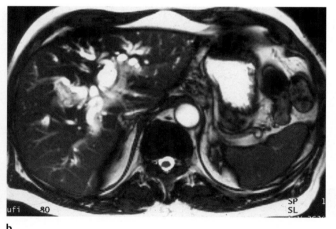

b

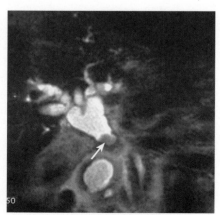

c

Fig. 17.**4 Cholangiocarcinoma (intraductal).** A dilated intrahepatic biliary system is seen. (**a**: spoiled GRE, coronal; **b**: T2WI [GRE], axial). An intraductal lesion (arrow) is evident in the common hepatic duct with prestenotic dilatation in (**c**) (MRCP).

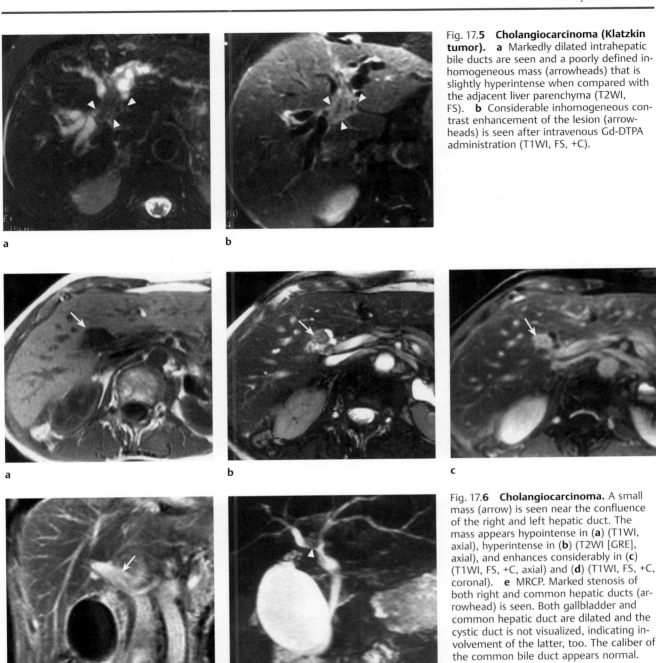

Fig. 17.**5** **Cholangiocarcinoma (Klatzkin tumor).** **a** Markedly dilated intrahepatic bile ducts are seen and a poorly defined inhomogeneous mass (arrowheads) that is slightly hyperintense when compared with the adjacent liver parenchyma (T2WI, FS). **b** Considerable inhomogeneous contrast enhancement of the lesion (arrowheads) is seen after intravenous Gd-DTPA administration (T1WI, FS, +C).

Fig. 17.**6** **Cholangiocarcinoma.** A small mass (arrow) is seen near the confluence of the right and left hepatic duct. The mass appears hypointense in (**a**) (T1WI, axial), hyperintense in (**b**) (T2WI [GRE], axial), and enhances considerably in (**c**) (T1WI, FS, +C, axial) and (**d**) (T1WI, FS, +C, coronal). **e** MRCP. Marked stenosis of both right and common hepatic ducts (arrowhead) is seen. Both gallbladder and common hepatic duct are dilated and the cystic duct is not visualized, indicating involvement of the latter, too. The caliber of the common bile duct appears normal.

Fig. 17.**7** **Cholangiocarcinoma (periampullary).** MRCP. A tight stenosis of the common bile duct is seen near the ampulla with marked prestenotic dilatation of both the extrahepatic and intrahepatic biliary system. Note the normal caliber of the major pancreatic duct (arrow).

Table 17.1 (Cont.) Bile duct disease

Disease	MRI Findings	Comments
Pancreatic carcinoma, metastases, and lymphoma (Figs. 17.8, 17.9)	Large soft-tissue mass with abrupt bile duct obstruction and prestenotic dilatation of the biliary system.	Besides carcinoma of the head of the pancreas and metastatic or lymphomatous adenopathy in the porta hepatis, direct invasion from a malignancy in a neighboring organ may also cause extrahepatic biliary obstruction.
Infective cholangitis	Dilated intrahepatic and extrahepatic ducts with thickened (edematous) bile duct walls. Often associated with biliary calculi and sludge. Pneumobilia may be found with gas-producing organisms. May proceed to multiple miliary hepatic abscess formations.	Presents characteristically with recurrent episodes of sepsis, fever, chills, jaundice, and abdominal pain. *Acute suppurative ascending cholangitis* is commonly associated with obstructing biliary stone or malignancy and most often caused by E. coli. *Recurrent pyogenic cholangitis* (oriental cholangiohepatitis) is frequently associated with liver fluke infestation, intrahepatic pigment stones, and sludge.
Sclerosing cholangitis	Beaded dilatation of both intrahepatic and extrahepatic bile ducts with thickened, often nodular walls and periportal inflammation. The latter can be differentiated from the dilated intrahepatic ducts on T2WI by a signal intensity intermediate between liver and bile. Both thickened bile duct walls and inflamed periportal triads enhance after intravenous Gd-DTPA. The enhanced high-signal periportal inflammation may produce a collar surrounding portal vein radicles. Enlarged portal lymph nodes are commonly associated.	Commonly presents with chronic or intermittent jaundice in middle-aged adults with 2:1 male predominance. History of previous biliary surgery (50%) and chronic pancreatitis (15%) may be present. Primary sclerosing cholangitis of unknown cause must be differentiated from a secondary form associated with inflammatory bowel disease (especially ulcerative colitis), cirrhosis, pancreatitis, retroperitoneal fibrosis, or retro-orbital pseudotumor. There is, however, no association with gallstones.
Cholelithiasis	Single or multiple, round or faceted, intraluminal foci of low or absent signal intensity surrounded by high signal intensity bile are seen on T2WI. On T1WI the signal intensity of gallstones varies depending on their composition, but they usually depict a very low signal intensity also. Intrahepatic biliary dilatation may not be present with extrahepatic obstruction.	Common cause of bile duct obstruction, especially in obese females in their forties and fifties. Other predisposing factors include hemolytic anemias, Crohn disease, diabetes, cirrhosis, cholestasis, and hyperparathyroidism.
Worm infestation	Single or multiple, hypointense intraluminal defects surrounded by hyperintense bile on T2WI with or without extrahepatic obstruction. *Ascaris* produce a long linear filling defect or discrete mass if coiled. Liver flukes produce multiple crescent or stiletto-shaped filling defects. A *hydatid cyst (echinococcus granularis)* of the liver may erode into the biliary system and discharge daughter cysts or cyst membranes into the bile.	*Ascaris* (25 to 35 cm long) and *liver flukes* (1 to 3 cm long) are nematodes ascending from the duodenum into the bile ducts. Liver fluke (clonorchis sinensis) infestation occurs by eating raw fish and is common in the Far East. Complications include bile duct obstruction, calculus and stricture formation, and bacterial superinfection with liver abscess formation.
Postoperative fistula or cystic duct remnant	Irregular cavity communicating with extrahepatic biliary system (fistula) or a tubular structure in patients who have undergone cholecystectomy (duct remnant)	Duct remnant is usually not associated with dilatation of the common bile duct, but may contain a stone.

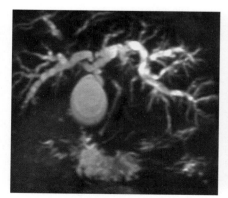

Fig. 17.8   **Pancreatic carcinoma.** MRCP. Abrupt obstruction of the common bile duct is seen with marked prestenotic dilatation of the extrahepatic and intrahepatic biliary system.

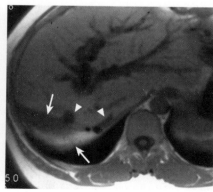

a

Fig. 17.9   **Lymph node metastases in porta hepatis from colon carcinoma.** Marked dilatation of the bile ducts is seen in the hypertrophied left hepatic lobe. Sequelae of right hepatic lobe resection for

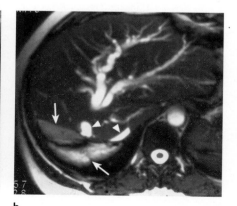

b

metastatic disease are also seen and include, besides two tiny gas bubbles evident as signal void foci, two biliomas (arrowheads) and two subcapsular hematomas (arrows) (**a**: T1WI; **b**: T2WI).

Table 17.**2** Gallbladder disease

Disease	MRI Findings	Comments
Adenomyomatosis (Figs. 17.10, 17.11)	*Generalized form*: Nonspecific gallbladder wall thickening with tiny intramural diverticula producing a "pearl necklace gallbladder". Visualization of the latter requires the intravenous administration of hepatobiliary chelates such as gadobenate dimeglumine (Gd-BOTA). *Localized form*: Adenoma presenting as smooth sessile mass outside the wall of the gallbladder fundus containing a diverticulum-like outpouching of the gallbladder lumen. *Annular form*: Hourglass configuration of the gallbladder with congenital transverse septum.	Hyperplasia of epithelial and muscular elements of the gallbladder wall with mucosal outpouching of epithelium-lined cystic spaces into or all the way through the thickened muscular layer (Rokitansky–Aschoff sinus). Develops with increasing age with 3:1 female predominance.
Cholesterolosis	Diffuse to micronodular thickening of the gallbladder wall ("strawberry gallbladder"). Associated with cholesterol stones in over 50 % of patients. *Cholesterol polyp*: Single or multiple, fixed intraluminal filling defects (< 1 cm) commonly located in the middle third of the gallbladder.	Abnormal deposits of cholesterol esters in macrophages (foam cells) and mucosal epithelium. Cholesterol polyps must be differentiated from *benign neoplasms* (e.g., papilloma, adenopapilloma) and other *inflammatory* and *hyperplastic polyps*.

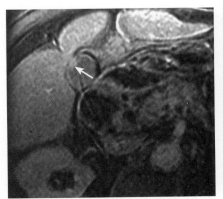

Fig. 17.**10** **Adenomatosis (localized form).** A small enhancing sessile mass (arrow) is seen originating from the wall of the gallbladder fundus (GRE, +C).

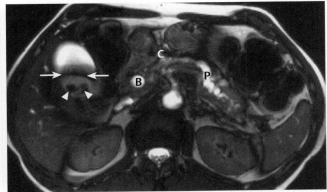

Fig. 17.**11** **Adenomatosis (annular form).** Hourglass deformity of the gallbladder with transverse septum (arrows) and gallstones (arrowheads) is seen. A pancreatic carcinoma (C) with dilated pancreatic (P) and common bile (B) duct is also present (T2WI).

Table 17.2 (Cont.) Gallbladder disease

Disease	MRI Findings	Comments
Gallbladder carcinoma (Figs. 17.12, 17.13)	Focal or diffuse thickening of the gallbladder wall of 1 cm and more or a polypoid mass of 2 cm and more is highly suggestive of malignancy. Other presentations include a fungating intraluminal mass with wide base or complete replacement of the gallbladder by tumor. On T2WI the mass is hypointense to the gallbladder bile and usually hyperintense to the adjacent liver. Contrast enhancement is variable, with cellular portions enhancing early and fibrous portions late. Tumor extension into the liver, porta hepatis, and pancreas is common. Liver involvement is best visualized on T2WI and after contrast enhancement, whereas extension into the pancreas and adjacent tissue is well depicted on fat-suppressed (FS) T1WI before and after Gd-DTPA administration. Biliary obstruction and regional lymph node involvement may also be present.	Most common biliary cancer. Usually occurring in patients over age 60 with 4:1 female predominance. Associated with chronic cholecystitis, including porcelain gallbladder and gallstones, ulcerative colitis, and familial polyposis coli. Histologically a well-differentiated adenocarcinoma of the scirrhous type is found in approximately 90% of cases. DD: After cholecystectomy, loops of bowel in the gallbladder fossa may simulate a gallbladder carcinoma or tumor recurrence, respectively.
Cholecystolithiasis (Fig. 17.14)	Gallstones generally present as round or faceted foci of low or absent signal intensity and are best visualized on T2WI, where they are contrasted by the high signal intensity bile. Rarely, calculi that contain lipid components may depict an increased signal intensity on T1WI, or may even have a rimmed or laminated appearance.	Two-thirds of the patients are asymptomatic and frequently gallstones are incidentally discovered in routine MRI. Symptomatic patients may present with biliary colics and or signs of cholecystitis. Peak age is the fifth and sixth decades with a 3:1 female predominance.

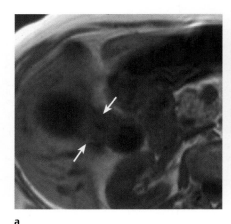

a

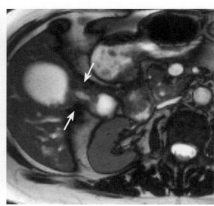

b

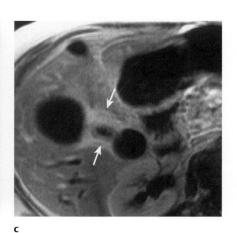

c

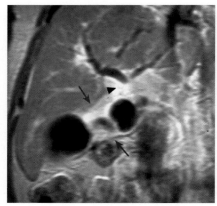

d

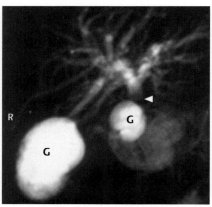

e

Fig. 17.12 Gallbladder carcinoma. A small mass (arrows) is seen encircling the gallbladder and causing a dumbbell deformity of the latter. The lesion has overall moderate signal intensity and, compared with bile, is hyperintense in (**a**) (T1WI, axial) and hypointense in (**b**) (T2WI [GRE], axial). Considerable contrast enhancement of the mass is seen in (**c**) (T1WI, FS, +C, axial) and (**d**) (T1WI, FS, +C, coronal). Tumor extension (arrowhead) into the porta hepatis is also evident in (**d**).
e MRCP shows the dumbbell deformity of the gallbladder (G) and the obstruction of the common hepatic duct (arrowhead) with prestenotic biliary dilatation.

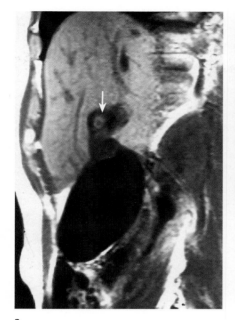

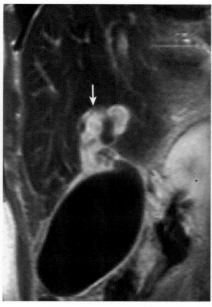

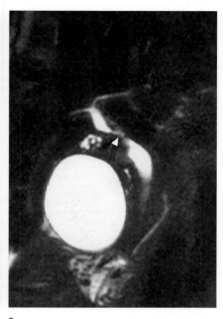

a

Fig. 17.**13** **Gallbladder carcinoma.** A mass (arrow) in the gallbladder neck is seen. The gallbladder is distended secondary to cystic duct obstruction. The lesion is hypointense to the surrounding liver parenchyma in (**a**)

b

(T1WI, sagittal) and depicts marked contrast enhancement in (**b**) (T1WI, FS, +C, sagittal). The tumor extends along the cystic duct and causes marked stenosis (arrowhead) of the common bile duct at its

c

confluence with the cystic duct. A second stenosis of the common bile duct is evident at its entrance into the pancreas (**c**: MRCP).

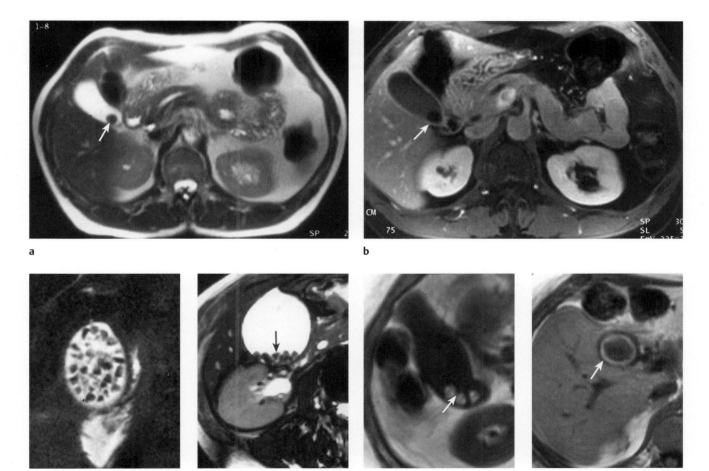

a

b

c   **d**   **e**   **f**

Fig. 17.**14** **Cholecystolithiasis.** Gallstones (arrows) are seen in four different patients. A solitary signal void gallstone is seen obstructing the gallbladder neck in (**a**) (T2WI, axial), causing cholecystitis evident by the enhanced and slightly thickened gallbladder wall in (**b**) (T1WI, FS, +C, axial). Multiple tiny faceted gall-

stones are seen in (**c**) (MRCP), producing a serrated appearance of the hyperintense bile in (**d**) (T2WI, axial). **e** Three small faceted gallstones of intermediate signal intensity are seen in the gallbladder fundus (T1WI, axial). **f** A rimmed gallstone is seen (T1WI, axial).

Table 17.2 (Cont.) Gallbladder disease

Disease	MRI Findings	Comments
Cholecystitis **(Figs. 17.15–17.17)**	Thickened gallbladder wall (>3 mm) with marked contrast enhancement is characteristically found in *acute cholecystitis*. Obstruction of the cystic duct due to calculous disease is present in the majority of patients. Intramural and/or pericholecystic fluid collections may be present in advanced cases. Intrahepatic periportal edema may also be found, but is nonspecific. In *chronic cholecystitis* a small irregular gallbladder with thickened, but only mildly enhancing wall is typically found. Gas within the wall or lumen of the gallbladder in the absence of surgical instrumentation or fistulization indicates *emphysematous cholecystitis*. Wall calcifications are virtually diagnostic for a *porcelain gallbladder*. In *xanthogranulomatous cholecystitis* an irregular thickened wall and invasion of the adjacent liver may be found simulating a gallbladder carcinoma. Demonstration of regular concentric rings in an enhanced or nonenhanced thickened gallbladder wall favors a benign condition.	Acute cholecystitis presents with abdominal pain in the right subcostal region that increases gradually in severity. About 20 % of patients present with mild jaundice. The disease has a preference for obese females in their fifth and sixth decades of life. Complications include gallbladder gangrene (shaggy, irregular wall with intraluminal hemorrhage), perforation with pericholecystic abscess formation and peritonitis, and empyema (*suppurative cholecystitis*) with signs of systemic toxicity. A *gallbladder hydrops* may result either from resolved acute cholecystitis or from cystic duct obstruction without inflammation. Emphysematous cholecystitis is usually found in patients with diabetes or debilitating disease and has a 5:1 male predominance.
Gallbladder trauma **(Fig. 17.18)**	Blood in the gallbladder in the hyperacute phase consists primarily of oxyhemoglobin and appears dark on T1WI and bright on T2WI. In the acute phase blood is in the deoxyhemoglobin state and appears hypointense on both T1WI and T2WI and is usually, but not always, homogeneous. In the subacute phase methemoglobin formation and hemolysis occur, resulting first in hyperintense bile on T1WI and subsequently on T2WI too. A hematocrit effect may be appreciated, especially on T2WI, with the supernatant fluid depicting a high signal intensity and the dependant portion containing the cellular elements a low signal intensity.	Unconcentrated bile has a low signal intensity on T1WI and high signal intensity on T2WI. With bile concentration the signal intensity increases on T1WI and sometimes a gradient is apparent with concentrated bile layering dependently. In both suppurative and hemorrhagic cholecystitis the bile may also appear hyperintense on T1WI.

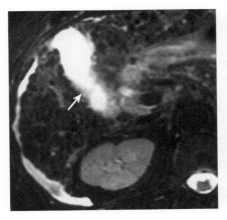

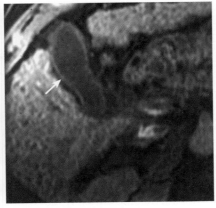

a

b

Fig. 17.**15** **Acute cholecystitis.** **a** A poorly defined edematous gallbladder wall with pericholecystic fluid accumulation (arrow) is seen in this patient with liver cirrhosis and ascites (T2WI, FS). **b** After intravenous Gd-DTPA administration considerable enhancement of the uniformly thickened gallbladder wall (arrow) is evident (GRE, +C).

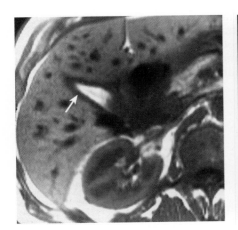

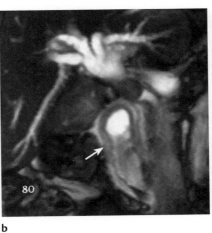

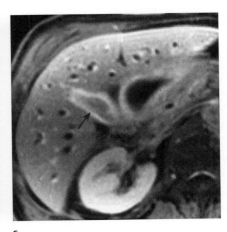

a

b

c

Fig. 17.**16** **Chronic cholecystitis in a patient with cholangiocarcinoma of the common bile duct.** A shrunken gallbladder (arrow) with markedly thickened wall is seen. **a** Note the high signal intensity of the thickened bile with high proteinaceous content (T1WI, axial).

b The thickened gallbladder wall surrounded by pericholecystic fluid produces an inner layer of intermediate signal intensity surrounded by an outer layer of high signal intensity (T2WI, coronal). The pericholecystic fluid accumulation may be caused by either cholecystitis or ascites in this case.

c Considerable contrast enhancement of the gallbladder wall is evident (T1WI, FS, +C, axial). Note also the prestenotic dilatation of the extrahepatic and intrahepatic biliary system due to the obstructing cholangiocarcinoma in the common bile duct.

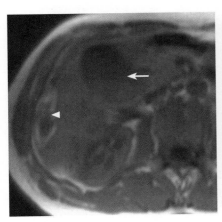

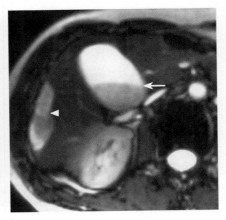

a

b

Fig. 17.**17** **Gallbladder trauma.** Blood is seen in the gallbladder, evident by the hematocrit effect (arrow) with the supernatant plasma depicting low signal intensity in (**a**) (T1WI) and high signal intensity in (**b**) (T2WI [GRE]). The cellular elements in the dependent portion appearing slightly hyperintense with regard to the serum on T1WI and hypointense on T2WI. Note also the subcapsular liver hematoma (arrowhead) with hemorrhaging into the posterior pararenal space.

18 Spleen

The spleen is an intraperitoneal organ of variable shape and size in the left upper quadrant lying between the fundus of the stomach and diaphragm. Its diaphragmatic surface is smooth and convex and faces upward, backward, and to the left. The diaphragm separates the spleen from the lowest part of the left lung and pleura and the ninth, tenth, and eleventh ribs of the left side. The costodiaphragmatic recess of the pleura may extend down as far as the inferior border of the spleen. One or more splenic clefts measuring up to 2 to 3 cm deep may be present on the diaphragmatic surface (Fig. 18.1). They have a sharp smooth margin and should not be confused with a splenic laceration, which displays a fuzzy margin and is associated with a perisplenic hematoma.

The visceral surface of the spleen is concave and directed towards the abdominal cavity with gastric, renal, pancreatic, and colonic impressions. Occasionally a medial splenic bulge (Fig. 18.2) is seen representing persistent fetal lobulation. It should not be mistaken for an ominous mass of the tail of the pancreas, left adrenal, or superior pole of the left kidney.

The spleen may be unusually mobile or even ectopic, in which case it is called *wandering spleen*. Torsion is a rare complication of a wandering spleen. Nodules of normal splenic tissue (*accessory spleens*) are found in approximately 20% of individuals, usually in the hilar region (Fig. 18.3). They have no pathologic significance, but may mimic mass lesions. Tissue characteristics and contrast enhancement patterns of accessory spleens are identical to that of the spleen itself. After splenectomy, accessory spleens may grow dramatically.

Peritoneal autotransplantation of splenic tissue that occurs after splenic trauma is called *splenosis*. Splenosis may be confused with other causes of peritoneal masses.

The spleen is almost entirely surrounded by peritoneum which is firmly adherent to its capsule. Recesses of the

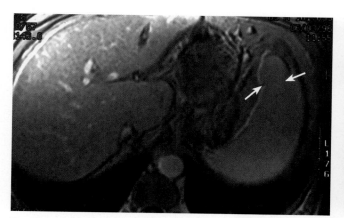

Fig. 18.**1 Splenic cleft (normal variant).** A sharply demarcated cleft (arrows) is evident on the anterior aspect of the spleen (spoiled GRE). Micronodular liver cirrhosis with enlarged caudate lobe is also present.

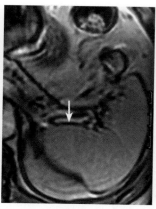

Fig. 18.**2 Medial splenic bulge (normal variant).** A medial splenic bulge (arrow) with identical signal characteristics and enhancement pattern as the spleen is seen (T1WI, FS, +C).

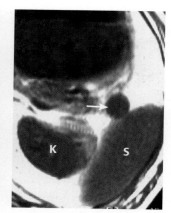

Fig. 18.**3 Accessory spleen (normal variant).** A round lesion (arrow) with identical signal characteristics and enhancement pattern (not shown) as the spleen (S) is seen (T1WI). A second accessory spleen was present in a more cephalad image (not shown). K: kidney.

greater sac intervene between the spleen and the stomach, and between the spleen and the left kidney. The spleen remains connected with the stomach and the posterior abdominal wall by two folds of the peritoneum, the gastrosplenic and the splenorenal ligaments, respectively. The splenic vessels enter the splenic hilum through the splenorenal ligament. The attachment of this ligament to spleen creates a 2 x 3 cm area on the medial aspect of the spleen that is void of peritoneal covering, a "bare area." The pancreatic tail transits the splenorenal ligament, thus, it can potentially serve as a conduit for pancreatic processes extending into the spleen.

The size of the spleen is variable. In the adult it is usually about 12 cm in length (craniocaudal diameter), 7 to 8 cm in width (anteroposterior diameter) and 3 to 4 cm in thickness. Splenic length of 15 cm and more is abnormal. Causes of *splenomegaly* include blood dyscrasias (hemolytic anemias, leukemias, myelofibrosis), infections (mononucleosis, brucellosis, typhoid, subacute bacterial endocarditis), infestations, (malaria, echinococcosis, kala-azar), neoplasms (lymphoma), splenic vein thrombosis, portal hypertension (including cirrhosis), trauma, and storage diseases (e.g. Gaucher disease).

The spleen has relatively long T1 and T2 relaxation times. Compared with the liver the spleen appears hypointense on T1WI and hyperintense on T2WI. The MR tissue characteristics of normal splenic tissue are similar to the average tissue characteristics of neoplastic diseases. Unenhanced MRI is therefore relatively insensitive for detection of splenic abnormalities. In infants the spleen may normally be isointense to the liver on both T1WI and T2WI.

Contrast enhancement of the *spleen* in the first 30 to 60 seconds after an intravenous bolus injection of Gd-DTPA is heterogeneous, spotty, or serpentine (Fig. 18.**4**). This early enhancement pattern of the spleen is transient and thought to represent differing blood flow rates between the red and white pulp of this organ. After 60 seconds the spleen has a uniformly increased signal intensity for several minutes and then gradually returns toward the baseline. If the spotty enhancement pattern is visible 1 minute or later after bolus injection, it is most likely caused by portal hypertension of any cause or by diffuse neoplastic or inflammatory infiltration of the spleen (Fig. 18.**5**). Absence of the normal heterogeneous enhancement immediately after a bolus injection may indicate a diffuse infiltration of the spleen by a disease process, but is not diagnostic, since it is also found with a variety of hepatic and pancreatic diseases without direct splenic involvement.

The differential diagnosis of splenic diseases is discussed in Table 18.**1**.

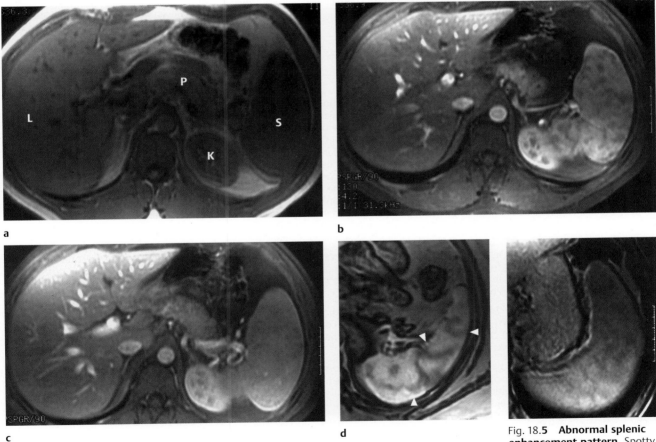

a

b

c

d

Fig. 18.**4** **Dynamic contrast enhancement patterns of normal spleen.** **a** (precontrast, T1WI): Note the uniform low signal intensity of the spleen (S). L: liver; P: pancreas; K: kidney. **b** (20 seconds post Gd-DTPA bolus.) A marked spotty contrast enhancement of the spleen is evident (T1WI, FS, +C). **c** (60 seconds post Gd-DTPA bolus.) The splenic enhancement has already become more or less uniform. **d** In a different patient a serpentine contrast enhancement pattern of the spleen (arrowheads) is found immediately after intravenous Gd-DTPA injection (T1WI, FS, +C).

Fig. 18.**5** **Abnormal splenic enhancement pattern.** Spotty contrast enhancement of the spleen is found 2 minutes and later after intravenous Gd-DTPA administration (T1WI, FS, +C). This finding is associated with portal hypertension and diffuse neoplastic or inflammatory infiltration of the spleen.

Table 18.1 Splenic diseases

Disease	MRI Findings	Comments
Asplenia syndrome (Ivemark syndrome)	Absent spleen, centrally located liver (hepatic symmetry), stomach on right or left side or in central position, annular pancreas, agenesis of the gallbladder, partial or total situs inversus, and both aorta and inferior vena cava on the same side of spine are characteristic features.	Associated with congenital heart disease and total anomalous pulmonary venous return. Bilateral trilobe lungs (bilateral minor fissures) are characteristic. Genitourinary anomalies are less common (15%) and include horseshoe kidney and double collecting system. Usually cyanotic infants with 80% mortality by the end of first year of life.
Polysplenia syndrome (bilateral left-sidedness)	Presence of two or more major spleens and indefinite number of splenules located on both sides of the mesogastrium and azygos/hemazygos continuation of the interrupted hepatic segment of the inferior vena cava is diagnostic. Associated findings include hepatic symmetry, malrotation of the bowel, midline aorta anterior to the spine, and preduodenal portal vein.	Associated chest anomalies include large azygos vein, bilateral superior venae cavae (50%), bilateral morphologic left lungs with absent middle lobe fissure (70%), dextrocardia (40%) with anomalous pulmonary venous return, and atrial/ventricle septum defects. Presents usually in infancy, but occasionally only in adulthood, with female predominance and a mortality rate of 90% by mid-adolescence.
Splenic cyst/pseudo-cyst	Solitary or less commonly multiple, nonenhancing, sharply marginated, homogeneous lesions with low signal intensity on T1WI and very high signal intensity on T1WI. May be multiloculated or septated. Curvilinear wall calcifications are rare except in hydatic (echinococcal) cysts. Infected and hemorrhagic cysts may depict a heterogeneous cyst content and/or a higher signal intensity on T1WI. Occasionally congenital cysts may contain fat or cholesterol crystals.	Most common benign splenic lesion. 80% of all splenic cysts are pseudocysts caused by trauma, infection, or infarct. *Congenital (epidermoid) cyst* (20%): Diagnosed usually in the second and third decades of life. Diameters of 10 cm and longer are not unusual. *Posttraumatic or postinfarct pseudocyst*: Results from cystic degeneration of splenic hematoma or infarct. *Pancreatic pseudocyst (intrasplenic)*: Associated with acute or chronic pancreatitis. *Hydatic (echinococcal) cyst*: Multiloculated cyst with enhancement of both cyst wall and septa surrounded by hypointense rim. DD: *Hemangioma, lymphangioma, cystic metastasis, granuloma, and abscess.*
Hemangioma (Fig. 18.6)	Solitary or, less commonly, multiple smoothly marginated well-defined round or lobulated homogeneous lesions which are hypointense on T1WI and hyperintense on T2WI. Larger (giant) hemangiomas may be heterogeneous secondary to hemorrhage, thrombosis, fibrosis, and hemosiderin deposition. Contrast enhancement occurs from the periphery towards the center and in the early phase appears more often ring-like than nodular. The enhanced hemangioma is hyperintense or, less commonly, hypointense relative to the surrounding spleen.	Second most common benign splenic tumor after splenic cysts. Multiple hepatic and splenic hemangiomas may be associated with the *Klippel–Trenaunay syndrome* (single lower limb overgrowth during adolescent growth spurt, port-wine nevus, and varicose veins on affected limb). In contrast to splenic hemangiomas a nodular peripheral enhancement pattern is virtually always found in large liver hemangiomas.
Lymphangioma	Presents as a cluster of homogeneous cysts, ranging from microcystic to macrocystic. High protein content and hemorrhage may alter the signal intensity of the cysts.	Spleen may be primary site of involvement or part of generalized abdominal lymphangiomatosis.
Hamartoma (splenoma)	Solid focal lesion that is isointense to the spleen on T1WI and hyperintense on T2WI. May contain cysts and calcifications. Prolonged enhancement after intravenous Gd-DTPA is characteristic.	Uncommon splenic lesion consisting of normal splenic tissue without trabeculae and follicles.
Angiosarcoma (Fig. 18.7)	Complex solitary mass with solid and cystic components and variable contrast enhancement or multiple inhomogeneous nodules of varying size in an enlarged spleen.	Rare tumor presenting in the sixth decade of life with poor prognosis (20% survival rate after 6 months). Usually not associated with thorotrast, vinylchloride, or arsenic exposure as opposed to liver angiosarcomas.

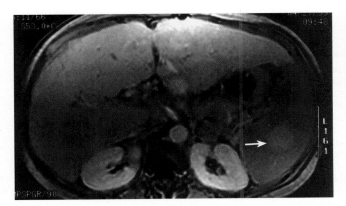

Fig. 18.**6** **Hemangioma.** A markedly enhanced lesion (arrow) is seen in the spleen in this late stage after intravenous Gd-DTPA administration (T1WI, FS, +C). The lesion was barely discernible on precontrast T1WI and T2WI (not shown). A micronodular cirrhotic liver with markedly enlarged lateral segment of the left hepatic lobe is also evident in this patient.

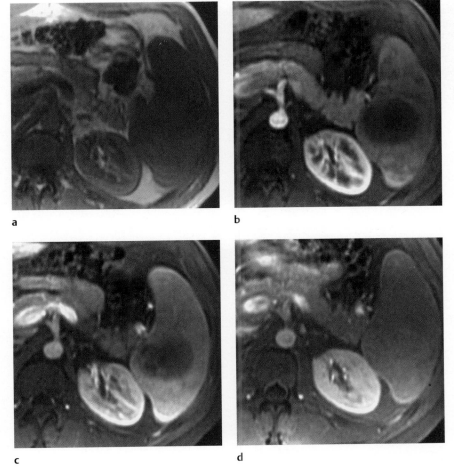

Fig. 18.**7** **Angiosarcoma.** Dynamic contrast enhancement study consisting of (**a**) (precontrast T1WI), (**b**) (T1WI, FS, 20 seconds after intravenous Gd-DTPA), (**c**) (60 seconds after Gd-DTPA), and (**d**) (120 seconds after Gd-DTPA) depicts a large and somewhat heterogeneous lesion in (**b**) and (**c**), whereas the lesion is barely recognizable in (**a**) and (**d**).

Table 18.1 (Cont.) Splenic diseases

Disease	MRI Findings	Comments
Lymphoma (non-Hodgkin and Hodgkin disease) (Fig. 18.8)	Presents as large solitary mass, diffuse infiltration, or multiple miliary to large (up to 10 cm) nodules in a normal-sized to massively enlarged spleen. MR characteristics of lymphoma and normal splenic tissue are relatively similar. Focal lesions tend to be hypointense on T1WI and T2WI. Associated central necrosis, hemorrhage, iron deposition, and fibrosis may alter the signal characteristics. After intravenous Gd-DTPA administration, the heterogeneous enhancement pattern of the spleen normally seen in the first minute may be absent and focal hypointense or even slightly hyperintense lesions may be seen subsequently in the later phase of enhancement.	Most common malignancy involving the spleen. Massive splenomegaly is likely to represent lymphomatous involvement. Spleen size is, however, an unreliable indicator of splenic involvement since it is present in about 30 % of patients without splenomegaly. On the other hand, in about one-third of lymphoma patients mild to moderate splenomegaly is caused by reactive hyperplasia or congestion alone. In non-Hodgkin lymphoma of the spleen bulky splenic hilar adenopathy is present in about half of the patients, whereas splenic hilar involvement is unusual with Hodgkin disease.
Leukemia	Diffuse infiltration of a slightly to markedly enlarged spleen with signal characteristics similar to normal splenic tissue. Absence of the normal heterogeneous enhancement pattern in the first minute after intravenous Gd-DTPA administration may be present, but is nonspecific.	Associated complications include splenic infarct, hemorrhage, and rupture with more characteristic MR findings. Generalized lymphadenopathy may also be present.
Metastases (Figs. 18.9–18.11)	Usually multiple nodules, commonly with similar signal characteristics as the normal splenic parenchyma and thus often difficult to visualize on precontrast examinations. After an intravenous Gd-DTPA bolus, metastases initially enhance less than the spleen and appear hypointense, but may become isointense within 2 minutes. Melanoma metastases sometimes depict a high signal intensity on T1WI because of the paramagnetic effect of their pigment. Necrotic (cystic) metastases have a hyperintense center on T2WI.	Metastases to the spleen are uncommon except in advanced disease where they usually are associated with liver metastases. They result from melanoma, breast, lung, ovary, and gastrointestinal primaries. Necrotic metastases originate most often from ovarian carcinomas and melanomas.

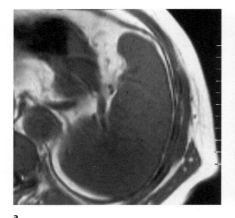

a

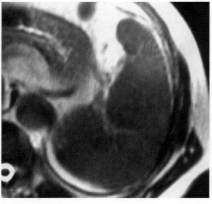

b

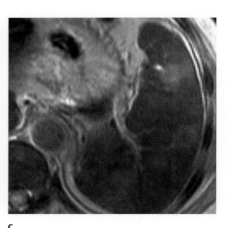

c

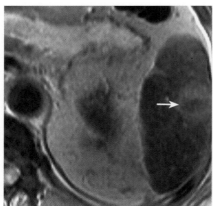

d

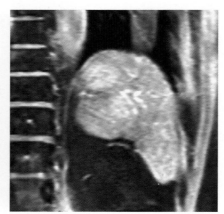

e

Fig. 18.8 **Hodgkin disease.** An enlarged spleen with somewhat inhomogeneous signal intensity is seen in both (**a**) (T1WI, axial) and (**b**) (T2WI, axial). After intravenous administration of Gd-DTPA, poorly defined nodular lesions, some with decreased central enhancement, are seen in (**c**) (T1WI, FS, +C, axial). In a more caudad image (**d**: T1WI, FS, +C, axial) another enhanced nodule (arrow) with central necrosis or fibrosis is better demonstrated. With heavy T2 weighted imaging in **e** (T2WI [GRE], coronal) the nodules appear slightly hyperintense with regard to the spleen.

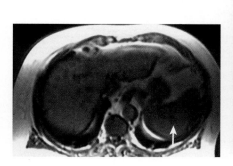

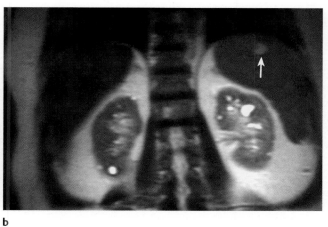

a   b

Fig. 18.**9   Splenic metastases from colon carcinoma.** Multiple liver metastases and a solitary splenic metastasis (arrow) with identical signal characteristics are seen. Compared with their surrounding parenchyma they appear hypointense in (**a**) (T1WI, axial) and hyperintense in (**b**) (T2WI, coronal). Note the significantly higher signal intensity of the renal cysts in (**b**).

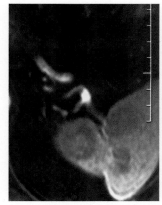

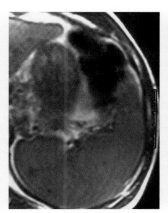

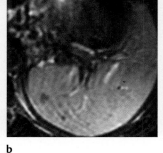

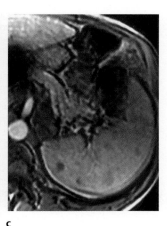

Fig. 18.**10   Splenic melanoma metastases.** In the early contrast enhancement phase after intravenous Gd-DTPA administration three hypointense lesions are visible within the spleen (T1WI, FS, +C). The slightly higher signal intensity in the center of the lesion may be caused by the paramagnetic effect of the melanin.

a   b   c

Fig. 18.**11   Splenic metastases from breast carcinoma.** At least two small hypointense metastases are seen in the spleen in (**a**) (T1WI]) and (**b**) (T2WI [GRE]). In the early stage after intravenous Gd-DTPA administration these hypointense metastases are better visualized and additional lesions are identified in (**c**) (T1WI, FS, +C).

Table 18.**1** (Cont.) Splenic diseases

Disease	MRI Findings	Comments
Abscess (Fig. 18.12)	Enlarged spleen with solitary or multiple, relatively poorly marginated cystic lesions which appear hypointense on T1WI and hyperintense on T2WI. After intravenous Gd-DTPA administration, they initially do not enhance and appear as hypointense lesions on FS T1WI. At a later stage, when the contrast agent is largely washed-out from the spleen, the abscesses may depict slight peripheral enhancement. Microabscesses are often best visualized on enhanced FS T1WI.	A pyogenic abscess results from hematogenous spread (75 %), trauma (15 %), or infarct (10 %) and is frequently associated with endocarditis, drug abuse, penetrating trauma, and sickle cell disease. Fungal microabscesses (*Candida, Aspergillus cryptococcus*) are much more common and usually found in immunocompromised patients with multiorgan involvement, including liver and kidneys.
Granulomatous disease (Fig. 18.13)	Splenomegaly with scattered or diffuse miliary to micronodular (< 1 cm) hypointense foci on both T1WI and T2WI. Nodules only minimally enhance or do not enhance at all, but their detection is improved after intravenous Gd-DTPA administration. Granulomas may calcify.	Infectious agents include *histoplasmosis, Mycobacterium tuberculosis, Mycobacterium avium intracellulare,* and *Pneumocystis carinii.* These granulomatous infections are frequently found in AIDS patients. Splenic involvement in *sarcoidosis* presents on MRI in similar fashion and is usually associated with pulmonary disease.
Gaucher disease	Massive splenomegaly with multiple nodules of variable signal intensity. The nodules are often best seen on T2WI as either hypointense or hyperintense lesions. Splenic infarcts, hemorrhages, fibrosis, and subcapsular fluid collections may also be associated.	Multisystemic hereditary disease caused by deficient glucocerebrosidase activity resulting in the accumulation of the glycolipoid glucosylceramide in macrophages (Gaucher cells) of the reticuloendothelial system of many organs, including the spleen.
Splenic trauma (Fig. 18.14)	*Subcapsular hematomas* appear as sharply demarcated, crescent- or lenticular-shaped lesions that flatten or indent the adjacent surface of the spleen. The signal intensity of the hematoma ranges from low to high on both T1WI and T2WI, depending on the stage of the hematoma. *Intraparenchymal hemorrhages* present in the acute stage as poorly defined, patchy, or streaky areas of increased signal intensity on T2WI and after contrast enhancement (Gd-DTPA extravasation). In the subacute stage (methemoglobin formation) the hemorrhage becomes hyperintense on T1WI. Rarely a space-occupying mass is formed by the hematoma within the splenic parenchyma. *Splenic laceration/fracture*: A cleft bisecting the spleen with interruption of the splenic margin or complete separation of the splenic fragments is seen, usually associated with a perisplenic hematoma and/or hemoperitoneum.	The spleen is the most frequently injured solid parenchymal organ in the abdomen. It is most frequently caused by blunt trauma and often associated with lower left rib fractures (40 %) and left renal injury. Hematomas may eventually calcify. Nontraumatic intraparenchymal hemorrhages frequently occur with tumors, infarcts, and coagulopathy. They may progress to a pseudocyst formation within 6 to 8 weeks. If the laceration is limited to the "bare area" of the spleen, blood will extravasate only into the left anterior pararenal space via the splenorenal ligament and will therefore not be detected by peritoneal lavage.
Splenic infarct (Fig. 18.15)	Multiple heterogeneous areas or massive focal lesions with variable signal intensity depending on the stage. Peripheral wedge-shaped lesions with the base abutting the splenic capsule and the apex pointing toward the hilum is characteristic but a less common presentation. With time infarcts progress from a poorly delineated lesion to a well-demarcated area. Healing with complete resolution may occur within a month. Late sequelae may include a residual contour defect, fibrosis, or pseudocyst formation. A splenic infarct is hemorrhagic and thus its heterogeneous signal characteristic is largely dependent on the age of the extravasated blood. After intravenous Gd-DTPA administration, contrast extravasation into the infarcted area resulting in a mottled enhancement pattern is only evident in the hyperacute phase. Total splenic infarct is rare and usually associated with torsion of an abnormally mobile spleen.	Most common cause of focal splenic defects. Splenic infarcts are associated with embolic disease, either septic (e.g., bacterial endocarditis) or atherosclerotic, splenic artery thrombosis (secondary to splenic artery aneurysm, pancreatitis, pancreas carcinoma, or splenic torsion), or thrombosis of the intrasplenic arterial or venous branches (e.g., sickle cell disease, myelolymphoproliferative disorders, and vasculitis such as periarteritis nodosa). In *sickle cell disease* the spleen has an overall decreased signal intensity due to iron overload secondary to multiple blood transfusion and/or fibrosis secondary to previous episodes of infarct. In this setting new infarcts present as hyperintense focal lesions on all imaging sequences.

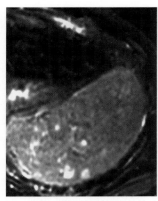

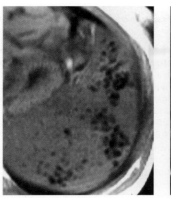
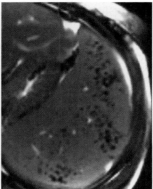

a   b

Fig. 18.**12   Splenic microab-scesses in septicemia.** Multiple tiny hyperintense lesions are seen scattered throughout the spleen (T2WI, FS).

Fig. 18.**13   Granulomatous disease.** Splenomegaly is seen with numerous miliary foci of low signal intensity on both T1WI (**a**) and T2WI (**b**). The findings in this case were caused by splenic schistosomiasis.

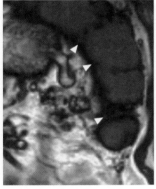

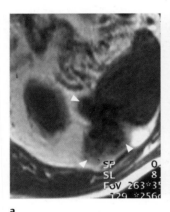
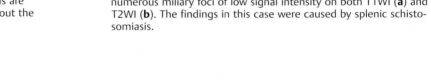

a   b

Fig. 18.**14   Splenic trauma (old).** A shattered spleen with three fibrotic fracture lines (arrowheads) presenting as serrated areas of signal void is seen (T2WI, coronal).

Fig. 18.**15   Splenic infarct.** Sequelae of an infarct are seen, mainly involving the posterior aspect of the spleen (arrowheads), in (**a**) (T1WI) and (**b**) (T2WI). The infarcted area is inhomogeneous, irregularly outlined, and shrunken.

Table 18.1 (Cont.) Splenic diseases

Disease	MRI Findings	Comments
Portal hypertension (Figs. 18.16, 18.17)	Demonstration of portosystemic venous collaterals is diagnostic. Splenomegaly is usually but not invariably present and may be massive. Siderotic nodules (*Gamna–Gandy bodies*) are found in the spleen in 13% of patients and represent organized foci of perifollicular and trabecular hemorrhage. The lesions appear as multiple (rarely single) 3–8-mm foci of low signal intensity and are best appreciated on GRE and T2WI images. The signal loss is caused by hemosiderin deposition and occasionally faint calcifications. Diffuse splenic hemosiderin deposition may also be encountered and presents with a generalized loss in signal intensity, especially on T2WI. Demonstration of ascites suggests sinusoidal (e.g., cirrhosis) or postsinusoidal portal hypertension (e.g., Budd–Chiari syndrome) and argues against presinusoidal obstruction (e.g., thrombosis of splenic or portal vein).	Prehepatic portal vein obstruction includes splenic vein thrombosis (e.g., secondary to pancreatitis or pancreas carcinoma) and portal vein thrombosis or compression. Intrahepatic presinusoidal portal obstruction is found with arterioportal fistulas, hepatic fibrosis (congenital, idiopathic, or toxic), biliary cirrhosis, $alpha_1$-antitrypsin deficiency, Wilson disease, cystic fibrosis, schistosomiasis, and chronic malaria. Intrahepatic sinusoidal/postsinusoidal portal obstruction is associated with Laennec (alcoholic) cirrhosis, postnecrotic cirrhosis secondary to hepatitis, and veno-occlusive disease of the liver. Posthepatic portal hypertension is usually caused by the Budd–Chiari syndrome.
Hemosiderosis and secondary hemochromatosis (Fig. 18.18)	Diffusely decreased signal intensity in both T1WI and particularly T2WI due to excessive iron deposition in the reticuloendothelial system of the spleen, liver, and bone marrow.	Iron overload results most often from multiple blood transfusions. DD: Primary (idiopathic) hemochromatosis, where the iron is primarily deposited in the hepatocytes and pancreatic parenchyma but not the spleen.

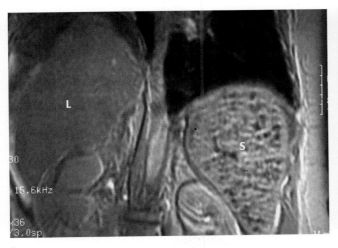

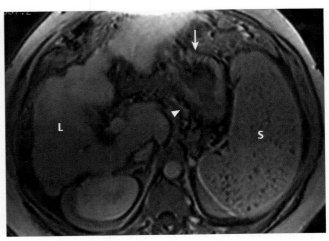

a

Fig. 18.16 Portal hypertension with Gamna–Gandy bodies in spleen. An irregularly shrunken cirrhotic liver (L) and an enlarged spleen (S) depicting numerous small foci (Gamna–Gandy bodies) of low signal intensity are seen in (**a**) (T2WI [GRE], coronal) and

b

after intravenous Gd-DTPA administration in (**b**) (T1WI, FS, +C, axial). Retroperitoneal collaterals (arrowhead) and gastric varices (arrow) are also evident in **b**. Ascites is also present and best appreciated about the liver.

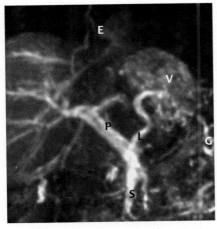

Fig. 18.17 Splenic vein thrombosis. Magnetic resonance angiography (MRA). Splenic vein is occluded and not visualized. Extensive portosystemic venous collaterals including large gastric varices (V) and small esophageal varices (E) are present. G: short gastric veins, L: left gastric vein, P: portal vein; S: superior mesenteric vein.

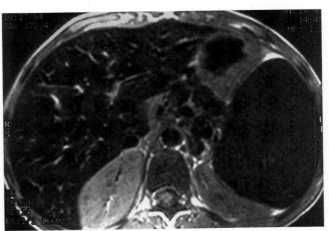

Fig. 18.18 Hemosiderosis. A markedly decreased signal intensity is seen in the spleen, liver, and bone marrow due to iron overload resulting from multiple blood transfusion in this patient with sickle cell disease (PDWI).

19 Pancreas

The size, shape, and position of the pancreas are quite variable. On axial images the pancreas appears as a thick, transversely oriented midline structure surrounded by retroperitoneal fat. It measures 12 to 15 cm in length and extends across the abdominal wall, behind the stomach, from the duodenum to the spleen (Fig. 19.1). The head of the pancreas, bordered right laterally and anteriorly by the duodenal loop, is thicker and more rounded than the rest of the organ. The diameter of the pancreatic head usually does not exceed the transverse diameter of the adjacent vertebral body. The head is connected to the main part, or body, by a slightly constricted neck. The body gradually narrows on its left side to become the tail. The body and tail appear on sections cephalad to the head, since they pass obliquely and slightly upward to the left. The posterior surface of the head of the pancreas is related to the inferior vena cava. The uncinate process of the head extends to the left and upward between the superior mesenteric vessels anteriorly and the inferior vena cava posteriorly. The superior mesenteric vein lies posterior to the neck of the pancreas and joins the splenic vein for the formation of the portal vein. The splenic vein is located on the posterior border of the body and tail of the pancreas. The lesser sac of the peritoneal cavity separates the anterior surface of the pancreas from the stomach. The main pancreatic duct (Wirsung) passes centrally within the pancreas from left to right. Most commonly the pancreatic duct unites with the common bile duct, which enters the pancreatic head from above and behind after passing the second portion of the duodenum posteriorly to form the ampulla of Vater near its duodenal orifice in the major duodenal papilla. Occasionally, the pancreatic and bile duct open separately into the duodenum. Frequently, an accessory pancreatic duct (Santorini) which communicates with the main duct drains primarily the lower portion of the pancreatic head through a separate opening at the more proximal lesser papilla in the duodenum.

The contour of the pancreas is smooth in the majority of cases, especially in younger individuals. With aging atrophy of the pancreas with fatty replacement of the glandular tissue may occur, resulting in a more lobulated appearance of the organ. *Fatty replacement (pancreatic lipomatosis)* (Fig. 19.2) is the most common tissue abnormality of the pancreas, but as such not necessarily indicative of disease. Fatty replacement is often uneven and may mainly involve the body and tail with relative sparing of the head. Focal fatty replacement may also be associated with an increase in size, especially in the head, resulting in lipomatous pseudohypertrophy. Fatty pancreatic replacement occurs, besides with aging as previously mentioned, also with obesity, diabetes mellitus, Cushing syndrome, chronic pancreatitis, and cystic fibrosis. Complete fatty replacement of the pancreas is found in the rare, congenital *Schwachman–Diamond syndrome* presenting with pancreatic insufficiency and dwarfism (metaphyseal dysostosis).

Anatomic variants of the pancreas are not uncommon. Pancreatic tissue completely encircling the second portion of the duodenum is called *annular pancreas* (Fig. 19.3).

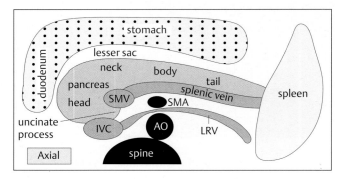

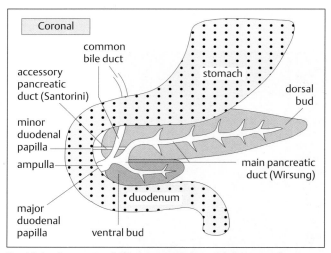

Fig. 19.**1** **Anatomy of the pancreas. (a**: axial. **b**: coronal) AO: aorta. IVC: inferior vena cava. LRV: left renal vein. SMA: superior mesenteric artery. SMV: superior mesenteric vein.

Failure of fusion of the ventral and dorsal bud results in *pancreas divisum* (Fig. 19.4), the most common congenital anomaly present at autopsy in about 10% of cases. In this condition the head of the pancreas is drained by the duct of Wirsung and the body and tail are drained by the duct of Santorini and there is no communication between these two ducts. An oblique fat cleft separating the head from the body is occasionally evident. Pancreas divisum is associated with an increased risk of recurrent pancreatitis. *Congenital absence* of either the *tail* or the *head of the pancreas* is occasionally encountered.

On conventional T1WI the pancreas is of intermediate signal intensity similar to the liver and hypointense to the surrounding retroperitoneal fat. With fat suppression the relative signal intensity of the pancreas increases markedly so that it becomes the brightest soft-tissue structure in the upper abdomen and appears hyperintense relative to the liver. On T2WI the pancreas is similar in signal intensity to the liver or slightly hyperintense. Fat around the pancreas has a similar signal intensity as the pancreas itself, resulting in poor demarcation of the pancreas from surrounding structures on T2WI.

A diffuse loss in signal intensity of the pancreas on both T1WI and T2WI is seen in *pancreatic fibrosis* and pancreatic

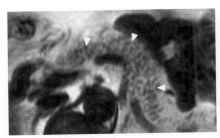

Fig. 19.**2** **Pancreatic lipomatosis.** Fatty replacement is evident in the body and tail (arrowheads) of the pancreas (T1WI).

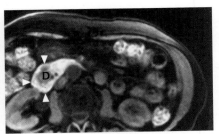

Fig. 19.**3** **Annular pancreas.** The markedly enhanced head of the pancreas (arrowheads) completely encircles the hypointense second portion of the duodenum (D) (T1WI, FS, +C).

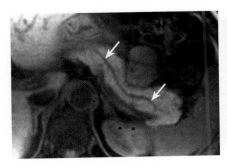

a

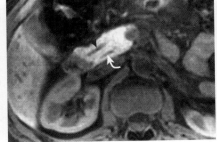

b

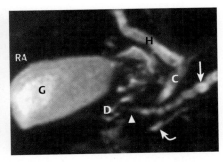

c

Fig. 19.**4** **Pancreas divisum.** The main pancreatic duct (arrows) drains both body and tail of the pancreas via an enlarged duct of Santorini (arrowhead) into the duodenum. The head of the pancreas is

largely drained by a hypoplastic duct of Wirsung (curved arrow) which does not communicate with the duct of Santorini in this condition. The hypoplastic duct of Wirsung corresponds to the portion that

embryogenically drains the ventral bud of the pancreas (see Fig. 19.**1b**). C: common bile duct; D: duodenum; G: gallbladder; H: common hepatic duct (**a** and **b**: T1WI, FS; **c**: MRCP).

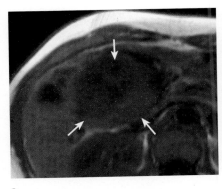

a

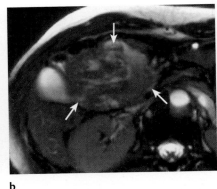

b

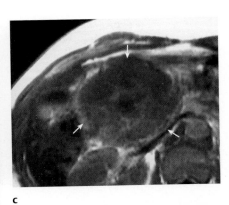

c

Fig. 19.**5** **Malignant fibrous histiocytoma of the retroperitoneum.** A large heterogeneous mass (arrows) with invasion of the head of the pancreas is seen. (**a**: T1WI. **b**: T2WI, [GRE]. **c**: T1WI, +C).

iron overload. Replacement of pancreatic parenchyma by fibrous tissue may occur in chronic pancreatitis and cystic fibrosis. *Pancreatic iron overload* is virtually diagnostic of primary (idiopathic) hemochromatosis, since excess iron deposition associated with hemolytic anemias and multiple blood transfusions are stored in the reticuloendothelial system of the liver, spleen, and bone marrow.

After an intravenous Gd-DTPA bolus injection, the pancreas enhances before the liver and reaches its maximum enhancement soon after peak aortic enhancement. Over the next few minutes the pancreas diminishes in signal intensity less rapidly than other organs of the upper abdomen. Oral contrast agents may be used to differentiate

stomach and small bowel from the pancreas and peripancreatic processes.

Mass lesions involving the pancreas may represent extension of disease from neighboring organs. Carcinomas originating from the stomach, duodenum, ampulla of Vater, bile duct, gallbladder, or liver, and malignancies originating from the retroperitoneum or the peripancreatic, splenic, and aortic lymph nodes may all invade the pancreas and thus mimic a primary pancreatic neoplasm (Fig. 19.5).

The differential diagnosis of pancreatic diseases is discussed in Table 19.**1**.

Table 19.1 Pancreatic diseases

Disease	MRI Findings	Comments
Pancreatic cyst (Fig. 19.6)	Solitary or multiple, homogeneous, sharply demarcated, nonenhancing lesion(s) with low signal intensity on T1WI and very high signal intensity on T2WI.	Congenital (true) cysts are rare. They are usually multiple in autosomal dominant (adult), polycystic kidney disease (associated with hepatic cysts), or in von Hippel–Lindau disease (associated with hepatic hemangiomas and adenomas).
Pancreatic pseudocyst (Figs. 19.7, 19.8)	Cystic lesion surrounded by an inflammatory/fibrotic pseudocapsule. An uncomplicated pseudocyst cannot be differentiated from a congenital cyst. It is low in signal intensity on T1WI and becomes brighter with progressive T2 weighting. Enhancement of the pseudocapsule is rarely appreciated. A hemorrhagic or superinfected pseudocyst generally depicts a higher signal intensity on T1WI and the cyst content may become heterogeneous, especially in the presence of debris. Cyst septation is extremely rare and indicates a complication, such as infection or hemorrhage.	Two-thirds of pseudocysts are located within the pancreas, the rest in the mesentery, retroperitoneum, liver, spleen, kidney, or mediastinum. Pseudocyst formation is a complication of pancreatic inflammation or trauma, but they are most commonly associated with chronic pancreatitis, where they are found in about 15 % of cases. *Retention cysts* are associated with pancreatic duct obstruction. They are usually multiple and rarely exceed several cm in diameter. They may communicate with adjacent ducts. *Mucinous ductal ectasia* due to pancreatic duct obstruction by mucous plugging may be massive and must be differentiated from a pseudocyst. *Extrapancreatic fluid collections* in acute pancreatitis differ from pseudocysts by the absence of a pseudocapsule. DD: Cystic pancreatic neoplasms. Mural nodules are inconsistent with pseudocysts.
Microcystic adenoma (serous cystadenoma) (Fig. 19.9)	Cystic neoplasm with greatly variable appearance ranging from a thin-walled unilocular or more commonly multilocular cyst to a well-demarcated lobulated mass with smooth or nodular contour containing innumerable small (usually <2 cm) cysts. The tumors range in size from 1 to 25 cm. After intravenous Gd-DTPA administration, considerable enhancement of the solid tumor component occurs. Delayed enhancement of the characteristic central stellate scar is rarely seen.	Benign cystic tumors occurring usually in the sixth and seventh decades of life with a 5:1 female predominance. Cysts contain proteinaceous fluid and are lined by a cuboidal epithelium with glycogen-rich cytoplasm. Central scar depicts amorphous ("sunburst") calcifications in 33 % of cases on plain film. May be associated with von Hippel–Lindau disease.

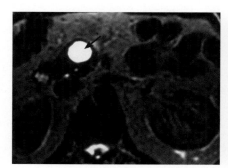

Fig. 19.**6** **Pancreatic cyst.** A sharply demarcated, homogeneous lesion with very high signal intensity is seen in the head of the pancreas (T2WI, FS).

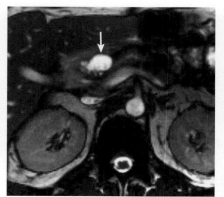

a

Fig. 19.**7** **Pancreatic pseudocyst.**
a A slightly inhomogeneous cystic lesion (arrow) with very high signal intensity is seen (T2WI).

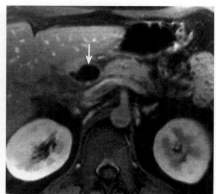

b

b After intravenous Gd-DTPA administration, an enhancing thin pseudocapsule surrounding the hypointense pseudocyst (arrow) is evident (T1WI, FS, +C).

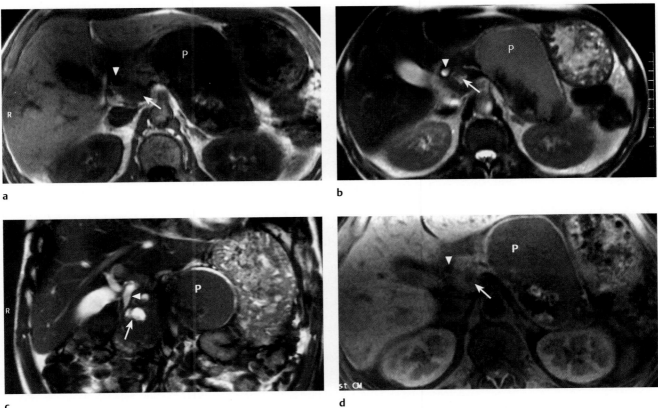

a

b

c

d

Fig. 19.**8** **Pancreatic pseudocyst.** A large pancreatic pseudocyst (P) is seen in the lesser sac. The signal intensity of the pseudocyst in T2WI is only intermediate, probably because of its high proteinaceous concentration. The inhomogeneous appearance of the cyst content adjacent to the pancreatic tail and in its most dependant portion is due to necrotic debris. A pseudocapsule surrounds the cyst and is best appreciated after contrast enhance-

ment (**d**). The pancreas has an inhomogeneous appearance due to chronic pancreatitis and depicts a smaller pseudocyst (arrow) within its head. The common bile duct (arrowhead) is dilated and its proximal end smoothly tapered (**c**) due to an inflammatory stenosis (**a**: T1WI, axial. **b**: T2WI, axial. **c**: T2WI [GRE], coronal. **d**: T1WI, FS, +C, axial).

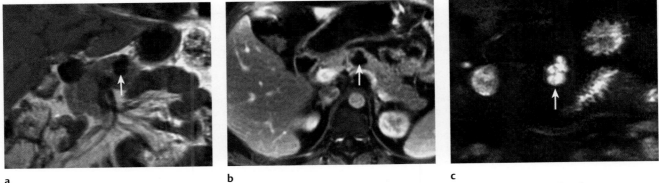

a

b

c

Fig. 19.**9** **Microcystic adenoma.** A multilocular cystic lesion (arrow) with somewhat heterogeneous appearance and without contrast enhancement is seen in the body of the pancreas (**a**: T1WI, coronal. **b**: T1WI, FS, +C, axial. **d**: MRCP).

Table 19.**1** (Cont.) Pancreatic diseases

Disease	MRI Findings	Comments
Macrocystic adenoma/ adenocarcinoma (mucinous cystic neoplasm) (Fig. 19.10)	Large, thick-walled, cystic lesion measuring 5 to 30 cm in diameter located in the tail or body (rarely head) of the pancreas. They are encapsulated and tend to be multiloculated with thick septa coursing between irregular cystic spaces. Both mural nodules and solid papillary excrescences protruding into the cyst lumen suggest malignancy. Signal intensity of the cysts is frequently relatively high on T1WI because of a high mucin content and/or frequent intracystic hemorrhage. Solid components of the lesions tend to enhance considerably after intravenous Gd-DTPA administration.	Premalignant/malignant neoplasm occurring typically in middle-aged women (8:1 female predominance) between age 40 and 70. Cysts are lined by a columnar mucin-producing epithelium. Benign lesions will eventually undergo malignant transformation. Hepatic metastases appear as thick-walled cystic lesions. Amorphous peripheral mural calcifications are evident on plain films in about 15% of cases.
Solid and papillary epithelial neoplasm of pancreas	Sharply defined inhomogeneous round or lobulated mass with solid and cystic components measuring 3 to 15 cm in diameter. May be completely cystic when complicated by extensive necrosis. Preferred location is the tail of the pancreas. Hemorrhage within the cyst is common rendering it hyperintense on T1WI and occasionally even hypointense on T2WI. The solid component of the lesion appears usually slightly hypointense on T1WI, slightly hyperintense on T2WI, and demonstrates marked contrast enhancement.	Rare low-grade malignant tumor often confused with cystadenoma or nonfunctioning islet cell tumor of the pancreas. Presents typically in young females (9:1 female predominance; age range 10 to 40 years) as a gradually enlarging abdominal mass.
Pancreatic islet cell tumor Figs. 19.11, 19.12)	Solitary or multiple, usually homogeneous pancreatic mass lesions of greatly variable sizes best visualized on fat suppressed (FS) T1WI, where they appear hypointense, and FS T2WI, where they are hyperintense relative to the surrounding pancreatic tissue. Marked contrast enhancement is evident immediately after intravenous Gd-DTPA administration. In smaller lesions (2 cm or less in diameter) the enhancement is uniform, whereas in larger lesions a peripheral ring enhancement is characteristic. *Insulinomas* (80% single benign, 10% multiple, 10% malignant) measure 1 to 2 cm in diameter and have no predilection for any part of the pancreas. *Gastrinomas* (75% solitary, 60% malignant) have an average tumor size of 4 cm at the time of diagnosis and are preferentially located in the pancreatic head. *Glucagomas, somatostatinomas,* (predominantly in head) and *VIPomas* (predominantly in body and tail) are solitary lesions with an average diameter of 6 cm at the time of detection. The majority of tumors are malignant. *Nonfunctioning islet cell tumors* (15%) are usually malignant, in the majority of cases measure 5 cm and more at time of detection, are preferentially located in the pancreatic head, and depict coarse nodular calcifications in 25%, which may be evident as foci of signal void on both T1WI and T2WI.	Derivatives of amine precursor uptake and decarboxylation (APUD) cells (also called APUDomas), of which 85% are functional. Occur in young to middle-aged adults with slight female predilection. *Multiple endocrine neoplasia (MEN)* MEN 1: Pituitary and parathyroid adenomas and pancreatic islet cell tumor. MEN II (or IIA): Parathyroid adenoma, medullary thyroid carcinoma, and pheochromocytoma. MEN III (or IIB): Medullary thyroid carcinoma, pheochromocytoma, and ganglioneuromatosis. Malignant islet cell tumors preferentially metastasize to regional lymph nodes and liver. Tumor calcification is highly suggestive of malignancy. *Insulinoma*: Most common functioning islet cell tumor presenting with hypoglycemia. Multiple tumors are frequently associated with MEN 1. *Gastrinoma*: Second most common islet cell tumor presenting with *Zollinger–Ellison syndrome* (severe recurrent peptic ulcer disease, hypokalemia, gastric hypersecretion, and diarrhea). Associated with MEN 1 in 25% of cases. Ectotopic gastrinomas (20%) are located in the duodenum (especially medial wall of second portion), stomach, jejunum, and peripancreatic nodes. *VIPoma* secrets *v*asoactive *i*ntestinal *p*eptides and is associated with the *WDHH syndrome* (watery diarrhea, hypokalemia, and hypochlorhydria).

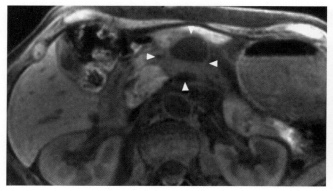

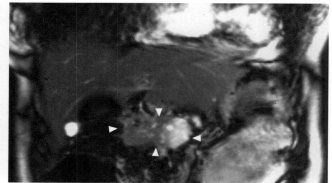

a   b   Fig. 19.**10 c, d** ▷

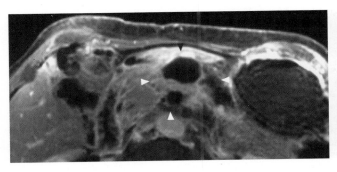

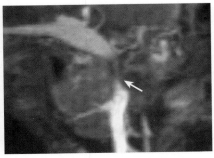

c

Fig. 19.**10**   **Macrocystic adenocarcinoma.** A large heterogeneous and poorly defined mass (arrowheads) with several different sized cystic components separated by irregular thick-walled septa is seen in (**a**) (T1WI, axial) and (**b**) (T2WI, [GRE], coronal). After intravenous Gd-DTPA administration considerable enhancement of

d

the solid components is evident in (**c**) (T1WI, FS, +C, axial). Magnetic resonance angiography (MRA) (**d**) depicts tumor invasion with marked stenosis of the most proximal segment of the superior mesenteric vein (arrow) with formation of numerous collaterals and nonvisualization of the occluded splenic vein.

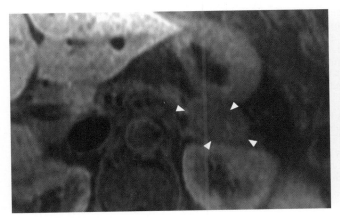

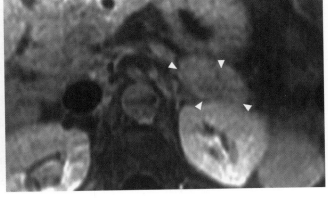

a

b

Fig. 19.**11**   **Pancreatic insulinoma.** A well-demarcated ovoid lesion (arrowheads) is seen in the tail of the pancreas depicting low signal intensity in (**a**) (T1WI, FS) and considerable contrast enhancement in (**b**) (T1WI, FS, +C).

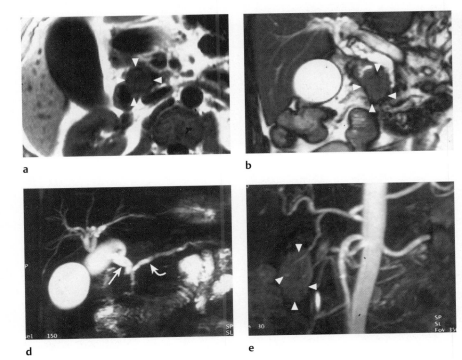

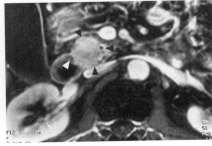

a

b

c

d

e

Fig. 19.**12**   **Malignant pancreatic islet cell tumor.** A mass lesion (arrowheads) is seen in the head of the pancreas with low signal intensity in (**a**) (T1WI, axial) and intermediate signal intensity in (**b**) (T2WI [GRE], coronal). After intravenous Gd-DTPA administration, marked enhancement is seen in (**c**) (T1WI, FS, +C, axial).   **d** MRCP. Obstruction of both common bile duct (arrow) and major pancreatic duct (curved arrow) within the head of the pancreas and prestenotic dilatation is evident.   **e** MRA. A considerable tumor blush (arrowheads) from the feeding pancreaticoduodenal artery is seen.

Table 19.**1** (Cont.) Pancreatic diseases

Disease	MRI Findings	Comments
Pancreatic adenocarcinoma (Figs. 19.13–19.15)	Poorly defined mass measuring 2 to 10 cm in diameter that is slightly hypointense on T1WI and isointense to slightly hyperintense on T2WI. Larger lesions with extensive central necrosis may depict a higher signal intensity in their center on T2WI. The tumor is best demonstrated as a hypointense lesion on fat suppressed T1WI. The tumor enhances less than normal pancreatic tissue and appears distinctly hypointense during the first few minutes after intravenous Gd-DTPA injection. After 5 to 10 minutes the lesion may become isointense or even hyperintense because of the slower contrast washout from the tumor as compared with the pancreas. Preferential location is the head of the pancreas (60%). Commonly associated findings include local tumor extension into splenic hilum, porta hepatis or retroperitoneum (70%), pancreatic and/or bile duct obstruction with prestenotic dilatation (60%), obliteration of the peripancreatic fat (50%), contiguous invasion of duodenum, stomach, left adrenal gland, or mesenteric root with encasement of the corresponding vessels (40%), splenic, superior mesenteric, and/or portal vein thrombosis with portosystemic collateral formation (30%), atrophy of the pancreatic body or tail (20%), and postobstructive pseudocyst formation (10%).	Accounts for 5% of cancer-related deaths in the United States (fourth most common cancer death cause). Presents commonly in the sixth and seventh decades of life (mean age: 55) with 2:1 male predominance. Painless jaundice is the classic clinical presentation for tumors originating in the head, whereas tumors originating from the body or tail present late with ill-defined symptoms such as back pain. Risk factors include hereditary pancreatitis (30% develop pancreatic carcinoma), alcohol abuse, smoking, and diabetes. At time of diagnosis 14% of patients have the tumor confined to the pancreas (stage 1), 21% have localized disease with regional lymph node metastases (stage 2), and 65% have distant metastases (stage 3). Distant metastases occur in the liver (33%), lymph nodes (20%), peritoneal seeding with ascites (10%), lungs, pleura, and bone. *Periampullary duodenal adenocarcinomas* and *cholangiocarcinomas of the intrapancreatic common bile duct* cannot be differentiated by magnetic resonance imaging (MRI) from a carcinoma of the pancreatic head, although obstruction of the pancreatic duct is uncommon with cholangiocarcinomas.
Extrapancreatic tumors, metastases, and lymphoma (see Fig. 19.5)	Secondary involvement of the pancreas by carcinomas originating in the stomach, duodenum, and gallbladder or by lymphoma (usually of the non-Hodgkin type) presenting as large mass with features similar to an advanced pancreatic adenocarcinoma. They also may be associated with peripancreatic nodal masses.	Metastases frequently originate from melanomas, carcinomas of the lung, breast, ovary, liver, and kidney, or from a variety of sarcomas. Primary lymphoma of the pancreas is rare (less than 1% of pancreatic neoplasms).

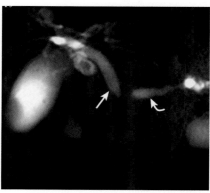

a

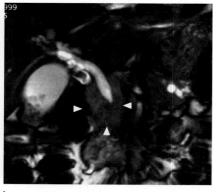

b

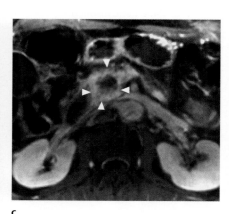

c

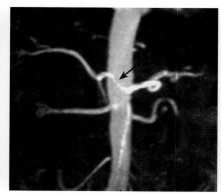

d

e

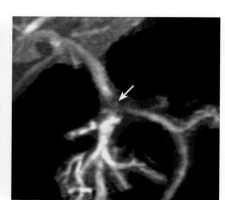

f

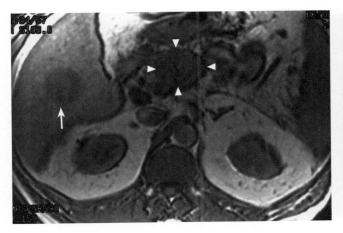

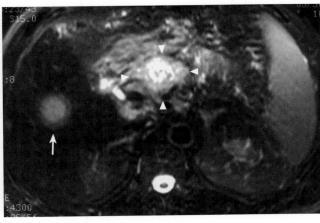

a

b

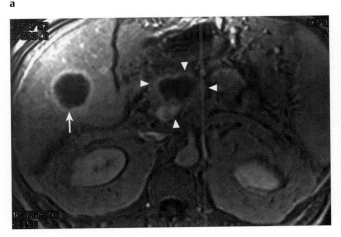

c

Fig. 19.**14   Pancreatic adenocarcinoma.** The signal characteristics and enhancement pattern of the primary tumor (arrowheads) in the pancreas and the metastatasis (arrow) in the liver are very similar and depict low signal intensity in (**a**) (T1WI), very high signal intensity in (**b**) (T2WI, FS), and marked peripheral enhancement after intravenous Gd-DTPA administration in (**c**) (T1WI, FS, +C). The very high signal intensity in T2WI is somewhat unusual and indicates complete necrosis with liquefaction in the center of the lesion.

◁ Fig. 19.**13   Pancreatic adenocarcinoma.** A poorly defined mass (arrowheads) of intermediate signal intensity is seen in both (**a**) (T1WI, axial) and (**b**) (T2WI [GRE], coronal). Note also in (**b**) the obstruction of the proximal common bile duct by the tumor with prestenotic dilatation, a larger calculus in dilated gallbladder neck, and numerous smaller calculi in the gallbladder fundus, the lumen of which appears constricted by localized wall thickening, indicating adenomyomatosis. After intravenous Gd-DTPA administration, an irregular peripheral enhancement of the tumor (arrowheads) is evident in (**c**) (T1WI, FS with contrast enhancment).   **d** MRCP. Complete obstruction of both the common bile duct (arrow) and major pancreatic duct (curved arrow) with prestenotic dilatation is evident. The mural thickening of the lateral wall of the gallbladder fundus is consistent with adenomyomatosis and the stone in the gallbladder neck is again seen.   **e** and **f** (MRAs) Tumor encasement of both the common hepatic artery (arrow) in **e** and the confluence (arrow) between the superior mesenteric, splenic, and portal vein in **f** is seen.

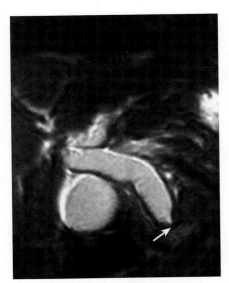

Fig. 19.**15   Periampullary pancreatic adenocarcinoma.** Complete tumor obstruction of the common bile duct (arrow) near the ampulla with prestenotic dilatation is seen. No tumor mass could be identified (MRCP).

Table 19.1 (Cont.) Pancreatic diseases

Disease	MRI Findings	Comments
Acute pancreatitis (Figs. 19.16, 19.17)	Early *edematous pancreatitis* cannot be diagnosed because of both considerable variability of the gland size in normal subjects and normal enhancement pattern. Diffuse or, less commonly, focal gland swelling and inflammatory strands extending from the pancreas into the peripancreatic fat evident as irregular hypointense lines on T1WI are the earliest signs. Progress to peripancreatic fluid collections with extension into the anterior pararenal space, the lesser sac, peripancreatic ligaments, and mesentery occurs. In severe pancreatitis small fluid collections appear within the pancreas itself. Peripancreatic/intrapancreatic fluid collections are best appreciated on fat suppressed (FS) T2WI as homogeneous foci of high signal intensity. Complications of acute pancreatitis include necrosis, hemorrhage, and abscess formation. Necrotic areas within the pancreas are best diagnosed by their failure to enhance immediately after intravenous Gd-DTPA administration. Occasionally, late enhancement of an infarcted area occurs. Hemorrhagic pancreatitis is characterized by inflammation, tissue necrosis, and hemorrhage. On FS T1WI subacute hemorrhage is high in signal intensity in contrast to the low signal intensity of nonhemorrhagic pancreatic fluid. Furthermore, extravasated blood may dissect throughout the retroperitoneum. Pancreatic and peripancreatic abscesses are difficult to differentiate from other fluid collections unless they contain gas, which occurs in less than half of the cases. Vascular complications include splenic vein thrombosis with collateral formation and pseudoaneurysm formation in the splenic artery.	Acute pancreatitis is defined as inflammatory disease of the pancreas with restoration of normal anatomy and function following resolution. Its hallmark is hyperamylasemia. The two most common causes are alcoholism (usually chronic pancreatitis) and cholelithiasis. Other causes include metabolic disorders (firstly, hypercalcemia, especially in hyperparathyroidism; secondly, hereditary pancreatitis characterized by large spherical pancreatic calcifications and a 30% risk of pancreatic carcinoma development; thirdly, hyperlipidemia types I and V; and fourthly malnutrition, including Kwashiorkor), infections and infestations (viral, such as mumps, hepatitis, and mononucleosis, or parasites, such as liver flukes), trauma (blunt or penetrating, and various surgical procedures including endoscopic cholangiopancreatography [ERCP]), penetrating ulcer disease, ischemia, and drug therapy. In 20% of cases pancreatitis is idiopathic. Edematous pancreatitis has a mortality rate of 4%. Necrotizing pancreatitis has a mortality rate of 80 to 90% and may be associated with hemorrhages (hemorrhagic pancreatitis) or bacterial infection (suppurative pancreatitis).
Chronic pancreatitis (Fig. 19.18)	Atrophic pancreas with diffuse low signal intensity of the entire organ on fat suppressed T1WI and diffusely diminished contrast enhancement is characteristic. Associated findings include irregular pancreatic duct dilatation (60%), intrapancreatic/peripancreatic pseudocysts (30%), pancreatic calcifications evident as punctate signal void foci (30%), splenic vein thrombosis with collateral formation (30%), and splenic artery pseudoaneurysm (rare). Focal enlargement of the pancreas may simulate a tumor. Superimposed acute pancreatitis may complicate the appearance of chronic pancreatitis.	Prolonged inflammatory disease of the pancreas characterized by irreversible damage to both anatomy and function of the organ. Histopathologically the destroyed pancreatic parenchyma is replaced by fibrous tissue. In *recurrent pancreatitis* a full morphologic and functional recovery occurs between acute exacerbations. Intrapancreatic/peripancreatic fluid collections associated with acute pancreatitis may resolve completely or develop a fibrous pseudocapsule within 6 to 8 weeks and thus transform to pseudocysts. Complications of chronic pancreatitis include development of pancreatic carcinoma (3%), obstructive jaundice, and development of pancreatic ascites.
Cystic fibrosis	Pancreas may be atrophic and largely replaced by fibrosis presenting with decreased signal intensity on fat suppressed T1WI (similar to chronic pancreatitis) or may be completely replaced by fat (lipomatous pseudohypertrophy) displaying an increased signal intensity on T1WI. Multiple small cysts representing dilated ducts and acini are occasionally seen.	Autosomal recessive multisystem disease occurring almost exclusively in Caucasians and characterized by mucous plugging of exocrine glands. Symptoms include sinusitis, chronic cough, recurrent pulmonary infections, progressive respiratory insufficiency, chronic obstipation, steatorrhea, and malabsorption.

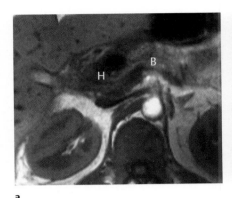
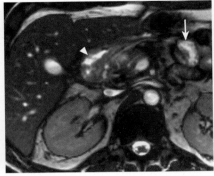
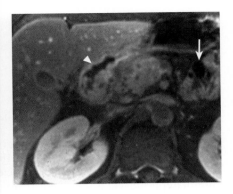

a

b

c

Fig. 19.16 Acute focal pancreatitis.
a Enlargement of the pancreatic head (H) is seen with heterogeneous and overall decreased signal intensity due to edema (spoiled GRE). The body of the pancreas (B) depicts an overall higher and more homogeneous signal intensity, indicating relative sparing.

b (T2WI [GRE].) Overall increased signal intensity in the edematous head with slightly hyperintense streaks extending into the anterior peripancreatic fat is evident. A larger irregular fluid collection (arrowhead) in the anterior peripancreatic fat is also seen. A small pancreatic pseudocyst (arrow) is evident anterior to the pancreatic body.

c (T1WI, FS, +C.) After intravenous administration of Gd-DTPA, a marked heterogeneous enhancement of the pancreatic head and peripancreatic tissue is seen. Patchy hypointense areas of under-perfusion in the head suggest beginning necrosis. The anterior peripancreatic fluid collection (arrowhead) is now evident as an area of signal void. The small pancreatic pseudocyst anterior to the pancreatic body (arrow) depicts a slightly enhancing smooth thin wall.

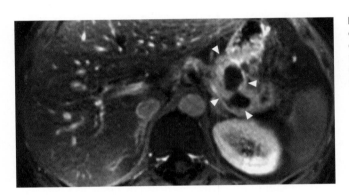

Fig. 19.17 Pancreatic abscess. A lesion (arrowheads) in the tail of the pancreas presents with a "figure 8"-shaped hypointense center and thick irregular and markedly enhancing wall after intravenous administration of Gd-DTPA. The inflammatory process extends anteriorly into the peripancreatic tissues and posterior wall of the stomach. (T1WI, FS, +C).

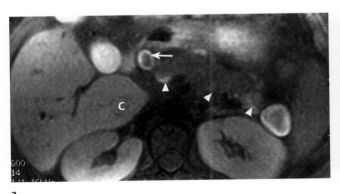
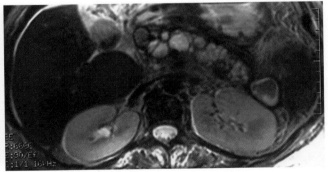

a

b

Fig. 19.18 Chronic pancreatitis. a Low signal intensity of the pancreas (arrowheads) is caused by fibrosis and multiple pancreatic/peripancreatic pseudocyst formation (T1WI). A thrombus in the portal vein (arrow) is also evident. Hypertrophy of the caudate lobe (C) of the liver secondary to alcoholic cirrhosis is also seen.

b The multiple pancreatic/peripancreatic pseudocysts are now easily recognizable as slightly heterogeneous hyperintense lesions in the distribution of the pancreas (T2WI). The decreased signal intensity in the liver is caused by hemosiderin deposition associated with cirrhosis.

20 Abdominal Wall

The abdominal wall is composed of the following layers: skin, subcutaneous tissue, muscles, a thin membrane termed the tranversalis fascia, extraperitonal fat, and the peritoneum. The anterior muscles of the abdominal wall are the paired rectus abdominal muscles. The oblique or anterolateral muscle group is formed by the external oblique, internal oblique, and tranversus abdominis muscles. At the linea semilunaris, the aponeurosis of the oblique muscles extends medially to form the fibrous rectus sheath. Superior to the arcuate line, the posterior layer of the internal oblique aponeurosis and the transversus aponeurosis pass posterior to the rectus muscle. Inferior to the arcuate line, the aponeuroses of all three muscle layers pass anterior to the rectus muscle. This transition forms an area of potential weakness along the linea semilunaris, which can become the site of a spigelian hernia. The posterior muscle group includes the latissimus dorsi, quadratus lumborum, and paraspinal muscles.

Congenital or acquired defects in the structure of the abdominal wall may result in hernias (Fig. 20.1). Physical diagnosis is most often diagnostic of hernias; however, MRI may be performed to differentiate hernias from mass lesions. In addition, hernias are frequently encountered as incidental findings during routine examinations.

Tumors and inflammatory conditions may originate in the abdominal wall or can affect it secondarily via direct extension or hematogenous dissemination. Most primary abdominal wall tumors are benign, with lipomas being the most frequently encountered. Malignant lesions occur much less commonly. The majority of primary malignant lesions are sarcomas of various types. Metastatic lesions are also observed, particularly with melanoma, lymphoma, ovarian, renal, and breast carcinoma. Inflammatory lesions in the abdominal wall most often arise from an infectious process. Peri-incisional abcesses and/or cellulitis may be seen in postsurgical patients. Direct extension of intra-

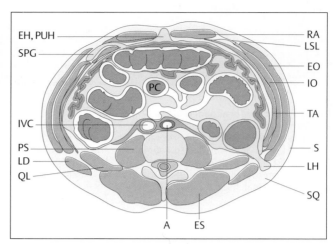

Fig. 20.**1** **Abdominal wall anatomy and potential sites of herniation.**
RA: rectus abdominus. LSL: linea semilunaris. EO: external oblique. IO: internal oblique. TA: transverses abdominus. S: skin. SQ: subcutaneous fat. LH: lumbar hernia. ES: erector spinae. A: aorta. IVC: inferior vena cava. PS: psoas. QL: quadratus lumborum. LD: latissimus dorsi. SPG: spigelian hernia. EH: epigastric hernia. PUH: paraumbilical hernia. PC: peritoneal cavity.

abdominal infections can be seen in the setting of inflammatory bowel disease, inflammation of a hollow viscus e. g. appendicitis, and much less commonly with fungal and parasitic infections.

Various abdominal wall abnormalities and their associated MRI findings are discussed in Table 20.1. Secondary changes in the abdominal wall related to primary intra-abdominal pathologies are discussed in other chapters and are only briefly, if at all, mentioned in this chapter.

Table 20.**1** Abnormalities of the abdominal wall

Disease	MRI Findings	Comments
Hernias		
Inguinal hernia (direct/indirect)	Mass containing fat or bowel in the subcutaneous tissue within the inguinal canal seen at the level of the pubic symphysis.	Most common hernia of the abdominal wall. Indirect inguinal hernias occur lateral to the inferior epigastric vessels. Large hernias may descend into the scrotum in males and into the labia majora in females. May be congenital via a patent processus vaginalis or acquired. Direct inguinal hernias occur medial to the inferior epigastric vessels. They tend to have a wider neck and thus are less likely to strangulate. Essentially all are acquired.
Femoral hernia	Hernia traversing the femoral canal. Does not emerge through the superficial inguinal ring, which distinguishes it from inguinal hernias.	More likely to strangulate than inguinal hernias. Always acquired.
Paraumbilical hernia	Midline hernia near the umbilicus contains fat and/or loops of bowel.	Acquired hernia in adults due to the separation of the rectus abdominus muscles. Secondary to obesity, multiple pregnancies, or other causes of increased intra-abdominal pressure.
True umbilical hernia	Midline hernia through the umbilicus in an infant.	Herniation through a weak umbilical scar. Usually resolves during childhood.
Epigastric hernia	Midline ventral hernia between the umbilicus and the xyphoid process. Usually only contains fat, rarely bowel.	Similar to paraumbilical hernia in etiology.
Incisional hernia	Usually contains small bowel, colon, or fat.	Delayed complication in approximately 4% of operations. Usually within 4 months after surgery.
Spigelian hernia	Herniation of fat and/or bowel through the linea semilunaris at the arcuate line between the umbilicus and the symphysis. The contents of the hernia characteristically lie between the internal and external oblique muscles. A narrow hernia neck is another characteristic sign.	Less than 2% of abdominal hernias are spigelian; these may be spontaneous or postoperative. Incarceration and strangulation are not uncommon.
Lumbar hernia	Superior lumbar herniation occurs through the lumbar triangle of Grynfelt–Lesshaft, which is bordered by the 12th rib, internal oblique muscle, and paraspinal muscles. The inferior lumbar triangle of Petit is bordered by the iliac crest, external oblique muscle, and the latissimus dorsi. Lumbar herniation may contain fat, bowel, or rarely kidney.	Uncommon. The hernia neck is usually wide and incarceration is rare. Most common between the ages of 50 and 70.
Infection/inflammation		
Cellulitis	Abnormal increased signal on T2WI limited to the skin and subcutaneous fat. May enhance mildly, which may assist in discrimination from noninfectious edema.	Most commonly from a wound infection.
Necrotizing fasciitis	Extensive necrosis of the subcutaneous tissues and fascia. Fluid may be seen tracking along fascial planes. Subcutaneous gas is often present but may be difficult to recognize.	Most commonly a complication of necrotizing pancreatitis. May extend to the abdominal wall from any adjacent tissue plane.
Pyomyositis	Abnormal enhancement and increased signal on T2WI in muscle and often, although to a lesser degree, in the adjacent subcutaneous fat.	Increased incidence with HIV infection, diabetes mellitus, and long term steroid therapy.

Table 20.1 (Cont.) Abnormalities of the abdominal wall

Disease	MRI Findings	Comments
Abscess (Fig. 20.2)	Most commonly a thick-walled cystic lesion, but may be ill defined; often with central necrosis. Low signal on T1WI and variable on T2WI with enhancement after Gd-contrast administration. The signal intensity of abscesses varies with general approximation of muscle signal to slightly lower on T1WI and high signal on T2WI.	May be a direct extension of an intra-abdominal process such as Crohn disease, diverticulitis, appendicitis, or perforated neoplasm.
Sebaceous cyst (Fig. 20.3)	Well-defined round lesion in the subcutaneous fat that is tangent to the skin. Homogenous low signal on T1WI and high on T2WI. With increased protein content some lesions have high signal on T1WI.	Benign subcutaneous lesion that develops after blockage of a sebaceous duct or gland. May occur in any location. Usually asymptomatic, but occasionally may become infected and form an abscess.
Benign neoplasms Lipoma (Fig. 20.4)	Well-defined lesion with signal characteristics identical to fat occasionally with thin low-signal fibrous septations or a capsule. Does not enhance significantly after contrast.	In the abdominal wall, may occur within the subcutaneous fat or within muscle.
Hemangioma	Heterogeneous, poorly marginated lesion on T1WI with linear, lace–like or coarse bands of high signal. These bands represent fat interspersed among low-signal regions corresponding to the vascular spaces that contain slowly flowing or stagnant blood and other connective tissues. On T2WI the lesion is typically well marginated and hyperintense, due to the stagnant blood, relative to subcutaneous fat. Phleboliths may be present as small foci of signal void. Contrast enhancement is marked. Feeding and draining vessels with rapid flow (signal void on spin echo [SE], hyperintense on gradient echo [GRE], vascular type enhancement with contrast) are only identified in a minority of cases.	*Cavernous hemangiomas* consist of large vascular channels. They also contain variable amounts of nonvascular tissues, the most common of which is fat, but also smooth muscle, fibrous tissue, and occasionally bone. *Capillary hemangiomas* are composed of capillary sized vascular channels, occur in infancy, grow rapidly in the first few months, and begin to regress spontaneously toward the end of the first year.

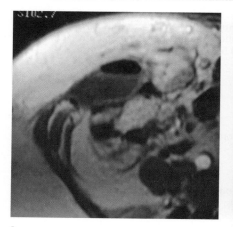

a

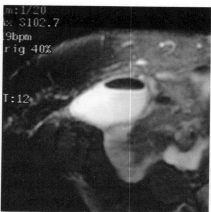

b

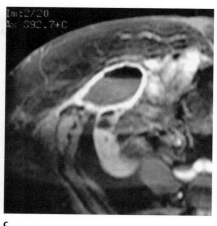

c

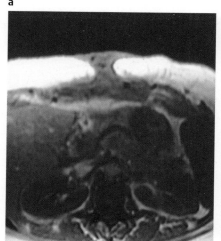

d

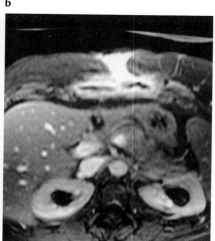

e

Fig. 20.2 **Abscess.** A fluid collection is present in the right lateral abdominal wall in the first example (**a–c**). Note the air–fluid level within the collection. After Gd-contrast administration, the thick capsule of the abscess enhances markedly. **d, e** The second case demonstrates a subincisional collection. (**a**: axial T1WI; **b**: axial T2WI, fat-suppressed [FS]; **c**: postcontrast axial T1WI, FS; **d**: axial T1WI; **e**: postcontrast axial T1WI, FS.)

Table 20.**1** (Cont.) Abnormalities of the abdominal wall

Disease	MRI Findings	Comments
Neurofibroma (Fig. 20.5)	Usually nodular masses that approximate muscle signal on T1WI and most often have high but variable signal intensity on T2WI within the subcutaneous fat and/or muscle. Enhancement varies from moderate to intense.	Associated with *neurofibromatosis type 1*. Spinal involvement or long plexiform neurofibromas of peripheral nerves may also be seen. Malignant degeneration may occur.

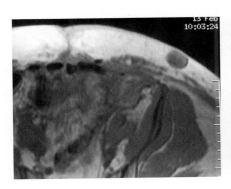

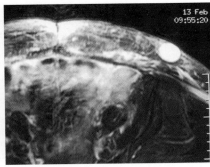

Fig. 20.**3** **Sebaceous cyst.** A well-defined spherical lesion in the subcutaneous fat, tangent to the skin. This lesion is approximately isointense to muscle on T1WI and has high signal on T2WI. (**a**: axial T1WI; **b**: axial T2WI, FS.)

a

b

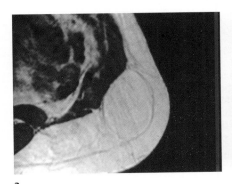

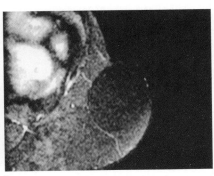

Fig. 20.**4** **Lipoma.** A sharply circumscribed lesion in the subcutaneous fat of the abdominal wall with a few thin septations. The signal characteristics of the lesion are identical to fat on the T1WI and FS T2WI. (**a**; axial T1WI; **b** axial T2WI, FS.)

a

b

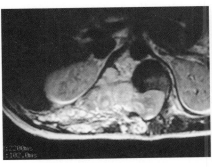

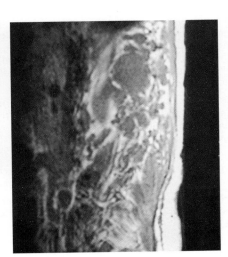

Fig. 20.**5** **Neurofibromatosis type 1.** Numerous round and lobulated lesions are present in the right posterior abdominal wall and paraspinal musculature. The lesions have high signal intensity on T1WI and intermediate signal intensity on T2WI. Note the lesion growing through and widening the right neural foramen at this level. (**a**: axial T1WI; **b**: sagittal T2WI.)

a

b

Table 20.**1** (Cont.) Abnormalities of the abdominal wall

Disease	MRI Findings	Comments
Malignant neoplasms		
Soft-tissue sarcomas (Fig. 20.6)	Large heterogeneous mass, often with hemorrhage and necrosis. Non-necrotic areas will enhance after Gd-contrast administration.	Rare in the abdominal wall as a primary site. Metastases and local recurrence after surgery are more common.
Lymphoma	Diffuse infiltration of muscle with tumor isointense to muscle or slightly lower on T1WI. On T2WI more often heterogeneous high and low signal areas, although may occasionally be homogeneously hyperintense.	Most often presents in the abdominal wall as direct extension from intra-abdominal disease. Primary abdominal wall lymphoma is very rare.
Desmoid tumor (Fig. 20.7)	Round well-defined mass, often large, may grow rapidly. Homogenous lesions usually low on T1WI and T2WI, but occasionally high on T2WI. Heterogenous signal on T1WI and T2WI often accompanies larger lesions. Marked enhancement after Gd-contrast administration.	Rare fibroblastic proliferation. Does not metastasize but frequently recurs and is locally invasive. More common in females between 20 and 40 years. In *Gardner syndrome*, almost 30% of patients will develop an abdominal-wall desmoid tumor.
Hematogenous metastases	Nodules in the skin, subcutaneous fat, or muscle. Melanoma is notable for its distinctive signal characteristics with high signal on T1WI and T2WI secondary to the paramagnetic effect of melanin.	Common primary tumors include melanoma, lymphoma, ovarian, renal, and breast carcinoma.
Contigous tumor extension (Fig. 20.8)	Infiltration of the abdominal musculature with obliteration of the adjacent fascial planes. May appear in a scar from a previous abdominal incision for resection of intra-abdominal malignancy.	Tumors from the superficial organs are most likely to extend to the abdominal wall. This includes malignancies of the transverse colon, gallbladder, urinary bladder, and omentum.
Trauma		
Hematoma	The appearance of hemorrhage changes with time. This is often complicated by the fact that some lesions will bleed intermittently. Many hematomas are therefore of heterogeneous signal intensity. Hyperacute hemorrhage has low signal on T1WI and high on T2WI. Acute hemorrhage has low signal on T1WI and T2WI. Subacute hemorrhage is high on T1WI and may be either high or low on T2WI. Chronic hemorrhage (hemosiderin) is low on T1WI and T2WI.	May be secondary to trauma, surgery, or anticoagulation. Can also occur spontaneously with muscle exertion. Muscle tears are associated with traumatic or exertional abdominal-wall hematomas and can be defined with MRI.
Rhabdomyolysis	Focal or diffuse areas of increased signal within the affected muscle on T2WI. Areas may enhance after contrast administration.	Release of myoglobin from traumatically or nontraumatically damaged muscle. May cause renal failure. MRI may be of great value in directing surgical fasciotomy, when this condition is associated with a compartment syndrome.
Focal muscular atrophy	Decreased muscle volume with or without fatty infiltration of the muscle or complete absence of the muscle. With fatty infiltration, high-signal fat is seen interspersed among the muscle bundles on T1WI.	Usually a delayed complication of tranverse or subcostal abdominal incision. Probably a denervation injury.
Miscellaneous abnormalities		
Varices	Increased number and caliber of veins in the subcutaneous fat. Signal voids with SE and high signal with GRE imaging. Vascular type enhancement. With portal venous hypertension recanalization of the umbilical vein and caput medusae of the dilated paraumbilical veins may be seen.	Portal hypertension is the most common cause. Occlusion of the central venous system in the abdomen, pelvis, or chest may also cause varices. The location of the collaterals may indicate the site of the underlying venous obstruction.
Endometriosis	Nodular or cystic mass in a surgical scar or near the umbilicus. High signal on T1WI and low signal on T2WI is classic, but signal characteristics vary with the menstrual cycle and/or presence of blood products.	A rare occurrence that may be difficult to distinguish from secondary malignancy without biopsy.
Tumoral ossification	Calcified conglomerates seen as signal voids in the soft tissues.	May occur anywhere. A rare occurrence in the abdominal wall.
Edema	Streaky and patchy foci of high signal on T2WI in the skin and subcutaneous tissues. Low to intermediate signal on T1WI.	Causes include heart failure, hypoproteinemia, and various systemic diseases.

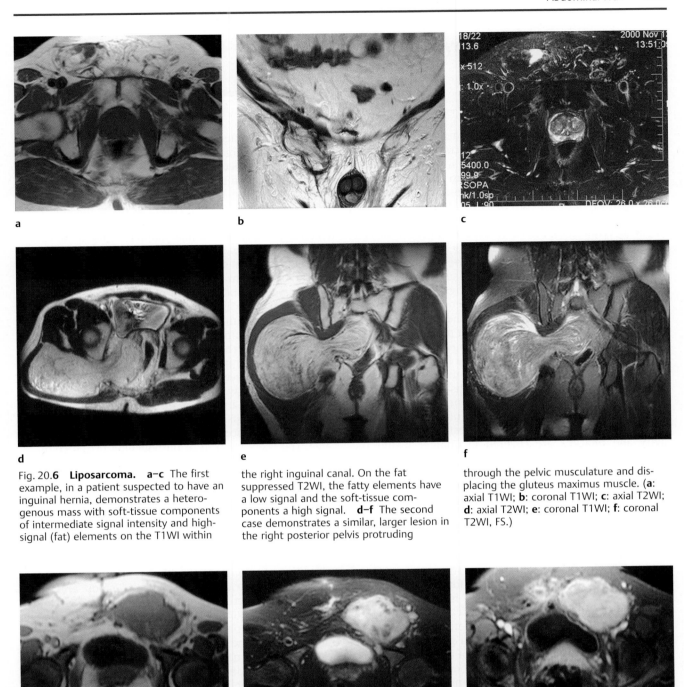

Fig. 20.6 Liposarcoma. a–c The first example, in a patient suspected to have an inguinal hernia, demonstrates a heterogenous mass with soft-tissue components of intermediate signal intensity and high-signal (fat) elements on the T1WI within the right inguinal canal. On the fat suppressed T2WI, the fatty elements have a low signal and the soft-tissue components a high signal. **d–f** The second case demonstrates a similar, larger lesion in the right posterior pelvis protruding through the pelvic musculature and displacing the gluteus maximus muscle. (**a**: axial T1WI; **b**: coronal T1WI; **c**: axial T2WI; **d**: axial T2WI; **e**: coronal T1WI; **f**: coronal T2WI, FS.)

Fig. 20.7   Desmoid tumor. A large lobulated mass in the left rectus abdominis muscle. The lesion has low signal intensity on T1WI and predominantly high signal intensity on T2WI. After contrast administration there is prominent, slightly heterogenous enhancement. (**a**: axial T1WI; **b**: axial T2WI, FS; **c**: T1WI, FS, with contrast enhancement.)

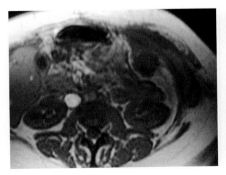

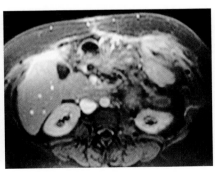

Fig. 20.8   Intra-abdominal metastasis from colonic adenocarcinoma growing into the abdominal wall. A poorly marginated mass in the left upper quadrant has infiltrated the adjacent transverse abdominis, internal oblique, and external oblique muscles and extends into the subcutaneous fat in the left lateral abdominal wall. The tumor is hypointense to muscle on T1WI and enhances after Gd-DTPA administration. (**a**: axial T1WI; **b**: axial T1WI, FS, with contrast enhancement.)

21 Gastrointestinal Tract

With the advent of increasingly faster acquisitions that reduce or eliminate bowel motion artifacts, MRI can investigate numerous pathologic conditions in the gastrointestinal tract. While endoscopy and barium examinations are the best modalities to visualize mucosal detail, mucosal abnormalities can be detected with MRI. Larger polyps, which may occur in isolation or in the spectrum of various polyposis syndromes, can be visualized. Mucosal thickening and distortion seen in inflammatory bowel disease and infectious conditions are detected as well. Larger mass lesions that develop with malignancies, such as adenocarcinoma or lymphoma, as well as benign tumors can be characterized. MRI also complements endoscopic and barium examinations by demonstrating the extraluminal extent of disease processes. In the patient presenting with an acute abdomen, an important caveat must be considered in the initial MRI examination. MRI has a low sensitivity for free intraperitoneal air and for the minute amounts of gas that occur in pneumotosis intestinalis or in the portal venous system. In such cases, CT scanning is the preferred modality. This chapter discusses the differential diagnosis for the abdominal and pelvic gastrointestinal tract; the oral cavity and pharynx are covered in Chapter 6 and the esophagus in Chapter 15.

In general, MRI of the gastrointestinal tract can be approached with a combination of T1, T2, and spoiled gradient-echo (GRE) sequences obtained during a single breath hold. Fat suppression is often beneficial. Gd-contrast, as in its other applications, can both increase the conspicuity of lesions and increase diagnostic specificity. Adequate luminal distention avoids the pitfall of mistaking coapted bowel wall for a mural lesion. There are numerous commercial formulations available for gastrointestinal contrast, although in practice water is often sufficient. Glucagon is an additional adjunct that can be employed to both increase distention and reduce peristaltic motion.

The thickness of the well-distended gastric wall is approximately 2–5 mm from the depth of a rugal fold. Rugal thickness is variable. The rugae in the body and fundus are usually more prominent than those in the antrum. Any measurement over 10 mm should be considered abnormal. Suspected gastric lesions may be better discerned with repeat scanning, depending on the location of the lesion, in either the decubitus, oblique, or prone position to isolate true lesions from redundant folds. It should be noted that normal gastric mucosa usually exhibits a greater degree of enhancement than small bowel or colon.

The wall of the normal fluid or contrast filled small bowel should be less than 3 mm thick. The mucosal folds, *valvulae conniventes*, in the small bowel are normally between 2–3 mm thick. Luminal diameter should not exceed 3 cm. The bowel wall should be sharply defined. The adjacent mesenteric fat should demonstrate homogeneous signal. The duodenum originates at the distal end of the pylorus, curves around the head of the pancreas, and meets the jejunum at the ligament of Treitz. Distal to the ligament of Treitz, the proximal two-fifths of the small bowel is considered the jejunum and the distal three-fifths the ileum. Small-bowel wall thickening is a nonspecific finding with numerous causes ranging from intrinsic mucosal disorders to reaction to adjacent inflammatory processes.

Normal colonic wall thickness is 3 mm or less. Measurements between 4 and 6 mm are suspicious in the absence of signal alterations. Wall thickness greater than 6 mm is abnormal. The ascending colon begins at the ileocecal valve. The cecum is a focal outpouching of the colon located just inferior to the ileocecal valve. The appendix usually arises from the posteromedial aspect of the cecum. At the hepatic flexure, the ascending colon becomes the tranverse colon, which travels to the left across the abdomen to become the descending colon at the splenic flexure. The sigmoid colon is the pelvic continuation of the descending colon. The rectum is the final segment of the colon.

The first portions of the duodenum, jejunum, ileum, cecum, transverse colon, and sigmoid colon are all intraperitoneal structures. The distal (second through fourth portions) duodenum, ascending colon, and descending colon are retroperitoneal structures. The position of the tranverse colon and sigmoid is variable depending on the extent of the mesocolon and sigmoid colon, respectively. The anterior and lateral surfaces of the rectum are covered by peritoneum, while the distal rectum is completely extraperitoneal.

The differential diagnosis of gastrointestinal disorders follows in Tables 21.**1**, 21.**2**, and 21.**3**.

Table 21.**1** Abnormal stomach

Disease	MRI Findings	Comments
Congenital		
Gastric duplication cyst	Rounded lesion in the left upper quadrant abutting the stomach. Signal approximates water, high on T2WI and intermediate to low on T1WI. Fluid–fluid levels are occasionally observed. Low signal foci of calcification may be seen in its wall.	Rare congenital abnormality. May be difficult to differentiate from pancreatic, omental or mesenteric cysts.
Gastric diverticulum	Thin outpouching of the gastric wall. May mimic a cyst when its neck is small.	May be acquired or congenital.
Neoplasms		
Gastric adenocarcinoma (Fig. 21.1)	Four morphologic presentations: 1) polyploid mass, which is lobulated and projects into the gastric lumen; 2) ulcerated mass, which may mimic benign peptic ulcer disease; 3) superficial spreading, which spreads along the mucosa and/or submucosa and produces nodular or distorted rugae; 4) linitis plastica, which describes diffuse infiltration and rigid thickening of the gastric wall. Tumors are typically isointense to the gastric wall on T1WI and moderately hyperintense on T2WI. Enhance after Gd-contrast administration.	Gastric carinoma may spread directly to adjacent omentum and viscera. Nodal and hepatic metastases are also seen. Intraperitoneal spread is a less common manifestation of metastatic disease.
Gastric polyps	Pedunculated or sessile mass projecting into the gastric lumen; does not cause thickening of the adjacent gastric wall.	Hyperplastic polyps (80%) are the most common polyps in the stomach; benign with no malignant potential. Adenomatous polyps (15%) are considered premalignant lesions. These may be sporadic but are also associated with *familial polyposis* syndrome and *Gardner syndrome.* Hamartomatous polyps are benign and occur with *Peutz–Jeghers syndrome.* *Cronkhite–Canada syndrome* produces hamartomatous polyps in the stomach, as well as in the small bowel and colon.
Leiomyoma, leiomyosarcoma	Lobulated mass arising within the gastric wall. Signal approximates smooth muscle on T1WI, but most lesions are heterogeneous. Central necrosis occurs commonly, resulting in heterogeneous signal due to presence of hemorrhage. Low signal foci of calcification are often present. May ulcerate. Enhances significantly with Gd-contrast administration.	Leiomyomas are most common in the antrum and body of the stomach, usually submucosal. Larger lesions may project into the lumen and/or into the peritoneal cavity. Leiomyosarcomas tend to be very large (greater than 10 cm) and frequently have regions of necrosis.

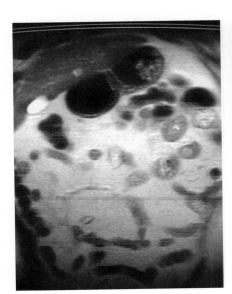

a

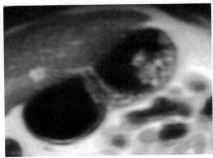

b

Fig. 21.**1** **Gastric adenocarcinoma.** A large, irregularly marginated lesion projects into the gastric lumen from the body of the stomach along the greater curvature. (**a, b**: T1WI spoiled GRE, coronal.)

Table 21.1 (Cont.) Abnormal stomach

Disease	MRI Findings	Comments
Lipoma	Well-defined lesion with signal characteristics identical to fat, occasionally with thin low-signal fibrous septatations or a capsule. No significant enhancement after contrast.	In the stomach, most commonly occur in the antral region.
Lymphoma (Fig. 21.2)	Thickening of the entire gastric wall (greater than 10 mm) or over a large region. Often markedly thickened (greater than 3 cm). Smoothly marginated or lobulated contours. Enhancement may be diffuse or heterogeneous.	Lymphoma represents 1–5% of all malignant tumors of the stomach, either in the setting of generalized lymphoma or as isolated primary disease (10%). Usually non-Hodgkin type.
Metastatic lesions	Usually submucosal. May ulcerate through the mucosa. Often multiple.	Ovary, breast, lung, melanoma, lymphoma, and thyroid are the most common primary malignancies to metastasize to the stomach.
Inflammatory lesions		
Peptic ulcer	Focal or regional thickening of the gastric wall with increased signal on T2WI. The ulcer crater may be difficult to perceive unless perpendicular to the imaging plane.	Can be difficult to distinguish from malignancy. Associated with *Helicobacter pylori* infection.
Gastritis	Edema and thickening of the gastric rugae. Can be regional or diffuse. Increased signal in affected areas on T2WI. The gastric wall may also be thickened.	The rugal pattern is usually preserved despite the edematous changes; destruction of the pattern suggests underlying malignancy. Crohn disease, postradiation effects, and infectious conditions, such as tuberculosis, may have a similar appearance. In the setting of AIDS, cytomegalovirus or *Cryptosporidium* infection should be considered.
Pancreatitis	Thickening of the gastric wall adjacent to the pancreas or a peripancreatic fluid collection.	Rarely associated with a pseduocyst of the gastric wall. See Chapter 19.
Gastric varices (Fig. 21.3)	Well-defined clusters of tubular or round lesions in the posteromedial fundus or gastric cardia. Varices with higher rates of flow are bright on GRE and create flow voids on spin echo (SE) sequences. Enhance markedly after Gd-contrast administration.	Most commonly occur in the setting of portal hypertension or splenic vein occlusion.

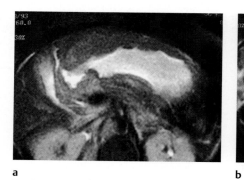
a
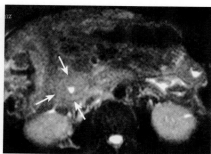
b
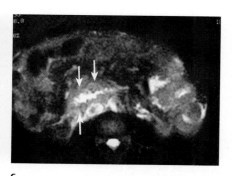
c

Fig. 21.2 **Lymphoma.** a A marked diffuse, smoothly lobulated wall thickening of the stomach is seen. b This is contiguous with extensive involvement in the duodenum, which is also markedly thickened with tumor involvement (arrows). (**a–c**: axial T2WI, FS.)

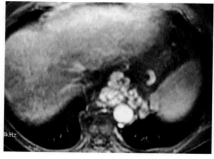
a
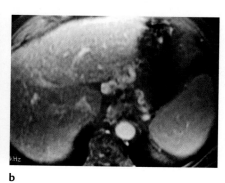
b

Fig. 21.3 **Gastric varices.** Several enhancing tubular structures are clustered at the gastroesophageal junction, gastric cardia, and gastric fundus. These prominent veins are conspicuous with contrast. (**a, b**: T1WI spoiled GRE with contrast, axial.)

Table 21.**2** Abnormal small bowel

Disease	MRI Findings	Comments
Congenital		
Annular pancreas	Ring of tissue with signal characteristics identical to normal pancreatic parenchyma encasing and narrowing the second portion of the duodenum. Often part of the ring is a fibrous band, which may be difficult to perceive.	Uncommon developmental anomaly.
Small bowel duplication cyst	Thin-walled, rounded or tubular lesion. Signal approximates water, high on T2WI and intermediate to low on T1WI. No enhancement after Gd-contrast administration.	Duplication cysts occur most commonly in the small bowel and esophagus. These usually do not communicate with the lumen. Spinal anomalies are often associated.
Meckel's diverticulum	Tubular outpouching of small bowel, usually within 2 feet (60 cm) of the ileocecal valve. Often (50%) contain ectopic gastric mucosa, which after Gd-contrast administration enhances to a greater degree than the adjacent small bowel mucosa.	Remnant of the embryologic omphalomesenteric (vitelline) duct. Can contain gastric, pancreatic, or colonic mucosa. May present with gastrointestinal bleeding when gastric mucosa is present.
Neoplasms		
Leiomyoma, leiomyo-sarcoma (Fig. 21.4)	Round or lobulated mass that typically grows extraluminally when encountered in the small bowel. Signal approximates smooth muscle on T1WI, but most lesions are heterogeneous. Central necrosis occurs commonly, resulting in heterogeneous signal due to the presence of hemorrhage. Low signal foci of calcification are often present. May ulcerate. Enhances significantly with Gd-contrast administration.	Leiomyoma is the most common benign neoplasm of the small bowel. Fifty percent are larger than 5 cm in diameter. Leiomyosarcomas of the small bowel occur most often in the ileum and least often in the duodenum.
Lymphoma (Fig. 21.2 b,c)	Large aneursymally dilated mass, often with ulceration. Multiple lesions may be seen. May also present with diffuse wall thickening or mural nodules. Moderate enhancement.	Primary sites of disease are in the ileum and jejunum with only 2% arising from the duodenum. Intussusception is not uncommon. Lymphadenopathy and splenomegaly are associated features.
Lipoma	Well-defined lesion with signal characteristics identical to fat, occasionally with thin low-signal fibrous septatations or a capsule. No significant enhancement after contrast.	Uncommon in the small bowel.

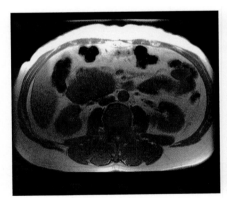

a

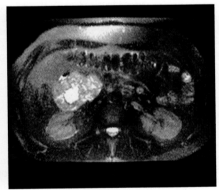

b

Fig. 21.**4** **Leiomyoma.** A large round mass with lobulated margins originating from the third portion of the duodenum. The lesion is isointense to muscle on T1WI. The central hyperintense region on T2WI reflects necrosis. After Gd-contrast administration, the thick peripheral margins of the tumor enhance prominently. (**a**: axial T1WI; **b**: axial T2WI, FS; **c**: T1WI spoiled GRE with contrast enhancement, axial; **d**: T1WI spoiled GRE, sagittal.)

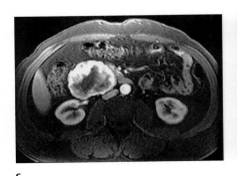

c

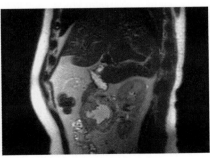

d

Table 21.**2** (Cont.) Abnormal small bowel

Disease	MRI Findings	Comments
Small bowel polyps	Multiple, usually small nodular mucosal lesions projecting into the lumen.	*Familial polyposis* and *Gardner syndrome* are associated with adenomatous polyps in the small bowel in about 5 % of cases; they are always associated with colonic polyps. Ninety percent of small bowel polyps in Gardner syndrome occur in the duodenum. *Peutz–Jeghers syndrome* is autosomal dominant and is associated with hamartomatous polyps in the small bowel, as well as the stomach and colon. About 50 % of cases of *Cronkhite–Canada syndrome* manifest hamartomatous small bowel polyps.
Carcinoid (Fig. 21.**5**)	Spiculated mass emanating from the bowel wall with retraction of adjacent bowel loops, which may become kinked, due to an induced desmoplastic reaction. Enhances after Gd-contrast administration.	The most common site for small bowel carcinoid is the ileum. May be multiple. Hepatic metastases typically markedly enhance.
Adenocarcinoma (Fig. 21.**6**)	Annular or lobulated mass. Usually isointense to the bowel wall on T1WI and slightly hyperintense on T2WI. Moderate, often heterogeneous enhancement.	Most commonly occur in the duodenum (50 %) and jejunum. Increased risk in patients with Crohn and celiac disease.
Metastases	Varied in appearance, ranging from nodules, scirrhous type lesions, intramural deposits, or polyploid masses that may project into the lumen.	Colon, stomach, breast, ovary, uterine, and melanoma are the most common malignancies to metastasize to the small bowel. Spread via peritoneal seeding is more common than hematogenous metastasis. In AIDS, *Kaposi sarcoma* commonly metastasizes to the small bowel and may hemorrhage.
Neurogenic tumor	Sessile or pedunculated masses that tend to be subserosal or submucosal, may project into the lumen. Low to intermediate signal on T1WI and high on T2WI. Enhance prominently with Gd-contrast administration, but may be heterogeneous in larger lesions.	Associated with neurofibromatosis type I, may be solitary or multiple. Plexiform neurofibromas may present as a mesenteric mass (see Table 22.**1**).
Inflammatory lesions		
Crohn disease	Small bowel wall thickening with or without luminal narrowing and stricture. The valvulae conniventes are lost or distorted. Involved areas are isointense to bowel wall on T1WI, variably hyperintense on T2WI, and enhance proportionately to disease activity. Skip lesions are areas of abnormality interspersed among normal bowel. Fistula formation is common in advanced disease and well demonstrated with MRI. Inflammatory changes, patchy areas of intermediate to high signal on T2WI, in the adjacent mesentery are often observed. Abscess formation is common in active disease.	The terminal ileum is the most common site of disease, but the entire gastrointestinal tract can be involved. Approximately one-third of cases are confined to the small bowel. Crohn disease can be associated with sclerosing cholangitis and inflammatory arthritis.
Hematoma	Thickening of the small bowel wall and valvulae conniventes. In the acute setting, low signal on T1WI and high on T2WI. Fluid–fluid levels are occasionally seen, particularly those associated with anticoagulation.	Intramural hematoma of the small bowel is most commonly due to blunt abdominal trauma (50 %), but also occurs in the setting of anticoagulation therapy, bleeding diathesis, or pancreatic disease.
Ischemia	Thickening of the bowel wall, occasionally with the classic "thumb printing" pattern. Dilatation of the bowel is often present. MR angiography (MRA) can demonstrate stenoses and occlusion of the superior mesenteric artery and celiac axis.	May be episodic or fulminant with infarction. Portal venous gas, an ominous finding in the setting of bowel infarction, is not easily seen on MRI. Similarly, *pneumatosis intestinalis* is very difficult to detect.
Diverticular disease	Focal outpouching of the small bowel wall that may be filled with fluid, food contents, or air.	The duodenum is the most common location. Most often asymptomatic, but occasionally may present with malabsorption or bleeding. Diverticulitis in the small bowel is very rare.
Graft versus host disease	Diffuse wall thickening affecting the entire small bowel. Inflammatory changes in the adjacent mesentery.	The most common complication of bone marrow transplantation affecting the gastrointestinal tract. Immunocompetent donor T cells attack host tissues and produce a profuse secretory diarrhea and malabsorption.

Table 21.**2** (Cont.) Abnormal small bowel

Disease	MRI Findings	Comments
Tuberculosis	Thickened bowel wall of the small bowel and colon. Common associated findings are adenopathy, hepatosplenomegaly, lesions in the liver and spleen. Tuberculous ascites may have slightly higher signal intensity than water on T1WI and can enhance after intravenous Gd-contrast administration.	Similar findings may occur with *mycobacterium avium intracellulare.*

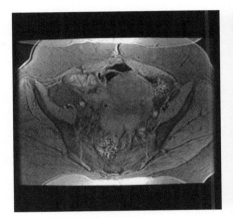

a

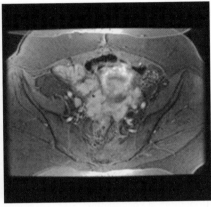

b

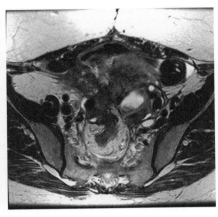

c

Fig. 21.**5** **Carcinoid.** A rounded mass with spiculated margins is seen anteriorly in the peritoneal cavity arising from the small bowel. The adjacent small bowel and sigmoid colon also have thickened walls with spiculations extending into the adjacent mesenteric fat. The mass and affected bowel walls enhance after contrast administration. (**a**: axial T1WI, FS; **b**: axial T1WI, FS, with contrast enhancement; **c**: axial T2WI.)

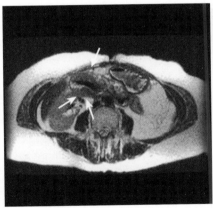

a

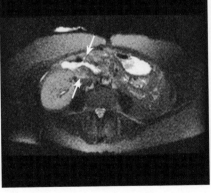

b

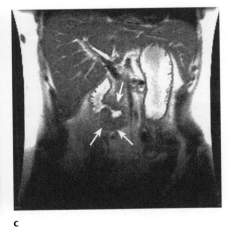

c

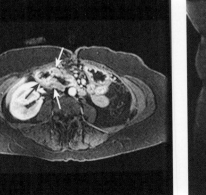

d

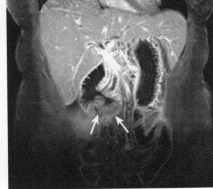

e

Fig. 21.**6** **Adenocarcinoma of the duodenum.** An annular lesion (arrows) narrows the junction of the second and third portions of the duodenum. The tumor is isointense to the normal bowel wall on T1WI and T2WI and enhances mildly with Gd-contrast administration. (**a**: axial T1WI; **b**: axial T2WI, FS; **c**: coronal T2WI; **d**: axial T1WI, FS, with contrast enhancement.)

Table 21.3 Abnormal colon

Disease	MRI Findings	Comments
Neoplasms		
Lipoma	Well-defined lesion with signal characteristics identical to fat, occasionally with thin low-signal fibrous septatations or a capsule. Does not enhance significantly after contrast.	The most common intramural tumor in the colon. The majority are encountered in the cecum and ascending colon.
Colonic polyps (Fig. 21.7)	Sessile or pedunculated intraluminal mass.	Adenomatous polyps may occur sporadically in the colon and are at risk for malignant degeneration. Fifty percent of polyps 2 cm or greater in size are malignant. When numerous adenomatous polyps are present, *familial polyposis, Gardner syndrome,* and the very rare *Turcot syndrome* can be considered. Hamartomatous polyps occur in the colon in approximately 30% of cases of *Peutz–Jeghers syndrome* and almost 100% of *Cronkhite–Canada syndrome*. *Juvenile polyposis* is usually limited to the rectum and most often (75%) consists of a large, solitary polyp.
Adenocarinoma (Figs. 21.8, 21.9)	Tumors may be polyploid or annular. Approximately isointense to the colonic wall on T1WI and variable signal on T2WI. Enhances with Gd-contrast administration. Perforated tumors can simulate diverticulitis.	The most common malignancy of the gastrointestinal tract. Risk factors include *ulcerative colitis, Crohn disease, familial polyposis, Gardner syndrome, the Lynch syndromes,* and *Turcot syndrome*.
Lymphoma	Bowel wall thickening with ulceration. Usually with mesenteric and retroperitoneal adenopathy.	The cecum is the most frequent site, but non-Hodgkin lymphoma rarely involves the colon (1.5%).
Metastasis	Lesions can constrict or invade in a way that mimics primary colonic adenocarcinoma.	Uterine, ovarian, pancreatic, gastric, renal, and prostate carcinoma may directly invade the colon or be disseminated with malignant ascites.
Carcinoid	Polyploid mass projecting into the lumen. Enhances after Gd-contrast adminstration.	The appendix and rectum are the two most common locations in the colon. In the appendix it is almost always benign. About one-third are multiple.
Mucocoele of the appendix	Rounded or elongated lesion arising from the appendix with homogeneous low to intermediate signal on T1WI and high signal on T2WI. Occasionally with mural calcification. No enhancement.	Rupture may result in *pseudomyxoma peritonei*. Associated with increased incidence of colonic adenocarcinoma and ovarian cystadenocarcinoma.

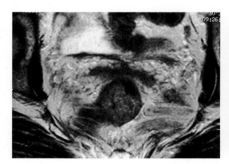

a

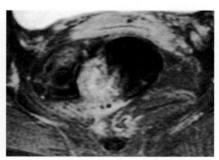

b

Fig. 21.**7 Villous adenoma of the rectum.** A mass lesion arising from the right lateral aspect of the rectal mucosa with enhancing frond-like projections. (**a**: axial T1WI; **b**: axial T1WI, FS, with contrast enhancement.)

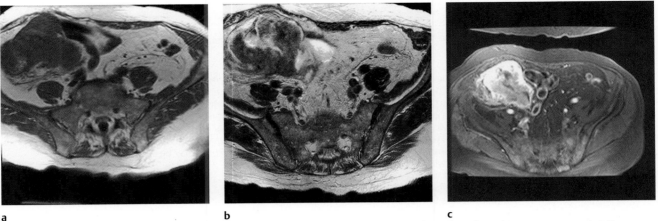

a   b   c

Fig. 21.**8** **Colonic adenocarcinoma.** A large lesion with indistinct borders arising from the right colon. This tumor recurred at the anastomotic site from a previous resection. (**a**: axial T1WI; **b**: axial T2WI; **c**: T1WI spoiled GRE with contrast enhancement, axial.)

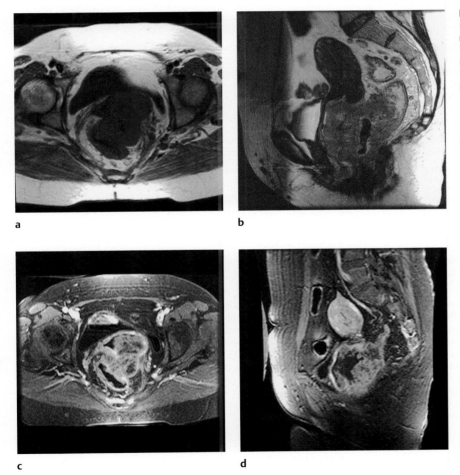

a   b

c   d

Fig. 21.**9** **Rectal adenocarcinoma.** The tumor extends from the left anterolateral rectum and invades the vagina. (**a**: axial T1WI; **b**: sagittal T2WI; **c**: T1WI spoiled GRE with contrast enhancement, axial; **d**: T1WI spoiled GRE with contrast enhancement, sagittal.)

Table 21.3 Abnormal colon

Disease	MRI Findings	Comments
Inflammatory disorders		
Crohn disease (Fig. 21.10)	Colonic wall thickening with or without lumenal narrowing and stricture formation. Involved areas are isointense to bowel wall on T1WI, variably hyperintense on T2WI, and enhance proportionately to disease activity. Skip lesions are areas of abnormality interspersed among normal bowel. Fistula formation is common in advanced disease and well demonstrated with MRI. Inflammatory changes, patchy areas of intermediate to high signal on T2WI, in the adjacent mesentery are often observed. Abscess formation is common in active disease.	The ascending colon is the most frequent site of involvement, while the sigmoid and rectum are usually uninvolved. Colonic mucosal involvement occurs in the early phase of the disease and is not well demonstrated on MRI, although occasionally deep apthous ulcers and fissures may be seen.
Ulcerative colitis	Thickened colonic wall with or without narrowing of the lumen and/or stricture formation. Loss of haustration. Affected regions enhance after Gd-contrast administration. *Backwash ileitis* is usually seen in advanced cases of ulcerative colitis. The terminal ileum is thickened and may be narrowed or mildly dilated. T2WI demonstrates intermediate to high signal in the wall of the terminal ileum and in the adjacent fat.	The rectum is almost always involved and is the first site of disease, which then spreads proximally. Extraluminal manifestations of the disease are uncommon, in contradistinction to Crohn disease. Associated with increased risk for colonic adenocarcinoma. Ulcerative colitis is the most common cause of toxic megacolon.
Ischemia/infarction	Bowel wall thickening, occasionally with "thumb printing." Usually with dilatation. Most often in the distribution of the inferior mesenteric artery.	May be segmental or diffuse. Risk factors include recent surgery, thromboembolic disease, and bowel obstruction.
Radiation enteritis (Fig. 21.11)	*Acute changes*: bowel wall thickening and infiltrative changes in the adjacent mesenteric fat. Mild to moderately increased enhancement. *Chronic Changes*: bowel wall thickening with luminal narrowing and/or stricture formation. The affected colon may become tubular with loss of its haustral pattern.	Generally observed after doses in excess of 40–50 Gy. Ulceration, bleeding, obstruction, and fistula formation are associated complications.
Typhlitis	Thickening of the cecum and often the ascending colon. Pericecal abscess formation may occur.	Transmural necrotizing process seen in neutropenic patients.
Tuberculosis	Thick-walled, distorted and contracted cecum.	Localized colonic tuberculosis is almost always limited to the cecum.
Appendicitis	Thickening of the appendiceal wall and often the cecal wall with infiltrative changes in the adjacent fat. Low to intermediate signal on T1WI and intermediate to high signal on T2WI. Variable enhancement with Gd-contrast administration. Appendicoliths are not easily seen as they appear as signal void within the lumen of the appendix.	Appendiceal abscess occurs in the right lower quadrant.
Diverticulosis/ diverticulitis (Fig. 21.12)	Diverticula are small (usually less than 1 cm in diameter) outpouchings of the colonic wall. A common incidental finding. With diverticulitis there is inflammation of a diverticulum with associated bowel wall thickening, often with spasm. Low to intermediate signal on T1WI and high on T2WI in the affected segment of colon as well as more patchy similar signal changes in the adjacent fat. An abscess may develop adjacent to the inflamed diverticulum or elsewhere in the peritoneal cavity.	Colonic diverticula are present in 6–8% of the population in the Western hemisphere. Incidence increases with age. The sigmoid is the most frequent location, but they can be seen throughout the colon. Diverticulitis develops secondary to occlusion of the diverticular neck with subsequent perforation. Fistula formation may occur.
Endometriosis	Rounded, occasionally septated lesions. High signal on T1WI and low signal on T2WI is classic, but signal character varies with the menstrual cycle and/or the presence of blood products.	Serosal implants most commonly encountered in the rectosigmoid.

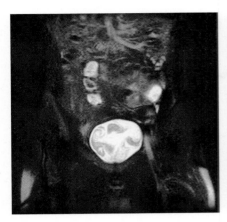

a

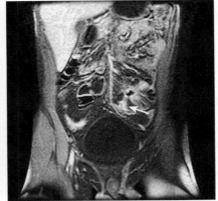

b

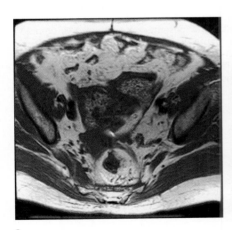

c

Fig. 21.**10** **Crohn disease.** A segment of the sigmoid colon demonstrates irregularity and thickening of its wall. The mildly increased signal in the adjacent mesocolon reflects edema on the T2WI. Note the small fistulous tract inferiorly (**b**, arrow). A barium enema performed shortly afterward redemonstrates the findings. (**a**: coronal T2WI, FS; **b**: T1WI spoiled GRE with contrast enhancement, coronal; **c**: double contrast barium enema.)

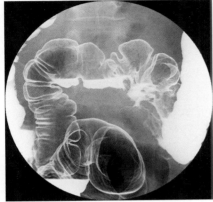

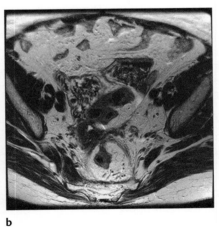

a

b

Fig. 21.**11** **Chronic radiation effects.** The rectum is narrowed and distorted. The rectal wall has low to intermediate signal intensity on all sequences. (**a**: axial T1WI; **b**: axial T2WI.)

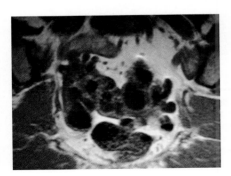

Fig. 21.**12** **Diverticulosis.** Several outpouchings of varying sizes of the sigmoid colon wall (coronal T1WI.)

22 Peritoneum and Mesentery

The peritoneal cavity consists of the greater and lesser sac. The greater sac comprises the majority of the cavity that extends from the diaphragm into the pelvis. The transverse mesocolon, which suspends the transverse colon from the peritoneum, divides the greater sac into supramesocolic and inframesocolic compartments. The lesser sac is a diverticulum of the greater sac, which forms a potential space posterior to the stomach and the lesser omentum. The peritoneal cavity can be further subdivided by peritoneal reflections into several compartments and recesses, which are anatomically interconnected (Figs. 22.1, 22.2). These peritoneal reflections, termed ligaments, along with the bowel mesenteries and omentum create barriers to the spread of infections, fluid collections, and tumors (Fig. 22.3). Paradoxically, the channels that these barriers form can serve as routes of dissemination for various disease processes.

The supramesocolic compartment, located superior to the transverse mesocolon, is the superior portion of the greater sac. It contains the liver, stomach, falciform ligament, lesser and greater omentum, and spleen. The lesser sac is bounded anteriorly by the stomach, duodenum, lesser omentum, and gastrocolic ligament, posteriorly by the body of the pancreas and the spleen, and inferiorly by the reflections of the greater omentum. The greater sac therefore envelops the lesser sac. The lesser sac communicates with the greater sac via the foramen of Winslow (epiploic foramen).

The inframesocolic space contains the jejunum, ileum, and the ascending, transverse, and descending colon. This space extends from the tranverse mesocolon to the level of the dome of the bladder and the anterior aspect of the rectum. The portion of the inframesocolic space distal to the pelvic brim is occasionally referred to as the pelvic peritoneal cavity. The inframesocolic space is further divided by the small bowel mesentery into the right and left inframesocolic spaces. The right and left paracolic gutters are lateral to the peritoneal attachments of the ascending and descending colon. On the right side, the right paracolic gutter extends into the posterior subhepatic space and Morison's pouch (hepatorenal space), which is the most dependent portion of the peritoneal cavity in the right upper quadrant as well as a frequent site of intraperitoneal collections. Collections in Morison's pouch can extend into the right subphrenic (supramesocolic) space if their volume is sufficient. The paracolic gutters also connect the inframesocolic space with the pelvis, where the pouch of Douglas and the lateral paravesical recesses are the most dependent parts and frequent sites of intraperitoneal collections.

The peritoneal ligaments can be difficult to identify on MRI since they are thin and often coapted against adjacent viscera or bowel. In the presence of ascites or other fluid collections they are more easily distinguished. The ligaments are discussed in anatomic order from superior to inferior.

At the superior margin of the supramesocolic space, the right triangular ligament forms from the superior and inferior reflections of the right coronary ligament at the right superolateral aspect of the right lobe of the liver to sepa-

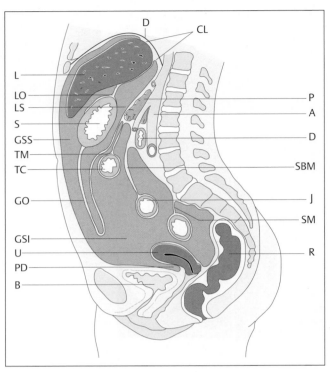

Fig. 22.1 Peritoneal spaces and ligaments, sagittal.
D: diaphragm. CL: coronary ligaments. P: pancreas. A: aorta. D: duodenum. SBM: small bowel mesentery. J: jejunum. SM: sigmoid mesocolon. R: rectum. U: uterus. B: bladder. PD: pouch of Douglas. GSI: greater sac inframesocolic space. GO:greater omentum. TC: transverse colon. TM: transverse mesocolon. S: stomach. GSS: greater sac supramesocolic space. LS: lesser sac. LO: lesser omentum. L: liver.

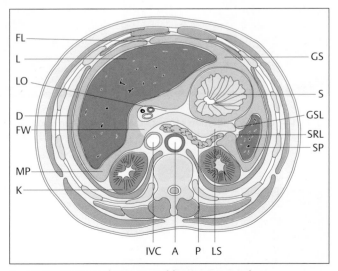

Fig. 22.2 Peritoneal spaces and ligaments, axial.
FL: falciform ligament. LO: lesser omentum. GS: greater sac. S: stomach. GSL: gastrosplenic ligament. SRL: splenorenal ligament. SP: spleen. LS: lesser sac. P: pancreas. A: aorta. IVC: inferior vena cava. K: kidney. FW: foramen of Winslow. MP: Morison's pouch. D: diaphragm. L: liver.

rate the right subphrenic space from Morison's pouch. The left triangular ligament forms from the superior and inferior reflections of the left coronary ligament to lie transversely along the superior aspect of the left lobe of the liver. The right and left coronary ligaments suspend the right and left lobes of the liver from the diaphragm, respectively. The falciform ligament lies between the right and left lobes of the liver. The ligamentum teres, the obliterated embryologic umbilical vein, lies within the falciform ligament and may be recanalized in the setting of portal hypertension. The gastrohepatic ligament is a part of the lesser omentum and connects the liver to the lesser curvature of the stomach. It contains the left gastric artery, left coronary vein, and lymph nodes. The hepatoduodenal ligament is continuous with the right lateral margin of the gastrohepatic ligament. Its free edge forms the anterior margin of the foramen of Winslow. The common hepatic duct, common bile duct, hepatic artery, and portal vein all lie within the hepatoduodenal ligament. The gastrophrenic ligament suspends the gastric fundus from the diaphragm just superior to the left kidney. The gastropancreatic plicae are peritoneal folds created by the branches of the celiac trunk. They attach the fundus to the retroperitoneum. The gastrosplenic ligament connects the greater curvature of the stomach to the splenic hilum. The phrenicocolic ligament is the superior border of the left paracolic gutter. It attaches to the spleen and the proximal descending colon. The greater omentum is the apron-like double peritoneal reflection that is folded over itelf and drapes anteriorly over the small bowel. The greater omentum is continous with the gastrocolic, gastrosplenic, and splenorenal ligaments. Extending from the ligament of Treitz to the ileocecal valve, the small bowel mesentery is a fan-shaped peritoneal fold that suspends the jejunum and ileum and harbors the superior mesenteric vessels. The sigmoid mesocolon bridges the sigmoid colon and the left iliac fossa.

The pelvic peritoneal ligaments are oriented differently in males and females and are considered separately.

In females, the peritoneum spreads anteriorly from the rectum onto the uterus. The anterior suspensory ligaments of the uterus are the broad and round ligaments. The broad ligaments contain the uterine vessels as well as nerves and lymphatics. In addition, the distal ureters course through the inferior aspects of the broad ligaments. The most inferior portion of the broad ligament is the cardinal ligament, which serves as the main support for the cervix and vagina. The round ligament travels into the inguinal canal and terminates in the labia majora. The ovarian ligaments connect the ovaries to the uterus.

In males, the peritoneum extends from the rectum over the seminal vesicles to the dome of the bladder. From the bladder the peritoneum climbs anteriorly and superiorly to the umbilicus and laterally to the pelvis sidewalls.

At the anterior abdominal wall in both males and females there are three groups of ligaments that stretch to the dome of the bladder: the median umbilical ligament, the remnant of the fetal urachus; the medial umbilical liga-

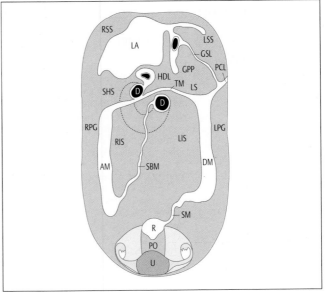

Fig. 22.3 Peritoneal spaces and ligaments, coronal.
LSS: left supramesocolic space. GSL: gastrosplenic ligament. PCL: phrenicocolic ligament. GPP: gastropancreatic plica. LS: lesser sac. TM: transverse mesocolon. HDL: hepatoduodenal ligament with portal vein. D: duodenum. SHS: subhepatic space. RSS: right supramesocolic space. LPG: left paracolic gutter. SM: sigmoid mesocolon. DM: descending mesocolon. LIS: left infracolic space. SBM: small bowel mesentery. RIS. right iniframesocolic space. AM: ascending mesocolon. RPG: right paracolic gutter. R: rectum. PD: pouch of Douglas. U: uterus.
(Modified from Kormano.)

ments, obliterated umbilical arteries; and the lateral umbilical ligaments, which are produced by the inferior epigastric arteries.

Peritoneal fluid collections tend to occur in the most dependent portions of the peritoneal cavity. In the supramesocolic space, this is usually Morison's pouch. In the inframesocolic space fluid often initially collects in the pouch of Douglas and may flow from there into the lateral paravesical space or into the paracolic gutters. It should be remembered that collections may be free flowing and can change location and distribution with changes in patient positioning. With larger fluid collections that fill or even distend the peritoneum, the bowel tends to cluster centrally in the least dependent portion of the peritoneal cavity. When bowel loops do not cluster in the typical fashion, adhesions should be suspected. Ascites may also become loculated due to benign or malignant causes and displace the bowel eccentrically.

Fluid collections are the most common peritoneal abnormality. These may be associated with multiple underlying diseases and are varied in character. Table 22.1 lists the differential diagnoses for various peritoneal pathologies.

Table 22.1 Peritoneal, mesenteric, and omental collections and masses

Disease	MRI Findings	Comments
Fluid collections/cysts		
Ascites (Fig. 22.4)	Commonly collects along the margins of the liver and spleen and in the pouch of Douglas. Collections gravitate to the most dependent portions of the abdomen and pelvis and may shift with changes in patient position. In larger ascitic collections the bowel rises to the least dependent location centrally within the abdomen. *Transudative ascites* essentially has signal characteristics identical to water with homogeneous low signal on T1WI and high signal on T2WI. *Exudative ascites* has a higher protein content than serum; thus the signal may appear with greater intensity than water on T1WI, but remains high on T2WI. *Chylous ascites* is composed of lipid material and proteins and thus appears as intermediate to high signal on T1WI. Usually high signal on T2WI.	Transudative ascites is produced in the setting of cirrhosis, congestive heart failure, renal insufficiency, or other hypoalbuminemic states. Exudative ascites is associated with neoplasms and infectious processes. An exception is *Meig syndrome* consisting of a benign, usually fibrous ovarian tumor, pleural effusion, and transudative ascites. Chylous ascites usually occurs in the setting of lymphatic obstruction, but can be seen occasionally with filiarial infections and in the nephrotic syndrome.
Peritonitis	*Acute*: Nonspecific peritoneal fluid. May have infiltrative changes in the mesenteric fat. *Chronic*: Thickening of the peritoneum with or without surface nodularity and adhesions. May enhance after Gd-contrast administration.	Most commonly occurs in the setting of infection within the abdominal cavity, but may also be caused by sterile inflammatory processes. Spontaneous bacterial peritonitis develops with seeding of the peritoneal cavity during bacteremia. *Tuberculous peritonitis* has the appearance of chronic peritonitis (see also *Inflammatory Masses* in this table).
Abscess (Fig. 22.5)	Most commonly a thick-walled cystic lesion, but may be ill defined; often with central necrosis. The wall has low signal on T1WI and variable signal on T2WI with enhancement after Gd-contrast administration. The signal intensity of abscesses varies with general approximation of muscle signal on T1WI and high signal on T2WI. Air–fluid levels may indicate fistulization with bowel.	May develop after perforation, inflammation, or surgery. Common locations include the right subphrenic space, the subhepatic space, and the pouch of Douglas.
Hematoma	The appearance of hemorrhage changes with time. This is often complicated by the fact that some lesions will bleed intermittently. Many hematomas are therefore of heterogeneous signal intensity. Hyperacute hemorrhage has low signal on T1WI and high on T2WI. Acute hemorrhage has low signal on T1WI and T2WI. Subacute hemorrhage has high signal on T1WI and either high or low on T2WI. Chronic hemorrhage (hemosiderin) has low signal on T1WI and T2WI.	Can result from blunt trauma, spontaneous rupture of a vascular tumor, ectopic pregnancy, or bleeding diathesis.
Biloma (Fig. 22.6)	Fluid collection occurring in the right upper quadrant, typically in the gallbladder fossa or adjacent to the liver. Signal intensity identical to water unless complicated by hemorrhage or infection.	Usually iatrogenic or post-traumatic, rarely spontaneous rupture of the gall bladder. Bile incites an inflammatory response in the peritoneal cavity, which may result in loculation of fluid in the porta hepatis.
Pseudomyxoma peritonei	Loculated, septated collections that classically scallop the margins of adjacent viscera or bowel. Bowel loops are displaced via mass effect. Low signal intensity on T1WI and high signal intensity on T2WI. Foci of calcification may develop in chronic cases. Does not enhance significantly.	Intraperitoneal accumulations of gelatinous material, usually from mucinous cystadenomas or cystadenocarcinomas. Commonly of the appendix or ovary. Can also occur in association with adenocarcinoma of the colon, ovary, or stomach.
Pancreatic pseudocyst (Fig. 22.7)	Thick-walled unilocular or multilocular collection that may contain debris and/or fluid–fluid levels. Occasionally may also contain hemorrhage or lipid. The walls enhance after Gd-contrast administration.	The most common cystic lesion of the lesser sac. May invade the mesentery.
Lymphangioma	Multiloculated and thin-walled, often with a lace-like pattern. Hyperintense on T1WI due to the presence of lipid materials. Intermediate to hyperintense on T2WI. Occasionally fluid–fluid levels are observed with hemorrhage. After ingestion of a fatty meal, the fat content of the fluid may increase.	Congenital malformation, which usually becomes symptomatic with abdominal pain in adolescence.

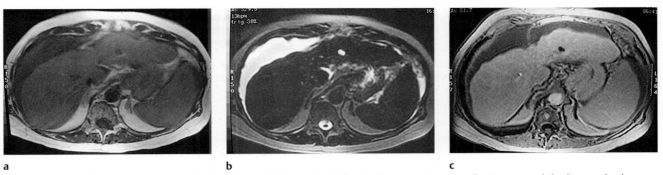

a   b   c

Fig. 22.**4   Transudative ascites.** Ascitic fluid with signal characteristic identical to water is seen collecting around the liver and spleen within the peritoneal cavity. Note the lobulated hepatic contour indicative of cirrhosis in this patient. A simple cyst is incidentally noted in the left lobe of the liver. (**a**: axial T1WI; **b**: axial T2WI FS; **c**: axial T1WI spoiled GRE with contrast.)

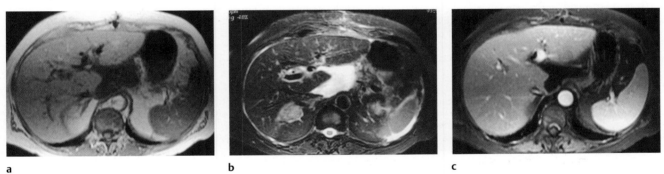

a   b   c

Fig. 22.**5   Abscess.** A multiloculated collection extends from Morison's pouch into the subhepatic space and the posterolateral abdominal wall. The thick, irregular septations enhance after Gd-contrast administration. (**a**: axial T1WI; **b**: axial T2WI, FS; **c**: T1WI, FS, with contrast enhancement.)

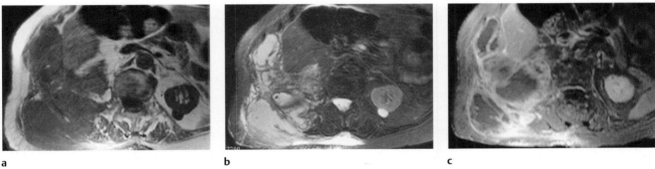

a   b   c

Fig. 22.**6   Biloma.** A well-defined fluid collection within the porta hepatis. There is no enhancement after contrast administration. This collection developed in a patient status post Whipple procedure. (**a**: axial T1WI; **b**: axial T2WI, FS; **c**: T1WI spoiled GRE with contrast enhancement, axial.)

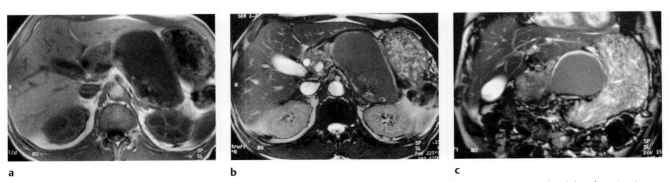

a   b   c

Fig. 22.**7   Pancreatic pseudocyst.** A sharply defined encapsulated fluid collection occupies the lesser sac. Note the debris layering in the dependent portion of the collection. After contrast administration, the thick capsule enhances prominently. (**a**: axial T1WI; **b**: axial T2WI; **c**: T1WI spoiled GRE with contrast enhancement, coronal.)

Table 22.1 (Cont.) Peritoneal, mesenteric, and omental collections and masses

Disease	MRI Findings	Comments
Duplication cyst, mesenteric cyst, mesothelial cyst, peritoneal inclusion cyst	Unilocular thin-walled or thick-walled rounded lesion. Low to intermediate signal on T1WI and high signal on T2WI. No significant enhancement.	Usually asymptomatic. Typically do not communicate with the bowel lumen.
Neoplasms		
Lymphoma	Variable morphology ranging from well-defined round or lobular masses to a poorly marginated mass, to a cake-like mass. Isointense to muscle on T1WI, intermediate on T2WI. Variable enhancement after Gd-contrast administration. When the tumor mass envelopes a mesenteric vessel, it may result in the "sandwich" sign.	The most common cause of mesenteric masses. The majority are non-Hodgkin lymphoma, which involve the mesentery in approximately 60% of cases.
Malignant mesothelioma (Fig. 22.8)	Peritoneal plaques with mural calcification in 70% of cases. The plaques may have nodular projections into the peritoneal cavity. Larger plaques may form omental cake. There is little ascites relative to the amount of peritoneal disease. The carcinomatous type occurs in 50% of cases with diffuse thickening of the peritoneum, multiple mesenteric and peritoneal nodules, and fixation of small bowel. The sarcomatous type occurs in 25% of cases and manifests with a large encapsulated mass. The carcinosarcomatous type occurs in the remaining 25% of cases with mixed features.	Associated with asbestos exposure. Typically a 20–40-year latency period. Associated bowel obstructions are common.
Cystic mesothelioma	Thin-walled and/or thinly septated lesion. Most commonly encountered in the pelvis, but may arise from any peritoneal surface. May encase or compress bowel, but usually does not create obstruction.	Unrelated to asbestos exposure. Nonmalignant but with a tendency for local recurrence. Female predominance.
Peritoneal carcinomatosis (Figs. 22.9, 22.10)	Develops in different patterns, ranging from small nodular projections to diffuse thickening of the peritoneum. In the omentum there may be nodules, plaques, or a thick, irregular blanket-like layer of tumor, termed cake. The mesentery may harbor nodules and plaques or adopt a stellate configuration. Ascites accompanies the majority (70%) of cases.	The most common malignancies to seed the peritoneal cavity are ovarian, colon, gastric, and pancreatic tumors.
Fibromatosis (desmoid tumor)	Round or ovoid lesions that may become very large. Homogeneous central necrosis is not usually a feature even with large lesions. Low signal intensity on T1WI and low to high signal intensity on T2WI. Tumors with a greater preponderance of low signal on T2WI tend to enhance only mildly, while those with higher signal on T2WI may enhance markedly.	The most common primary solid tumor of the mesentery. Locally invasive with frequent recurrence after resection, but does not metastasize. Associated with *Gardner syndrome*.

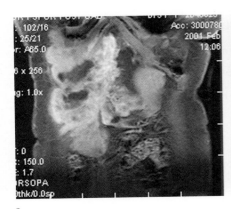

a

Fig. 22.8   Malignant mesothelioma. A large plaque-like lesion arising from the right anterior peritoneal surface has in-

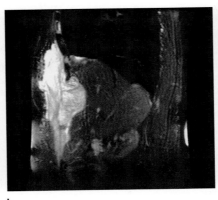

b

vaded the abdominal wall. The mass enhances after contrast administration. (**a**: T1WI spoiled GRE with contrast enhance-

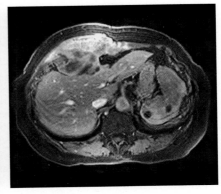

c

ment, coronal; **b**: T1WI spoiled GRE with contrast enhancement, sagittal; **c**: T1WI spoiled GRE with contrast enhancement, axial.)

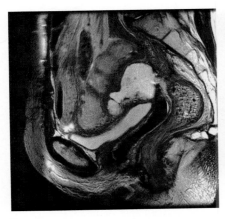

a

Fig. 22.9   Peritoneal carcinomatosis in ovarian carcinoma. A round lesion with a thick irregular margin lies superior to the

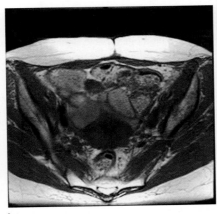

b

dome of the bladder. Thick irregular bands of tumor, which mildly enhance after contrast administration, have grown along the

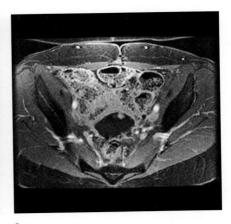

c

adjacent mesentery and small bowel. (**a**: sagittal T2WI; **b**: axial T1WI; **c**: axial T1WI, FS, with contrast enhancement.)

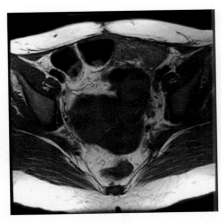

a

Fig. 22.10   Peritoneal metastases from wolffian duct carcinoma. Posterior to the bladder are several rounded lesions that have homogeneously low to intermediate

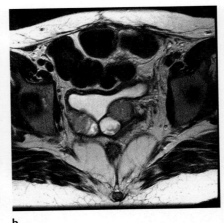

b

signal intensity on T1WI and are heterogenous with low and high signal intensity regions on T2WI. There is moderate heterogenous enhancement after contrast ad-

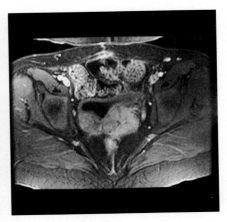

c

ministration. (**a**: axial T1WI; **b**: axial T2WI; **c**: T1WI spoiled GRE with contrast enhancement, axial.)

Table 22.**1** (Cont.) Peritoneal, mesenteric, and omental collections and masses

Disease	MRI Findings	Comments
Fibrosing mesenteritis (retractile mesenteritis, mesenteric lipodystrophy, mesenteric panniculitis) (Fig. 22.11)	Lobulated or stellate mass that separates and distorts adjacent small bowel loops. May also present as small scattered masses. Slightly hypointense to mesenteric fat on T1WI and T2WI with interspersed bands or patches of low signal fibrous material. Foci of calcification may be present. Mild enhancement with Gd-contrast administration.	Associated with *Gardner syndrome* and fibrosing mediastinitis. On rare occasions may induce thrombosis of the mesenteric vasculature.
Lipoma (Fig. 22.12)	Well-defined lesion with signal characteristics identical to fat, occasionally with thin low-signal fibrous septatations or a capsule. Does not enhance significantly after contrast.	The second most common primary solid tumor of the mesentery. Liposarcomas are rare in the peritoneum, but do occur.
Leiomyoma, leiomyosarcoma	Round or lobulated mass. Signal approximates smooth muscle on T1WI, but most lesions are heterogeneous. Central necrosis occurs commonly, resulting in heterogeneous signal due to presence of hemorrhage. Low-signal foci of calcification are often present. Air–fluid levels signify fistulization with bowel. The solid components enhance significantly after Gd-contrast administration.	Can arise from the mesentery itself or from adjacent small bowel. Benign and malignant lesions are not reliably distinguished with imaging.
Neurofibroma	Usually nodular masses that approximate muscle signal on T1WI; most often high but variable signal intensity on T2WI within the mesentery. Plexiform neurofibromas may attain large proportions. Enhancement varies from moderate to intense.	May occur as an isolated lesion or with multiple lesions in association with Neurofibromatosis type 1.
Splenosis	Spherical nodules with signal characteristics identical to splenic tissue. Most common in the splenic bed, but can become widely disseminated in the peritoneal cavity.	Autotransplantations of splenic tissue after trauma or splenectomy. Usually asymptomatic. Rarely may cause hemorrhage or abdominal pain.
Mesenteric teratoma	Solitary rounded lesion, often predominantly cystic with or without sepatation. Fatty, osseous, and dermal (hair) elements are present to varying degrees.	Very rare pediatric tumor. Eighty-five percent of cases occur in infants below 1 year.
Inflammatory masses		
Tuberculosis	Mesenteric adenopathy that may become stellate lesions or confluent masses. May form omental cake, mimicking carcinomatosis. The peritoneum is usually involved and may be diffusely thickened with or without nodular projections. Tuberculous ascites has a high protein content and is slightly hyperintense to water on T1WI.	Usually encountered with pulmonary tuberculosis. Increased incidence with AIDS.
Crohn disease (See Fig. 21.11)	Inflammatory changes, patchy areas of low signal on T1WI and intermediate to high signal on T2WI, are often observed in the mesentery adjacent to affected areas of bowel. Mesenteric adenopathy is often present. Abscess formation is common in active disease. See also Tables 21.**2** and 21.**3** for gastrointestinal manifestations.	Extensive mesenteric involvement is characteristic of Crohn disease and assists in differentiating it from other entities, particularly ulcerative colitis.
Mesenteric lymphadenitis	Enlarged mesenteric nodes, occasionally with mild enhancement. May be seen with mild wall thickening of the ileum and or cecum.	Benign inflammation of the mesenteric lymph nodes, most often related to an infectious process such as *Salmonella*, *Campylobacter*, *Yersinia*, or various viruses.

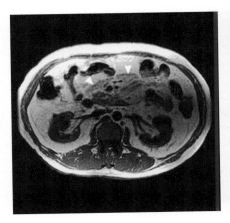

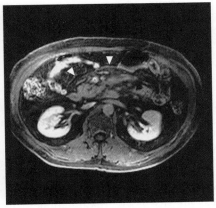

a

b

Fig. 22.**11** **Fibrosing mesenteritis.** On the precontrast T1WI, a poorly defined region of subtle decreased signal intensity is seen centrally within the small bowel mesentery. There is slight distortion of the mesenteric architecture. This region enhances mildly after contrast administration (arrowheads). (**a**: axial T1WI; **b**: T1WI, FS, with contrast enhancement.)

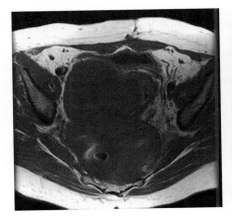

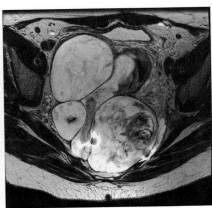

a

b

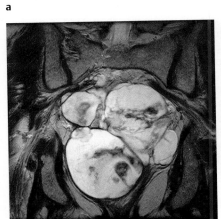

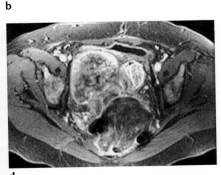

c

d

Fig. 22.**12** **Liposarcoma.** A conglomerate of large lobulated lesions within the pelvic peritoneal cavity. Liposarcomas can vary considerably in their signal characteristics depending on the relative proportions of fatty and stromal elements. This particular lesion has homogeneously low to intermediate signal intensity on T1WI and predominantly high signal intensity on T2WI with some heterogeneous low-signal elements. The lesion enhances significantly after Gd-contrast administration. (**a**: axial T1WI; **b**: axial T2WI; **c**: coronal T2WI; **d**: axial T1WI with contrast enhancement.)

23 Retroperitoneum

The retroperitoneum lies posterior to the peritoneal cavity and anterior to the spine and paraspinal musculature. Numerous pathologic processes originate in the retroperitoneum and an understanding of its anatomical divisions is necessary for providing an accurate radiologic assessment. This chapter details the differential diagnosis for lesions occurring in the retroperitoneum. Pathology intrinsic to the kidneys, adrenal glands, and pancreas are discussed separately in other chapters.

The anterior border of the retroperitoneum is formed by the posterior peritoneum. The transversalis fascia forms the posterior border. The anterior and posterior renal fasciae (Gerota's fascia) fuse behind the colon and form the lateroconal fascia, which delineates its lateral border. Within this framework of fascia, the retroperitoneum is subdivided into three compartments: the anterior pararenal space, the perirenal space, and the posterior pararenal space (Fig. 23.1).

The *anterior pararenal space* extends from the posterior parietal peritoneum to the anterior renal fascia. The lateroconal fascia is its lateral border. It contains the ascending and descending colon at its extreme right and left, respectively, and the duodenal loop and the pancreas centrally. Fluid collections in the anterior pararenal space are commonly confined to their site of origin, but they may extend into the lesser sac, into small bowel mesentery, and along the transverse mesocolon.

The *perirenal space* encompasses the kidney, adrenal glands, and their investing fat. The perirenal spaces are not continuous across the midline, although the anterior renal fascia occasionally continues across the midline below the renal hila. The normal thickness of the renal fascia is 1–2 mm. Abnormally thick renal fascia (greater than 2–3 mm) can be caused by edema, hyperemia, fibrosis, lipolysis, inflammation, malignancy, or trauma.

The *posterior pararenal space* extends from the posterior renal fascia to the tranversalis fascia. This relatively thin layer of fat continues without interruption as properitoneal fat of the abdominal wall, lying external to the lateroconal fascia. It is medially limited by the margin of the psoas muscle and contains no organs.

Normal retroperitoneal lymph nodes are assessed by size criteria. The upper limit of normal node diameter is 10 mm. Nodal enlargement may be secondary to neoplastic or inflammatory processes, but distinguishing between the two in the absence of other findings remains problematic since signal characteristics for normal and pathologic nodes are variable. On T1WI lymph nodes are isointense to muscle and thus easily discerned from surrounding high signal retroperitoneal fat. On T2WI nodes are typically high signal, approximating that of fat. With T2 weighting and fat suppression (FS) technique or with STIR, the high signal nodes can also be detected. MRI can easily discriminate nodes from vessels. With spin echo (SE) sequences, vessels appear as signal voids and with gradient echo (GRE) sequences they have a high signal intensity.

The abdominal aorta measures less than 3 cm in diameter and tapers gradually in caliber before bifurcating into the common iliac arteries at the level of L3–4. The origins of the celiac, superior mesenteric, renal, and inferior mesenteric arteries are all within the retroperitoneum. Abnormalities of the aorta and its branches such as aneurysms, thrombi, or dissection can be studied with standard sequences, but MR angiographic (MRA) techniques create far superior images. Dynamic Gd-DTPA injection with 3D GRE sequencing, often with a high dose administration, and 2D or 3D time of flight (TOF) acquisitions are commonly employed in dedicated vascular cases.

The inferior vena cava is formed by the junction of the right and left common iliac veins just caudal to the aortic bifurcation and runs on the right side of the abdominal aorta. The diameter of the inferior vena cava varies from a slit-like structure to a rounded vessel 2–3 cm wide. Respiration causes changes in diameter of the inferior vena cava. A collapsed inferior vena cava at multiple levels may indicate severe hypovolemia, and a dilated inferior vena cava may indicate heart failure. Flow-sensitive and contrast-enhanced sequences can be employed to detect thrombi within the inferior vena cava or other venous structures.

Table 23.1 discusses the differential diagnosis of various retroperitoneal abnormalities.

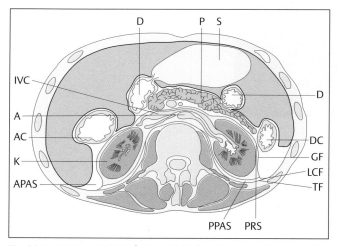

Fig. 23.**1** **Retroperitoneal spaces.** D: duodenum. S: stomach. P: pancreas. DC: descending colon. GF: Gerota's fascia. LCF: lateroconal fascia. TF: transversalis fascia. PRS: perirenal space. PPAS: posterior pararenal space. APAS: anterior pararenal space. K: kidney. AC: ascending colon. IVC: inferior vena cava. A: aorta. (Modified from Amis.)

Table 23.**1** Retroperitoneal Abnormalities

Disease	MRI Findings	Comments
Lymphadenopathy **Lymphoma** **(Fig. 23.2)** **(Fig. 23.2*)**	Enlarged lymph nodes, occasionally several centimeters in diameter, which can coalesce into a large mass. Untreated lymphoma is homogeneous and isointense to slightly hyperintense to muscle on T1WI. On T2WI it can be homogenously hyperintense (approximating fat signal) or heterogeneous with areas of high and low signal intensity. After therapy, involved nodes may become hypointense to muscle or heterogeneous. Signal voids from calcifications are seen in treated disease, but these can be difficult to detect in lymph nodes.	Involvement of only one (stage I) or two (stage II) lymph node chains on the same side of the diaphragm carries a better prognosis than involvement of lymph node chains on both sides of the diaphragm with or without involvement of extralymphatic organs (stages III and IV).

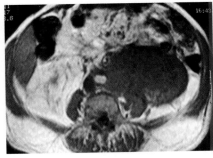

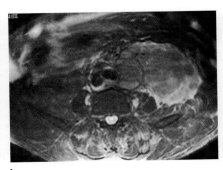

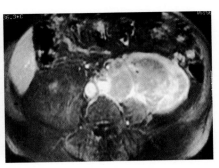

a

b

c

Fig. 23.**2**   **Non-Hodgkin lymphoma.** A well-defined mass lesion is seen in the left retroperitoneum, partially encasing the abdominal aorta. There is heterogeneous enhancement after Gd-contrast administration. (**a**: axial T1WI; **b**: axial T2WI, FS; **c**: axial T1WI, FS, with contrast enhancement.)

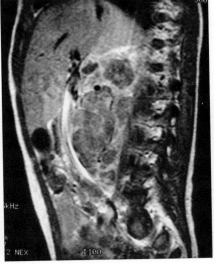

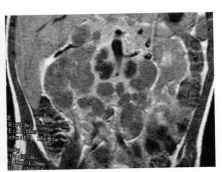

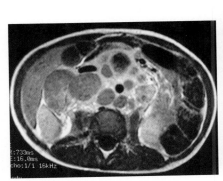

23.2*a

23.2*b

23.2*c

Fig. 23.**2***   **Hodgkin lymphoma.** The retroperitoneum is filled with numerous enlarged lymph nodes. The nodes are slightly hyperintense to skeletal muscle. Note the displacement of the intraperitoneal viscera. (**a**: T1WI, axial; **b**: T1WI, sagittal; **c**: T1WI, coronal.)

Table 23.1 (Cont.) Retroperitoneal Abnormalities

Disease	MRI Findings	Comments
Testicular neoplasms (Fig. 23.3)	Enlarged para-aortic lymph nodes near the renal hilum is a characteristic finding.	Testicular neoplasms are the most common malignancy in men aged 20 to 34. About 95 % are germ cell tumors including seminoma, embryonal cell tumor, choriocarcinoma, teratocarcinoma, and mixed-element tumors.
Other metastatic tumors	Enlarged retroperitoneal lymph nodes in the abdominal and pelvic regions. Any node larger than 1 cm is suspicious.	Cervical, prostatic, bladder, uterine, and renal and ovarian carcinomas frequently metastasize to retroperitoneal lymph nodes. Nodes containing metastases may not be enlarged. Other primaries include lung and gastrointestinal tract carcinomas.
Benign lymphadenopathy (HIV, immunosuppression)	Reactively enlarged lymph nodes can reach 2 cm in size, especially in immunosuppressed patients.	Benign lymphadenopathy is relatively rare.
Tuberculosis	Lymphadenopathy in mesenteric and peripancreatic lymph nodes. Necrotic nodes may have increased signal on T2WI. May have peripheral rim enhancement with Gd-contrast.	Complicates pulmonary disease in 6–38 % of immunocompromised patients. May be secondary to *Mycobacterium tuberculosis* or *Mycobacterium avium intracellulare*.
Sarcoidosis	Lymphadenopathy associated with hepatosplenomegaly in the absence of signs of portal hypertension. The lymph nodes tend to remain distinct unlike malignant lymphoma where they tend to coalesce.	Usually associated with pulmonary sarcoidosis (75 %). Differentiation from lymphoma is difficult without biopsy.
Amyloidosis	Lymphoma-like lymph node enlargement may occur. Involvement of the gastrointestinal tract is a more common manifestation.	Deposition of protein-polysaccharide material in various organs. Can be primary or secondary to rheumatoid arthritis, multiple myeloma, hematogenous malignancy, chronic infection, or advanced age.
Cyst-like masses		
Lymphocele	Rounded or ovoid well-circumscribed thin-walled lesion, occasionally with septations. Usually low to intermediate on T1WI and high onT2WI, but varies with its protein content.	May occur days or weeks after surgery, most commonly after renal transplantation or retroperitoneal or pelvic lymph node dissection.
Urinoma, seroma	Can be a discrete thin-walled mass-like lesion or a poorly defined collection of fluid tracking through the fascial planes into the pelvis. Low on T1WI and high on T2WI; mimics water signal characteristics.	May be post-traumatic or iatrogenic. Infected and sterile collections cannot be reliably distinguished from one another.
Abscess	Most commonly a thick-walled cystic lesion, but may be ill defined; often with central necrosis. The wall has low signal on T1WI and variable signal on T2WI, with enhancement after Gd-contrast administration. The signal intensity of abscesses varies with general approximation of muscle signal on T1WI and high signal on T2WI.	The most common causes are colonic perforation, pancreatic abscess, unsuspected duodenal perforation, and surgical contamination. Common in immunocompromised patients.
Hematoma (Fig. 23.4)	The appearance of hemorrhage changes with time. This is often complicated by the fact that some lesions will bleed intermittently. Many hematomas are therefore of heterogeneous signal intensity. Hyperacute hemorrhage has low signal on T1WI and high on T2WI. Acute hemorrhage has low signal on T1WI and T2WI. Subacute hemorrhage has high signal on T1WI, may be either high or low on T2WI. Chronic hemorrhage (hemosiderin) has low signal on T1WI and T2WI.	May be spontaneous or secondary to trauma, anticoagulation, vascular tumors, leaking aneurysms, or long-term hemodialysis. Usually contained within well-defined muscle groups and resolves spontaneously.
Pancreatic pseudocyst (See Fig. 22.6)	Thick-walled rounded fluid collection with low signal intensity on T1WI and high on T2WI; may have debris layering in its dependent portions. The wall may enhance after Gd-contrast administration. If the cyst is hemorrhagic, signal characteristics are altered with high T1WI and high T2WI occurring in the setting of acute pancreatitis.	Occurs as a complication of acute or chronic pancreatitis or pancreatic trauma. May invade the retroperitoneal space, but usually remains outside of Gerota's fascia.

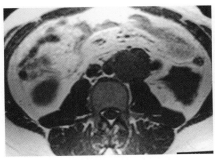

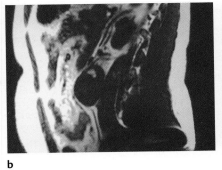

a

b

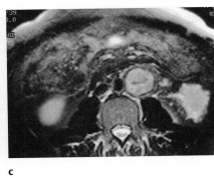

c

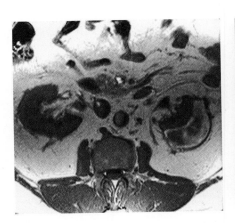

d

Fig. 23.**3 Metastatic seminoma.** A discrete lesion in the left para-aortic lymph node chain; low signal intensity on T1WI, high signal intensity on T2WI, and peripheral enhancement. (**a**: axial T1WI; **b**: sagittal T1WI; **c**: axial T2WI, FS; **d**: T1WI spoiled GRE, axial, with contrast enhancement.)

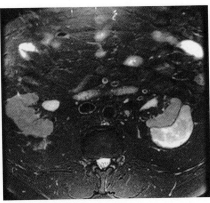

a

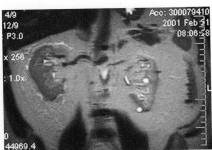

b

Fig. 23.**4 Perinephric hematoma.**
a, b A crescentic heterogeneous signal hematoma along the lateral aspect of the left kidney.   **c, d** Follow-up images demonstrate complete resolution after several weeks. (**a**: axial T1WI; **b**: axial T2WI, FS; **c**: axial T1WI; **d**: coronal T2WI, FS.)

c

d

Table 23.**1** (Cont.) Retroperitoneal Abnormalities

Disease	MRI Findings	Comments
Vascular abnormalities		
Abdominal aortic aneursym and branch artery aneurysms (Figs. 23.5, 23.6)	Saccular or fusiform dilatation of the aorta with a diameter greater than 3 cm. May contain thrombus. Calcification, when present, creates signal voids within the thrombus or vessel wall.	Common in the Western population (1–3%) secondary to atherosclerosis; mycotic and traumatic aneurysms are much less common. The risk of rupture correlates with the diameter and the rate of enlargement of the aneurysm.
Stenosis of abdominal aortic branch arteries (Figs. 23.7, 23.8)	Smooth or irregular narrowing of an artery origin typically at or near the ostium, but segmental narrowing along the course of a vessel is very common. In general, stenoses of the celiac and superior mesenteric artery predispose to bowel ischemia and renal artery stenosis may cause hypertension that is refractory to medical therapy. Focal or segmental regions of dilatation may be seen with vasculitis.	The most common cause is atherosclerosis. *Fibromuscular dysplasia* is most commonly seen in females and, when it affects the renal arteries, may cause severe hypertension. Vasculitis, including *Takayasu disease* and *polyarteritis nodosa*, are rare causes.
Aortic dissection (Fig. 23.9, see also Fig. 15.9)	Visualization of an intimal flap is diagnostic. Dilatation of the aorta may or may not be present. The false lumen more commonly has slower flow and/or thrombus.	In general, Stanford type A (DeBakey I and II) involves the ascending aorta and requires surgical treatment. Stanford type B (DeBakey III) affects the descending aorta and is medically managed.
Caval transposition	On caudal sections, the inferior vena cava is seen to the left of the aorta. It crosses over to the right side either anterior or posterior to the aorta at the level of the renal veins.	The incidence of this anomaly is 0.2–0.5%.
Duplication of the inferior vena cava	A second left-sided inferior vena cava originates from the left common iliac vein and ascends to the level of the renal veins, where it anastomoses with the normally positioned vena cava.	The incidence of this anomaly is 0.2–3%. A duplicated inferior vena cava can mimic a prominent left gonadal vein. The latter can be traced to the level of the inguinal canal or ovary, whereas a duplicated inferior vena cava anastomoses to the left common iliac vein.

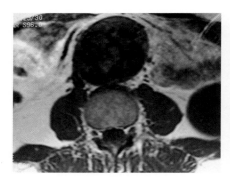

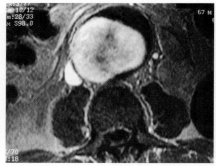

Fig. 23.**5** **Abdominal aortic aneurysm.** A large fusiform infrarenal abdominal aortic aneurysm. Note the crescentic low-signal thrombus present anteriorly within the lumen in (**b**). Bilateral common iliac artery aneurysms are also present in (**c**). The infrarenal origin of the aneurysm is detailed in (**d**). (**a**: axial T1WI; **b**: T1WI spoiled GRE, axial, with contrast enhancement; **c**: maximum intensity projection T1WI spoiled GRE, postcontrast; **d**: maximum intensity projection T1WI spoiled GRE, postcontrast.)

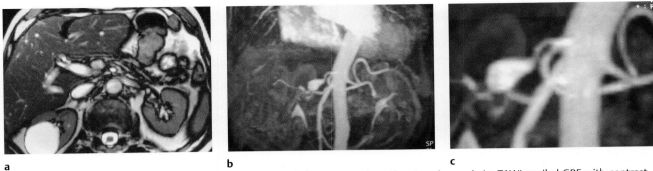

a

b

c

Fig. 23.6   Hepatic artery aneursym. A fusiform aneurysm of the common hepatic artery (arrows). (**a**: T1WI spoiled GRE with contrast enhancement, axial; **b, c**: maximum intensity projection T1WI spoiled GRE, postcontrast.)

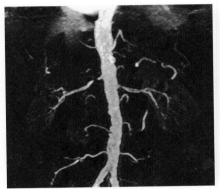

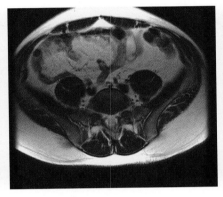

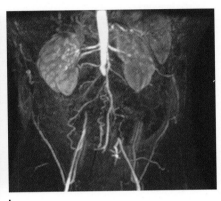

Fig. 23.7   Renal artery stenosis. A solitary right renal artery with a markedly stenotic segment proximally. (Maximum intensity projection T1WI spoiled GRE with contrast enhancement.)

a

Fig. 23.8   Leriche syndrome. The distal abdominal aorta and bilateral common iliac arteries are occluded. Note the distal reconstitution of the iliac arterial systems

b

bilaterally via collateralization.(**a**: axial T1WI; **b**: maximum intensity projection T1WI spoiled GRE, postcontrast.)

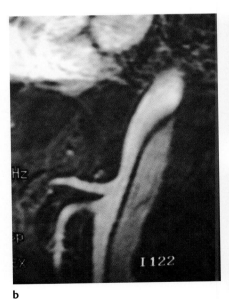

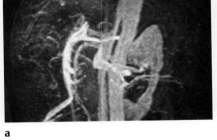

a

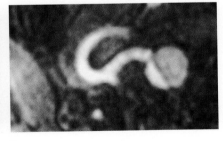

c

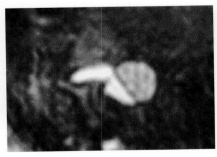

d

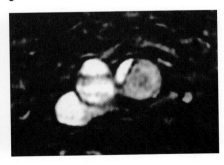

e

b

Fig. 23.9   Aortic dissection (Stanford type B, DeBakey III). The true lumen enhances brightly with contrast, while the false lumen with slower flow enhances moderately. The maximum intensity projection provides an overview of the extent

of the dissection (**a**). The origins of the celiac and superior mesenteric arteries are well seen in the sagittal plane (**b**) arising from the true lumen, but should be evaluated in the axial plane as well (**c** details the celiac origin, **d** details the superior

mesenteric artery origin). In this case the dissection extends into the common iliac arteries bilaterally (**e**). (**a**: Maximum intensity projection T1WI spoiled GRE with contrast enhancement; **b–e**: T1WI spoiled GRE, axial, with contrast enhancement.)

Table 23.**1** (Cont.) Retroperitoneal Abnormalities

Disease	MRI Findings	Comments
Anomaly of the left renal vein	The left renal vein can occur on both the anterior and posterior sides of the aorta or only posterior to the aorta.	The circumaortic left renal vein is seen in 1.5–8.7 % of the population and a retroaortic renal vein in 1.8–2.4 %. A retrocaval ureter is rare (0.09 %).
Azygos continuation of the inferior vena cava	The intrahepatic inferior vena cava is absent, and enlarged azygos and hemiazygos veins are demonstrated in the retrocrural space.	Incidence is 0.2–4.3 %. This anomaly is associated with congential heart disease. Left pulmonary isomerism, polysplenia, dextrocardia, and abdominal situs inversus are also commonly associated.
Thrombosis of the inferior vena cava (Figs. 23.10, 23.11)	Focal caval enlargement with an intraluminal thrombus. TOF or GRE sequencing with Gd-contrast demonstrate the low-signal thrombus outlined within the high signal lumen. Collateral vessels are often present in chronic thrombosis.	May be secondary to bland or septic thrombosis, but is more commonly a result of tumor extension from malignancies of the kidney, adrenal gland, or liver.
Miscellaneous		
Mesodermal tumors (Fig. 23.12)	Tend to present as a large mass that may be solid, cystic, or mixed. Generally the solid component is isointense to muscle. Foci of hemorrhage may be present. If fat is detected within the lesion, liposarcoma should be considered.	Primary retroperitoneal tumors are uncommon. Eighty-five percent are malignant. Liposarcoma, leiomyosarcoma, malignant fibrous histiocytoma, fibrosarcoma, malignant hemangiopericytoma, and malignant mesechymoma are the most commonly encountered.

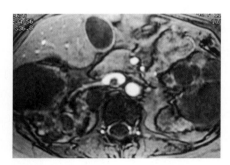

Fig. 23.**10 Thrombus within the inferior vena cava.** A nonocclusive thrombus as indicated by the arrow. (T1WI spoiled GRE, axial, with contrast enhancement.)

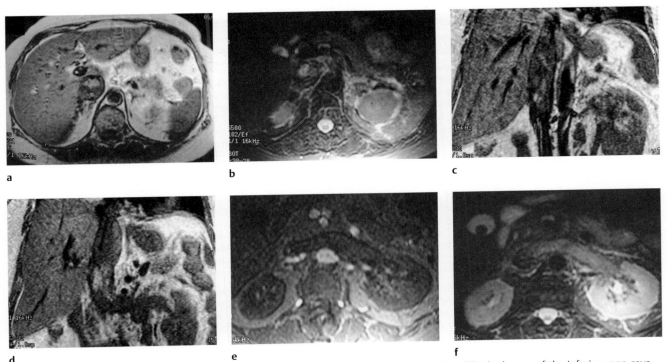

Fig. 23.11 Tumor thrombus within the inferior vena cava. A large heterogeneous thrombus fills the lumen of the inferior vena cava extending from the left renal vein in a patient with renal cell carcinoma. (**a**: axial T1WI; **b**: axial T2WI; **c, d**: coronal T1WI; **e**: axial T1WI; **f**: axial T2WI.)

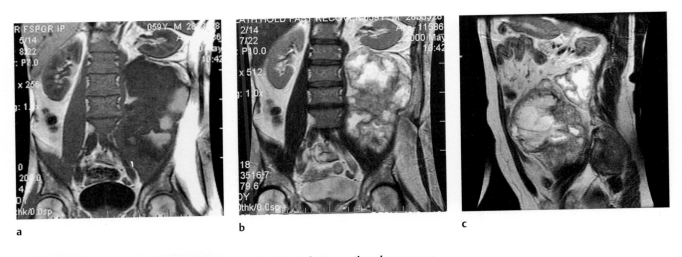

Fig. 23.12 Soft-tissue chondrosarcoma. A large, lobulated mass is seen arising in the left perirenal space displacing the left kidney superiorly. (**a**: coronal T1WI; **b**: coronal T2WI; **c**: sagittal T2WI; **d**: T1WI spoiled GRE with contrast enhancement, coronal.)

Table 23.1 (Cont.) Retroperitoneal Abnormalities

Disease	MRI Findings	Comments
Neurogenic tumors (Fig. 23.13)	Lobulated mass with well-defined or ill-defined borders occurring along the course of a nerve. Low to intermediate signal on T1WI and usually high on T2WI. Most enhance significantly after Gd-contrast administration. Larger lesions may enhance heterogeneously. See Chapter 8 for more detailed descriptions.	About one-third of primary retroperitoneal tumors are of neurogenic origin, usually in patients below age 30. *Ganglioneuroma, pheochromocytoma,* and *neurofibroma* are the most common benign tumors. *Neuroblastoma* is a common maligancy below the age of 6. Patients with *von Hippel–Lindau syndrome, tuberous sclerosis,* or *neurofibromatosis* have a genetic predisposition to neurogenic tumors.
Undescended testes (cryptorchidism)	In younger children, an ovoid structure that is isointense to muscle on T1WI and has a high signal on T2WI. With increasing age, the undescended testicle becomes increasingly fibrotic and has a low signal on T1WI and T2WI. It can be discovered anywhere along the path of testicular migration from the level of the renal vein to the inguinal canal, usually paralleling the course of the gonadal vein.	Eighty percent of maldescended testes are located distal to the inguinal ring. The remaining 20% are above the ring and usually are found adjacent to the iliac vessels. Ectopically located testis and congenital absence of the testis do occur. Undescended testes are associated with increased risk of malignancy (most commonly seminoma), infertility, and torsion.
Retroperitoneal fibrosis (Figs. 23.14, 23.15)	Dramatically enhancing fibrous sheet or broad-based bulky mass that envelops the aorta, inferior vena cava, iliac vessels, and ureters. Most often low to isointense to muscle on both T1WI and T2WI, but can be heterogeneous. Retroperitoneal fibrosis displaces the ureters medially, unlike retroperitoneal lymphadenopathy, which displaces them laterally.	Proliferation of fibrous and inflammatory tissue in the retroperitoneum. Primary or idiopathic in 70% and secondary in 30% where it may be associated with malignancies or abdominal aortic aneurysms. Methysergide and ergotamine are known causative agents.

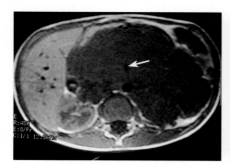

a

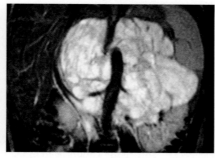

b

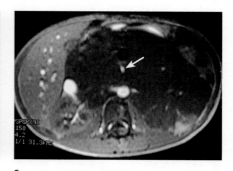

c

Fig. 23.**13** **Ganglioneuroma.** A large heterogeneous mass occupies most of the retroperitoneum and encases the abdominal aorta and superior mesenteric artery (arrow). The inferior vena cava is displaced laterally. (**a**: axial T1WI; **b**: coronal T2WI, FS; **c**: axial T1WI FSPGR with contrast enhancement.)

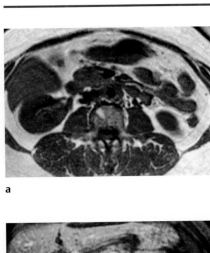
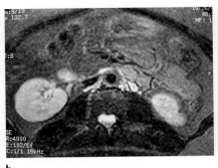
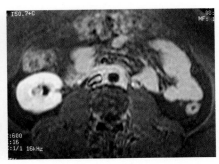

a

b

c

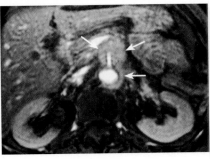

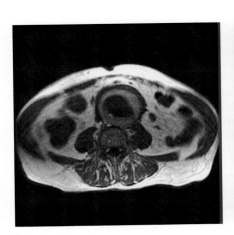

d

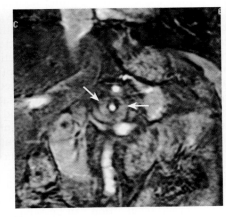

e

Fig. 23.**14 Retroperitoneal fibrosis.** In the first example (**a–c**), a mantle of intermediate signal intensity material envelops the abdominal aorta and inferior vena cava. There is moderate enhancement after GD-contrast administration. In the second example (**d, e**), a thick band of fibrous tissue (arrows) encases the abdominal aorta and the superior mesenteric artery. (**a**: T1WI, axial; **b**: T2WI FS, axial; **c**: T1WI FS with contrast, axial; **d**: T1WI spoiled GRE with contrast, axial; **e**: T1WI spoiled GRE with contrast, coronal).

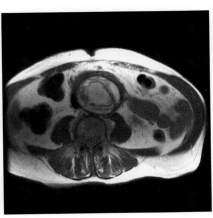

a

b

Fig. 23.**15 Inflammatory abdominal aortic aneurysm.** A thick band of inflammatory tissue surrounds the aneurysmally dilated abdominal aorta. (**a**: axial T1WI; **b**: double inversion recovery [IR], axial.)

24 Kidneys

The kidneys are embedded in the perinephric fat of the *perirenal space* (Fig. 24.**1**). This space is bounded anteriorly and posteriorly by the *renal (perirenal) fascia*. The anterior renal fascia is also referred to as Gerota's fascia and the posterior renal fascia as Zuckerkandl's fascia. The renal fascia is better seen on T1WI than T2WI and its normal width does not exceed 2 mm. Its two layers fuse behind the ascending or descending colon to form the lateroconal fascia.

The pararenal compartments are located outside the renal fascia. The *anterior pararenal space* contains the ascending and descending colon, the descending and transverse portions of the duodenum and the pancreas. The anterior boundary of the pararenal space is the parietal peritoneum. The *posterior pararenal space* contains only fat and is bound posteriorly by the fascia transversalis. Although these retroperitoneal compartments are anatomically well defined, an infectious or tumorous process can easily spread from one space to the other. Furthermore, pelvic disease, especially involving the rectosigmoid, may spread cephalad into the perirenal and pararenal compartments.

The renal parenchyma is tightly invested by a rigid *renal capsule* composed predominantly of fibrous tissue. The renal capsule is normally not visible on MRI. Chemical shift artifacts may, however, produce a band of low signal intensity along one margin of the kidney and a band of high signal intensity along the opposite margin. Because of the rigidity of the renal capsule a *subcapsular process* such as a hematoma compresses primarily the adjacent renal parenchyma, which becomes flattened by the pathologic fluid collection that often assumes a lenticular shape.

The *renal arteries* arise at the level of the first or second lumbar vertebra and lie posterior to the corresponding *renal veins*, which are usually somewhat larger. The right renal artery crosses posterior to the inferior vena cava, whereas the left renal vein crosses anterior to the aorta. A left retroaortic or circumaortic renal vein occurs in 2% and 5% of cases, respectively. On spin echo (SE) sequences the renal arteries and veins appear as tubular structures devoid of signal.

On T1WI the renal cortex, including columns of Bertin, has an intermediate signal intensity and can be differentiated from the hypointense renal medulla. The corticomedullary differentiation can be enhanced with fat suppression. It is decreased or absent in patients with impaired renal function. On T2WI the renal cortex and medulla are both of high signal intensity and usually cannot be differentiated from each other.

Gadolinium chelates such as Gd-DTPA are filtered by the renal glomeruli and concentrated in the renal tubules and ducts. The signal intensity of gadolinium in the urine depends on its concentration. When dilute, it enhances T1 relaxation and produces a high signal intensity in the urine; when highly concentrated, it induces magnetic susceptibility signal loss and causes urine to have a low signal intensity. With SE sequences a corticomedullary differentiation can be seen on T1WI immediately after intravenous Gd-DTPA administration, whereas shortly thereafter the enhancement of cortex and medulla becomes equal resulting in uniform renal enhancement.

MRI appears as equally effective as CT for detecting and staging renal cancer. Because of its higher cost MRI is currently limited to patients in whom CT is contraindicated or has yielded equivocal results. Indications for MRI include: 1) evaluation of the intravascular extent of tumor thrombosis; 2) characterization of renal masses in which CT is indeterminate (e. g., cyst-like lesions with thick walls, calcifications, multiple septa, indistinct interface with renal parenchyma, attenuation of cyst content of 25 Hounsfield units and higher, and/or some contrast enhancement); 3) hypersensitivity to intravenous iodinated contrast agents; 4) impaired renal function that contraindicates use of iodinated contrast agents; and 5) patients in whom radiation dose may be a major concern (e. g., serial tumor evaluation in children or in pregnancy).

Renal transplant complications include parenchymal diseases (acute rejection, acute tubular necrosis, cyclosporine nephrotoxicity, infection), vascular lesions (renal artery or vein stenosis or occlusion and pseudoaneurysm), ureteral obstruction or leak, and peritransplant fluid collections (urinoma, lymphocele, abscess, and hematoma). The normal renal allograft demonstrates corticomedullary differentiation on T1WI similar to a normal native kidney. In acute rejection the renal transplant is enlarged and loss of corticomedullary differentiation is found on T1WI. Loss of corticomedullary differentiation is, however, nonspecific and is also observed in severe, long-standing cyclosporine toxicity. However, in the early stage of cyclosporine toxicity and acute tubular necrosis the corticomedullary differentiation is usually preserved and the transplant is not enlarged. Vascular lesions (such as renal artery occlusion or renal vein thrombosis) and ureteral obstruction can be readily diagnosed by MRI and thus differentiated from other causes of transplant dysfunction. Peritransplant fluid

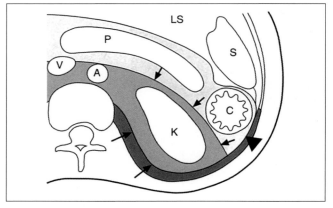

Fig. 24.1   Extraperitoneal anatomy of the left flank.
Light gray area: anterior pararenal space. Medium gray area: perirenal space. Dark gray area: posterior pararenal space. Short arrows: anterior renal fascia (Gerota's fascia). Long arrows: posterior renal fascia (Zuckerkandl's fascia). Arrowhead: lateroconal fascia. A: aorta. C: colon. K: kidney. LS: lesser sac. P: pancreas. S: spleen. V: inferior vena cava.

collections are well depicted by MRI. Urinomas and lymphoceles are homogeneous cystic lesions with identical signal intensity. However, urinomas tend to occur in the first week after transplantation and contrast extravasation into the lesion may be evident on late images after intravenous Gd-DTPA administration. Lymphoceles are the most common peritransplant fluid collections, and, compared with urinomas, tend to be larger, may be septated, and usually do not occur before the third week post transplantation. Peritransplant hematomas and abscesses depict more variable, heterogeneous signal intensity when compared with urinomas and lymphoceles.

The differential diagnosis of lesions in the kidney and perinephric space is discussed in Tables 24.1 and 24.2, respectively.

Table 24.1 Focal and diffuse renal disease

Disease	MRI Findings	Comments
Renal ectopy (Fig. 24.2)	Malpositioned kidneys are readily located and identified because of their characteristic corticomedullary differentiation best seen on precontrast fat suppressed T1WI and immediately after enhancement with Gd-DTPA. At a later stage the contrast-enhanced kidney appears as a uniformly hyperintense mass. In *horseshoe kidneys* the lower poles of both kidneys are fused across the midline immediately anterior to the spine.	In *longitudinal ectopy* the kidney is malpositioned in any location from the thorax to the sacrum. Pelvic kidney is the most common location and frequently associated with vesicoureteral reflux, hydronephrosis, hydrospadia, and contralateral renal agenesis. In *crossed ectopy* the malpositioned kidney is commonly fused with the contralateral kidney. In *renal fusion* the fused kidneys are located in the midline and may assume the shape of a horseshoe, disk, or pancake. Ureteral obstruction by aberrant arteries is frequently associated. In *renal malrotation* the collecting system is usually positioned anteriorly.
Renal duplication	Two separate renal sinuses and pelves are seen, separated by a parenchymal bridge. Upper pole moiety is subject to obstruction and may simulate an upper pole mass on excretory urography when completely obstructed. Hydronephrosis and hydroureter of the obstructed upper collecting system is readily diagnosed by MRI. Lower pole moiety is subject to vesicoureteral reflux.	In complete renal and ureteral duplication the ureter draining the upper system inserts ectopically medial and below the orthotopic ureter into the bladder trigonum or urethra and may be associated with an ectopic ureterocele. Other congenital renal anomalies include partial duplication, supernumery kidney, and renal hypoplasia or agenesis.

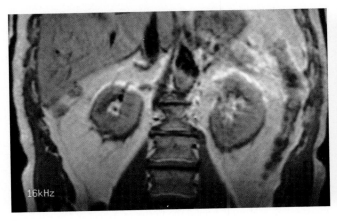 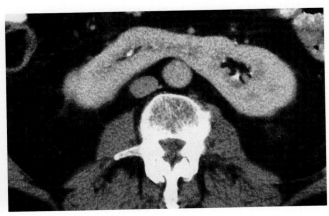

a   b

Fig. 24.2 Horseshoe kidney. **a** Abnormal axis and rotation of both kidneys is evident in the coronal plane (T1WI). **b** Fusion of the lower poles of both kidneys across midline is best appreciated in the axial plane (CT).

Table 24.1 (Cont.)   Focal and diffuse renal disease

Disease	MRI Findings	Comments
Renal sinus lipomatosis (Fig. 24.3)	Extensive proliferation of fat with characteristic high signal intensity on both T1WI and T2WI in the renal sinus associated with loss of renal parenchyma. May result in concentric encroachment of the renal collecting system ("trumpet-like" pelvocaliceal system on intravenous urography) but without obstruction.	Etiology: 1) normal increase of sinus fat with aging and obesity; 2) vicarious proliferation of sinus fat with renal atrophy of any cause; 3) fibrolipomatosis induced by extravasation of urine into the renal sinus (e.g. in chronic prostatism).
Hydronephrosis (Fig. 24.4)	Dilated collecting system with signal characteristics of water is evident within a normal or enlarged kidney on precontrast images. After intravenous Gd-DTPA administration a persistent nephrogram with delayed and decreased contrast medium excretion is characteristic. In chronic obstruction the kidney decreases in size and depicts decreased enhancement, but the collecting system remains dilated. In endstage obstruction the kidney appears as a fluid-filled cyst with a rim of renal tissue draped around it.	Early hydronephrosis can only be differentiated from an extrarenal pelvis and postobstructive uropathy by the persistent nephrogram and delayed urinary Gd-DTPA excretion. Level of obstruction can easily be identified with MRI by following the dilated ureter in the axial plane to the point of obstruction. *Ureteral calculi* are the most frequent cause of obstruction and, regardless of their composition, are signal void on MRI. They are best visualized when the urine is enhanced by Gd-DTPA. Other freely mobile filling defects in the collecting system include *blood clots* and *fungus balls*.
Renal cyst (Fig. 24.5)	Single or multiple well-defined, homogeneous, round lesions of low signal intensity on T1WI and high signal intensity on T2WI. Typically the cyst wall is very thin or not detectable when projecting beyond the renal outline. No enhancement is found after intravenous Gd-DTPA administration. Complicated cysts contain blood, septa, or calcifications. Hemorrhagic cysts frequently are high in signal intensity on both T1WI and T2WI because of methemoglobin formation. They may appear homogeneous, demonstrate a fluid–fluid level or hematocrit effect due to settling of the red blood cells.	Most common renal mass in the adult. Infected cysts usually occur in elderly females, presenting with leukocyturia and a history of unresponsiveness to antibiotic treatment for acute pyelonephritis. On MRI a cystic lesion with thickened irregular wall, internal septation, and inhomogeneous signal intensity may be seen. It may not be possible to differentiate this lesion from an abscess, hematoma, or cystic tumor. Cyst puncture is usually required for a definitive diagnosis.

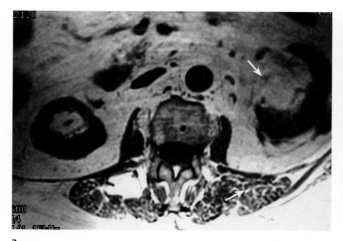

a

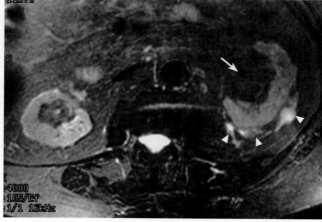

b

Fig. 24.3   Renal sinus lipomatosis. Atrophy of the left renal parenchyma with increased fatty tissue (arrow) in the renal sinus demonstrating high signal intensity in (**a**) (T1WI) and low signal intensity in (**b**) (T2WI, FS). Three small renal cysts (arrowheads) are also present, scattered around the posterior aspect of the left kidney.

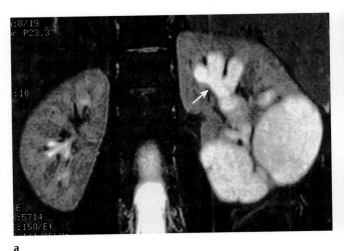

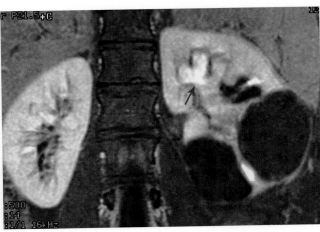

a

b

Fig. 24.**4** **Hydronephrosis and renal cysts.** **a** A dilated upper collecting system (arrow) and two large renal cysts in the lower pole both present with high signal intensity (T2WI, FS, coronal). **b** After intravenous Gd-DTPA administration the hydronephrotic upper collecting system (arrow) enhances, whereas the two renal cysts in the lower pole do not (T1WI, FS, +C, coronal).

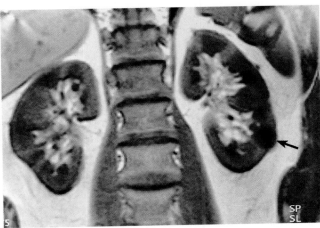

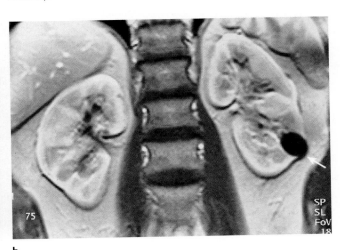

a

b

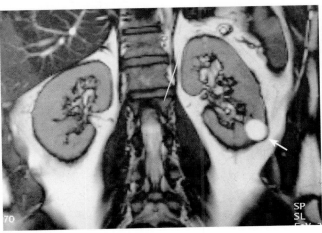

c

Fig. 24.**5** **Renal cyst.** A hypointense lesion (arrow) is seen in the lower pole of the left kidney (**a**: T1WI, coronal). The cyst (arrow) does not enhance and is better delineated after intravenous Gd-DTPA administration (**b**: T1WI, +C) and is hyperintense in **c** (T2WI [GRE], coronal).

Table 24.**1** (Cont.) Focal and diffuse renal disease

Disease	MRI Findings	Comments
Parapelvic cyst (renal sinus cyst)	Features of simple renal cyst, but located in the renal sinus. Differentiation from an ectatic renal pelvis may require intravenous Gd-DTPA administration demonstrating lack of enhancement of the cyst.	Occurs frequently in the fifth and sixth decade of life and is almost always asymptomatic. Very rare complications may include obstructive caliectasis and renal vascular hypertension due to compression of renal arteries.
Autosomal dominant polycystic kidney disease (Fig. 24.6)	Bilateral, often markedly enlarged kidneys with lobulated contours, but often not symmetrically involved. Multiple cysts of varying sizes cause splaying and distorting of the collecting system and characteristically demonstrate varying signal intensity due to blood products of different ages. Unilateral involvement is exceedingly rare.	Also referred to as *adult polycystic kidney disease*. Cysts are often also present in the renal, pancreas, spleen, and lung. Progressive renal failure and hypertension is usually evident in the fourth decade, but occasionally as early as childhood or young adulthood.
Autosomal recessive polycystic kidney disease	Symmetric, slightly enlarged kidneys with numerous tiny cysts (usually 1–2 mm, occasionally larger but always smaller than 1 cm). They represent abnormally proliferated and dilated collecting tubules and do not produce calyceal or renal pelvis distortion. After intravenous Gd-DTPA administration a prolonged and increasingly hyperintense, heterogeneous nephrogram is seen with delayed and decreased urinary contrast medium excretion.	Also referred to as *infantile polycystic kidney disease*. Occurs in neonates and young children below 5 years. Associated with dilated bile ducts, periportal fibrosis, and pancreatic fibrosis. Poor prognosis with death from renal failure or portal hypertension.
Multicystic dysplastic kidney	Unilateral involvement consisting of a small or large single-chamber or multiloculated cystic mass. No functional renal parenchyma is seen after intravenous Gd-DTPA administration (unlike multilocular cystic nephroma or polycystic kidney disease).	Radiographically central or peripheral calcifications are often present. Frequent cause of palpable abdominal mass in an otherwise healthy infant or child, resulting from failed fusion of the metanephros and ureteric bud. Compensatory hypertrophy of the contralateral kidney is normally present, often with an element of ureteropelvic obstruction.
Multilocular cystic nephroma (Fig. 24.7)	Single or multiple fluid-filled cysts measuring up to 10 cm. Cysts are separated by thick septa and are sharply demarcated from the renal parenchyma. Cyst wall and septa enhance after intravenous Gd-DTPA administration. The cyst content is usually hypointense on T1WI and hyperintense on T2WI. Occasionally the cysts depict a high signal intensity on T1WI due to the presence of proteinaceous material or methemoglobin.	Occurs most commonly in boys below 5 years and women between 40 and 70 years. Radiographically peripheral and central calcifications of circular, stellate, flocculent, or granular nature are seen in up to 50% of cases. On ultrasound, multiple cystic masses with highly echogenic septa are characteristic. *Cystic Wilms' tumor* and *cystic renal cell carcinoma* must be differentiated. Nodular thickening of the cyst wall and/or septa may be the clue.
Medullary cystic disease	Bilateral small kidneys with multiple small medullary cysts that do not extend to the renal margins are characteristic.	Rare, usually inherited disorder manifesting itself in adolescents and young adults with progressive renal failure.
Medullary sponge kidney	Bilateral, unilateral, or segmental ectasia of the tubules in often enlarged papillae presenting after intravenous Gd-DTPA administration as tubular structures radiating from the calyx into the papilla.	Usually asymptomatic. In almost half of the cases small calculi measuring up to 5 mm may be present in the ectatic tubules.

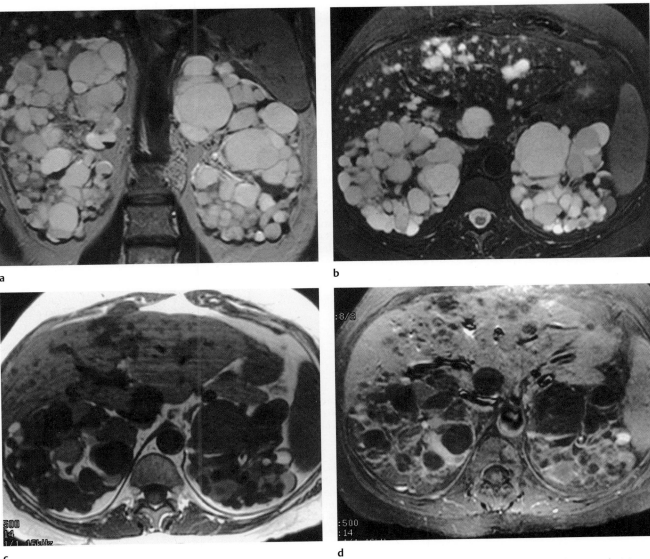

a

b

c

d

Fig. 24.**6** **Autosomal dominant polycystic kidney disease.** Bilateral, markedly enlarged kidneys with multiple cysts of varying sizes are seen presenting with high signal intensity in (**a**) (T2WI, coronal) and (**b**) (T2WI, axial), low signal intensity in (**c**) (T1WI, axial) and no enhancement after intravenous Gd-DTPA administration in (**d**) (T1WI, FS, +C). Multiple hepatic and pancreatic cysts are also present.

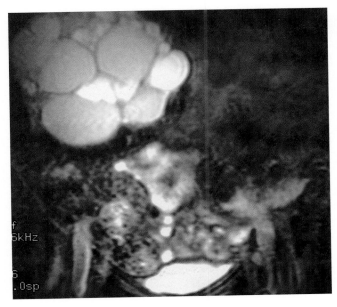

Fig. 24.**7** **Multilocular cystic nephroma.** A multiloculated cystic mass is seen originating from the lower pole of the right kidney (T2WI, coronal).

Table 24.1 (Cont.) Focal and diffuse renal disease

Disease	MRI Findings	Comments
Acquired cystic disease of dialysis (Fig. 24.8)	Small kidneys with largely preserved contours as the cysts, varying from 0.5 to 2 cm in diameter, are mostly intrarenal. Complications include hemorrhage and development of renal adenomas and carcinomas.	Up to 50% of patients on chronic dialysis. Incidence increases with time, particularly after the third year. In 7% of patients renal carcinomas are associated.
Von Hippel–Lindau disease (Fig. 24.9)	Combination of multiple renal cysts and solid tumors (carcinomas, adenomas, and hemangiomas) is characteristic. Renal carcinomas are often small, less than 2 cm in size, and may occur within the cysts themselves. Involvement usually is bilateral and multicentric.	Inherited (autosomal dominance) neurocutaneous dysplasia complex with onset in the second or third decade. Retinal angiomatosis, cerebellar and spinal hemangioblastomas, pheochromocytomas, pancreatic tumors and cysts, and hepatic adenomas and hemangiomas may be associated.
Renal pseudotumor	Focal enlargement of normal renal parenchyma simulating a tumor on other imaging studies. On MRI the mass has all the characteristics of normal renal tissue, including enhancement after intravenous Gd-DTPA administration.	These anomalies include: *Fetal lobations*: cortical bulges centered over corresponding calices. *Dromedary hump*: in the mid-portion of the left kidney due to prolonged pressure by the spleen during fetal development. *Column of Bertin*: focal hypertrophy of the septal cortex in the mid-portion of the kidney causing deformation of the adjacent calices and infundibula. *Hilar lip*: suprahilar and infrahilar cortical bulge above and below the renal sinus. *Nodular compensatory hypertrophy*: hypertrophied normal renal tissue secondary to focal renal scarring.
Renal adenoma (Fig. 24.10)	Solitary or, less commonly, multiple cortical nodules measuring by definition less than 3 cm in diameter. MRI appearance similar to renal cell carcinoma of the same size.	Most common cortical lesion at autopsy. Might be a precursor of a renal cell carcinoma.
Oncocytoma	Solid, noninvasive renal mass averaging 6 cm in diameter (range 1 to 26 cm) and sharply demarcated from the renal cortex. A central stellate scar secondary to infarction and hemorrhage may be seen in larger lesions (greater than 3 cm) and does not enhance after intravenous Gd-DTPA administration.	The majority of lesions are asymptomatic and occur in middle-aged patients with slight male predominance. Histologically this benign tumor may be mistaken for a well-differentiated renal cell carcinoma with oncocytic features.

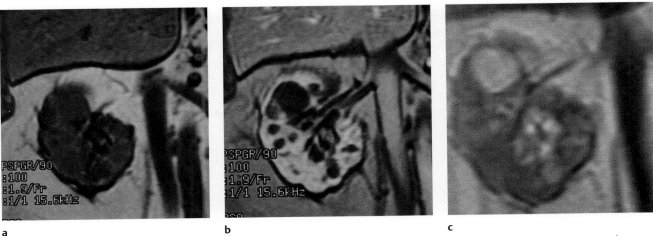

Fig. 24.8 Acquired cystic disease of dialysis. Numerous small intrarenal cysts without distortion of the renal contour are seen (**a**: spoiled GRE, coronal; **b**: spoiled GRE, +C, coronal; **c**: T2WI, coronal).

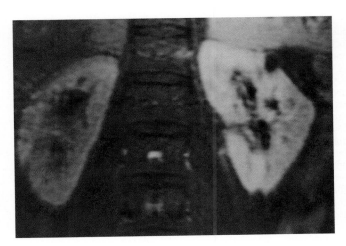

Fig. 24.9 Von Hippel–Lindau disease. Multiple small solid and cystic lesions are seen in the kidneys after intravenous Gd-DTPA administration (T1WI, FS, +C, coronal).

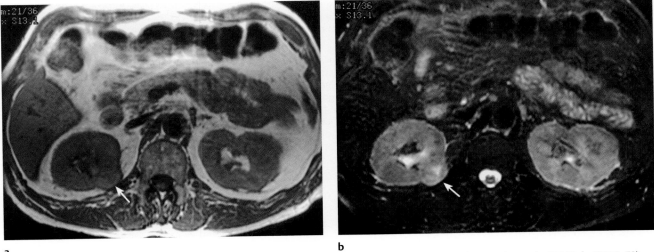

Fig. 24.10 Renal adenoma. A small cortical nodular lesion (arrow) is seen isointense to the renal parenchyma (**a**: T1WI; **b**: T2WI, FS).

Table 24.**1** (Cont.) Focal and diffuse renal disease

Disease	MRI Findings	Comments
Angiomyolipoma (renal hamartoma) (Fig. 24.**11)**	Single or multiple renal masses ranging from 1 to 8 cm in diameter with heterogeneous signal intensity on all sequences depending on the tissue composition of the tumor and the presence of intratumoral hemorrhage. The demonstration of intratumoral fat is virtually diagnostic. After intravenous Gd-DTPA administration inhomogeneous tumor enhancement is seen sparing the fatty tissue and areas of necrosis.	Tumor is composed of blood vessels, smooth muscle, and fat. Radiographically scattered calcifications may be evident in 6% of cases. Occurs as isolated lesion mainly in middle-aged females, often presenting with acute flank pain and macrohematuria after minor trauma, or as renal manifestation of *tuberous sclerosis*, where the lesions commonly are multiple and bilateral. Although the MRI diagnosis of angiomyolipoma is highly specific, occasionally rare tumor such as renal lipomas, liposarcomas, and Wilms' tumors containing small amounts of fatty tissue cannot be absolutely excluded.
Mesenchymal renal tumors	No characteristic features except for the demonstration of fatty tissue in lipomas (see also under angiomyolipoma), the homogeneous low signal intensity of fibromas on all pulse sequences, and the highly inhomogeneous contrast enhancement pattern of cavernous hemangiomas progressing from the periphery (discontinuous nodular ring) to complete enhancement of the lesion with or without its center.	Variety of very rare, benign, or malignant renal tumors.
Renal cell carcinoma (Figs. 24.**12 and** 24.**13)**	Homogeneous or heterogeneous, irregularly shaped, poorly demarcated mass producing an irregular or lobulated contour and distortion of the collecting system. The signal intensity is variable and depends on the degree of tumor vascularity and the presence of hemorrhage and necrosis. In the absence of hemorrhage and necrosis the signal intensity of the tumor tends to be isointense to normal renal parenchyma on both T1WI and T2WI. After intravenous Gd-DTPA administration inhomogeneous enhancement that is more intense in the tumor periphery is usually seen, but homogeneous enhancement may occur in smaller lesions. Compared to the normal surrounding renal parenchyma the tumor overall enhances, however, considerably less. Rarely, renal cell carcinomas are largely to completely cystic. Tumor thrombi in the renal vein and inferior vena cava are isointense to the primary lesion and usually enhance, whereas blood clots do not. On GRE sequences tumor clots depict an intermediate signal intensity, whereas blood clots are usually low in signal due to the presence of hemosiderin. Regional lymph nodes measuring more than 1 cm in diameter are considered abnormal, but the demonstration of a necrotic center is more specific for metastatic involvement.	Most common malignant renal tumor, accounting for 85% of all renal primaries. Twice as frequent in males than females and rare in patients below 40 years (peak age: 55). Gross hematuria (60%) and flank pain (50%) are the most common clinical presentations. Bilateral involvement in 2% of cases. *Robson staging:* I: tumor confined to kidney. II: tumor spread to perinephric fat but confined within renal fascia (MRI cannot reliably differentiate between stages I and II since the renal capsule is not visualized). IIIA: tumor spread to renal vein or cava. IIIB: tumor spread to local lymph nodes. IIIC: tumor spread to both local vessels and lymph nodes. IVA: tumor spread to adjacent organs (except ipsilateral adrenal). IVB: distant metastases.
Renal transitional cell carcinoma	Small tumors may present as smooth or irregular (frond-like), often eccentric filling defects of intermediate signal intensity outlined by urine of low signal intensity on T1WI and of high signal intensity on T2WI. Contrast enhancement of the tumor is only moderate. Larger tumors cause hydronephrosis, obliterate the peripelvic fat, and invade the renal vessels and parenchyma without affecting the renal contour.	Most common uroepithelial tumor (90%), multiple in one-third of cases. Majority are males above 60 years presenting with hematuria and flank pain. *Squamous cell carcinomas* (10%) are frequently associated with preceding chronic renal infection including leukoplakia and renal calculi.

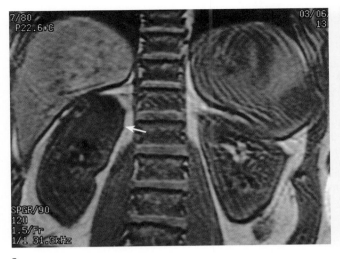

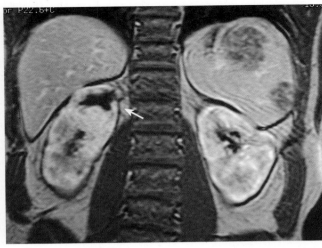

a

b

Fig. 24.**11** **Angiomyolipoma.** **a** A mass (arrow) is seen in the upper pole of the right kidney containing only a small amount of fatty tissue (spoiled GRE, coronal). **b** After intravenous adminis-

tration of Gd-DTPA the lesion (arrow) enhances except for an eccentric necrotic area (spoiled GRE, +C, coronal). Two cavernous hemangiomas are evident in the spleen.

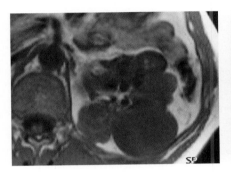

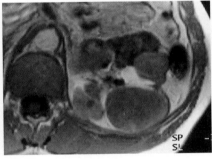

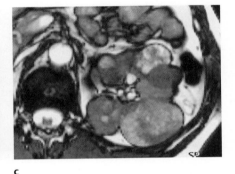

a

b

c

Fig. 24.**12** **Renal cell carcinoma.** A large lobulated mass with variable signal intensity and moderate contrast enhancement is seen in the left kidney. (**a**: T1WI; **b**: T1WI, +C; **c**: T2WI [GRE]).

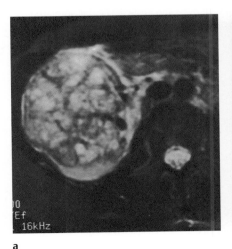

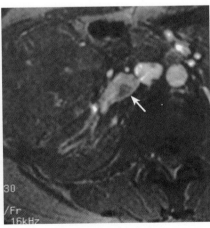

Fig. 24.**13** **Renal cell carcinoma.** **a** A large heterogeneous mass with high signal intensity is seen in the right kidney (T2WI, FS). **b** A tumor thrombus (arrow) of intermediate signal intensity partially occludes the enlarged renal vein (spoiled GRE).

a

b

Table 24.**1** (Cont.) Focal and diffuse renal disease

Disease	MRI Findings	Comments
Wilms' tumor (nephroblastoma) (Figs. 24.14 and 24.14*)	Usually large heterogeneous mass of intermediate signal intensity on T1WI and high signal intensity on T2WI and marked but inhomogeneous contrast enhancement. Focal areas of hemorrhage and necrosis are frequently present. Rarely a large cyst with irregularly thickened wall and septa is the dominant feature. Tumor invasion into the renal vein occurs in one-third of cases. Bilateral involvement occurs in 5%. In the adult the tumor is virtually indistinguishable from a renal cell carcinoma, except for a large central necrosis which is more typical of the latter.	Occurs most often in asymptomatic children between 1 and 5 years, presenting usually with an asymptomatic abdominal mass. Hypertension, hematuria, aniridia, and hemihypertrophy may be associated. Metastases to lungs, lymph nodes, and liver occur. In contrast to neuroblastomas, bone metastases and tumor calcifications are rare. DD: *Mesoblastic nephroma:* benign intrarenal mass in neonates with MRI appearance similar to Wilms' tumor, but without venous extension. *Nephroblastomatosis:* Multiple nodules of primitive metanephric tissue. Benign condition with unilateral or bilateral renal involvement predisposing to the development of Wilms' tumor.
Renal lymphoma (Fig. 24.15)	Homogeneous infiltrate or mass without necrosis. Isointense or slightly hypointense to the renal cortex on T1WI, hypointense on T2WI, and poor contrast enhancement. Bilateral involvement is common with a variety of manifestations: 1) Renal enlargement caused by diffuse infiltration with maintenance of the normal renal contour. 2) Multiple soft-tissue nodules. 3) Solitary intrarenal mass. 4) Retroperitoneal disease extending into the renal pelvis. 5) Compression of the collecting system or vascular structures causing hydronephrosis or a nonfunctioning kidney.	Late manifestation of the disease, caused by hematogenous spread or direct extension from adjacent pararenal lymphomatous tissue. Absence of clinical symptoms in over 50% of patients. *Leukemia* can also produce bilateral renal enlargement due to diffuse infiltration or intrarenal masses (chloromas).
Renal metastases (Fig. 24.16)	Usually multiple, bilateral renal nodules, or, less commonly, a solitary renal lesion with variable signal intensity and contrast enhancement corresponding to the primary tumor. Metastases are usually small and do not distort the renal contour or the collecting system.	Most common renal malignancy at autopsy, but infrequently diagnosed ante mortem. Lung and breast carcinomas are the most common primaries, but stomach, colon, pancreas, cervix, gonads, melanomas, and sarcomas are other sites of origin.
Pyelonephritis (acute)	Renal involvement may be diffuse or, more commonly, focal. Affected kidney or lobe may depict edematous swelling, loss of corticomedullary differentiation on T1WI, inflammation of the adjacent perinephric fat, and thickening of the renal fascia. After intravenous administration of Gd-DTPA a diminished and prolonged nephrogram with inhomogeneous, often streaky appearance extending from the papilla to the periphery or even wedge-shaped defects are seen.	Most commonly an ascending *E coli* infection presenting with fever, chills, and flank pain. Hematogenous route of infection accounts for 15% of cases. May occur at any age with marked female predisposition. Presents with fever, chills, and flank pain. Diabetics are at particularly high risk. *Chronic atrophic pyelonephritis* (Fig. 24.17) is usually associated with vesicoureteral reflux. Calyceal dilatation with overlying cortical scarring, preferentially located in the polar regions, is characteristic.

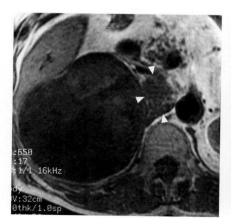

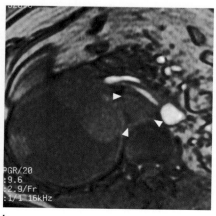

Fig. 24.**14 Wilms' tumor. a** A large, relatively homogeneous mass is seen in the right kidney with extension into the right renal hilum (arrowheads) (T1WI). **b** The hilar extension of the tumor (arrowheads) causes extrinsic compression and anterior displacement of the right renal vein and inferior vena cava without invasion (spoiled GRE).

a   b

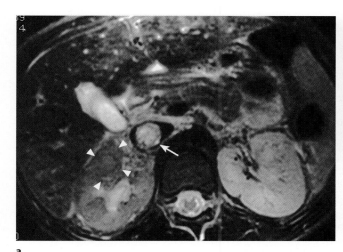

a

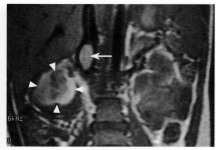

b

Fig. 24.**14*** **Wilms' tumor.**
A heterogeneous mass (arrowheads) with variable signal intensity is seen in the right kidney with a tumor thrombus (arrows) of the same signal intensity extending into the right renal vein in (**a**) (T2WI, axial) and the inferior vena cava in (**b**) (T1WI, coronal).

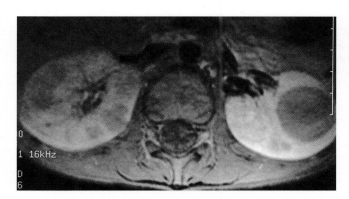

Fig. 24.**15** **Renal non-Hodgkin lymphoma.** Bilateral enlarged kidneys with well to poorly defined homogeneous lesions of intermediate signal intensity, but hypointense compared to the enhanced kidneys are seen after intravenous Gd-DTPA administration (T1WI, FS, +C).

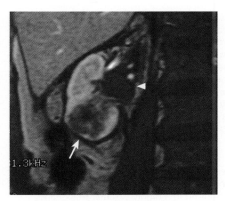

Fig. 24.**16** **Renal metastasis from bronchogenic carcinoma.** An inhomogeneously enhancing, hypointense lesion (arrow) is seen in the lower pole of the right kidney after intravenous Gd-DTPA administration (T1WI, FS, +C, coronal). The nonenhancing, homogeneous, hypointense lesion (arrowhead) in the renal pelvis represents an obstructed collecting system.

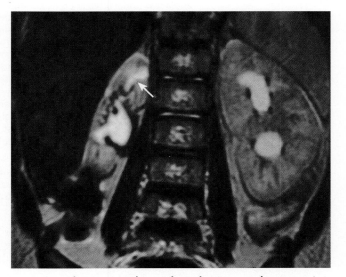

Fig. 24.**17** **Chronic atrophic pyelonephritis secondary to vesicoureteral reflux.** A markedly shrunken right kidney with dilated collecting system including the right upper pole calyx (arrow) is seen. Dilation of the left collecting system is also caused by vesicoureteral reflux (T2WI, coronal).

Table 24.**1** (Cont.) Focal and diffuse renal disease

Disease	MRI Findings	Comments
Renal abscess (Fig. 24.18)	Cavitating mass with thick irregular wall and liquified center, presenting with heterogeneous signal intensity simulating a necrotic neoplasm. Inflammation of the adjacent perinephric fat is usually more conspicuous in abscess than tumor and often associated with thickening of the renal fascia. Demonstration of gas (signal void) as bubbles or gas–fluid level is diagnostic but rarely present. After intravenous administration of Gd-DTPA the marked enhancement is limited to the abscess wall.	Usually a complication of acute pyelonephritis, often associated with ureteral obstruction. Hematogenous abscesses (20%) may be bacterial, tuberculous, or fungal and most frequently originate from pulmonary infections or endocarditis. May be found with intravenous drug abuse. Are occasionally multiple.
Xanthogranulomatous pyelonephritis	Diffuse or, much less commonly, focal renal enlargement of mixed heterogeneous signal intensity with lobulated contour and frequent extension into the perinephric space and adjacent organs. A large central calculus devoid of signal and a pyonephrotic collecting system, which may be distorted or partially replaced by inflammatory masses, are characteristically present. After intravenous Gd-DTPA administration the single or multiple masses depict inhomogeneous, but overall poor enhancement. Urinary Gd-DTPA excretion is poor or absent.	Chronic suppurative granulomatous infection in a chronically obstructed kidney (usually due to nephrourolithiasis, occasionally by stricture or tumor). The majority of cases are associated with proteus infections. All ages may be affected (peak fourth to fifth decade) with a 3:1 female predominance. Involvement is diffuse (90%) or focal (tumefactive form).
Renal hematoma	Signal intensity varies with stage (*acute*: low on T1WI, high on T2WI, decreases with intracellular deoxygemoglin formation; *subacute*: high on T1WI and T2WI; *chronic*: low on T1WI and T2WI). No enhancement occurs after intravenous Gd-DTPA unless acutely bleeding. *Intrarenal* (renal contusion): poorly defined focus of abnormal signal intensity and loss of corticomedullary differentiation on T1WI. *Subcapsular*: lenticular lesion compressing the renal parenchyma medially and bulging the renal capsule laterally.	Renal biopsies, extracorporeal shock-wave lithotripsy and trauma are common causes. Spontaneous hematomas in the absence of bleeding diathesis should raise suspicion of an underlying malignancy or angiomyolipoma. Classification of renal trauma: 1) Limited to renal parenchyma: renal contusion or subcapsular hematoma without disruption of calyceal system and renal capsule. 2) Complete laceration or renal fracture with involvement of renal capsule and/or calyceal system. 3) Shattered kidney (multiple separate renal fragments) or injury to the renal vascular pedicle.
Renal ischemia and infarction (Fig. 24.19)	Thromboembolism in the renal artery or vein displays a high signal intensity on SE sequences that is contrasted by the flow void of circulating blood and a low signal intensity on GRE sequences as opposed to the high signal intensity of flowing blood. Acute ischemia results in a normal or slightly enlarged kidney, whereas a chronic ischemic kidney is small with smooth contours. After intravenous Gd-DTPA administration diminished enhancement and persistence of the corticomedullary differentiation is seen in ischemia. Renal infarcts from embolic events tend to occur between calyces and produce a well-defined wedge-shaped peripheral defect. In total renal artery occlusion the contrast enhancement is limited to a peripheral rim supplied by the capsular arteries.	Renal infarction may be secondary to trauma (avulsion or occlusion of renal artery), embolism (originating from the heart, aorta, or catheters), thrombosis (arteriosclerosis or vasculitis), or sudden complete renal vein thrombosis. *Renal vein thrombosis* develops in association with nephrotic syndrome, glomerulonephritis, dehydration (especially in infants), sepsis, trauma, extrinsic compression, and tumor invasion. Most often renal vein thrombosis develops gradually and remains asymptomatic. In acute renal vein thrombosis a markedly enlarged edematous and hemorrhagic kidney is seen on MRI besides the thrombosis.
Arteriovenous malformation (AVM)	Intrarenal mass with large feeding and draining vessel depicting a flow void on SE sequences and enhancement equal to the aorta after intravenous Gd-DTPA administration is diagnostic.	May be congenital or acquired (trauma, biopsy, or spontaneous rupture of an aneurysm). Arteriovenous shunting in a highly vascular malignancy must be differentiated. Intrarenal *aneurysm* or *pseudoaneurysm* also produce a flow void on SE sequences unless the blood flow in them is sluggish or the lesions are thrombosed.

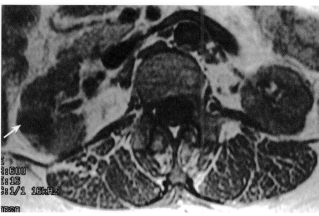

a

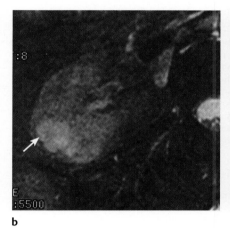

b

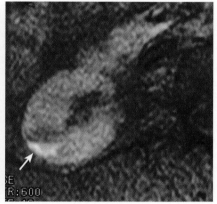

c

Fig. 24.**18** **Renal abscess.** Bilaterally shrunken kidneys due to lupus nephritis are seen. In the right lower pole a poorly marginated hypointense focus (arrow) is seen in (**a**) (T1WI), which becomes hyperintense in (**b**) (T2WI, FS) and depicts a fluid level in (**c**) (spoiled GRE). Note also the complete loss of corticomedullary junction.

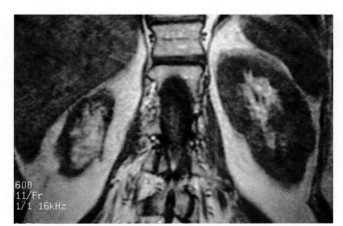

Fig. 24.**19** **Chronic renal infarction.** Symmetrically shrunken right kidney with compensatory increase in renal sinus fat is seen (T1WI, coronal).

Table 24.2 Focal lesions in the perinephric space

Disease	MRI Findings	Comments
Perinephric lipoma and fibroma (Fig. 24.20)	Small, homogeneous, well-circumscribed lesions originating from the perinephric fat or renal capsule or fascia. Lipomas depict high signal intensity and fibromas low signal intensity on both T1WI and T2WI.	Usually incidental findings. Benign mesenchymal tumors are even rarer than their malignant counterparts.
Perinephric liposarcomas	Variable appearance ranging from a predominantly fatty, somewhat heterogeneous mass with irregularly thickened linear or nodular septa (well-differentiated liposarcoma) to a cystic lesion (myxoid liposarcoma). Larger tumors tend to displace rather than invade the renal parenchyma and have a smooth interface.	Most common mesenchymal sarcoma originating from the perinephric fat or renal capsule and fascia. Other rare primary perinephric malignancies include *malignant fibrous histiocytomas, leiomyosarcoma,* and *angiosarcoma.*
Perinephric metastases and lymphoma	Signal intensity and contrast enhancement correspond to the primary lesion.	Usually direct extension or local metastases from primary renal and adrenal malignancies. Rarely hematogenesis or lymphangitic spread from more distant organs.
Perinephric hematoma (Fig. 24.21)	Well to poorly defined mass that may displace the adjacent kidney. Acute hematomas are of low signal intensity on T1WI and of high or intermediate (deoxyhemoglobin) signal intensity on T2WI. Subacute hematomas depict a hyperintense periphery on both T1WI and T2WI, with heterogeneous increase in signal intensity centrally over the following weeks, especially on T1WI. Chronic hematomas develop a low signal peripheral rim (secondary to hemosiderin deposition and fibrosis), more prominent on T2WI than T1WI, around a central region of high signal intensity.	Traumatic causes include blunt or penetrating trauma, renal biopsy, percutaneous nephrostomy and nephrolithotomy, and extracorporeal shock-wave lithotripsy. Nontraumatic causes include nephritis, arteritis, lupus, polyarteritis nodosa, acquired cystic disease of dialysis, renal tumors, blood dyscrasia, anticoagulation, and aneurysms of the renal artery or abdominal aorta.
Perinephric urinoma (See Fig. 24.20)	Localized or diffuse cystic lesion of low signal intensity on T1WI and high signal intensity on T2WI (similar to urine). Gadolinium extravasation into the fluid collection may be seen on late images after intravenous Gd-DTPA administration. Large urinomas may dissect along tissue planes into the pelvis.	Small urinomas may resolve spontaneously within 3 to 4 days. Larger urinomas may induce a fibroblastic encapsulation within 3 to 6 weeks. Caused by tear in the collecting system with continuing renal function. Tear may be traumatic, iatrogenic, or infectious (nonobstructive urinoma) or caused by ureteral or bladder outlet obstruction.
Perinephric lymphocele	Homogeneous cystic, occasionally septated lesion of low to intermediate signal intensity on T1WI and high signal intensity on T2WI.	Develops usually 2 weeks or later after lymph node dissection.
Perinephric abscess (Fig. 24.22)	Poorly defined, heterogeneous mass of low to intermediate signal intensity on T1WI and high signal intensity on T2WI. Surrounding edema and inflammation in the perinephric space may extend to the renal fascia. Gas presenting as bubbles devoid of signal or air–fluid levels within the lesion is virtually diagnostic, but only rarely present. After intravenous Gd-DTPA administration enhancement of the abscess wall sparing the necrotic or liquified center is characteristic.	Usually an extension of underlying renal disease, especially a concomitant renal abscess. Diabetes mellitus and nephrourolithiasis are common predisposing factors. Other inflammatory conditions such as pancreatitis, diverticulitis, and appendicitis may also spread into the perinephric space.

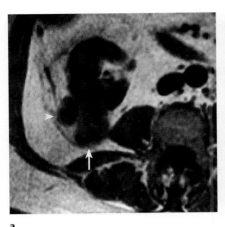
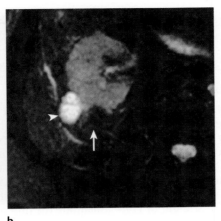

a **b**

Fig. 24.**20** **Perinephric fibroma and urinoma.** Two small round lesions are seen in the posterior perinephric space. The more posterior lesion (arrow) is of low signal intensity in both (**a**) (T1WI) and (**b**) (T2WI, FS), demonstrates minimal contrast enhancement (not shown), and is consistent with a fibroma originating from the renal capsule. The second more anterior lesion (arrowhead) is of low signal intensity in (**a**) and high signal intensity in (**b**), did not enhance, and is consistent with a small urinoma.

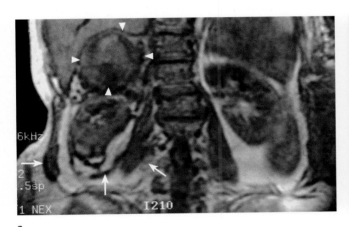
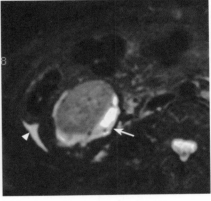

a **b**

Fig. 24.**21** **Perinephric hematoma.** **a** Rupture of a pheochromocytoma (arrowheads) resulted in perinephric and paranephric hemorrhage (arrows), evident as irregularly decreased signal intensity in the corresponding spaces (T1WI, coronal). **b** The hemorrhage presenting with increased signal intensity is seen in the perinephric space (arrow) and right paracolic gutter (arrowhead) (T2WI, FS, axial).

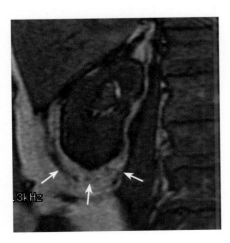

Fig. 24.**22** **Perinephric abscess.** Extension of a right kidney abscess into the posterior perinephric space is evident by an irregular and poorly defined decrease in signal intensity (arrows) in the perinephric fat (T1WI, coronal).

25 Adrenal Glands

Adrenal glands are small retroperitoneal structures located lateral to the spine at the level of the eleventh and twelfth rib and embedded in the perinephric fat that separates the kidney from the anterior (Gerota) and posterior (Zuckerkandl) renal (perirenal) fascia. On axial MRI normal adrenals extend 2–4 cm in a caudocranial direction and display a variety of shapes. The limbs of the adrenal glands have a uniform thickness of 5–8 mm with straight or concave margins. A limb thickness of 10 mm is highly suggestive of adrenal disease, with the exception of sites where two limbs converge.

On axial images the right adrenal gland usually has an oblique linear configuration, paralleling the crus of the diaphragm, and rarely an inverted V, an inverted Y, and X, H, or triangular shape. The right adrenal usually lies 1–2 cm superior to the cranial pole of the right kidney and immediately posterior to the inferior vena cava. The right adrenal is also sandwiched between the right crus of the diaphragm medially and the right lobe of the liver laterally.

The left adrenal most often has an inverted V or an inverted Y shape and occasionally assumes a triangular shape on axial images. The left adrenal lies lateral to the crus of the left diaphragm and posterior and slightly medial to the tail of the pancreas and the stomach. The lower portion of the left adrenal may be in contact with the anteromedial aspect of the upper pole of the left kidney. The left adrenal is generally slightly caudal to the right adrenal.

On MRI the normal adrenal appears as a homogeneous structure of low to intermediate signal intensity on all pulse sequences. The signal intensity difference between adrenal gland and surrounding fat is greater on T1WI than T2WI. With proper technique normal adrenals can be visualized in virtually every case.

Differentiation of adrenal metastases from benign adenomas remains a challenge. On T2WI metastases usually have a higher signal intensity than adenomas, but a significant overlap exists. Fat suppression techniques further facilitate the differentiation between these two conditions. The approach that appears to be most promising is the combined use of an in-phase and out-of-phase gradient echo (GRE) technique. This chemical shift imaging method allows assessment of the intracellular fat content. Benign adenoma containing intracytoplasmic lipids (steroids) lose signal on out-of-phase images. Metastases do not contain intracytoplasmic lipids and thus do not lose signal on out-of-phase images. However, adenomas that do not contain lipids in sufficient quantities and other benign masses cannot be differentiated from metastases with this technique.

After intravenous administration of Gd-DTPA, metastases enhance to a greater extent and retain the contrast medium for a longer period than benign adenomas. However, because of the substantial variability in the vascularity of metastases ranging from hypovascular to hypervascular, benign and malignant lesions cannot reliably be differentiated based on their difference in contrast medium uptake and washout rates. When the combination of various MRI techniques is inconclusive in the assessment of adrenal metastatic disease, CT-guided biopsy must be considered if clinically indicated.

The differential diagnosis of focal and diffuse adrenal enlargement is discussed in Table 25.1.

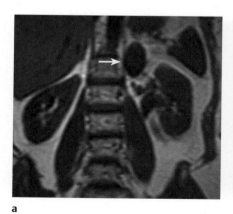
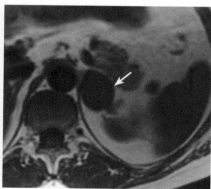
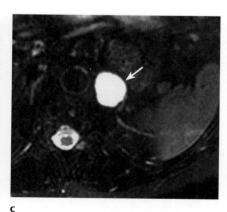

a   b   c

Fig. 25.**1** **Hemorrhagic pseudocyst.** A homogeneous adrenal lesion (arrow) is seen, which is hypointense in (**a**) (T1WI, coronal) and (**b**) (T1WI, axial) and very bright in (**c**) (T2WI, FS, axial).

Table 25.1 Focal or diffuse adrenal enlargement

Disease	MRI Findings	Comments
Adrenal pseudotumors	Normal anatomic structures can simulate an adrenal mass, especially on the left side. Such structures include medial lobulation of the spleen, accessory spleen, outpouching of adjacent stomach or small bowel, and colonic interposition between kidney and liver. A normal adrenal gland can be found in these conditions.	Vascular structures including tortuous renal vessels, tortuous splenic artery, and portosystemic venous collaterals in portal hypertension (e.g. spontaneous splenorenal shunt) are differentiated from an adrenal lesion by their signal characteristics (signal void on SE sequences). Tumors arising from the kidneys, liver, pancreas, or retroperitoneum can mimic a primary adrenal mass.
Adrenal cyst and pseudocyst (Fig. 25.1)	Small to very large, usually unilateral, round lesion with smooth homogeneous well-defined contour; low signal intensity on T1WI, high signal intensity on T2WI, no contrast enhancement. Hemorrhagic pseudocysts depict a variable signal intensity on T1WI and T2WI depending on the stage of blood degradation.	Rare. True cysts are endothelial (e.g. lymphangiomatous or angiomatous), epithelial, or parasitic in origin. Rim calcification is unusual except in echinococcal cysts. Pseudocysts are more common and result from adrenal hemorrhage or necrosis. Rim calcifications are relatively common in hemorrhagic pseudocysts.
Adrenal cortical hyperplasia (Fig. 25.2)	Diffuse homogeneous bilateral adrenal enlargement with preservation of the normal glandular shape. Hyperplastic glands usually have a smooth outline and normal signal intensity on T1WI and T2WI. Less commonly the enlarged adrenals may have a nodular or lumpy appearance with nodules up to 2 cm in diameter (macronodular hyperplasia).	Cushing syndrome (hypercortisolism) is caused by bilateral adrenal cortical hyperplasia in 80%, but in one-third of the cases the adrenals are normal by CT or MRI criteria. The syndrome is four times more common in females, with the highest incidence between 20 and 40 years of age. *Conn syndrome* (primary aldosteronism) presents in 20% of cases with bilateral nodular adrenal hyperplasia and is characterized by mild hypertension, hypokalemia, sodium retention, and reduced plasma renin levels. *Congenital adrenal cortical hyperplasia* (inborn block of adrenal cortical steroid production) causes in utero virilization of females and precocious puberty in males. Adrenal hyperplasia may also be found in systemic illness, acromegaly, hyperthyroidism, hypertension, diabetes, and malignant disease.

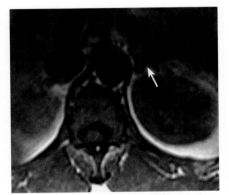

Fig. 25.2 Adrenal cortical hyperplasia.
A slightly enlarged, nodular adrenal gland (arrow) is seen (T1WI). The histologic diagnosis was micronodular hyperplasia in Conn syndrome.

Table 25.1 (Cont.) Focal or diffuse adrenal enlargement

Disease	MRI Findings	Comments
Adrenal cortical adenoma (Fig. 25.3)	Usually unilateral homogeneous mass measuring 2–4 cm in diameter of low to intermediate signal intensity similar to normal adrenal tissue. On T2WI adenomas usually are isointense to the liver. After intravenous Gd-DTPA administration the enhancement typically is mild to moderate and the contrast washout is rapid. The most characteristic feature is loss of signal with fat suppression techniques such as out-of-phase GRE images, in which the loss of signal in the lesion parallels the loss of signal in the bone marrow of the adjacent vertebral body and corresponds to the intracellular lipid content of the adenoma. Bilateral in 10% of cases.	Most common adrenal mass and most frequently nonhyperfunctioning and incidentally diagnosed. Increased occurrence in elderly, obese, or hypertensive patients or with carcinomas of the bladder, kidney, or endometrium. Hyperfunctioning adrenal adenomas are responsible for 15% of cases with Cushing syndrome. *Aldosteronomas* (Fig. 25.4) are responsible for 80% of Conn syndrome. The tumor averages less than 2 cm in diameter (range 0.5–3.5 cm) and is located twice as frequently on the left than the right side. Compared with nonhyperfunctioning adenomas its signal intensity is typically increased on T2WI.
Pheochromocytoma (Figs. 25.5, 25.6)	Usually unilateral large heterogeneous soft-tissue mass measuring 3–12 cm in diameter, with low signal intensity on T1WI and high signal intensity on T2WI (hyperintense to liver). Marked contrast enhancement with slow washout is seen after intravenous Gd-DTPA administration. Hemorrhage and central necrosis are commonly present in larger tumors and may progress to a cystic pheochromocytoma that may be difficult to differentiate from a true cyst or pseudocyst.	Secretion of high amounts of catecholamines results in paroxysmal attacks characterized by hypertension, diaphoresis, tachycardia, and anxiety. Elevated urinary metanephrine and vanillylmandelic acid levels are characteristic. Approximately 10% are bilateral, 10% malignant, 10% extra-adrenal (organ of Zuckerkandl at origin of inferior mesenteric artery, para-aortic sympathetic chain, gonads, urinary bladder, and mediastinum), and 10% familial (associated with Sipple or MEN II syndrome, mucosal neuroma or MEN III syndrome, von Hippel–Lindau syndrome, or neurofibromatosis). Radiographically calcifications are present in almost 10% of cases.
Myelolipoma (Fig. 25.7)	Unilateral, usually small lesion with high signal intensity on both T1WI and T2WI. Rarely large tumors measuring up to 12 cm in diameter are encountered. Foci of calcifications are seen as areas of signal void within the tumor in 20% of cases. Less commonly, the tumor displays soft-tissue signal characteristics with small regions of fatty tissue.	Rare benign asymptomatic tumor consisting of myeloid (megakaryocytes), and erythroid elements and mature fat cells. Flank or abdominal pain may develop secondary to hemorrhage (retroperitoneal) or necrosis.

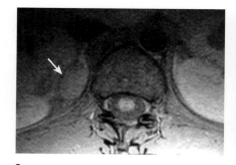 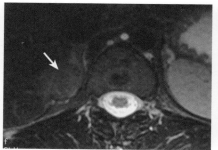 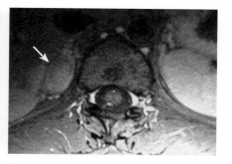

a   b   c

Fig. 25.3 **Adrenal cortical adenoma (nonhyperfunctioning).** An enlarged hypointense adrenal is seen in (**a**) (T1WI) and (**b**) (T2WI, FS). After intravenous Gd-DTPA administration only slight contrast enhancement is evident in (**c**) (T1WI, FS, +C).

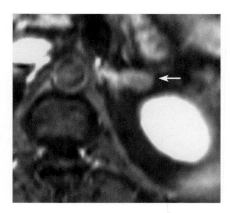

Fig. 25.**4** **Aldosteronoma.** Considerable contrast enhancement is seen in the small left adrenal lesion after intravenous Gd-DTPA administration (T1WI, FS, +C).

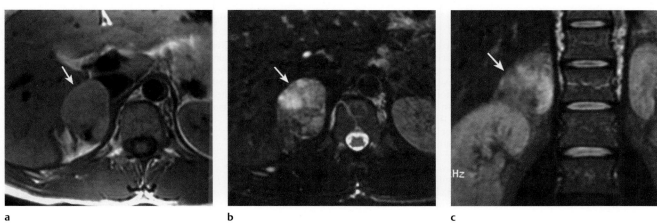

a   b   c

Fig. 25.**5** **Pheochromocytoma.** A right adrenal mass (arrow) is seen with homogeneous intermediate signal intensity in (**a**) (T1WI, axial) and heterogeneous high signal intensity in (**b**) (T2WI, FS, axial) and (**c**) (T2WI, FS, coronal).

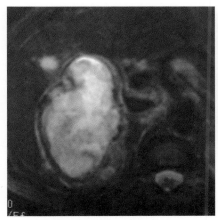

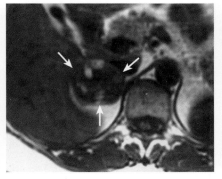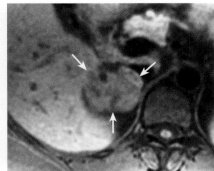

a   b

Fig. 25.**7** **Myelolipoma.** A right adrenal mass (arrows) is seen with small foci of fatty tissue appearing hyperintense in (**a**) (T1WI) and hypointense in (**b**) (T1WI, FS).

Fig. 25.**6** **Pheochromocytoma with intratumoral hemorrhage.** A large adrenal mass with heterogeneous and markedly increased signal intensity is seen (T2WI, FS).

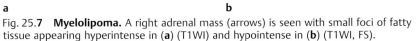

Table 25.**1** (Cont.) Focal or diffuse adrenal enlargement

Disease	MRI Findings	Comments
Mesenchymal adrenal tumors	MRI findings not characteristic (hypointense on T1WI and hyperintense on T2WI), except for the low signal intensity of fibromas on all pulse sequences and the contrast enhancement pattern of cavernous hemangiomas (peripheral discontinuous ring of nodules immediately after intravenous Gd-DTPA administration).	Extremely rare. Besides hemangiomas and fibromas other lesions occur such as lymphangiomas, neurofibromas, myomas, and hamartomas as well as their malignant counterparts.
Neuroblastoma (Fig. 25.8)	Unilateral, usually large, heterogeneous mass of intermediate signal intensity on T1WI and high signal intensity on T2WI. Marked inhomogeneous enhancement occurs after intravenous Gd-DTPA administration. Punctate to coarse calcifications are present in up to 50% of cases, but frequently are difficult to appreciate by MRI as foci of signal void. Invasion of the kidney and retroperitoneum with extension across the midline and encasement of the inferior vena cava, aorta, and its major vessels is quite characteristic in the advanced stage.	Approximately 80% occur in children below 3 years. Vanillylmandelic acid and homovanillic acid in urine is characteristic. Metastases (bone 60%, lymph nodes 40%, liver 15%, intracranial 14%, and lungs 10%) are already present in the majority of children at the time of diagnosis. Histologic spectrum ranges from the highly malignant *sympathicogonioma* to the relatively benign *ganglioneuroma*. *Adult neuroblastoma* is rare, extra-adrenal sites are more frequent (e.g., mediastinum, retroperitoneum, and pelvis), and calcifications are uncommon.
Adrenal cortical carcinoma (Fig. 25.9)	Unilateral heterogeneous mass with low signal intensity on T1WI and high signal intensity on T2WI, usually measuring more than 5 cm in diameter at time of diagnosis. Tumor diameter in excess of 10 cm is common. Inhomogeneous contrast enhancement with delayed washout is seen after intravenous Gd-DTPA administration. Frequent complications, especially in larger lesions, include tumoral hemorrhage (hyperintense on T1WI) and central necrosis (absent central contrast enhancement). Functional carcinomas may lose signal intensity on out-of-phase GRE images. The lack of uniform loss of signal intensity may differentiate these tumors from adenomas.	Radiographically dystrophic calcification is occasionally seen. Occurs at any age and presents commonly with abdominal pain and palpable mass. About 50% of adrenal cortical carcinomas are hormonally active (twice as common in females) and patients may develop Cushing syndrome.

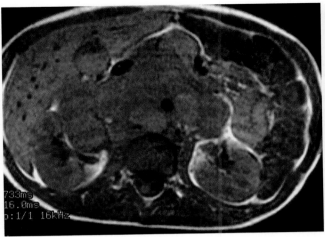
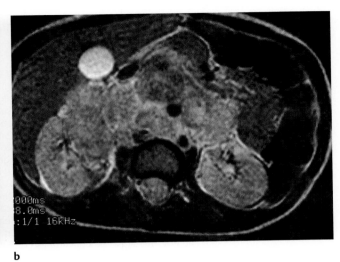

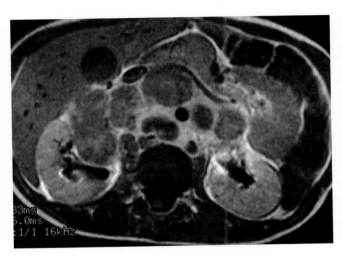

Fig. 25.**8** **Neuroblastoma.** A bulky abdominal mass is seen extending from the right kidney across the midline to the left kidney and almost reaching the anterior abdominal wall. The heterogeneous mass demonstrates low signal intensity in (**a**) (T1WI), high signal intensity in (**b**) (T2WI), and considerable, but inhomogeneous contrast enhancement in (**c**) (T1WI, +C).

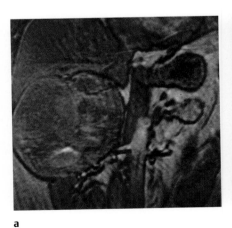
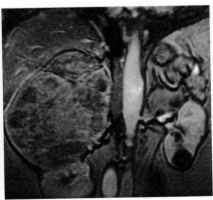

Fig. 25.**9** **Adrenal cortical carcinoma.** **a** A large, relatively well-defined, heterogeneous mass is seen between the right kidney and liver (spoiled GRE, coronal). **b** Inhomogeneous enhancement of the lesion occurs after intravenous Gd-DTPA administration. Note also the small renal cyst in the lower pole of the left kidney (T1WI, FS, +C, coronal).

Table 25.1 (Cont.) Focal or diffuse adrenal enlargement

Disease	MRI Findings	Comments
Adrenal metastases (Figs. 25.**10**, 25.**11**)	Unilateral or bilateral. Usually relatively small lesions, but may attain any size. Signal intensity is variable but usually low on T1WI and high on T2WI. The signal intensity of metastases is usually similar to the primary tumor or other metastatic deposits, provided they are of comparable size. Small metastases appear to be homogeneous, but with increase in size intratumoral hemorrhage and necrosis occur more frequently. Marked contrast enhancement with delayed washout is typical after intravenous Gd-DTPA administration. Direct extension occurs from renal and pancreatic carcinomas. Small adrenal metastases can be differentiated from adrenal adenomas by the fact that metastases do not lose signal on out-of-phase GRE images.	Hematogenous adrenal metastases originate in order of decreasing frequency from carcinomas of the lung, breast, gastrointestinal tract, or thyroid and melanomas. A small adrenal mass in a tumor patient is, however, more likely an adenoma than metastatic deposit. Primary *adrenal lymphoma* is exceedingly rare and of the non-Hodgkin variety. In secondary lymphoma retroperitoneal lymphadenopathy is usually present. Adrenal lymphoma depicts low to intermediate signal intensity on T1WI and intermediate to high signal intensity on T2WI. Contrast enhancement is variable but usually minimal.
Adrenal granulomas	Unilateral or, more commonly, bilateral adrenal enlargement. Signal intensity varies with stage of disease. Granulomas without necrosis and calcifications tend to be hypointense on T1WI and hyperintense on T2WI. Central necrosis increases the signal intensity on T2WI. Granulomas with extensive calcifications and fibrosis present with low signal intensity on all pulse sequences. Contrast enhancement is usually rather modest.	Tuberculosis, histoplasmosis, and blastomycosis are the most frequent infectious sources. *Adrenal abscesses* are rare in adults but occur more frequently in neonates secondary to meningococcal infections. *Addison disease* (adrenal insufficiency) may be a late sequela of granulomatous disease, especially histoplasmosis. Autoimmune disease (idiopathic) or pituitary insufficiency are, however, the most common causes.
Adrenal hemorrhage (See Figs. 25.**1**, 25.**6**)	Unilateral or bilateral mass, usually not exceeding 3 cm in diameter. With time the lesion decreases in size and displays change in signal intensity. In the acute stage the hematoma is hypointense on T1WI and hyperintense on T2WI. In the subacute stage an increased signal intensity is seen in both T1WI and T2WI due to methemoglobin formation. The hemorrhage may appear as an area of low signal intensity on all pulse sequences after fibrosis, hemosiderin deposition and/or calcifications develop.	Secondary to autocoagulation, bleeding diathesis, sepsis, shock, trauma, surgery, and pregnancy. Posttraumatic adrenal hemorrhage occurs on the right side in 85% of cases. Right adrenal hemorrhage is also a complication of liver transplantation. Bilateral involvement may result in acute adrenal insufficiency that is potentially fatal. If not fatal, Addison disease may be a late sequela. In the neonate adrenal hemorrhage may be associated with birth trauma, hypoxia (prematurity), septicemia, and bleeding disorders.

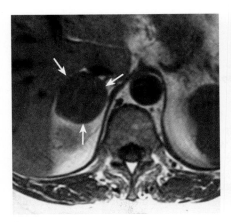

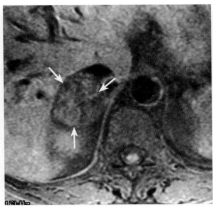

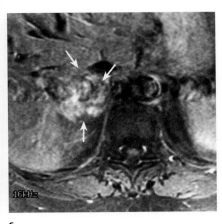

a

b

c

Fig. 25.**10** **Adrenal metastasis (broncho-genic carcinoma).** An enlarged right adrenal (arrows) is seen demonstrating ho- mogeneous and low signal intensity in (**a**) (T1WI), heterogeneous and increased sig- nal intensity in (**b**) (T1WI, FS), and con- siderable inhomogeneous contrast en- hancement in (**c**) (T1WI, FS, +C).

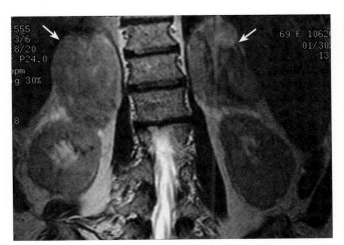

Fig. 25.**11** **Adrenal metastases (breast carcinoma).** Huge bilateral adrenal metastases (arrows) are seen, which are isointense to the kidneys (T2WI, coronal).

26 Pelvis

The boundaries of the pelvis are defined by the osseous ring formed by the innominate bones and sacrum. Lesions within the pelvic cavity may arise from this bony framework or its attached muscles, but will not be covered here since they have been discussed in detail in Tables 9.2 and 12.1 of the musculoskeletal section. The pelvis is also the most dependent portion of the peritoneal cavity. Its peritoneal reflections delineate the midline cul-de-sac or pouch of Douglas (rectovesical pouch in males and rectovaginal pouch in females) and the lateral paravesical recesses. Besides ascites, intraperitoneal spread of infections and tumors consistently seek the pouch of Douglas, the most caudal and posterior part of the peritoneal cavity. These disease processes have been covered in Table 22.1. This chapter is limited to the MRI anatomy and pathology of the internal pelvic organs.

T1WI provides, similar to CT, a high contrast between internal pelvic organs and surrounding fat. It is well suited to display the pelvic anatomy, assess tumor extension into the adjacent fat, and detect lymphadenopathy. T2-weighted pulse sequences depict the morphology of internal pelvic organs and are essential for the delineation and staging of tumors still limited to the involved organ.

The normal *urinary bladder* wall consists of the mucosa, lamina propria, and detrusor muscle. Normal mucosa and lamina propria are not visualized by MRI. On T2WI the bladder wall may depict an inner dark layer, a central intermediate layer, and an outer dark layer, all of which are believed to reside within the detrusor muscle. This difference is caused by the less dense packing of the central muscle fibers as opposed to more densely packed inner and outer muscle fibers.

The *rectum* depicts five layers with alternating high and low signal intensity on T2WI. The bright inner layer of the bowel represents luminal fluid and mucus coating the mucosal surface. The actual bowel wall consists of the mucosa presenting as a hypointense thin line, a brighter submucosa, a hypointense muscularis propria, and the hyperintense perirectal fat.

The *vagina* is sandwiched between the urethra and bladder anteriorly and rectum posteriorly. On axial images the collapsed vagina has a characteristic H-shape. On T2WI a thin layer of hyperintense mucus is seen between the apposed low-density walls of the vagina consisting of mucosa, lamina propria, and smooth muscle. The perivaginal venous plexus is evident as a layer of high signal intensity surrounding the vagina.

The *cervix* is divided by the vaginal fornices into supravaginal and vaginal portions. On axial T2WI the cervix appears as a cylinder or ring with a central lumen of high signal intensity representing mucus in the endocervical canal. The cervix consists of a low-signal-intensity inner layer surrounding the endocervical canal and an intermediate-signal-intensity outer layer.

The *uterus,* consisting of fundus body and cervix, is a pear-shaped organ measuring 7–9 cm in length in the reproductive age. On T2WI a zonal anatomy is recognized consisting, from the inside out, of endometrium, junctional zone, and myometrium. The central high-signal-intensity stripe represents the normal endometrium and endometrial cavity. It is thinnest during menstruation and reaches maximum width during midsecretory phase, averaging 5–7 mm. The junctional zone appears as a band of low signal intensity bordering the hyperintense central stripe. The junctional zone averages 5 mm in width and does not vary during the menstrual cycle. The junctional zone represents the innermost layers of the myometrium. The outer myometrium is of intermediate signal intensity on T2WI. Changes in myometrial width parallel changes in endometrial width. The myometrium reaches a maximum width of approximately 2.5 cm in the midsecretory phase that is accompanied by an increase in signal intensity. Occasionally a serosal layer can be depicted as a thin line of low signal intensity adjacent to the myometrium. In the postmenopausal woman, the myometrium no longer shows these cyclic changes and usually has a diffusely low signal intensity on T2WI. With increasing age the uterus atrophies and decreases overall in size.

On T2WI the almond-shaped *ovaries* measure up to 5 cm in length and demonstrate multiple hyperintense small follicles located preferentially in the periphery of an inhomogeneous stroma with intermediate to high signal intensity. The capsule may be evident as a dark line surrounding the discrete well-defined follicles. In the postmenopausal woman the involuted and atrophic ovaries contain fewer, smaller, or no cysts and may become difficult to identify.

The *prostate*, measuring approximately 3 cm craniocaudad, 3 cm anteroposterior, and 5 cm in width, is located inferior to the urinary bladder between the pubic symphysis anteriorly and the rectum posteriorly. It is shaped like an inverted cone; the cephalic end is called the base and the caudal end is the apex. On T2WI a central zone (25 % of prostatic tissue) of low signal intensity can be differentiated from a peripheral zone (70 % of prostatic tissue) of high signal intensity. The transition zone (5 % of prostatic tissue) surrounds the periurethral gland and usually cannot be distinguished from the central zone by MRI. The central zone is conical in configuration, with the base parallel to that of the prostate. A fibromuscular capsule surrounds the prostate and blends anteriorly with the anterior fibromuscular stroma and the puboprostatic ligaments. The neurovascular bundle is located in the retroprostatic fat at 5 and 7 o'clock position at the prostatic base and at 3 and 9 o'clock position at the apex. It appears hypointense to the surrounding fat on T1WI and is more difficult to differentiate from the fat on T2WI.

Benign prostatic hypertrophy preferentially affects the transition zones that may become the largest prostatic zone, whereas *prostatic carcinomas* tend to occur in the peripheral zone.

The *seminal vesicles* are located cephalad to the prostate, between bladder and rectum. On T2WI the hyperintense content within the lumens sharply contrasts with the hypointense walls of these tubular structures. The confluence of the corresponding seminal vesicle and vas deferens, which forms the ejaculatory duct, is sometimes evident on MRI.

The *testes* are sharply demarcated, homogeneous oval glands of intermediate signal intensity on T1WI and high signal intensity on T2WI. The mediastinum testis, containing the rete testis and efferent ductules and part of the testicular blood supply, appears as an area of lower signal intensity in the superoposterior aspect of the testis. The tunica albuginea forms a fibrous covering for the testis and presents as a band of low signal intensity surrounding the testis. It is covered by the visceral layer of the tunica vaginalis, except at the head and tail of the epididymis and along the posterior border of the testis, where the testicular vessels and nerve enter the gland. The tunica vaginalis is an extension of the peritoneum and frequently contains a small amount of fluid between its visceral and parietal layers. An increase in this fluid is termed a hydrocele. The *epididymis* consists of a superior head, a central body, and an inferior tail. It appears as an inhomogeneous structure of intermediate signal intensity on T2WI extending along the lateroposterior aspect of the hyperintense testis. The head is connected with the cranial pole of the testis by the efferent ductules of the gland and the tail is attached to the caudal pole. A recess of the tunica vaginales lies between the body of the epididymis and testis. The spermatic cord containing the vas deferens and spermatic vessels suspends the testis in the scrotum.

In *cryptorchism* MRI may facilitate locating an undescended testicle (Fig. 26.1). It may be located anywhere from the renal hilum to the superior scrotum or be congenitally absent. Testes located proximal to the inguinal canal and atrophic testes distal to the inguinal canal are usually not palpable. Localization accuracy is lowest for intra-abdominal testes. Because of their intense enhancement intravenous administration of Gd-DTPA combined with fat suppression may be the best suited imaging technique.

Ectopic organs, such as pelvic kidneys (Fig. 26.2), are readily identified by MRI. Hernias containing bowel, fat, or both are easily diagnosed and differentiated from true mass lesions. After abdominoperineal resection of the rectum, the uterus or the prostate and seminal vesicles may be located in the presacral space and can easily be differentiated from presacral recurrent tumor. Other common *presacral masses* (Figs. 26.3 and 26.4) include abscess formation (secondary to rectal perforation or sacral osteomyelitis), hematoma (secondary to sacral fracture), benign or malignant bone lesions (e. g., giant cell tumor, metastasis, plasmacytoma, chordoma), rectal carcinoma, and teratogenic and neurogenic tumors.

Midline or lateral surgical transposition of the ovaries prior to radiation therapy for lymphoma or cervix carcinoma, respectively, is sometimes performed to preserve ovarian function and must be differentiated from metastatic implants. Other *iatrogenic pseudolesions* include intestinal urinary reservoirs in patients with urinary diversions, tissue expanders to displace bowel from radiation ports, and implanted reservoirs for penile prostheses and artificial sphincters.

Renal and *pancreatic transplants* are usually placed within the pelvis. The pancreatic transplant is often connected to the bladder by a segment of bowel to allow drainage of exocrine fluids. It should not be mistaken for an abnormal peritransplant collection, such as hematoma, seroma, abscess, urinoma, lymphocele or pancreatic pseudocyst.

MRI of the pelvis can be useful in the *differentiation* of *postoperative* and *postradiation fibrosis from tumor recurrence*. These conditions tend to be of low signal intensity with T1WI, but may demonstrate different signal intensity

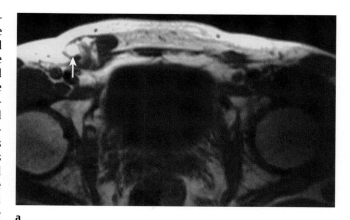

a

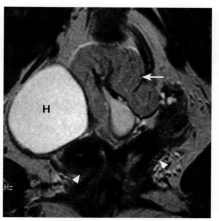

b

Fig. 26.**1 Cryptorchism.** The undescended testis (arrow) is in the right inguinal canal and demonstrates low signal intensity in (**a**) (T1WI, axial) and high signal intensity in (**b**) (T1WI, coronal).

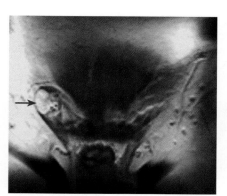

Fig. 26.**2 Pelvic kidney, uterus didelphys, and hydrosalpinx.** A pelvic kidney (arrow) of intermediate signal intensity with slightly dilated renal pelvis, a large hyperintense cystic lesion (right hydrosalpinx [H]), and a uterus didelphys (arrowheads) are seen (T2WI, coronal).

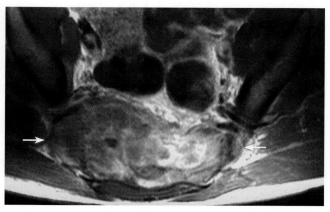

Fig. 26.**3 Ewing sarcoma of sacrum.** A large presacral mass (arrows) with inhomogeneous contrast enhancement is seen (T1WI, +C).

in spin-echo (SE) and gradient-echo (GRE) T2WI. During the first year after treatment only an enlarging mass is indicative of recurrence. At this time the inflammatory and granulomatous changes induced by the therapy have a signal intensity similar to viable tumor, and considerable contrast enhancement may be seen in all conditions. In an uncomplicated case 1 year and later after treatment the inflammatory and granulomatous changes have usually progressed to fibrosis, which has a low signal intensity on T2WI and does not enhance appreciably after intravenous Gd-DTPA administration. In contrast, a recurrent malignancy tends to be relatively high in signal intensity on T2WI and enhances substantially with Gd-DTPA. Unfortunately exceptions in signal behavior exist between these two entities. Recurrent tumors may be low in signal intensity on all pulse sequences if they incite a desmoplastic reaction. On the other hand, fibrosis complicated by either hemorrhage or infection may depict a high signal intensity on all imaging sequences and considerable contrast enhancement.

In *obstetrics* MRI may supplement ultrasonography, which remains the imaging modality of choice. Accurate pelvimetry without ionizing radiation can be obtained. Maternal complications, such as growing fibroids and ovarian cysts or ovarian and pelvic vein thrombosis, are readily diagnosed by MRI.

The placenta can be identified as early as 10 weeks of gestational age, depicting high signal intensity on T2WI. Gestational trophoblastic disease (Fig. 26.5) presents as a heterogeneous mass and can be differentiated into benign hydatidiform moles and invasive moles, depending on the presence or absence of endometrial invasion with disruption of the zonal anatomy of the uterus. Choriocarcinomas are invasive moles with distant metastases. MRI is also able to accurately locate the gestational sac in ectopic pregnancy. In the third trimester fetal presentation, anatomy, and pathology are readily depicted by MRI.

The differential diagnosis of pelvic lesions is discussed in Table 26.1. Female reproductive system lesions are discussed in Table 26.2 and male reproductive system lesions in Table 26.3.

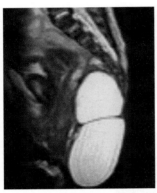

Fig. 26.**4**   **Cystic teratoma of coccyx.** A large homogeneous, hyperintense lesion with septation is seen anterior to the sacrum and coccyx (T2WI, sagittal).

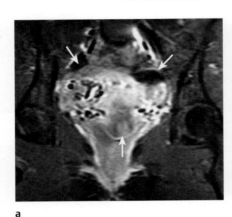

a

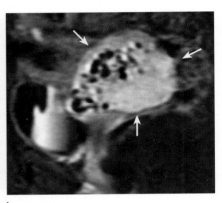

b

Fig. 26.**5**   **Gestational trophoblastic disease.** After intravenous Gd-DTPA administration an enlarged, markedly enhancing uterus (arrows) with numerous tiny cysts is seen. Endometrial infiltration with disruption of the zonal anatomy of the uterus is present, indicative of an invasive mole (T1WI, FS, +C). (**a**: coronal; **b**: sagittal.)

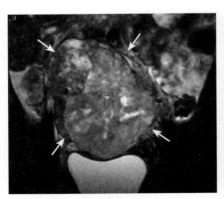

Fig. 26.**6**   **Embryonal rhabdomyosarcoma.** A large inhomogeneously enhanced mass (arrows) is seen arising from the urogenital ridge outside the urinary bladder (T1WI, FS, +C, coronal).

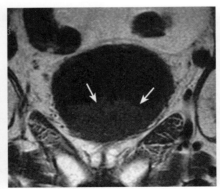

a

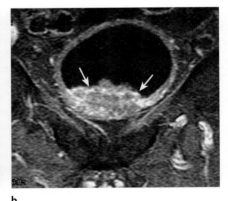

b

Fig. 26.**7**   **Bladder carcinoma.** An irregular mass (arrows) is seen in the floor of the bladder that does not extend into the perivesical fat (**a**: T1WI, coronal). After intravenous Gd-DPTA administration inhomogeneous enhancement of the tumor (arrows) is seen in (**b**) (T1WI, FS, +C, coronal).

Table 26.**1** Pelvic lesions

Disease	MRI Findings	Comments
Lesions of female reproductive system	See Table 26.**2**	
Lesions of male reproductive system	See Table 26.**3**	
Urinary bladder		
Bladder endometriosis	Focal, irregular bladder wall thickening with intravesical and/or extravesical component, containing solitary or multiple hemorrhagic cysts with blood products of different ages causing mixed, but at least in part high signal intensity on both T1WI and T2WI. Preferred location is posterior bladder wall.	In 30–40-year-old women, characteristically presenting with cyclic bladder irritability and hematuria. History of previous gynecologic or abdominal surgery is frequent.
Mesenchymal bladder tumors	Small polypoid to large, often fungating mass lesions. Benign and malignant varieties cannot be differentiated unless there is evidence of wall infiltration. Pedunculated lesions tend to be benign.	Rare. *Leiomyoma, rhabdomyoma, neurofibroma, hemangioma,* and *fibrosarcomas* occur. Bladder *pheochromocytoma* (benign or malignant) are usually located at the bladder base and characteristically present with sudden episodic hypertension, tachycardia, and flushing during micturition. *Embryonal rhabdomyosarcoma (botryoid sarcoma)* (Fig. 26.**6**) is the most common bladder tumor in children.
Bladder carcinoma (Figs. 26.**7**, 26.**8**)	Pedunculated sessile or infiltrative mass of slightly higher signal intensity than the bladder wall and lower signal intensity than the urine on T2WI. Partial disruption of the detrusor muscle, which normally presents on T2WI as three layers of low, intermediate and low signal intensity, indicates muscle infiltration. Complete disruption of all three layers indicates perivesical tumor extension. Tumor invasion into the perivesical fat and regional lymph node involvement (lymph node size greater than 1.5 cm) are best demonstrated on T1WI. Contrast enhancement of the tumor may improve its delineation.	Usually in patients above 50 years with male predominance. Over 90 % are *transitional cell carcinomas*. Squamous cell carcinomas are associated with inflammatory conditions such as schistosomiasis and adenocarcinomas with urachal remnants. Bladder *papillomas* (solitary or multiple) are histologically benign polypoid lesions without wall infiltration. Because of their high rate of recurrence they are often classified as grade I transitional cell carcinomas.

Staging

Jewett–Marshall	TNM	
O	Tis	Carcinoma in situ
A	T1	Submucosal invasion
B1	T2	Superficial muscle invasion
B2	T3a	Deep muscle invasion
C	T3b	Perivesical invasion
D	T4	Spread to contiguous organ or lymph nodes.

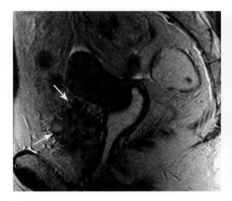
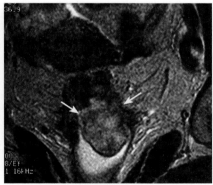

a   b

Fig. 26.**8** **Bladder carcinoma.** A heterogeneous mass (arrows) originating from the bladder roof extends into the perivesical fat (**a**: T2WI, sagittal; **b**: T2WI [GRE], coronal).

Table 26.1 (Cont.) Pelvic lesions

Disease	MRI Findings	Comments
Urachal carcinoma	Midline, partially to completely cystic lesion originating in the anterior bladder dome. After intravenous Gd-DTPA administration enhancement occurs in the solid parts of the tumor or the irregularly thickened wall of the cyst.	Usually a mucin-producing adenocarcinoma resulting from malignant transformation within urachal remnants. Occurs in patients above 40 years with male predominance. *Urachal cysts* are benign, thin-walled cystic lesions in the same location.
Bladder lymphoma and metastases (Fig. 26.9)	Solid focal mass or diffuse thickening of the bladder wall resulting from direct extension from adjacent malignancy (e.g., carcinoma of rectum, prostate, cervix, uterus, and rectosigmoid or pelvic lymphoma) or metastatic spread.	Canalicular bladder metastases originate from the kidney or ureter and the rare hematogenous metastases usually derive from carcinomas of lung or breast or melanomas.
Cystitis (Fig. 26.10)	Thickened, smooth or irregular bladder wall often associated with nodular masses protruding into the bladder lumen. Perivesical fat infiltration may also be present. Signal intensity usually is low on T1WI and high on T2WI, but varies depending on the presence of calcifications, fibrosis, cysts, hemorrhage, or gas.	Bladder wall calcifications occur in schistosomiasis, tuberculous and postirradiation cystitis. A shrunken fibrotic bladder is found with chronic interstitial cystitis, tuberculous cystitis, cystitis cystica, schistosomiasis, and after radiation therapy. Cystitis cystica is associated with multiple cysts protruding into the bladder lumen. Hemorrhagic and abacterial cystitis are associated with blood clots within the bladder lumen. In emphysematous cystitis (usually in diabetics) both intramural and intraluminal gas may be evident.
Malacoplakia	Single or multiple focal plaques or nodules of less than 3 cm in diameter, preferentially located on the bladder floor. Central necrosis or cyst formation occurs occasionally.	Uncommon chronic granulomatous response to Gram-negative infection (usually *E. coli*). Often found in diabetic patients with female predominance.
Bladder amyloidosis	Focal irregular bladder wall thickening of intermediate signal intensity similar to skeletal muscle on both T1WI and T2WI. Lateral bladder wall is the preferred location, whereas the trigone is rarely involved.	In primary amyloidosis as part of systemic involvement or limited to bladder secondary to chronic infection.
Intramural bladder hematoma	Focal wall thickening that may be associated with perivesical involvement and intraluminal blood clots. In the acute stage the hematoma has a low signal intensity on T1WI and a high signal intensity on T2WI. With methemoglobin formation a high signal intensity can be found on both T1WI and T2WI. May eventually result in localized bladder wall fibrosis with low signal intensity on both T1WI and T2WI.	Occurs after surgery, instrumentation and trauma. In the setting of blunt trauma, extraperitoneal bladder rupture is often associated with pelvic fractures and intraperitoneal bladder rupture typically occurs with a fully distended bladder.
Ureterocele (Fig. 26.10*)	Small unilateral or bilateral cystic lesions adjacent to the normal ureteral orifices caused by the prolapsed distal ureters (simple ureteroceles). Or cystic lesion of varying size and shape at the base of the bladder (ectopic ureterocele) associated with an ectopic ureteral orifice distal to the trigone within or outside the bladder.	Simple ureteroceles may be congenital or acquired and predispose to obstruction, infection, and stone formation. Are often discovered incidentally. Ectopic ureteroceles are commonly associated with a duplicated system draining the upper nonfunctioning or hydronephrotic segment.
Intraluminal pseudo-mass of the bladder (Fig. 26.11)	Position-dependent, mobile intraluminal masses of varying signal intensity may be caused by bladder calculi, blood clots, fungus balls, and foreign objects including Foley catheters.	Calculi are most frequently associated with prostatism and neurogenic bladders. Blood clots commonly occur with tumor, trauma, instrumentation, vascular malformations, hemorrhagic cystitis, and bleeding diathesis. Fungus balls are most often caused by candida albicans in patients with debilitating diseases or diabetes.
Bladder diverticula	Usually multiple outpouchings of bladder wall presenting as cystic perivesical lesions that communicate with the bladder lumen. Acquired diverticula due to bladder outlet obstruction are associated with diffuse thickening of the bladder wall.	Congenital (primary) diverticula may be solitary and usually located near a ureteral orifice (e.g. Hutch diverticulum). An *everted ureterocele* may occasionally simulate a small diverticulum near the ureteral orifice. Acquired (secondary) diverticula are associated with bladder outlet obstruction and neurogenic bladders. Benign prostatic hyperplasia is by far the most common cause.

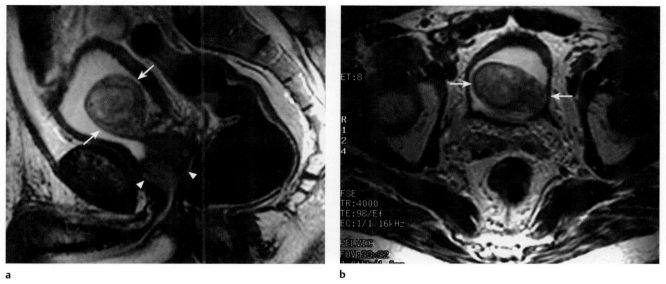

Fig. 26.**9**   **Bladder metastasis.** A prostate carcinoma (arrowheads) extends into the urinary bladder (arrows). (**a**: T2WI, sagittal; **b**: T2WI, axial).

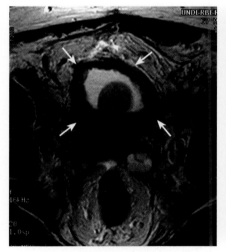

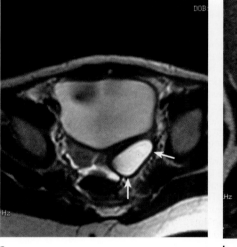

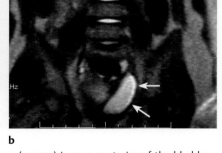

Fig. 26.**10**   **Chronic cystitis in prostatism.** A markedly thickened bladder wall (arrows) is seen in a patient with benign prostatic hypertrophy including an intravesical adenomatous nodule requiring chronic urinary bladder catheterization (T2WI).

Fig. 26.**10** *   **Ectopic ureterocele.** A cystic mass (arrows) is seen posterior of the bladder representing a dilated distal left ureter with insertion into the urethra (T2WI) (**a**): axial, (**b**): coronal.

Table 26.1 (Cont.) Pelvic lesions

Disease	MRI Findings	Comments
Extrinsic bladder mass (Fig. 26.11)	Perivesical tumors (benign and malignant), fistulas, abscesses, hematomas, and fluid collections (urinomas and lymphoceles) may produce extrinsic compression of the bladder wall and at times be difficult to differentiate from an intrinsic bladder wall lesion.	Prostatic enlargement due to benign hyperplasia or carcinoma represents the most common cause of extrinsic bladder mass affecting the bladder floor.
Colon and rectum		
Colorectal duplication cyst	Thin-walled, tubular or cystic lesions within or adjacent to the bowel wall.	Duplication cysts may communicate with the bowel lumen and become a source of infection.
Endometriosis of the rectosigmoid (Fig. 26.12)	One or several focal mural implants with variable signal intensity, but usually hyperintense on T1WI and mixed, intermediate to high on T2WI. Common implant sites are rectosigmoid wall, cul-de-sac (pouch of Douglas), and rectovaginal septum. Rectal tethering producing a pear-shaped rectum with the point directed toward the uterus is classic.	In 30–40-year-old women who may present with cyclic rectal bleed and/or rectal pain while defecating during menses.
Colonic polyps	Single or multiple intratumoral mass lesions of varying size that demonstrate enhancement after intravenous Gd-DTPA administration. Invasion through bowel wall is evident as bowel wall disruption at the attachment site of the polyp. The frond-like projections of villous adenomas are best appreciated on Gd-DTPA-enhanced fat suppressed images.	Adenomatous polyps are the most common colic neoplasm. Tubular, tubulovillous, and villous adenomas are differentiated. Malignant potential increases in this order and with the size of the adenoma. Lesions exceeding 2 cm should be considered malignant. DD: hyperplastic polyps that are always benign and rarely exceed 5 mm in diameter.
Colonic lipoma	Polypoid lesion with characteristic high signal intensity on all pulse sequences.	Other benign and malignant mesenchymal neoplasm such as leiomyoma and leiomyosarcomas are rare in the colon and rectum.
Carcinoid	Because of its small size, the primary tumor may not be evident on MRI. The tumor-induced desmoplastic reaction in the mesentery, producing kinking and separation of the adjacent bowel loops, typically demonstrates low signal intensity on all pulse sequences. After intravenous Gd-DTPA administration the tumor and its liver metastases enhance, the latter often depicting a characteristic ring enhancement pattern.	Location frequency in gastrointestinal tract: appendix 45%, small bowel (especially distal ileum) 35%, rectum 15%, colon 5%.
Colorectal carcinoma (Fig. 26.13)	Presents as polypoid mass and/or segmental wall thickening with low signal intensity on T1WI and intermediate signal intensity on T2WI. After intravenous Gd-DTPA administration considerable enhancement occurs. Perirectal lymph node involvement is best evaluated with T1WI. Correlation between lymph node size and likelihood of malignancy exists. Lymph nodes exceeding 15 mm in diameter are considered malignant but lymph nodes as small as 5 mm in diameter may be metastatic.	*TNM staging* Tis Carcinoma in situ T1 Limited to mucosa/submucosa T2 Extension into muscularis propria T3 Extension into perirectal fat T4 Extension into adjacent organs N0 No lymph nodes involved N1 1–3 regional nodes involved N2 4 or more regional nodes involved N3 Distant lymph node(s) involved M0 No metastases (other than lymph nodes) M1 Distant metastases Stage 0: Tis, N0, M0 Stage 1: T1 or 2, N0, M0 Stage 2: T3 or T4, N0, M0 Stage 3: any T, N1 to 3, M0 Stage 4: any T, any N, M1
Colorectal lymphoma and metastases	Single or multiple focal lesions to diffuse bowel nodularity and wall thickening, all with considerable enhancement after intravenous Gd-DTPA.	Primary colonic lymphoma is rare. It is relatively frequent in AIDS patients with predilection for the rectum. Secondary lymphoma is usually associated with massive mesenteric adenopathy. Colonic metastases usually occur from direct tumor extension from a neighboring organ.

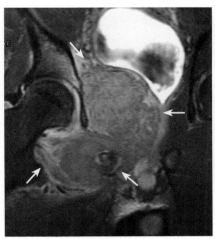

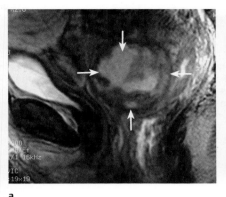

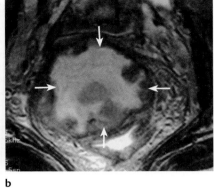

Fig. 26.**12** **Endometriosis.** A heterogeneous mass is seen in the cul-de-sac (arrows) with inhomogeneous and variable signal intensity (**a**: T2WI, sagittal; **b**: T2WI, axial).

Fig. 26.**11** **Intraluminal bladder blood clot.** Ewing sarcoma (arrows) originating from the right superior pubic ramus displaces the hyperintense bladder containing gadolinium concentrated urine that outlines an irregular hypointense blood clot (T1WI, FS, +C, coronal).

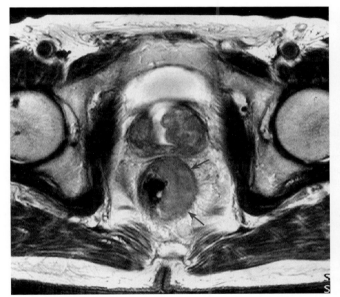

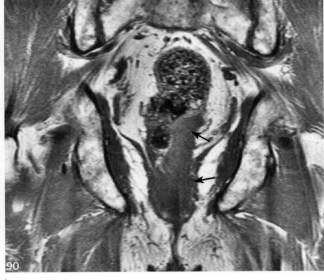

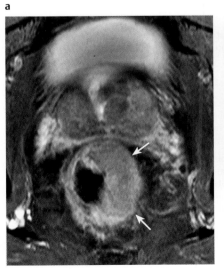

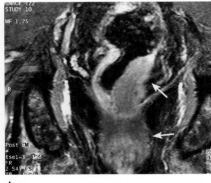

Fig. 26.**13** **Rectal carcinoma.**
a, b Asymmetric thickening of the rectal wall (arrows) by a relatively homogeneous hypointense mass with extension into the perirectal fat is seen (T1WI, axial and coronal). **c, d** After intravenous Gd-DTPA administration marked contrast enhancement of the tumor is seen (T1WI, FS, +C, axial and coronal). Sequelae of previous transurethral resections of the prostrate (TURP) are also evident on the axial images.

Table 26.1 (Cont.) Pelvic lesions

Disease	MRI Findings	Comments
Diverticulitis (Fig. 26.14)	Segmental colonic wall thickening associated with inflammatory changes in the pericolonic fat. Focal pericolonic abscesses, fistulas, and intramural sinuses may also be evident. Inflammatory changes demonstrate low signal intensity on T1WI, high signal intensity on T2WI, and marked contrast enhancement. Abscesses may depict a nonenhancing necrotic center. Preferential location is the sigmoid colon, where usually multiple diverticula are seen.	Other infectious processes with similar MRI features primarily involving the rectosigmoid include *schistosomiasis, lymphogranuloma venereum,* and *gonorrheal proctitis.* A diffuse infectious colitic process is found in *pseudomembranous colitis* and *cytomegalovirus colitis* (in AIDS and renal transplant recipients). Infectious enterolitides primarily involving the terminal ileum and cecum include *tuberculosis, Yersinia colitis,* and *amebiasis* (terminal ileum is spared). The inflammatory changes in *appendicitis* and *periappendiceal abscess* formation are indistinguishable by MRI from diverticulitis.
Inflammatory bowel disease	Segmental or diffuse bowel wall thickening; hypointense on T1WI, hyperintense on T2WI, and marked enhancement after intravenous Gd-DTPA administration. Bowel wall involvement may be circumferential or asymmetric. Extension into the perienteric fat is common. Ancillary findings include sinus tracts, fistulas, and abscess formations, all of which are particularly common in Crohn disease. Disease activity may be assessed by the length of bowel involvement, bowel wall thickness, and degree of contrast enhancement.	In *Crohn disease* the most common appearance is a thickened terminal ileum with asymmetric involvement of the cecum. In a more advanced stage skip areas, stricture formations with or without proximal bowel dilatation, mesenteric fibrofatty proliferation, and enlarged mesenteric lymph nodes are frequently associated. In *ulcerative colitis* rectal involvement with continuous proximal extension to a variable degree is always evident on MRI after intravenous contrast enhancement. *Graft versus host disease:* MRI findings are similar to ulcerative colitis, but both small and large bowel are usually involved. *Radiation enterocolitis* is characteristically limited to the field of irradiation. In *ischemic colitis* the left colon including splenic flexure and sigmoid ("watershed areas") are most commonly involved.
Pelvis		
Pelvic lipomatosis	Nonmalignant overgrowth of adipose tissue with characteristic fatty signal characteristics compressing the pelvic organs. Narrowing, elongation, and elevation of the rectosigmoid and urinary bladder, producing an inverted pear-shape appearance of the latter, are characteristic.	Often an incidental finding occurring at any age (peak 25–60 years) with 10:1 male predominance. Obesity is not a contributing factor. Recurrent urinary tract infections and ureteral obstruction may be associated.
Pelvic fibrosis	Dense fibrous tissue with low signal intensity on all pulse sequences and without contrast enhancement enveloping the pelvic organs.	May be idiopathic, associated with retroperitoneal fibrosis or, more commonly, secondary to pelvic irradiation, inflammation, or hemorrhage. Ureteral obstruction is a frequent complication.
Pelvic edema	Diffuse soft tissue edema causing an overall decrease in signal intensity on T1WI and an increase in signal intensity on T2WI without mass effect. Often associated with edema in the lower extremities.	Occlusion of the inferior vena cava by tumor or thrombosis may be evident on MRI.
Pelvic carcinomatosis and lymphoma (Figs. 26.15, 26.16)	Extensive tumor infiltration with encasement or invasion of the pelvic organs. High signal intensity on T2WI and substantial contrast enhancement differentiates tumor from fibrosis (e.g. postoperative or postradiation scarring).	Metastatic and lymphomatous disease is the most common pelvic malignancy.
Pelvic lymphocele	Large cystic fluid collection, often with internal septation occurring after lymphadenectomy or associated with renal transplants.	Lymphoceles are the most common peritransplant fluid collection. Compared with urinomas, lymphoceles tend to be larger, may be septated, and occur later (2 weeks or later after transplantation).
Pelvic urinoma	Urine containing pseudocyst secondary to a tear in the distal ureter or bladder presenting as a thin-walled homogeneous fluid collection with low signal intensity on T1WI and high signal intensity on T2WI. After intravenous Gd-DTPA administration extravasation of the contrast agent into the lesion may be evident on late images.	In the pelvis urinomas are frequently the sequelae of trauma or surgery (e.g., urinary diversions, radical prostatectomy) or are associated with *renal transplants*, tending to occur in the first week after transplantation.

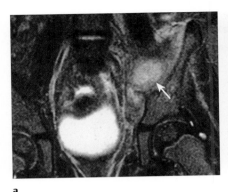

a

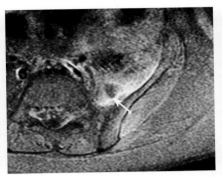

b

Fig. 26.**14** **Diverticular abscess.**
a A poorly defined hyperintense lesion (arrow) is seen in the left pelvis (T2WI, FS, coronal).

b After intravenous Gd-DTPA administration a nonenhancing center (arrow) is surrounded by a markedly enhancing periphery (T1WI, FS, +C, axial).

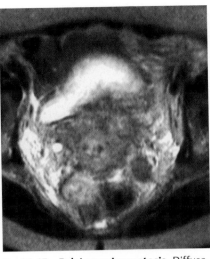

Fig. 26.**15** **Pelvic carcinomatosis.** Diffuse tumor infiltration with encasement or infiltration of all organs in the pelvic floor is secondary to metastatic cervical carcinoma (T2WI).

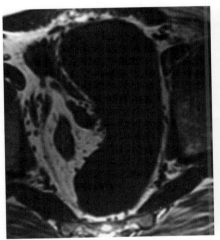

a

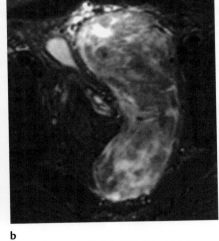

b

Fig. 26.**16** **Pelvic leiomyosarcoma.** A large well-defined mass is seen extending from the sacrum to the pubis. The mass is homogeneous and hypointense in (**a**) (T1WI, axial) and heterogeneous and hyperintense in (**b**) (T2WI, FS, axial). After intravenous Gd-DTPA administration the lesion demonstrates marked contrast enhancement in (**c**) (T1WI, FS, +C, axial) and (**d**) (T1WI, FS, +C, sagittal).

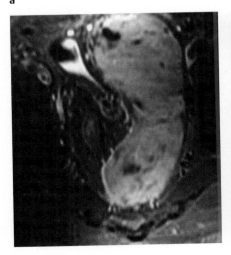

c

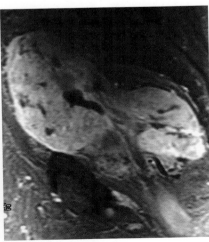

d

Table 26.1 (Cont.) Pelvic lesions

Disease	MRI Findings	Comments
Pelvic hematoma (Fig. 26.17)	Poorly marginated, asymmetric soft-tissue abnormality or relatively sharply marginated focal lesion with mass effect depicting low signal intensity on T1WI and high signal intensity on T2WI in the acute stage. Sedimentation may occur within an acute hematoma, causing a hematocrit effect or fluid–fluid level. Deoxyhemoglobin formation may cause a temporary decrease in signal intensity on T2WI. After a few days the hematoma progresses to extracellular methemoglobin formation with high signal intensity on both T1WI and T2WI and eventually to fibrosis, with or without hemosiderin deposition, causing low signal intensity on both T1WI and T2WI. Occasionally a "concentric ring" sign is seen in the subacute stage on T1WI, consisting of liquified blood degradation products in the center with intermediate signal intensity, surrounded by an inner ring of methemoglobin producing high signal intensity and an outer hypointense ring of macrophages laden with hemosiderin.	Usually caused by trauma, postoperative bleeding, anticoagulation, hemophilia, or neoplasia.
Pelvic abscess (Fig. 26.18)	Irregularly defined, heterogeneous mass with low signal intensity on T1WI and high signal intensity on T2WI. After intravenous Gd-DTPA the abscess wall enhances whereas the necrotic center does not. Air bubbles within the lesion are highly suggestive of an abscess presenting with signal void on all image sequences.	Most often associated with appendicitis, diverticulitis, or previous pelvic surgery, but may also be found with inflammatory adnexal disease, Crohn disease, carcinoma, trauma, and colonic perforation or as renal transplant complication.
Fistula	On T2WI fluid-filled tracks connecting the involved visceras may be seen. Fat suppression may highlight the fistula by suppressing the high signal intensity of the adjacent fat. Fistulas containing gas are devoid of signals. Focal discontinuity of the involved organ walls at the site of fistula penetration may also be evident.	*Vesicointestinal fistulas* occur secondary to diverticulitis (51%), colorectal carcinomas (16%), Crohn's disease (12%), bladder carcinoma (5%), and rarely after surgical injury and irradiation. *Vesicovaginal fistulas* occur most commonly after hysterectomy, but also after radiation therapy, urogenital malignancies, and pelvic fractures. *Vesicouterine fistulas* are rare and usually secondary to caesarean section. *Vesicocutaneous* and *vesicoretroperitoneal sinuses* usually are postoperative sequelae.

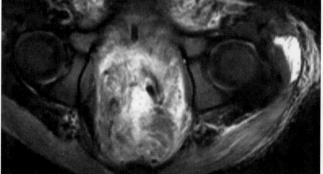

Fig. 26.**17** **Pelvic hematoma (subacute).** A heterogeneous, relatively poorly defined lesion with mixed intermediate to high signal intensity is seen (T2WI). A second hyperintense hematoma is evident in the left gluteus medius muscle.

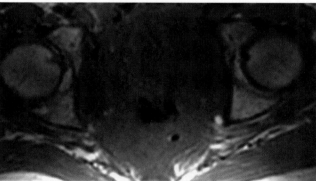

a

b

Fig. 26.**18** **Pelvic abscess (postoperative).** a A large zone of ▷ low signal intensity is seen in the pelvis involving rectal wall, perirectal fat, and surrounding tissues (T1WI). b After intravenous Gd-DTPA administration marked enhancement of the region occurs, except for several necrotic abscess centers that do not enhance (T1WI, FS, +C).

Table 26.**2** Female reproductive system lesions

Disease	MRI Findings	Comments
Vagina and vulva		
Congenital anomalies (Fig. 26.19)	Malformations include vaginal absence, persistent urogenital sinus, cloacal malformation, vaginal duplication, and atresia. The latter may be caused by transverse vaginal septum or imperforate hymen leading to the accumulation of fluid (hydrocolpos), blood (hematocolpos), or pus (pyocolpos) within the distended, cystic-appearing vagina.	Acquired vaginal obstructions are exceedingly rare. Vaginal obstruction may be associated with fluid, blood, or pus retention within the uterus resulting in a hydro-, hemato-, or pyometrocolpos, respectively.
Gartner's duct cyst	Inclusion cyst lateral to the vagina and uterus wall.	Vestigial remnant of wolffian duct.
Bartholin's cyst	Vulvovaginal gland cyst measuring up to 5 cm in diameter.	Occur at all ages. May result from stenosis or occlusion of the duct of a Bartholin's gland secondary to a prior infection such as gonorrhea.
Vulvar and vaginal carcinoma (Figs. 26.20, 26.21)	Poorly marginated focal or diffuse area of mixed low signal intensity on T1WI and intermediate to high signal intensity on T2WI. Invasion of the ischiorectal fat and pelvic walls as well as regional lymph node metastases (lymphatic drainage of proximal two-thirds of vagina occurs to deep pelvic nodes and distal one-third of vagina to inguinal nodes) are best depicted on T1WI.	95 % of primary vaginal and vulvar malignancies are squamous cell carcinomas. Clear-cell vaginal adenocarcinomas are associated with in-utero diethylstilbestrol (DES) exposure. Direct vaginal invasion from a cervical carcinoma is common. Benign neoplasms (rare) and endometriosis can mimic a vaginal malignancy.

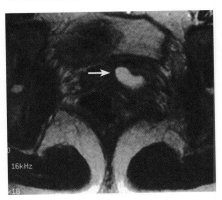

Fig. 26.**19** **Hydrocolpos.** A didelphic uterus, including two separated vaginas, were present. The left vagina (arrow) was occluded and retained high signal intensity fluid (T2WI, oblique axial).

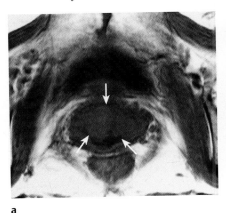

a

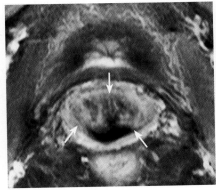

b

Fig. 26.**20** **Vaginal carcinoma.** A low signal intensity, slightly inhomogeneous lesion (arrows) is seen in the anterior wall of the vagina (**a**: T1WI). After intravenous Gd-DTPA administration, the lesion does not extend into the perivaginal plexus seen as a hyperintense layer surrounding the vagina (**b**: T1WI, FS, +C).

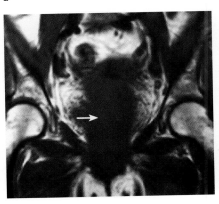

c

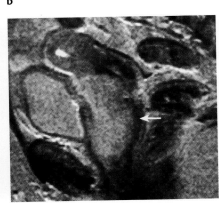

d

Fig. 26.**21** **Vaginal non-Hodgkin lymphoma.** A homogeneous mass (arrow) is seen in the vagina. The mass is hypointense in (**a**) (T1WI, coronal) and hyperintense in (**b**) (T2WI, sagittal).

Table 26.2 (Cont.) Female reproductive system lesions

Disease	MRI Findings	Comments
Vaginal embryonal rhabdomyosarcoma	Polypoid, bulky mass with grape-like appearance (botryoid sarcoma) of low signal intensity on T1WI and mixed high signal intensity on T2WI. Local invasion is frequent and usually extensive.	Usually in children below 5 years.
Cervix and uterus		
Congenital anomalies (Figs. 26.22–26.26)	Uterine anomalies are readily identified: *Unicornuate uterus*: elongated banana-like shape. *Bicornuate uterus*: fundal notch or indentation. *Septate uterus*: outwardly convex fundal contour with complete midline septum extending into endocervical canal (*uterus septus*) or partial septum limited to endometrial canal (*uterus subseptus*). *Didelphic uterus*: two separate uteri and cervices are present. *Arcuate uterus*: heart-shaped endometrial cavity and flat fundal contour. *Hypoplastic, T-shaped uterus.*	Embryologically, the paired müllerian ducts fuse at gestational age of 10–17 weeks to form the uterus, cervix, fallopian tubes, and upper two-thirds of the vagina. Failure of development of both müllerian ducts leads to uterine agenesis or hypoplasia. In utero DES exposure may be associated with a hypoplastic, T-shaped uterus. Congenital (cervical dysgenesis, vaginal agenesis) or acquired (secondary to tumor, infection, instrumentation, or irradiation) obstruction of the endocervical canal results in dilatation of the uterus by retention of fluid (hydrometra), blood (hematometra), or pus (pyometra).
Nabothian cyst (Fig. 26.27)	Single or multiple well-defined fluid-filled structures in the cervix, which occasionally is mildly enlarged.	Represent obstructed cervical glands. Small cervical myomas typically presenting with low signal intensity on both T1WI and T2WI must be differentiated.
Adenomyosis (Fig. 26.28)	Presents on T2WI as focal, ill-defined, oval, or elongated lesions within the junctional zone or diffuse widening of the junctional zone exceeding 5 mm in width, causing a smooth uterine enlargement. Adenomyosis generally depicts a low signal intensity on all pulse sequences but may contain areas of high signal intensity to the presence of endometrial glands and/or hemorrhages. Contrast enhancement is similar to the normal myometrium.	Focal or diffuse invasion of the myometrium by endometrium, inciting myometrial hyperplasia (endometriosis interna). Occurs in multiparous women in their later reproductive years and may be asymptomatic or present with pelvic pain, menorrhagia, and dysmenorrhea.

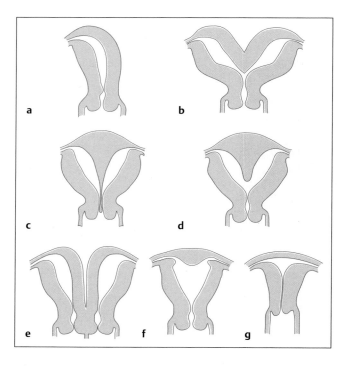

Fig. 26.22 **Uterine anomalies. a** Unicornuate uterus. **b** Bicornuate uterus. **c** Completely septate uterus. **d** Partially septate uterus. **e** Didelphic uterus. **f** Arcuate uterus. **g** Hypoplastic T-shaped uterus.

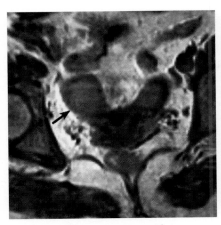

Fig. 26.**23**   **Bicornate uterus.** The enlarged right horn (arrow) of the bicornuate uterus contained an endometrial carcinoma (PDWI, oblique axial).

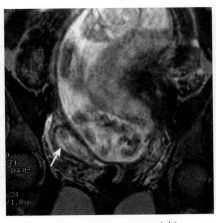

Fig. 26.**24**   **Bicornuate uterus.** A bicornuate uterus is seen with a small right horn (arrow) and large left horn containing an 18-week-old fetus and placenta (T2WI, coronal).

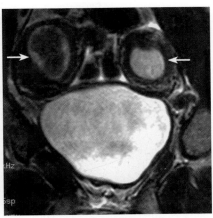

Fig. 26.**25**   **Didelphic uterus.** Obstruction of both uteri (arrows) containing blood on the right (hematometra) and fluid on the left (hydrometra) is seen (T2WI, coronal).

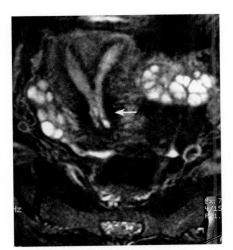

Fig. 26.**26**   **Completely septated uterus.** A septum divides the uterine cavity and continues into the cervix (arrow). The tiny hyperintense foci in the cervical wall are nabothian cysts (T2WI, FS, oblique axial).

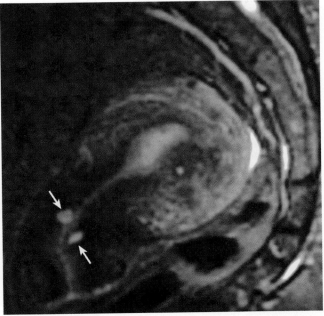

Fig. 26.**27**   **Nabothian cysts.** Two hyperintense foci (arrows) are seen adjacent to the endocervical canal. An enlarged myomatous uterus with slight deformity of the uterine cavity is also evident (T2WI, FS, sagittal).

Table 26.2 (Cont.) Female reproductive system lesions

Disease	MRI Findings	Comments
Uterine leiomyoma (fibroid) **(Figs. 26.29–26.31)**	Enlarged lobulated uterus with nodular distortion of the outline presenting with single or, more frequently, multiple mass lesions in intramural, subserosal, or submucosal location. Subserosal fibroids may be pedunculated. Uncomplicated tumors appear homogeneous, round, well-defined and of low signal intensity on T1WI and T2WI. Highly cellular leiomyomas and those with hemorrhagic or hyaline degeneration depict an inhomogeneous and increased signal intensity on T1WI and T2WI. Degenerating myomas may approach the signal intensity of fluid on T2WI. Contrast enhancement of uncomplicated myomas is similar to the myometrium.	Most common uterine mass usually occurring after 30 years in 25% of all women. Myomas grow during pregnancy and shrink in puerperium and after menopause. Leiomyomas are asymptomatic in 75% of cases, but may present with infertility, bladder or rectal pressure, pelvic pain, and hypermenorrhea. *Leiomyosarcomas* are uncommon, but cannot be differentiated by MRI from a benign leiomyoma. After menopause an enlarging uterine mass is never a benign leiomyoma and, besides carcinoma and leiomyosarcoma, other malignant mesenchymal tumors must be considered. *Lymphoma* and *metastases* may cause diffuse uterine enlargement and mimic fibroids.

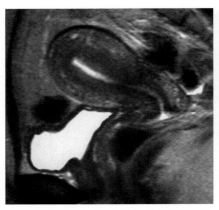

Fig. 26.**28   Adenomyosis.** Smooth enlargement of the uterus with diffuse widening of the hypointense functional zone is diagnostic (T2WI, sagittal).

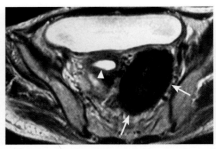

Fig. 26.**29   Subserosal uterine leiomyoma.** A large, relatively homogeneous, hypointense lesion (arrows) originates from the adjacent uterus with retained hyperintense secretions (arrowhead) due to obstruction of the endocervical canal by a cervical carcinoma (T2WI).

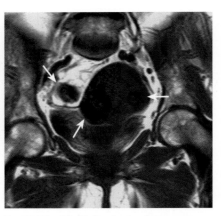

Fig. 26.**30   Multiple uterine leiomyomas.** An enlarged uterus with multiple nodules (arrows) is seen. Compared with the uterus, the nodules demonstrate heterogeneous hypointense signal intensity due to partial calcifications (T1WI, coronal).

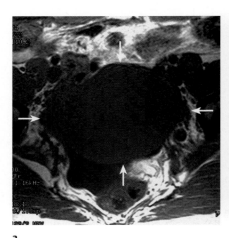

a

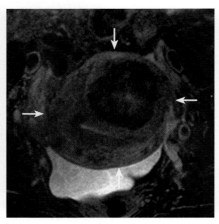

b

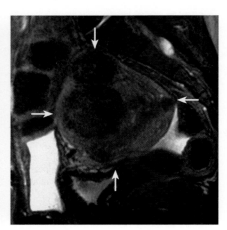

c

Fig. 26.**31   Necrotic uterine leiomyomas.** An enlarged uterus (arrows) with nodular contour is seen presenting with homogeneous low signal intensity in (**a**) (T1WI, axial) and heterogeneous slightly increased signal intensity in (**b**) (T2WI, FS, axial) and (**c**) (T2WI, FS, sagittal), indicating partial necrosis of the leiomyomas. Hyperintense ascites in the cul-de-sac is also evident in (**c**).

Table 26.**2** (Cont.) Female reproductive system lesions

Disease	MRI Findings	Comments
Endometrial polyp (Fig. 26.**32)**	On T2WI a round mass of intermediate signal intensity measuring 2–4 cm in diameter may be found within the endometrial cavity, usually in the fundus. The stalk can occasionally be identified in the periphery of the lesion as a band of low signal intensity due to fibrous tissue.	Endometrial polyps are focal areas of hyperplasia of glands and stroma. In most cases MRI cannot reliably differentiate these lesions from a noninvasive or superficial endometrial carcinoma. Small endometrial polyps and endometrial hyperplasia may increase the width of the endometrial cavity focally or diffusely, but increased endometrial fluid or blood retention may produce the same finding.

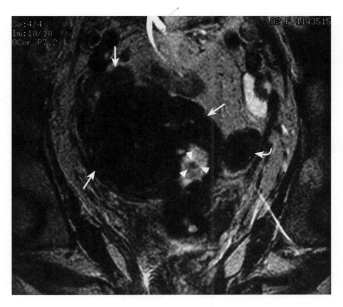

Fig. 26.**32** **Endometrial polyp in myomatous uterus.** An eccentrically enlarged myomatous uterus (arrows) with a subserosal fibroid (curved arrow) is seen. The uterine cavity contains a round lesion (arrowheads) of intermediate signal intensity surrounded by endometrial blood or fluid of high signal intensity (T2WI, FS, coronal).

Table 26.2 (Cont.) Female reproductive system lesions

Disease	MRI Findings	Comments
Cervical carcinoma (Figs. 26.33–26.36)	Heterogeneous mass of low signal intensity on T1WI (isointense to cervical stroma) and of high signal intensity on T2WI (hyperintense to cervical stroma). Retained secretions in the uterine cavity, due to obstruction of the endocervical canal, may be evident. Parametrial invasion is diagnosed when the tumor extends through the entire cervical cylinder. Pelvic side wall invasion and lymph node involvement (abnormal >1.5 cm, suspicious >1.0 cm) are best evaluated with T1WI. Considerable tumor enhancement is evident after intravenous Gd-DTPA administration.	95 % are squamous cell carcinomas, frequently occurring in younger women (peak age 45–55 years) of low socioeconomic standing. *Staging* TNM FIGO Tis 0 — Carcinoma in situ T1 I — Confined to cervix T2 II — Extension beyond cervix, but not to pelvic side wall or lower third of vagina T3 III — Extension to pelvic wall, lower third of vagina, or hydronephrosis T4 IVA — Invasion of bladder or rectum M1 IVB — Distant metastases
Endometrial carcinoma (Figs. 26.37, 26.38)	On T2WI the tumor is slightly hypointense to the endometrium and variable, but more or less isointense to the myometrium. After intravenous Gd-DTPA injection the tumor enhances considerably less than the surrounding myometrium and becomes hypointense. Contrast medium administration also allows differentiation between nonenhancing clot and polypoid tumor within the endometrial canal. The endometrium and endometrial canal are usually widened, the maximal normal width in postmenopausal women not under estrogen replacement should not exceed 3 mm. Disruption or absence of the hypointense junctional zone indicates myometrial invasion. Invasion of adjacent bladder or bowel is suggested when no fat plane separates the tumor from the neighboring organ and is definite when there is an increased signal intensity within the wall of these organs on T2WI. Involvement of the pelvic and para-aortic lymph nodes is best assessed on T1WI.	95 % are adenocarcinomas, usually occurring in women above 55 years. Risk factors include multiparity, unopposed estrogen therapy, obesity, and diabetes mellitus. *Staging* TNM FIGO Tis 0 — Carcinoma in situ T1 I — Limited to myometrium of uterine fundus and body T2 II — Invasion of cervix T3a IIIA — Involvement of serosa, adnexa, and/or positive peritoneal cytology T3b IIIB — Involvement of vagina N1 IIIC — Pelvic and/or para-aortic lymph node involvement T4 IVA — Bladder and/or bowel involvement M1 IVB — Distant metastases.

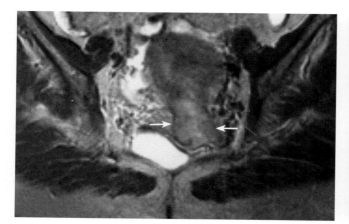

a

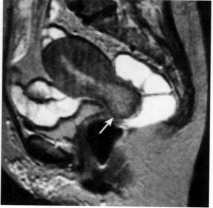

b

Fig. 26.33 Cervical carcinoma. A heterogeneous mass (arrows) of intermediate signal intensity is seen limited to the cervix (T2WI, axial and sagittal).

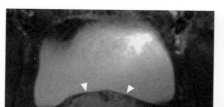

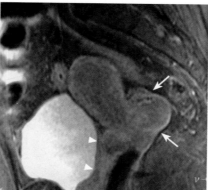

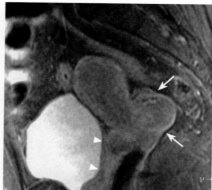

a

b

Fig. 26.34 Cervical carcinoma. After intravenous Gd-DTPA administration there is no visible differential enhancement between uterus and cervical tumor, which extends posteriorly into the rectouterine space (arrows) and anteriorly into the vesicouterine fold (arrowheads) without invasion of either bladder or rectum (T1WI, FS, +C, axial and sagittal).

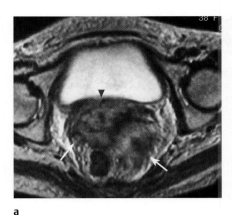

a

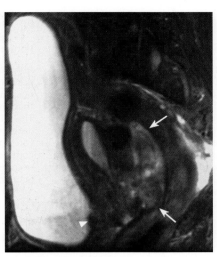

b

Fig. 26.**35 Cervical carcinoma.** A heterogeneous, poorly defined cervical mass is seen between bladder and rectum with infiltration of the perirectal tissue planes (arrows) and posterior bladder wall (arrowhead). Obstruction of the endocervical canal is evident from the fluid retention in the uterine cavity (T2WI, axial and sagittal).

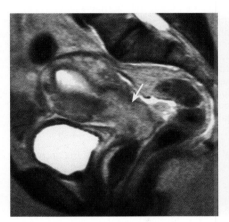

a

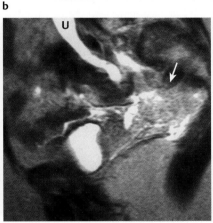

b

Fig. 26.**36 Cervical carcinoma.** A large, rather poorly defined cervical mass (arrow) is seen with inhomogeneous, intermediate to high signal intensity. It extends into the uterus with obstruction of the uterine cavity in (**a**) (T2WI, sagittal) and spreads into the perivesical and perirectal soft-tissue planes with ureteral (U) and vascular obstruction in (**b**) (T2WI, sagittal).

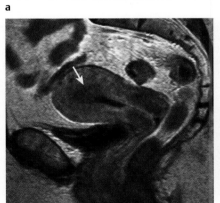

a

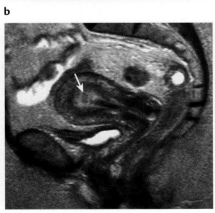

b

Fig. 26.**37 Endometrial carcinoma.**
a A small hypointense lesion (arrow) is seen with slight widening of the endometrial canal (T1WI, sagittal).   **b** The inhomogeneous lesion (arrow) is isointense to the myometrium, from which it is separated by the hypointense junctional zone (T2WI, sagittal).

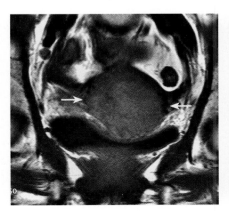

a

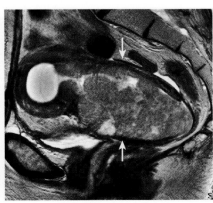

b

Fig. 26.**38 Endometrial carcinoma.**
a A markedly enlarged, slightly inhomogeneous mass (arrows) of intermediate signal intensity is seen (T1WI, coronal).   **b** After intravenous Gd-DTPA administration inhomogeneous contrast enhancement of the large tumor (arrows) is seen. Accumulation of fluid in the obstructed endometrial canal of the fundus is also evident (T2WI, +C, sagittal).

Table 26.**2** (Cont.) Female reproductive system lesions

Disease	MRI Findings	Comments
Gestational tropho-blastic disease (GTD) **(Fig. 26.39)**	On T2WI a hydatidiform mole appears as a heterogeneous mass of high signal intensity that distends the endometrial cavity. Grapelike clusters of thin-walled cysts are frequently evident within the lesion. Tortuous dilated vessels devoid of signals are occasionally seen. Invasive moles and choriocarcinomas present as heterogeneous masses invading the endometrium and distorting the zonal architecture of the enlarged uterus. Contrast enhancement is inhomogeneous in all forms of GTD. Enlarged ovaries due to theca lutein cyst formation may be associated.	Abnormal elevation of serum β-human chorionic gonadotropin (β-HCG) is diagnostic and usually, but not always, associated with a uterus that is larger than expected for the duration of the pregnancy. The GTD spectrum ranges from benign hydatidiform mole (90%) to invasive mole (8%) and choriocarcinoma (2%). The latter two conditions most commonly follow a hydatidiform mole, but may occur to any gestational event including abortion, ectopic or term pregnancy. Choriocarcinoma metastases may be found in the lungs (80%), vagina (30%), bone marrow (20%), liver, and brain.
Uterine infection **(Fig. 26.40)**	Endometritis may lead to pus accumulation in the obstructed and distended endometrial cavity (pyometra), presenting with low signal intensity on T1WI and high signal intensity on T2WI. Differentiating the retention of pus from sterile fluid (hydrometra) or fresh blood (hematometra) is only possible with the demonstration of gas evident as signal void. Endometritis may progress to myometritis and eventually abscess formation within the uterine wall.	In child-bearing age acute endometritis occurs following abortion, delivery, instrumentation, or surgery. Gas within the uterus is highly suggestive of an anaerobic infection, but it may normally be found in the immediate period following vaginal delivery, caesarian section, surgery, and instrumentation. In pelvic *inflammatory disease* the infection spreads from the vagina upward to the cervix, uterus, fallopian tubes, and adjacent pelvic structures. It may be caused by a variety of organisms including *Neisseria gonorrhoeae* and *Chlamydia trachomatis*. In the postmenopausal woman uterine infections are usually associated with malignancies.
Adnexa		
Congenital parovarian cysts **(Fig. 26.41)**	*Paroöphoron*: cyst in the suspensory ligament of the ovary between ovary and fallopian tube in medial location. *Epoöphoron*: cyst in the suspensory ligament of the ovary between ovary and fallopian tube in lateral location. *Hydatids of Morgagni*: one or more vesicles attached to the fringes of the fallopian tube.	Vestigial remnants of wolffian duct in the mesosalpinx.
Ovarian cysts **(Fig. 26.42)**	Usually solitary, thin-walled cystic lesion without septation measuring less than 4 cm in diameter. However larger, multiple or bilateral cysts occur. Nevertheless both a cyst size exceeding 4 cm in diameter and internal septation favor a cystic neoplasm. Serous ovarian cysts are homogeneous and isointense to urine on all pulse sequences. Hemorrhagic cysts containing blood products of different ages demonstrate an inhomogeneous high signal intensity on both T1WI and T2WI, sometimes layering and/or a hematocrit effect, and occasionally a signal void hemosiderin rim.	"Retained" functional cysts include follicular and corpus luteum cysts. *Polycystic ovarian disease (Stein–Leventhal syndrome)* classically presents with hirsutism, menstrual irregularity, and reduced fertility. On T2WI multiple small cysts (<8 mm) of high signal intensity are seen in a ring-like configuration in the periphery of usually both ovaries; the ovaries are either normal in size or symmetrically enlarged.

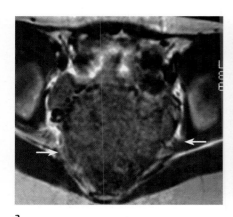

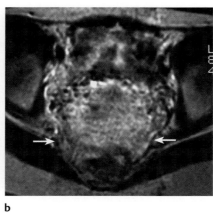

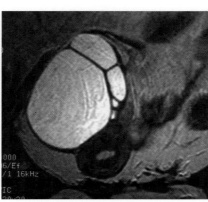

Fig. 26.**39** **Invasive mole.** An enlarged uterus (arrows) consisting of grape-like clusters of tiny, thin-walled cysts distorting the normal zonal architecture of the uterus is seen in (**a**) (PDWI) and (**b**) (T2WI).

a

b

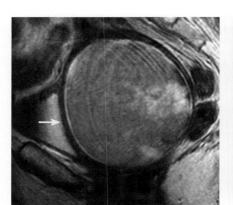

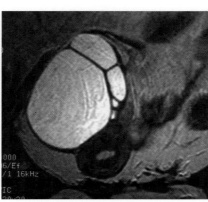

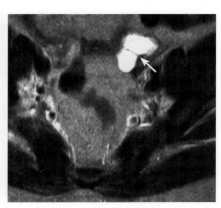

Fig. 26.**40** **Endometritis with pyometra.** The endometrial cavity (arrow) is markedly distended by pus and debri secondary to occlusion of the endocervical canal (T2WI, sagittal).

Fig. 26.**41** **Adnexal cyst.** A large hyperintense cystic lesion and four daughter cysts are seen (T2WI, coronal).

Fig. 26.**42** **Ovarian cysts.** Two small cystic lesions (arrow) are seen (T2WI).

Table 26.2 (Cont.) Female reproductive system lesions

Disease	MRI Findings	Comments
Ovarian endometriosis (Figs. 26.43, 26.44)	One or more, usually multilocular cystic lesions with signal intensity reflecting varying stages of hemorrhage. Most commonly, a high signal intensity is seen within the cystic lesion on both T1WI and T2WI. However, lesions may be hypointense on both T1WI and T2WI, or even hyperintense on T1WI and hypointense on T2WI. Central ill-defined areas of low signal intensity within hyperintense endometrial cyst, described as shading, may be seen on T2WI, possibly related to change in viscosity and protein concentration within the intracystic fluid. Signal void areas and/or a signal void rim due to fibrosis and/or accumulation of hemosiderin-laden macrophages may also be present. The edges of the lesion are often hazy or angular because of adhesions.	Affects women in the third and fourth decades of life and depends on normal hormonal stimulation. Presenting symptoms include infertility, acquired dysmenorrhea, pelvic pain, dyspareunia, and abnormal uterine bleeding. The pain characteristically is cyclic, beginning premenstrually and ceasing after menstruation.
Dermoid and teratoma	Well-defined lesion containing fatty and cystic components with or without gravity-dependent layering. The fat may form a fat–fluid level, or a compact mass of fat may be seen surrounded by intracystic fluid producing a chemical shift artifact. A nodule of varying histologic composition (dermoid plug or Rokitansky nodule) may arise from the cyst wall and project into its lumen. Globular calcifications representing abortive teeth or bones and rim calcifications may be evident as areas devoid of signal on all pulse sequences.	Common ovarian neoplasms, usually diagnosed during reproductive life. Dermoid cysts predominantly derive from the ectodermal germ cell layer, whereas teratomas are derivatives from all three germ cell layers. Most cystic teratomas are benign, with less than 3% undergoing malignant transformation. Primary *malignant teratomas*. A loss of surrounding tissue fat planes and invasion of the bladder, bowel, or pelvic muscles may be evident.
Benign ovarian neoplasms (Fig. 26.45)	Well-demarcated solid or mixed solid and cystic masses without invasion of neighboring fat planes and organs. Absence of local invasion does not, however, exclude malignancy. Lesions may be bilateral.	Solid lesions include fibroma, leiomyoma, Brenner tumor (estrogenic and calcifications), thecoma (estrogenic), and Sartoli–Leydig cell tumor (androgenic). Mixed solid and cystic lesions include serous and mucinous cystadenomas, granulosa cell tumor (estrogenic), and arrhenoblastoma.

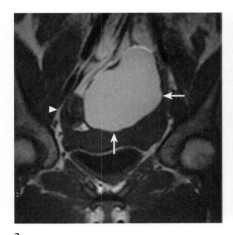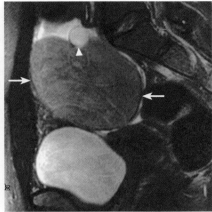

a   b

Fig. 26.**43** **Ovarian endometriosis.** A large cystic mass (arrows) is seen cephalad to the urinary bladder. The cystic lesion depicts high signal intensity in (**a**) (T1WI, coronal) and intermediate signal intensity in (**b**) (T2WI, sagittal), indicating that the cyst content is hemorrhagic and contains methemoglobin. The right ovary (arrowhead) is adherent to the cyst in (**a**). A hyperintense focus (arrowhead) is seen in the superior cyst wall in (**b**) consistent with a focus of intracystic endometriosis. A didelphic uterus is sandwiched between the posterior aspect of the bladder and cystic lesion, evident as areas of low signal intensity on both imaging sequences.

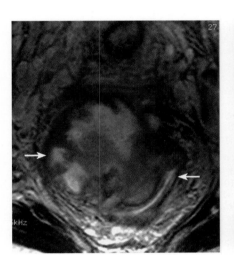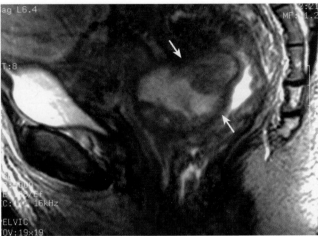

a   b

Fig. 26.**44** **Ovarian endometriosis.** A heterogeneous lesion (arrows) with greatly variable signal intensity is seen in the cul-de-sac (T2WI, axial and sagittal).

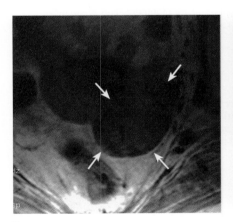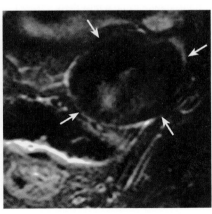

a   b

Fig. 26.**45** **Ovarian fibroma.** A well-defined, slightly inhomogeneous lesion (arrows) is seen with overall low signal intensity in both (**a**) (PDWI, coronal) and (**b**) (T2WI, FS, coronal).

Table 26.2 (Cont.) Female reproductive system lesions

Disease	MRI Findings	Comments
Ovarian carcinoma Fig. 26.46)	Typically large complex masses exceeding 5 cm in diameter and ranging in nature from predominantly cystic to mixed solid cystic and predominantly solid. The tumors appear heterogeneous, hypointense on T1WI and hyperintense on T2WI. Cystic fluid containing methemoglobin or a high protein concentration depicts a high signal intensity on all pulse sequences. Contrast enhancement is considerable, but limited to the solid tumor components. Demonstration of metastases or invasion of neighboring fat planes and organs unequivocally indicate malignancy. The presence of heterogeneous soft-tissue component, irregular septation, indistinct tumor margins, and ascites favor malignancy, but are not diagnostic. In pseudomyxoma peritonei, a complication of either mucinous cystadenoma or cystadenocarcinoma, peritoneal implants of high signal intensity on T2WI are seen.	Common primary ovarian malignancies include papillary or undifferentiated adenocarcinomas, serous or mucinous cystadenocarcinomas, and endometrioid carcinomas. Relatively rare primary malignancies include malignant teratomas, endodermal sinus tumors, mixed mesenchymal tumors, malignant thecomas, malignant arrhenoblastomas, and dysgerminomas. *Staging* TNM / FIGO TI — I — Limited to ovary TIa — IA — Limited to one ovary TIb — IB — Limited to both ovaries TIc — IC — + ascites (malignant) TII — II — Limited to pelvis TIIa — IIA — Involvement of uterus/fallopian tubes TIIb — IIB — Involvement of other pelvic structures TIIc — IIC — + ascites (malignant) TIII ± NI — III — Limited to abdomen except liver MI — IV — Hematogenous metastases or spread beyond abdomen
Ovarian metastases	Solid or cystic, often bilateral ovarian lesions that may antedate the discovery of the primary tumor. Massive enlargement of the ovaries may be seen.	Ovaries are the most frequent metastatic site in the female pelvis. Metastases frequently originate from pelvic organs and gastrointestinal tract. *Krukenberg tumor* refers to ovarian metastases from colon, stomach, pancreatic and biliary primaries.
Tubo-ovarian abscess	Thick-walled, usually multiloculated cystic mass that may contain gas or fluid–fluid levels. The lesion characteristically has indistinct margins and causes an inflammatory reaction in the adjacent fat planes. It may extend into the cul-de-sac and is frequently bilateral.	Often an anaerobic bacterial infection secondary to sexually transmitted disease, IUD, pelvic infections, and surgery. *Hydrosalpinx* and *pyosalpinx* refer to ampullary or infundibular obstruction of the fallopian tube, which is filled with sterile fluid or pus, respectively, and present as cystic or tubular structure in extraovarian location.
Ovarian torsion	In the acute stage the involved ovary is enlarged, edematous, and hemorrhagic with multiple enlarged peripheral follicles measuring up to 12 mm in diameter due to transudation of fluid into them. Engorged blood vessels with decreased flow and absence of contrast enhancement may also be evident. Small amount of intraperitoneal fluid is frequently present. If not corrected ovarian torsion progresses to hemorrhagic necrosis and eventually ovarian fibrosis and atrophy.	Presents with acute abdominal pain, nausea, vomiting, and fever. Prepubertal girls are frequently affected. Other risk factors include ovarian mass or cyst, hypermobility of adnexa, and pregnancy.
Ectopic pregnancy	Cystic or complex lesion in the adnexa, most commonly in the isthmus of the fallopian tube. Blood in the cul-de-sac is frequently associated.	Presents by the seventh week of menstrual age or later with positive pregnancy test, pelvic pain, abnormal vaginal bleeding, and often palpable adnexal mass.

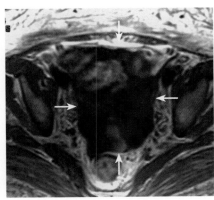 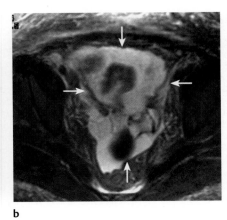

a

b

Fig. 26.**46** **Ovarian cystadenocarcinoma.** A complex, mixed solid cystic lesion (arrows) is seen, which predominantly demonstrates low signal intensity in (**a**) (T1WI) and high signal intensity in (**b**) (T2WI).

Table 26.**3** Male reproductive system lesions

Disease	MRI Findings	Comments
Prostate		
Prostatic cysts (Fig. 26.47)	Homogeneous cystic structures of usually low or, in case of methemoglobin formation or high protein concentration, intermediate to high signal intensity on T1WI and high signal intensity on T2WI. Congenital cysts include: *Utricular cyst*: arises in midline from verumontanum, in posterosuperior direction without extension above the prostate. *Müllerian duct cyst*: arises from region of verumontanum slightly lateral to midline with cephalad extension above the prostate. *Ejaculatory duct cyst*: intraprostatic along expected course of ejaculatory duct due to congenital or acquired obstruction of the latter.	Acquired cysts include: *Cystic degeneration of benign prostatic hypertrophy*: most common cystic prostatic lesion located in the transition zone. *Retention cyst*: dilatation of glandular acini due to glandular ductule obstruction. *Cavitary/diverticular prostatitis*: "Swiss cheese" appearance caused by dilated acini and ductules secondary to fibrosis in chronic or tuberculous prostatitis. *Prostatic abscess*: irregular cyst wall, often with septation. *Surgical defects*: secondary to transurethral resection of prostate (TURP).
Benign prostatic hypertrophy (Fig. 26.48)	Diffuse prostatic enlargement with smooth outline caused by hyperplasia of the transition zone. On T2WI the transition and central zones, which normally depict a homogeneous low signal intensity, become heterogeneous and may increase in signal intensity and blur the demarcation from the hyperintense peripheral zone. The hyperplastic transition zone may even demonstrate a diffuse nodular pattern, ranging in signal intensity on T2WI from low to high depending on the prevalence of glandular tissue.	Benign prostatic hypertrophy cannot be reliably differentiated by MRI from small prostatic carcinomas. Furthermore, both conditions may coexist in the same patient. The prostatic weight can be estimated assuming a specific gravity for prostatic tissue of 1.05 by the formula 0.55 x length x depth x width. The weight of normal prostates amounts to less than 30 g.
Prostate carcinoma (Figs. 26.49–26.51)	Typical presentation on T2WI is a low-signal-intensity lesion in the hyperintense peripheral zone producing an asymmetric prostatic enlargement with deformed or nodular contour. Prostate carcinoma confined to the central gland cannot be differentiated from benign prostatic hypertrophy. The rare mucin-producing, cystic prostate carcinoma is hyperintense on T2WI. Disruption of the prostate capsule posterolaterally results in infiltration of the retroprostatic fat near the neurovascular bundles. Invasion of the seminal vesicles may be evident by thickening of the seminal vesicle tubules and subsequent complete tumor replacement. Invasion of bladder and rectum indicates a further advanced stage. Postbiopsy changes may hamper both tumor detection and staging for several weeks by either underestimating or overestimating the tumor presence or tumor extent, depending on the time interval between biopsy and MRI scan.	Prostate specific antigen (PSA) is usually elevated (normal range 0.1–4 ng/ml). An annual PSA increase of more than 20% or more than 0.75 ng/ml is suspicious for carcinoma, since each gram of malignant prostatic tissue results in about 10 times as much serum PSA as its benign counterpart. *Staging* (modified Jewitt–Whitmore) A Nonpalpable A1 Well-differentiated tumor smaller than 1.5 cm; less than 5% of TURP chips positive A2 Diffuse, poorly differentiated tumor; more than 5% of TURP chips positive B Tumor palpable, confined to prostate B1 Tumor smaller than 1.5 cm B2 Tumor greater than 1.5 cm C Localized tumor with capsular involvement C1 Capsular invasion C2 Capsular penetration C3 Seminal vesicle involvement D Distant metastases D1 Pelvic lymph node involvement D2 Extrapelvic lymph node involvement D3 Metastases to bone, soft tissues, and other organs

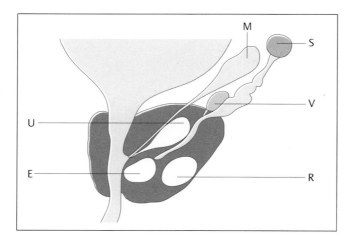

Fig. 26.47   Prostatic cysts.
E: ejaculatory duct cyst. M: müllerian duct cyst. R: retention cyst (congenital or acquired). S: seminal vesical cyst. U: utricular cyst. V: vas deferens cyst.

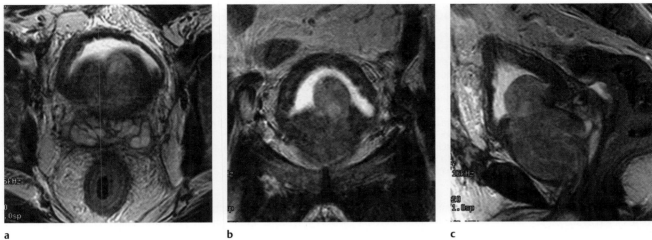

a   b   c

Fig. 26.**48** **Benign prostatic hypertrophy.** Marked diffuse and nodular enlargement of the prostatic gland is seen with elevation of the bladder floor (T2WI) (**a**): axial; (**b**) coronal; (**c**): sagittal.

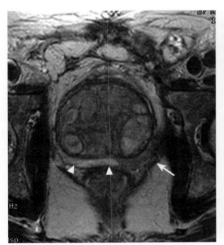

Fig. 26.**49** **Prostate carcinoma.** The hyperintense peripheral zone (arrowheads) is compressed by a markedly enlarged central gland (transition zone) owing to benign prostatic hypertrophy. Loss of normal signal intensity in the peripheral zone is evident left posterolaterally (arrow), caused by a prostate carcinoma. The carcinoma extends into the adjacent left neurovascular bundle and its enveloping retroprostatic fat, which also appears hypointense when compared with the normal right side (T2WI).

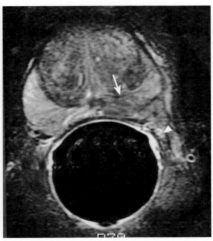

Fig. 26.**50** **Prostate carcinoma.** Compared with the normal high signal intensity seen in the right peripheral zone, a marked decrease in signal intensity is seen in the left peripheral zone (arrow). The tumor extends into the left retroprostatic fat and neurovascular bundle (arrowhead) (T2WI).

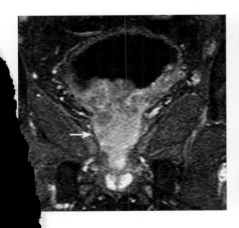

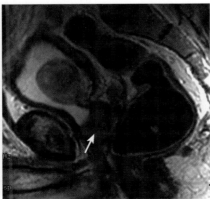

b

Fig. 26.**51** **Prostate carcinoma with bladder infiltration (two cases).** A large prostatic lesion (arrow) extending into the urinary bladder is seen (**a**: T1WI, FS, +C, coronal; **b**: T2WI, sagittal).

Table 26.3 (Cont.) Male reproductive system lesions

Disease	MRI Findings	Comments
Prostatitis (Figs. 26.52, 26.53)	Manifestations depend on stage. Acute prostatitis presents with edematous swelling of the gland, resulting in increased signal intensity on T2WI. An irregular, occasionally septated cavity suggests abscess formation. In chronic prostatitis a diffuse or focal loss of signal intensity may be seen in the peripheral zone on T2WI. Irregular dilation of ductules and glandular acini due to fibrosis may produce small cystic lesions throughout the prostate ("Swiss cheese" appearance).	*Granulomatous prostatitis.* Granulomas may be nonspecific (inflammatory reaction to the accumulation of inspissated secretion or necrotic tissue secondary to acute or chronic prostatitis) or tuberculous. On MRI they may present as low signal intensity foci in the peripheral zone, mimicking a prostate carcinoma. In tuberculous prostatitis multiple small cavitary/cystic lesions may also be evident.
Seminal vesicles		
Seminal vesicle cyst (Fig. 26.54)	Unilateral or bilateral, homogeneous cystic mass cephalad to the prostate, between bladder and rectum. Appears hypointense on T1WI and hyperintense on T2WI.	Congenital cysts are frequently associated with ipsilateral mesonephric duct anomalies including ectopic ureter insertion, renal dysgenesis, and duplication of the collecting system. Acquired cysts result from infections or tumorous obstruction (e.g. prostate carcinoma).
Seminal vesicle neoplasms	Metastatic prostate carcinoma is by far the most common malignancy presenting as unilateral or, less commonly, bilateral thickening of the seminal vesicle tubes or obstructing mass of typically low signal intensity on T2WI.	The differential diagnosis of low-signal-intensity seminal vesicle lesions includes senile amyloidosis and chronic infection and hemorrhage. Metastatic bladder and rectum carcinomas as well as the rare primary benign or malignant seminal vesicle tumors tend to have a higher signal intensity on T2WI.
Seminal vesicle infection and hemorrhage (Fig. 26.55)	Variable signal intensity depending on stage of the disease.	Frequently superimposed on seminal vesical neoplasms or obstruction.
Testes and epididymis		
Benign mass lesions	*Epidermoids* are intratesticular or extratesticular lesions appearing slightly hypointense to the testis on T1WI and slightly hyperintense on T2WI. *Benign teratomas* cannot be differentiated from the malignant variety. *Adenomatoid tumors* tend to occur in the epididymis and, because of their fibrosis, usually depict a low signal intensity.	*Cysts* located in the testis or tunica are a frequent incidental finding, measuring less than 2 cm in diameter and depicting water signal intensity without contrast enhancement. *Dilated seminiferous tubules* present as a mass of dilated tubules in the mediastinum testis associated with an ipsilateral spermatocele. *Intratesticular varicocele* presents as a markedly enhancing mass of dilated tubules in the mediastinum testis associated with an ipsilateral varicocele.
Testicular carcinoma	Well-demarcated, bulky mass that tends to be isointense to the testis on T1WI and inhomogeneous and hypointense to the testis on T2WI. A rim of normal testicular tissue typically remains, even in large lesions. Compared with seminomas, nonseminatous tumors are much more heterogeneous and tend to have a fibrous tumor capsule evident as a band of low signal intensity circumscribing the lesion. Invasion of the epididymis, spermatic cord, or scrotum may be evident. Primary lymphatic spread occurs to the high para-aortic lymph nodes near the renal hilus. Pelvic lymph node metastases are only found with local tumor extension beyond the testis.	Germ cell tumors (97%) include seminoma (50%), embryonal cell carcinoma including yolk sac tumor (25%), malignant teratoma including teratocarcinoma (20%), and choriocarcinoma (2%). They are usually diagnosed in the first 4 decades of life (peak age 20–40 years). Stromal cell tumors (3%) include Leydig cell tumor and Sertoli cell tumor. Ninety percent are benign. They may arise at any age but frequently occur in the first 5 years of life. *Staging* I Limited to testis and spermatic cord II Nodal metastases below diaphragm IIA Nonpalpable IIB Bulky mass III Nodal metastases above diaphragm or extranodal metastases IIIA Confined to lymphatic system IIIB Extranodal
Testicular lymphoma and leukemia	Unilateral or bilateral diffuse, poorly demarcated infiltration of the testis and/or epididymis. The testes may be enlarged but maintain normal configuration. On T2WI the infiltrates appear relatively homogeneous and hypointense to normal testicular tissue.	Lymphoma and leukemia are the most common testicular malignancy in men above 50 years. Testicular lymphoma may be primary, the manifestation of occult disease seated elsewhere, or, more commonly, part of disseminated disease. The testis is a frequent site of leukemia relapse, especially in children. *Testicular metastases* are very rare.

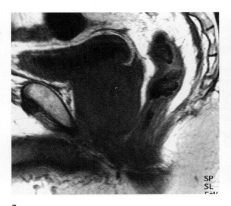

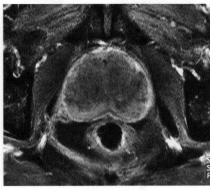

Fig. 26.**52** **Prostatitis (acute). a** diffuse enlargement of the prostatic gland is seen (T1WI, sagittal). **b** After intravenous Gd-DTPA administration marked, fairly homogeneous enhancement of the prostatic gland without evidence for abscess formation is seen (T1WI, FS, +C, axial).

a **b**

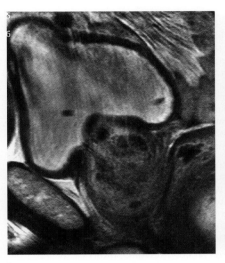

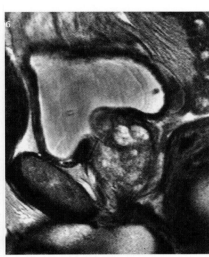

Fig. 26.**53** **Prostatitis with multiple abscess formation.** A diffusely enlarged prostatic gland is seen with multiple abscesses presenting as hypointense foci in (**a**) (spoiled GRE, sagittal), and hyperintense foci in (**b**) (T2WI [GRE], sagittal).

a **b**

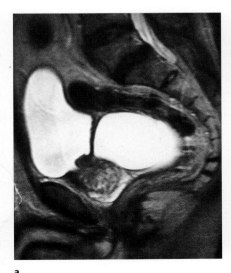

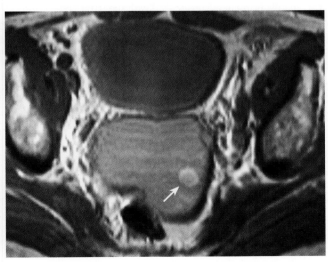

a **b**

Fig. 26.**54** **Seminal vesical cyst. a** A large cystic lesion is seen posterior to the bladder. Agenesis of the left kidney, left ureter, and both seminal vesicles was also present (T2WI, sagittal).

b A small hyperintense focus (arrow) is seen within the seminal vesical cyst, representing a serous cystadenoma (PDWI, axial).

Table 26.3 (Cont.) Male reproductive system lesions

Disease	MRI Findings	Comments
Epididymitis	In the acute stage diffuse or focal enlargement of the epididymis with increased signal intensity on T2WI approaching the signal intensity of a normal testis. Complications include abscess formation, hemorrhage, and orchitis. Frequently associated findings include edematous swelling and hypervascularity of the spermatic cord and a sympathetic hydrocele. Inguinal adenopathy may also be present. In chronic epididymitis an overall decreased signal intensity compared to the normal epididymis is seen on T2WI.	Common intrascrotal infection in adolescent and young males secondary to ascending infection (usually beginning as prostatitis). Common bacteria include *E. coli, S. aureus, N. gonorrhoeae,* and *Mycobacterium tuberculosis.* *Orchitis* is usually the sequela of epididymitis. Testicular involvement may be diffuse or focal, acute or chronic. On MRI the signal intensity varies accordingly. Pure orchitis without epididymitis suggests viral etiology.
Testicular hematoma	Inhomogeneous intratesticular signal intensity of great variability depending on the age of the hematoma. In testicular rupture or fracture the tunica albuginea is completely disrupted. A hematocele with signal intensity commensurable to the testicular hematoma is frequently associated.	Spontaneous testicular hematomas may occur in patients with bleeding diathesis or on anticoagulation therapy. Spontaneous rupture of an underlying tumor that may be masked by the hematoma should also be considered.
Testicular torsion	Hemorrhagic swelling of both epididymis and testis, enlarged proximal spermatic cord with diminished or absent blood flow and demonstration of the twisted cord are diagnostic. The point of twist is seen as a small, low-signal-intensity focus from which several curvilinear lines of varying signal intensity emanate representing various spiralling structures of the twisted stalk (whirlpool pattern). A hematocele is also frequently associated.	Occurs in patients below 30 years presenting with sudden scrotal swelling, tenderness, and severe pain. Requires immediate surgical correction since testes with completely interrupted blood supply remain viable for only 3–6 hours. Mechanism: occlusion of the veins in the twisted cord results in progressive testicular swelling until the intratesticular pressure exceeds the arterial pressure and the blood flow ceases, resulting in hemorrhagic necrosis.
Testicular infarct	Presentation of acute/subacute infarct depends on both type of vascular occlusion (partial versus complete, arterial versus venous) and degree of blood degradation. In chronic infarct the testis are small and of low signal intensity on all imaging sequences.	Common causes of testicular infarct include torsion, trauma, leukemia, bacterial endocarditis, and various types of vasculitis. *Torsion of testicular and epididymal appendices* (vestigial remnants) results in hemorrhagic infarct of these structures presenting as a small attached round mass.
Hydrocele (Fig. 26.56)	Abnormal fluid accumulation within the tunica vaginalis, presenting as a cystic lesion draped around the anterior, medial, and lateral border of the testis. May extend along the spermatic cord and communicate with the peritoneal cavity. A hernia is frequently associated with the latter condition.	May be secondary to trauma, testicular torsion, tumor, epididymitis, or orchitis. May contain blood (hematocele) or pus (pyocele). *Spermatocele* is a round cystic lesion arising from the head of the epididymis and is typically located posterosuperior to the testis.
Varicocele	Collection of dilated serpiginous veins posterolateral to the testis near the epididymal head and extending into the spermatic cord. The velocity of the blood is usually too slow to produce a flow void on SE sequences and frequently depicts intermediate signal intensity on T1WI and high signal intensity on T2WI due to sluggish flow.	Abnormal dilatation and tortuosity of the veins of the pampiniform plexus, occurring most commonly on the left side. It may be idiopathic or secondary to compression of the testicular vein from abdominal disease and lead to infertility.

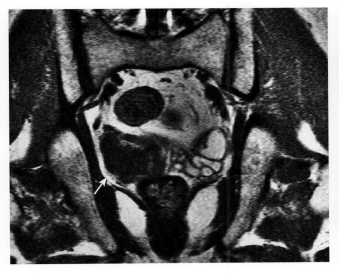

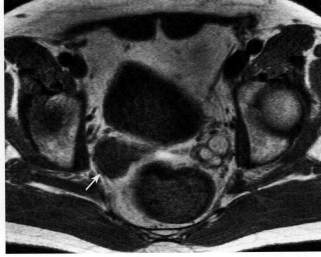

a

b

Fig. 26.**55** **Staphylococcal infection of right seminal vesicle.**
Edema and inflammation mask the right seminal vesicle (arrow) in
(**a**) (T1WI, sagittal) and (**b**) (T1WI, axial). In (**c**) (T2WI, axial) the
right seminal vesicle (arrow) appears engorged and depicts a
slightly higher signal intensity, when compared with the left side.

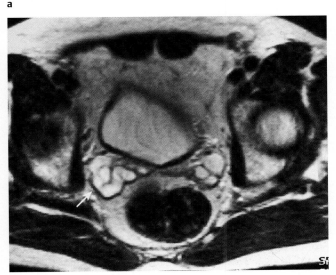

c

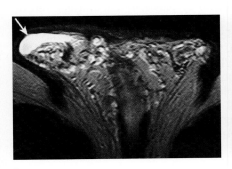

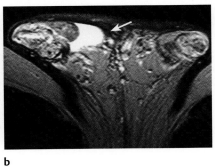

a

b

Fig. 26.**56** **Hydrocele.** Fluid accumulation
(arrow) is seen around the anterior, medial,
and lateral border of the right testis (**a, b**:
T2WI).

References

Amis ES, Newhouse JH. Essentials of uroradiology. Boston: Little Brown, 1991.

Berquist TH. MRI of the musculoskeletal system. 4th ed. Philadelphia: Lippincott Raven, 2001.

Braunwald E, Fauci AS, Kasper DL, Hauser SL, Longo DL, Jameson JL. Harrison's principles of internal medicine. 15th ed. NY: McGraw Hill, 2001.

Burgener FA, Kormano M. Differential diagnosis in conventional radiology. 2nd ed. Stuttgart: Thieme, 1991.

Burgener FA, Kormano M. Differential diagnosis in computed tomography. Stuttgart: Thieme, 1996.

Cotran RS, Kumar V, Collins T. Robbins pathologic basis of disease. 6th ed. Philadelphia: Saunders, 1998.

Dähnert W. Radiology review material. 4th ed. Baltimore: Williams and Wilkins, 1999.

Davidson AJ, Choyke P, Wagner BJ, Hartman D, Bralow L. Davidson's radiology of the kidney and genitourinary tract. 3rd ed. Philadelphia: Saunders, 1998.

Ebel K-D, Blickmann H. Differential diagnosis in pediatric radiology. Stuttgart: Thieme, 1999.

Edelman RR, Zlatkin MB, Hesselink JR. Clinical magnetic resonance imaging. 2nd ed. Philadelphia: Saunders, 1996.

Fraser RG, Paré PD, Fraser RS, Generaux GP. Diagnosis of diseases of the chest. 3rd ed. Philadelphia: Saunders, 1991.

Gray HL, Bannister LH, Williams PL. Gray's anatomy. 38th ed. Edinburgh: Churchill Livingstone, 1995.

Harnsberger HR. Handbook of head and neck imaging. 2nd ed. Chicago: Mosby-Yearbook, 1995.

Higgins CB, Hricak H, Helens CA. Magnetic resonance imaging of the body. 3rd ed. Philadelphia: Lippincott Raven, 1996.

Hosten N, Winter P. Imaging of the globe and orbit: A guide to differential diagnosis. Stuttgart: Thieme, 1998.

Kawashima A, Fishman EK, Kuhlman JE. CT and MR evaluation of posterior mediastinal masses. Critical Reviews in Diagnostic Imaging 1992; 33:311û367.

Kirks DR. Practical pediatric imaging. 3rd ed. Philadelphia: Lippincott Raven, 1998.

Krestin GPP, Choyke PL. Acute abdomen: Diagnostic imaging in the clinical context. Stuttgart: Thieme, 1996.

Lee JKT, Heiken JP, Sagel SS, Stanley RJ. Computed body tomography with MRI correlation 3rd ed. New York: Raven Press, 1997.

Lenz M. CT and MRI of head and neck tumors. Stuttgart: Thieme, 1993.

Meyers MA. Dynamic radiology of the abdomen: normal and pathologic anatomy. 5th ed. New York: Springer, 2000.

Mirowitz SA. MR pitfalls and variants in the extrahepatic abdomen. Magn Reson Imaging Clin N Am. 3(1):23û37, 1995.

Moss AA, Gamsu G, Genant HK, eds. Computed tomography of the body with magnetic resonance imaging. 2nd ed. Philadelphia: Saunders, 1992.

Osborne AG. Diagnostic neuroradiology. St. Louis: Mosby, 1994.

Radü EW, Kendall BE, Moseley IF. Computertomographie des Kopfes. 3rd ed. Stuttgart: Thieme, 1994.

Reeder MM. Reeder and Felson's gamuts in radiology. 4th ed. New York: Springer, 1996.

Reeders JW, Mathieson JR. AIDS imaging. Philadelphia: Saunders, 1997.

Resnick D. Diagnosis of bone and joint disorders. 4th ed. Philadelphia: Saunders, 2001.

Sabiston DC, Jr. Textbook of surgery: the biological basis of modern surgical practice. 16th ed. Philadelphia: Saunders, 2000.

Silverman F. Caffey's pediatric x-ray diagnosis: a textbook for students and practitioners of pediatrics, surgery and radiology. 9th ed. Chicago: Mosby-Yearbook, 1993.

Som PM, Bergeron RT. Head and neck imaging. 3rd ed. St. Louis: Mosby, 1996.

Stark DD, Bradley WG. Magnetic resonance imaging. 3rd ed. St. Louis: Mosby, 1999.

Stoller DW. Magnetic resonance imaging in orthopaedics and sports medicine. Philadelphia: Lippincott Raven, 1997.

Swartz JD, Harnsberger HR. Imaging of the temporal bone. 3rd ed. Stuttgart: Thieme, 1997.

Taybi H, Lachman RS. Radiology of syndromes, metabolic disorders and skeletal dysplasia. 4th ed. Chicago: Mosby, 1996.

Valvassori GE, Mafee MF, Carter BL. Imaging of the head and neck. 2nd ed. Stuttgart: Thieme, 1995.

Webb WR, Brant WE, Helms CA. Fundamentals of body CT. 2nd ed. Philadelphia: Saunders, 1997.

Wegener OH. Whole body computed tomography. 2nd ed. Berlin: Blackwell, 1993.

White CS. MR imaging of the thoracic veins. Magn Reson Imaging Clin N Am 8(1); 17û32, 2000.

Index

Page numbers in *italics* refer to illustrations

M